Redox-Active Molecules as Therapeutic Agents

Redox-Active Molecules as Therapeutic Agents

Editor

Ana Sofia Fernandes

MDPI • Basel • Beijing • Wuhan • Barcelona • Belgrade • Manchester • Tokyo • Cluj • Tianjin

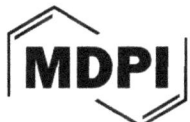

Editor
Ana Sofia Fernandes
CBIOS—Universidade Lusófona's Research
Center for Biosciences & Health Technologies,
Campo Grande 376,
1749-024 Lisboa, Portugal

Editorial Office
MDPI
St. Alban-Anlage 66
4052 Basel, Switzerland

This is a reprint of articles from the Special Issue published online in the open access journal *Antioxidants* (ISSN 2076-3921) (available at: https://www.mdpi.com/journal/antioxidants/special_issues/Redox-Active_Molecules_Therapeutic_Agents).

For citation purposes, cite each article independently as indicated on the article page online and as indicated below:

LastName, A.A.; LastName, B.B.; LastName, C.C. Article Title. *Journal Name* **Year**, *Volume Number*, Page Range.

ISBN 978-3-0365-4381-9 (Hbk)
ISBN 978-3-0365-4382-6 (PDF)

Cover image courtesy of Ana Sofia Fernandes.

© 2022 by the authors. Articles in this book are Open Access and distributed under the Creative Commons Attribution (CC BY) license, which allows users to download, copy and build upon published articles, as long as the author and publisher are properly credited, which ensures maximum dissemination and a wider impact of our publications.

The book as a whole is distributed by MDPI under the terms and conditions of the Creative Commons license CC BY-NC-ND.

Contents

About the Editor vii

Ana Sofia Fernandes
Redox-Active Molecules as Therapeutic Agents
Reprinted from: *Antioxidants* **2022**, *11*, 1004, doi:10.3390/antiox11051004 1

Sepideh Mirzaei, Ali Zarrabi, Farid Hashemi, Amirhossein Zabolian, Hossein Saleki, Negar Azami, Soodeh Hamzehlou, Mahdi Vasheghani Farahani, Kiavash Hushmandi, Milad Ashrafizadeh, Haroon Khan and Alan Prem Kumar
Nrf2 Signaling Pathway in Chemoprotection and Doxorubicin Resistance: Potential Application in Drug Discovery
Reprinted from: *Antioxidants* **2021**, *10*, 349, doi:10.3390/antiox10030349 5

Rita Manguinhas, Ana S. Fernandes, João G. Costa, Nuno Saraiva, Sérgio P. Camões, Nuno Gil, Rafael Rosell, Matilde Castro, Joana P. Miranda and Nuno G. Oliveira
Impact of the APE1 Redox Function Inhibitor E3330 in Non-Small Cell Lung Cancer Cells Exposed to Cisplatin: Increased Cytotoxicity and Impairment of Cell Migration and Invasion
Reprinted from: *Antioxidants* **2020**, *9*, 550, doi:10.3390/antiox9060550 31

Sandra Ferreira, Nuno Saraiva, Patrícia Rijo and Ana S. Fernandes
LOXL2 Inhibitors and Breast Cancer Progression
Reprinted from: *Antioxidants* **2021**, *10*, 312, doi:10.3390/antiox10020312 49

Tzu-Jung Yu, Jen-Yang Tang, Li-Ching Lin, Wan-Ju Lien, Yuan-Bin Cheng, Fang-Rong Chang, Fu Ou-Yang and Hsueh-Wei Chang
Withanolide C Inhibits Proliferation of Breast Cancer Cells via Oxidative Stress-Mediated Apoptosis and DNA Damage
Reprinted from: *Antioxidants* **2020**, *9*, 873, doi:10.3390/antiox9090873 65

Kimberly J. Nelson, Terri Messier, Stephanie Milczarek, Alexis Saaman, Stacie Beuschel, Uma Gandhi, Nicholas Heintz, Terrence L. Smalley, Jr., W. Todd Lowther and Brian Cunniff
Unique Cellular and Biochemical Features of Human Mitochondrial Peroxiredoxin 3 Establish the Molecular Basis for Its Specific Reaction with Thiostrepton
Reprinted from: *Antioxidants* **2021**, *10*, 150, doi:10.3390/antiox10020150 81

Saniya Ossikbayeva, Marina Khanin, Yoav Sharoni, Aviram Trachtenberg, Sultan Tuleukhanov, Richard Sensenig, Slava Rom, Michael Danilenko and Zulfiya Orynbayeva
Curcumin and Carnosic Acid Cooperate to Inhibit Proliferation and Alter Mitochondrial Function of Metastatic Prostate Cancer Cells
Reprinted from: *Antioxidants* **2021**, *10*, 1591, doi:10.3390/antiox10101591 99

Joshua J. Scammahorn, Isabel T. N. Nguyen, Eelke M. Bos, Harry Van Goor and Jaap A. Joles
Fighting Oxidative Stress with Sulfur: Hydrogen Sulfide in the Renal and Cardiovascular Systems
Reprinted from: *Antioxidants* **2021**, *10*, 373, doi:10.3390/antiox10030373 123

Luigi Di Luigi, Guglielmo Duranti, Ambra Antonioni, Paolo Sgrò, Roberta Ceci, Clara Crescioli, Stefania Sabatini, Andrea Lenzi, Daniela Caporossi, Francesco Del Galdo, Ivan Dimauro and Cristina Antinozzi
The Phosphodiesterase Type 5 Inhibitor Sildenafil Improves DNA Stability and Redox Homeostasis in Systemic Sclerosis Fibroblasts Exposed to Reactive Oxygen Species
Reprinted from: *Antioxidants* **2020**, *9*, 786, doi:10.3390/antiox9090786 143

Kihae Ra, Hyun Ju Oh, Eun Young Kim, Sung Keun Kang, Jeong Chan Ra, Eui Hyun Kim, Se Chang Park and Byeong Chun Lee
Comparison of Anti-Oxidative Effect of Human Adipose- and Amniotic Membrane-Derived Mesenchymal Stem Cell Conditioned Medium on Mouse Preimplantation Embryo Development
Reprinted from: *Antioxidants* **2021**, *10*, 268, doi:10.3390/antiox10020268 163

Antonella Angiolillo, Deborah Leccese, Marisa Palazzo, Francesco Vizzarri, Donato Casamassima, Carlo Corino and Alfonso Di Costanzo
Effects of *Lippia citriodora* Leaf Extract on Lipid and Oxidative Blood Profile of Volunteers with Hypercholesterolemia: A Preliminary Study
Reprinted from: *Antioxidants* **2021**, *10*, 521, doi:10.3390/antiox10040521 179

Regina Menezes, Alexandre Foito, Carolina Jardim, Inês Costa, Gonçalo Garcia, Rita Rosado-Ramos, Sabine Freitag, Colin James Alexander, Tiago Fleming Outeiro, Derek Stewart and Cláudia N. Santos
Bioprospection of Natural Sources of Polyphenols with Therapeutic Potential for Redox-Related Diseases
Reprinted from: *Antioxidants* **2020**, *9*, 789, doi:10.3390/antiox9090789 191

Rita Crinelli, Carolina Zara, Luca Galluzzi, Gloria Buffi, Chiara Ceccarini, Michael Smietana, Michele Mari, Mauro Magnani and Alessandra Fraternale
Activation of NRF2 and ATF4 Signaling by the Pro-Glutathione Molecule I-152, a Co-Drug of N-Acetyl-Cysteine and Cysteamine
Reprinted from: *Antioxidants* **2021**, *10*, 175, doi:10.3390/antiox10020175 215

Gabriela Krausova, Antonin Kana, Marek Vecka, Ivana Hyrslova, Barbora Stankova, Vera Kantorova, Iva Mrvikova, Martina Huttl and Hana Malinska
In Vivo Bioavailability of Selenium in Selenium-Enriched *Streptococcus thermophilus* and *Enterococcus faecium* in CD IGS Rats
Reprinted from: *Antioxidants* **2021**, *10*, 463, doi:10.3390/antiox10030463 235

About the Editor

Ana Sofia Fernandes

Ana Sofia Fernandes graduated with a degree in Pharmaceutical Sciences in 2004 and a PhD in Pharmacy (specialty of Toxicology) in 2010 and is currently a European Registered Toxicologist (2018). She is an Associate Professor of Pharmacology and Toxicology at Universidade Lusófona. She is also the Scientific Director for Innovation and the coordinator of the Laboratory of Pharmacology and Therapeutics of CBIOS—Research Center for Biosciences & Health Technologies. Ana Fernandes participated in the COST actions EU-ROS and NutRedOx. She has received 5 international awards, including an Early Research Career Prize (Society for Free Radical Research Europe, 2010). Her main research interest is to explore the impact of reactive oxygen species and of redox modulators on cancer etiology and progression.

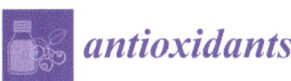

Editorial

Redox-Active Molecules as Therapeutic Agents

Ana Sofia Fernandes

CBIOS, Universidade Lusófona's Research Center for Biosciences & Health Technologies, Campo Grande 376, 1749-024 Lisbon, Portugal; ana.fernandes@ulusofona.pt

Citation: Fernandes, A.S. Redox-Active Molecules as Therapeutic Agents. *Antioxidants* **2022**, *11*, 1004. https://doi.org/10.3390/antiox11051004

Received: 19 April 2022
Accepted: 18 May 2022
Published: 20 May 2022

Publisher's Note: MDPI stays neutral with regard to jurisdictional claims in published maps and institutional affiliations.

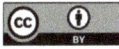

Copyright: © 2022 by the author. Licensee MDPI, Basel, Switzerland. This article is an open access article distributed under the terms and conditions of the Creative Commons Attribution (CC BY) license (https://creativecommons.org/licenses/by/4.0/).

Oxidative stress and altered redox signaling have been described in a plethora of pathological conditions, such as inflammation, cardiovascular diseases, diabetes, cancer, and neurodegenerative disorders, among others [1]. The concept of redox-active therapeutics explores the potential usefulness of redox-active molecules to modulate the etiology/progression of such diseases. Although the therapeutic potential of many natural and synthetic compounds has been suggested for decades, recent advances in molecular biology and pharmacology have strengthened this field of research by providing novel mechanistic insights, especially regarding the redox modulation of critical signaling pathways. The scope of this Special Issue is to give a broad and updated overview of the therapeutic potential of redox-active molecules, covering from fundamental science to clinical research, focused on the potential effects of either natural or synthetic compounds on different redox-related diseases.

Redox-modulating strategies have been widely explored in the cancer pharmacology field. Some classical chemotherapeutic drugs, such as doxorubicin, are known to increase intracellular ROS levels [2]. A review paper by Mirzaei et al. [3] addresses the role of nuclear factor erythroid 2-related factor 2 (Nrf2) signaling in doxorubicin resistance. Furthermore, the modulation of Nrf2 as a strategy to ameliorate the side effects of doxorubicin is discussed. Another combinational therapy is proposed in a research paper by Manguinhas et al. [4], in a study on non-small-cell lung cancer cells. The authors explored the combination of cisplatin with E3330, an inhibitor of the redox function of the apurinic/apyrimidinic endonuclease 1. This compound was able to increase cytotoxicity and impair cell migration and invasion, boosting cisplatin's anti-cancer effects. An emerging class of drugs for anticancer therapy are the inhibitors of lysyl oxidase enzymes. Ferreira et al. [5] reviewed the role of LOXL2, a member of this family of enzymes, on cancer development and metastases, with a special focus on breast cancer. The recent advances in the development of LOXL2 inhibitors are also described.

Along with synthetic drugs, many natural compounds have shown noteworthy results in cancer pharmacology. Yu et al. [6] investigated the effects of Withanolide C in breast cancer cells. The authors found that the compound exerts oxidative stress-mediated cytotoxicity, apoptosis and DNA damage in breast cancer cell lines. Another natural product with anticancer properties is the antibiotic Thiostrepton. Nelson et al. [7] explored the mechanistic basis for the interaction of Thiostrepton with peroxiredoxin 3, which is the molecular target of this drug. Plant (poly)phenols have also demonstrated anticancer activities in various models of neoplasia. Ossikbayeva et al. [8] suggest that the combination of curcumin and carnosic acid synergistically suppresses the proliferation of metastatic prostate cancer cells, and they describe the underlying mechanisms.

Besides oncology, other therapeutic areas may benefit from redox interventions. A review article from Scammahorn et al. [9] describes the current research of therapeutic strategies based on H_2S, which displays powerful antioxidant properties, against renal and cardiovascular pathologies. Di Luigi et al. [10] proposes that the phosphodiesterase type 5 inhibitor sildenafil could be a therapeutic candidate for systemic sclerosis treatment, as it protects against oxidative damage in human dermal fibroblasts isolated from patients.

In addition to small molecules, redox-active interventions may also include cell therapy products. Oxidative stress is a major cause of damage to the quantity and quality of embryos produced in vitro. A research paper by Ra et al. [11] studied the conditioned medium of amniotic membrane-derived mesenchymal stem cells as a novel antioxidant intervention for assisted reproduction.

This Special Issue also includes a clinical study carried out by Angiolillo et al. [12]. The authors evaluated the effects of *Lippia citriodora* leaf extract on lipid and oxidative blood profile of volunteers with hypercholesterolemia and suggested that dietary supplementation with such an extract could be beneficial in this condition. In fact, plants constitute an incredible and still underexplored reservoir of molecules with potential therapeutic applications. Menezes et al. [13] developed a strategy combining metabolomics, statistics, and the evaluation of (poly)phenols' bioactivity using a yeast-based discovery platform to allow the bioprospection of natural sources of (poly)phenols with therapeutic potential for redox-related diseases.

Disturbances in glutathione homeostasis are implicated in several diseases. Therefore, different approaches aimed at replenishing glutathione levels have been suggested. The compound I-152 combines two pro-GSH molecules, N-acetyl-cysteine and cysteamine. Crinelli et al. [14] explored the molecular mechanisms of I-152 and demonstrated that not only does it supply GSH precursors, but it also activates the Nrf2 and the activating transcription factor 4 signaling pathways. Another novel antioxidant approach consists of selenium enrichment of yeasts and lactic acid bacteria, which combines the beneficial effects of these microorganisms and of selenium supplementation. A research paper by Krausova et al. [15] studied the bioavailability and effects of Se-enriched strains in a rat model.

This Special Issue has highlighted the vast possibilities of redox-active interventions. However, in most cases, many questions still need to be answered during the drug development journey, before these molecules could reach clinical use. The articles published in this Special Issue represent some more steps in this direction. I would like to acknowledge all the authors for their contributions.

Funding: No external funding was received.

Conflicts of Interest: The author declares no conflict of interest.

References

1. Egea, J.; Fabregat, I.; Frapart, Y.M.; Ghezzi, P.; Görlach, A.; Kietzmann, T.; Kubaichuk, K.; Knaus, U.G.; Lopez, M.G.; Olaso-Gonzalez, G.; et al. European Contribution to the Study of ROS: A Summary of the Findings and Prospects for the Future from the COST Action BM1203 (EU-ROS). *Redox Biol.* **2017**, *13*, 94–162. [CrossRef] [PubMed]
2. Flórido, A.; Saraiva, N.; Cerqueira, S.; Almeida, N.; Parsons, M.; Batinic-Haberle, I.; Miranda, J.P.; Costa, J.G.; Carrara, G.; Castro, M.; et al. The Manganese(III) Porphyrin MnTnHex-2-PyP5+ Modulates Intracellular ROS and Breast Cancer Cell Migration: Impact on Doxorubicin-Treated Cells. *Redox Biol.* **2019**, *20*, 367–378. [CrossRef] [PubMed]
3. Mirzaei, S.; Zarrabi, A.; Hashemi, F.; Zabolian, A.; Saleki, H.; Azami, N.; Hamzehlou, S.; Farahani, M.V.; Hushmandi, K.; Ashrafizadeh, M.; et al. Nrf2 Signaling Pathway in Chemoprotection and Doxorubicin Resistance: Potential Application in Drug Discovery. *Antioxidants* **2021**, *10*, 349. [CrossRef] [PubMed]
4. Manguinhas, R.; Fernandes, A.S.; Costa, J.G.; Saraiva, N.; Camões, S.P.; Gil, N.; Rosell, R.; Castro, M.; Miranda, J.P.; Oliveira, N.G. Impact of the APE1 Redox Function Inhibitor E3330 in Non-Small Cell Lung Cancer Cells Exposed to Cisplatin: Increased Cytotoxicity and Impairment of Cell Migration and Invasion. *Antioxidants* **2020**, *9*, 550. [CrossRef] [PubMed]
5. Ferreira, S.; Saraiva, N.; Rijo, P.; Fernandes, A.S. LOXL2 Inhibitors and Breast Cancer Progression. *Antioxidants* **2021**, *10*, 312. [CrossRef] [PubMed]
6. Yu, T.-J.; Tang, J.-Y.; Lin, L.-C.; Lien, W.-J.; Cheng, Y.-B.; Chang, F.-R.; Ou-Yang, F.; Chang, H.-W. Withanolide C Inhibits Proliferation of Breast Cancer Cells via Oxidative Stress-Mediated Apoptosis and DNA Damage. *Antioxidants* **2020**, *9*, 873. [CrossRef] [PubMed]
7. Nelson, K.J.; Messier, T.; Milczarek, S.; Saaman, A.; Beuschel, S.; Gandhi, U.; Heintz, N.; Smalley, T.L.; Lowther, W.T.; Cunniff, B. Unique Cellular and Biochemical Features of Human Mitochondrial Peroxiredoxin 3 Establish the Molecular Basis for Its Specific Reaction with Thiostrepton. *Antioxidants* **2021**, *10*, 150. [CrossRef] [PubMed]
8. Ossikbayeva, S.; Khanin, M.; Sharoni, Y.; Trachtenberg, A.; Tuleukhanov, S.; Sensenig, R.; Rom, S.; Danilenko, M.; Orynbayeva, Z. Curcumin and Carnosic Acid Cooperate to Inhibit Proliferation and Alter Mitochondrial Function of Metastatic Prostate Cancer Cells. *Antioxidants* **2021**, *10*, 1591. [CrossRef] [PubMed]

9. Scammahorn, J.J.; Nguyen, I.T.N.; Bos, E.M.; van Goor, H.; Joles, J.A. Fighting Oxidative Stress with Sulfur: Hydrogen Sulfide in the Renal and Cardiovascular Systems. *Antioxidants* **2021**, *10*, 373. [CrossRef] [PubMed]
10. di Luigi, L.; Duranti, G.; Antonioni, A.; Sgrò, P.; Ceci, R.; Crescioli, C.; Sabatini, S.; Lenzi, A.; Caporossi, D.; del Galdo, F.; et al. The Phosphodiesterase Type 5 Inhibitor Sildenafil Improves DNA Stability and Redox Homeostasis in Systemic Sclerosis Fibroblasts Exposed to Reactive Oxygen Species. *Antioxidants* **2020**, *9*, 786. [CrossRef] [PubMed]
11. Ra, K.; Oh, H.J.; Kim, E.Y.; Kang, S.K.; Ra, J.C.; Kim, E.H.; Park, S.C.; Lee, B.C. Comparison of Anti-Oxidative Effect of Human Adipose- and Amniotic Membrane-Derived Mesenchymal Stem Cell Conditioned Medium on Mouse Preimplantation Embryo Development. *Antioxidants* **2021**, *10*, 268. [CrossRef] [PubMed]
12. Angiolillo, A.; Leccese, D.; Palazzo, M.; Vizzarri, F.; Casamassima, D.; Corino, C.; di Costanzo, A. Effects of Lippia Citriodora Leaf Extract on Lipid and Oxidative Blood Profile of Volunteers with Hypercholesterolemia: A Preliminary Study. *Antioxidants* **2021**, *10*, 521. [CrossRef] [PubMed]
13. Menezes, R.; Foito, A.; Jardim, C.; Costa, I.; Garcia, G.; Rosado-Ramos, R.; Freitag, S.; Alexander, C.J.; Outeiro, T.F.; Stewart, D.; et al. Bioprospection of Natural Sources of Polyphenols with Therapeutic Potential for Redox-Related Diseases. *Antioxidants* **2020**, *9*, 789. [CrossRef] [PubMed]
14. Crinelli, R.; Zara, C.; Galluzzi, L.; Buffi, G.; Ceccarini, C.; Smietana, M.; Mari, M.; Magnani, M.; Fraternale, A. Activation of NRF2 and ATF4 Signaling by the Pro-Glutathione Molecule I-152, a Co-Drug of N-Acetyl-Cysteine and Cysteamine. *Antioxidants* **2021**, *10*, 175. [CrossRef] [PubMed]
15. Krausova, G.; Kana, A.; Vecka, M.; Hyrslova, I.; Stankova, B.; Kantorova, V.; Mrvikova, I.; Huttl, M.; Malinska, H. In Vivo Bioavailability of Selenium in Selenium-Enriched Streptococcus Thermophilus and Enterococcus Faecium in CD IGS Rats. *Antioxidants* **2021**, *10*, 463. [CrossRef] [PubMed]

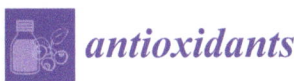

Review

Nrf2 Signaling Pathway in Chemoprotection and Doxorubicin Resistance: Potential Application in Drug Discovery

Sepideh Mirzaei [1], Ali Zarrabi [2], Farid Hashemi [3], Amirhossein Zabolian [4], Hossein Saleki [4], Negar Azami [4], Soodeh Hamzehlou [4], Mahdi Vasheghani Farahani [4], Kiavash Hushmandi [5], Milad Ashrafizadeh [2,6], Haroon Khan [7] and Alan Prem Kumar [8,9,*]

1. Department of Biology, Faculty of Science, Islamic Azad University, Science and Research Branch, Tehran 1477893855, Iran; sepidehmirzaei.smv@gmail.com
2. Sabanci University Nanotechnology Research and Application Center (SUNUM), Tuzla 34956, Istanbul, Turkey; alizarrabi@sabanciuniv.edu (A.Z.); milad.ashrafizadeh@sabanciuniv.edu (M.A.)
3. Department of Comparative Biosciences, Faculty of Veterinary Medicine, University of Tehran, Tehran 1417466191, Iran; faridhashemi172@gmail.com
4. Young Researchers and Elite Club, Tehran Medical Sciences, Islamic Azad University, Tehran 1477893855, Iran; ah_zabolian@student.iautmu.ac.ir (A.Z.); h.saleki@student.iautmu.ac.ir (H.S.); n.azami@student.iautmu.ac.ir (N.A.); ss.hamzehlou@gmail.com (S.H.); Mahdi.vf.1997@gmail.com (M.V.F.)
5. Department of Food Hygiene and Quality Control, Division of Epidemiology, Faculty of Veterinary Medicine, University of Tehran, Tehran 1417466191, Iran; houshmandi.kia7@ut.ac.ir
6. Faculty of Engineering and Natural Sciences, Sabanci University, Orta Mahalle, Üniversite Caddesi No. 27, Orhanlı, Tuzla 34956, Istanbul, Turkey
7. Department of Pharmacy, Abdul Wali Khan University, Mardan 23200, Pakistan; haroonkhan@awkum.edu.pk
8. Cancer Science Institute of Singapore, Department of Pharmacology, Yong Loo Lin School of Medicine, National University of Singapore, Singapore 117599, Singapore
9. NUS Centre for Cancer Research, Yong Loo Lin School of Medicine, National University of Singapore, Singapore 117597, Singapore
* Correspondence: apkumar@nus.edu.sg

Abstract: Doxorubicin (DOX) is extensively applied in cancer therapy due to its efficacy in suppressing cancer progression and inducing apoptosis. After its discovery, this chemotherapeutic agent has been frequently used for cancer therapy, leading to chemoresistance. Due to dose-dependent toxicity, high concentrations of DOX cannot be administered to cancer patients. Therefore, experiments have been directed towards revealing underlying mechanisms responsible for DOX resistance and ameliorating its adverse effects. Nuclear factor erythroid 2-related factor 2 (Nrf2) signaling is activated to increase levels of reactive oxygen species (ROS) in cells to protect them against oxidative stress. It has been reported that Nrf2 activation is associated with drug resistance. In cells exposed to DOX, stimulation of Nrf2 signaling protects cells against cell death. Various upstream mediators regulate Nrf2 in DOX resistance. Strategies, both pharmacological and genetic interventions, have been applied for reversing DOX resistance. However, Nrf2 induction is of importance for alleviating side effects of DOX. Pharmacological agents with naturally occurring compounds as the most common have been used for inducing Nrf2 signaling in DOX amelioration. Furthermore, signaling networks in which Nrf2 is a key player for protection against DOX adverse effects have been revealed and are discussed in the current review.

Keywords: doxorubicin; chemoresistance; oxidative stress; redox signaling; nuclear factor erythroid 2-related factor 2 (Nrf2); cancer therapy

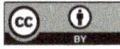

1. Introduction

Doxorubicin (DOX) is an anthracycline isolated from Streptomyces with proficiency in treatment of various cancers such as thoracic cancers, reproductive cancers, gastrointestinal and brain tumors [1]. Three major mechanisms are followed by DOX in suppressing progression and proliferation of cancer cells, including inhibiting DNA topoisomerase II activity, DNA intercalation and enhancing production of free radicals, especially reactive oxygen species (ROS) that are of importance in triggering apoptosis through mitochondrial pathway [2]. After its discovery, DOX was considered as the first option in treatment of cancer patients and showed promising clinical results. However, these ideal findings disappeared with development of DOX resistance [3–6].

Currently, two major obstacles are considered for cancer chemotherapy with DOX including A) DOX resistance, and B) dose-dependent toxicity [7–9]. The toxicity of DOX against normal cells has a negative impact on its efficacy in cancer therapy, since high dose of DOX cannot be administered to cancer patients to overcome resistance. In order to reverse DOX resistance, a combination of DOX with other compounds such as selenium is utilized to induce apoptosis and necrosis in cancer cells, leading to their enhanced sensitivity to DOX chemotherapy [10]. Mitochondrial transcription factor A (TFAM) stimulates mitochondrial dysfunction and AMP-activated protein kinase (AMPK) in suppressing DOX resistance [11]. That is why molecular pathways that promote cancer cell growth and viability, can induce DOX resistance. For instance, in non-small cell lung cancer, vasohibin2 (VASH2) functions as a tumor-promoting factor in enhancing proliferation that subsequently, stimulates DOX resistance [12]. Identification of such factors is of importance in suppressing DOX resistance by developing potential therapeutics for their targeting [13].

One of the processes contributing to DOX resistance is glycolysis. Cancer cells demonstrate enhanced glucose uptake and, to have enough energy, they induce glycolysis as a way of reaching a high amount of energy in a low time. In osteosarcoma cells, sphingosine kinase 1 (Sphk1) undergoes up-regulation due to hypoxia and activation of hypoxia-related molecular pathway, known as hypoxia-inducible factor 1α (HIF-1α) [14,15]. Then, an increase occurs in glycolysis, providing condition for DOX resistance [16]. Non-coding RNAs (ncRNAs) such as long non-coding RNAs (lncRNAs) and microRNAs (miRNAs) also participate in development of DOX resistance due to their regulatory effects on biological mechanisms and molecular pathways [17–21]. In addition to recognition of tumor-promoting molecular pathways and using combination chemotherapy, another strategy that utilizes nanostructures for DOX delivery has been developed. This strategy is ideal for in vitro and in vivo experiments and nanoparticles can provide a platform for co-delivery of DOX with other anti-tumor agents, leading to targeted delivery at tumor site and reversing chemoresistance [22]. Therefore, the DOX resistance is an increasing challenge, and more experiments are required to find novel strategies in reversing chemoresistance.

Another obstacle in using DOX in cancer chemotherapy is its dose-dependent toxicity. Clinical studies have confirmed this issue. Cardiomyopathy, gastrointestinal (GI) side effects and hematological abnormalities result from using DOX alone or in combination with other chemotherapeutic agents in cancer therapy [23–25]. Increased level of oxidative stress and subsequent apoptosis induction are responsible for DOX toxicity [26]. Furthermore, DOX can stimulate matrix metalloproteinase-2 (MMP-2) for mediating cardiotoxicity. Application of MMP inhibitors is associated with inhibiting intracellular and extracellular matrix remodeling and ameliorating DOX toxicity [27]. What is noteworthy is that a number of plant-derived natural compounds such as alpha-tocopheryl succinate [28], naringenin [29] and atorvastatin [30] have been applied in DOX side effect alleviation. These compounds mainly diminish oxidative stress, inflammation and apoptosis.

These studies demonstrate that free radical generation is the most important way that DOX follows in cancer therapy. However, free radicals can negatively affect major organs in the body such as kidney, liver and brain. In the present review, we focus on a molecular pathway which involves nuclear factor erythroid 2-related factor 2 (Nrf2) as a regulator of oxidative stress in cells. Although activation of Nrf2 signaling protects cells against oxidative damage [31], it can induce chemoresistance via suppressing oxidative-mediated cell death in cancer cells [32].

2. Materials and Methods

In searching and collecting data for the current review, we used databases such as Pubmed, Google Scholar and Science Direct. Keywords such as "Nrf2 + Doxorubicin", "Nrf2 + resistance", and "Nrf2 + chemoprotection" were used. Furthermore, most of the experiments and articles are from 2020.

3. Nrf2 Signaling Pathway

Counteracting oxidative stress and inflammation is the main aim of Nrf2 signaling in cell protection [33–44]. Sequestration of Nrf2 occurs in normal conditions by Kelch-like ECH-associated protein 1 (Keap1), when ROS and oxidative levels are at standard limit [45]. For providing proteasomal degradation of Nrf2, preventing its accumulation in cytoplasm and subsequent translocation to nucleus, Keap1 as a ubiquitin ligase adaptor protein, represents Nrf2 to Cullin-3 (Cul3)/RBX1 complex [46]. In contrast, electrophiles and oxidative stress are considered as inducers of Nrf2 signaling. In this way, Keap1 dissociation from Cul3 occurs via structural modification of Keap1 at cysteine 151 [47]. Furthermore, glycogen synthase kinase-3β (GSK-3β) prevents Nrf2 degradation by Nrf2 phosphorylation at serine 335 and 338. Then, Nrf2 polyubiquitination and its identification by β transducin repeat containing E3 ubiquitin-protein ligase (βTrCP) occur that are in favor of preventing Nrf2 degradation and providing CUL3/RBX1-induced degradation [48,49].

As a result, high levels of Nrf2 accumulate in cytoplasm that is followed by nuclear translocation and targeting genes containing antioxidant response element (ARE) region [50]. These genes include heme oxygenase-1 (HO-1), NAD(P)H dehydrogenase quinone 1 (NQO1), γ-glutamyl cysteine ligase modulatory and catalytic subunits (GCLM and GCLC, respectively), and ferritin accounting for inducing oxidant and antioxidant balance in cells [51–55]. Noteworthy, Nrf2 activation can be beneficial in reducing inflammation via activating HO-1, and subsequent inhibition of NF-κB signaling, which generally acts as a tumor-promoting factor [56–58]. Nrf2 down-regulation is associated with an increase in inflammatory response via NF-κB activation [59]. Furthermore, it has been reported that Nrf2 activation is in favor of reducing levels of pro-inflammatory cytokines in cells (Figure 1) [60–65].

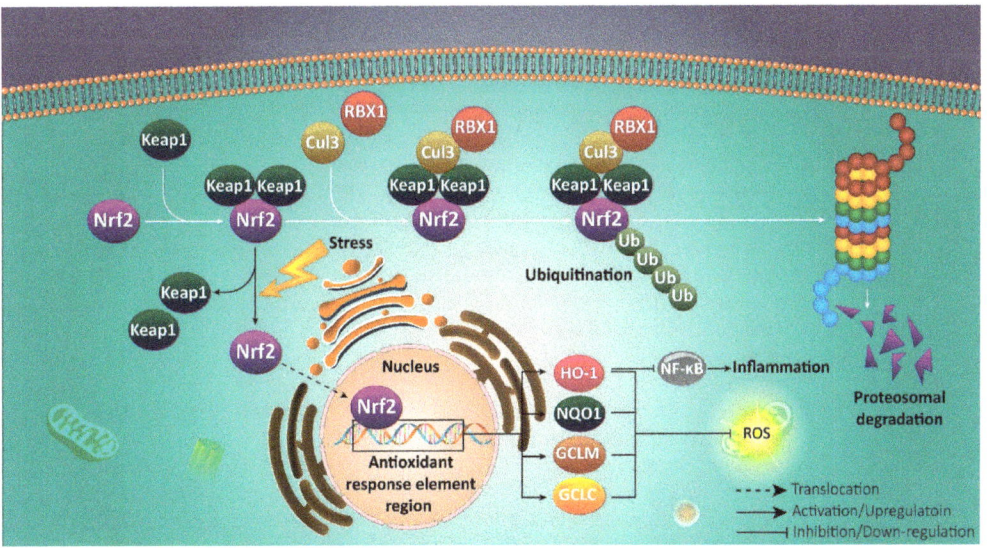

Figure 1. A schematic presentation of Nrf2 signaling pathway. Oxidative stress induces nuclear translocation of Nrf2 to promote antioxidant activity via up-regulating HO-1, NQO1, and GCLM.

4. Nrf2 in Protection and Chemoresistance

Chemoresistance remains a major challenge for cancer therapy [66–70]. The dual role of Nrf2 during cancer chemotherapy has been investigated in a variety of experiments. First, activation of Nrf2 signaling is advantageous in reducing side effects of chemotherapeutic agents. For instance, paclitaxel exposure is associated with induction of mechanical allodynia, while stimulation of Nrf2 signaling by oltipraz significantly reduces this adverse impact via HO-1 induction [71]. Furthermore, peroxisome proliferator-activated receptor gamma (PPARγ) can function as an upstream inducer of Nrf2 signaling in alleviation of paclitaxel-induced mechanical allodynia [72]. Exposing cells to cisplatin enhances levels of oxidant parameters such as malondialdehyde (MDA) and reduces activity and levels of antioxidant enzymes such as superoxide dismutase (SOD), catalase (CAT) and glutathione (GSH). Nrf2, as a cytoprotective mechanism, supports kidney cells against oxidative stress and apoptosis via reinforcing antioxidant defense system [73]. Furthermore, Nrf2 activation is of importance in reducing cisplatin-mediated toxicity in reproductive system. In this way, tadalafil diminishes apoptosis and oxidative stress via Nrf2 up-regulation [74]. It has been reported that activation of Nrf2/HO-1 signaling is in favor of enhancing cell survival upon chemotherapy [75]. What is noteworthy is that phytochemicals such as curcumin [76] and formononetin [77] induce Nrf2/HO-1 signaling in reducing toxicity of oxaliplatin against liver and brain cells. These studies clearly demonstrate that Nrf2 signaling is of importance for alleviation of chemotherapy-mediated side effects.

Although Nrf2 signaling activation is of interest in reducing chemotherapy-mediated side effects, increasing evidence demonstrates association of Nrf2 activation with chemoresistance. Tumor-promoting factors such as bone morphogenetic proteins (BMP) induce Nrf2 signaling in promoting cancer cells survival and triggering chemoresistance [78]. It seems that Nrf2 can enhance tumor-initiating cell lineage that subsequently, mediates chemoresistance [79]. The p53 can provide proteasomal degradation of Keap1 via inducing Nrf2/ARE signaling to promote proliferation and apoptosis inhibition, resulting in chemoresistance [80]. Upon Nrf2 activation, glutamine metabolism increases to induce chemoresistance, and is associated with poor prognosis of cancer patients [81]. Furthermore, Nrf2 can positively interact with TAZ member of Hippo signaling in providing chemoresistance [82]. Anti-tumor compounds such as ailanthone [83] and kaempferol [84] decrease Nrf2 expression in promoting oxidative damage and ROS levels as well as triggering apoptosis, leading to enhanced cancer sensitivity to chemotherapy. Overall, studies are in agreement with the fact that Nrf2 activation induces chemoresistance [85] and its inhibition can be considered as an ideal strategy in reversing drug resistance.

5. Natural Compounds in Ameliorating Doxorubicin-Mediated Toxicity

As it was discussed earlier, plant derived-natural compounds are able to regulate Nrf2 signaling in exerting their protective effect against oxidative stress-mediated diseases [86–88]. Pristimerin (Pris) is a natural triterpenoid compound derived from Celastraceae plant with different pharmacological activities such as anti-tumor, anti-inflammatory and antioxidant [89,90]. In respect of the potential of Pris in regulating Nrf2 signaling, it can be beneficial in ameliorating DOX-mediated cardiotoxicity that could be developed due to increased oxidative stress and ROS levels as the main risk factors. In this way, Pris enhances expression of Nrf2 at mRNA and protein levels, resulting in an increase in expression of its downstream targets including NQO1, HO-1 and GCL. Then, oxidative stress parameters undergo a decrease, while antioxidant defense system is reinforced, leading to decreased DOX-mediated cardiotoxicity [91]. In addition to heart, kidney and liver are negatively affected following DOX administration due to an increase in oxidative stress and inflammation [92,93]. Asiatic acid (AA) is another phytochemical that has been under attention due to its efficacy in preventing ageing, improving wound healing and exerting anti-tumor activity [94–97]. Recently, it has been shown that AA possesses high antioxidant potential that is of importance in reducing toxic effects of DOX against major organs of body. For this purpose, AA increases Nrf2 expression that diminishes necrosis, hyaline degeneration and congestion in heart. Hepatoprotective effects include reducing leukocyte inflammation, necrosis and apoptosis. Finally, kidney is protected against DOX toxicity via decreasing necrosis and inflammation [98]. These studies reveal that Nrf2 not only protects cells against DOX-mediated oxidative stress, but also decreases inflammation, and is therefore responsible for reducing cell death.

AMPK is considered as upstream mediator of Nrf2 signaling. It seems that AMPK activation is vital for inducing Nrf2 signaling [99]. By stimulating Nrf2 signaling, AMPK protects against oxidative stress and enhances expression of downstream targets such as HO-1 [100]. β-LAPachone (B-LAP) as a protective agent, targets AMPK/Nrf2 signaling in reducing DOX-mediated cardiotoxicity. B-LAP promotes expression of AMPK to induce Nrf2 signaling for elevating expression levels of SOX, CAT and GPX, leading to amelioration of DOX-mediated cardiotoxicity [101]. Following Nrf2 activation by phytochemicals, ROS levels decrease, preventing mitochondrial dysfunction and subsequent induction of apoptosis in cells exposed to DOX [102].

Cardamonin (CAR), a flavone exclusively found in Alpinia plant, has demonstrated potential in reducing oxidative stress via regulating Nrf2 signaling. It is noteworthy that CAR activates Nrf2 signaling that is of importance in reducing Th2 cytokine generation and preventing dermatitis [103]. In vivo experiment on mice demonstrates that CAR alleviates myocardial contractile dysfunction via enhancing Nrf2 expression [104]. These studies reveal that Nrf2 is a potential target of CAR in cell protection, and similarly, CAR follows a same pathway in reducing DOX-mediated toxicity. Both inflammation and oxidative stress are inhibited by CAR administration. This is mediated by activating Nrf2 signaling and subsequent up-regulation of SOD, GSH, CAT and reduced levels of ROS [105]. Chitosan oligosaccharide (COS) is a hydrolyzed form of chitosan that is found in exoskeleton of crustaceans and walls of fungi and insects [106]. A wide variety of biological activities including immune response regulation, anti-tumor, antimicrobial and anti-apoptosis are considered for COS [107–111]. A recent study has shown that COS can prevent oxidative damage and induce heart growth upon exposure to DOX. COS reduces ROS levels, mitochondrial dysfunction and apoptosis in cells. Mechanistically, COS induces AMPK in triggering Nrf2/ARE axis [112]. This study demonstrates that complicated signaling networks are involved in protecting against DOX-mediated toxicity in which Nrf2 signaling is the key player. The aim of Nrf2 activation is to up-regulate expression of downstream targets such as HO-1 and NQO1 that participate in improving antioxidant/oxidant balance and ameliorating DOX-mediated toxicity [113,114].

The *p*-coumaric acid (*p*CA) is a phenolic compound that functions as a ROS scavenger in reducing oxidative stress and protecting cells against drug toxicity [115]. Different molecular pathways are affected by *p*CA in exerting its protective effects and Nrf2 is among them. In this way, *p*CA promotes Nrf2 expression to prevent ROS generation and inflammation caused by lipopolysaccharide (LPS) [116]. It seems that *p*CA inhibits acute lung injury via AMPK/Nrf2/HO-1 axis activation to induce antioxidant response [117]. These studies advocate the fact that *p*CA has potential modulatory effects on Nrf2 signaling. *p*CA significantly increases cell survival and prevents apoptosis via caspase-3 down-regulation. It has been reported that ROS generation inhibition and preventing mitochondrial dysfunction are major mechanisms for protecting against DOX-mediated cardiotoxicity. Consequently, *p*CA induces Nrf2 signaling to inhibit ROS overgeneration, preventing subsequent mechanisms that are essential for DOX-mediated cardiotoxicity [118]. Therefore, using compounds inducing Nrf2 signaling can protect against DOX-mediated cardiotoxicity [119].

Tanshinone IIA (Tan IIA) is a potent antioxidant agent exclusively found in Radix *Salvia miltiorrhiza* [120]. Similar to other phytochemicals with antioxidant activity, Tan IIA targets Nrf2 signaling. Tan IIA administration is associated with improvement in silica-mediated pulmonary inflammatory response, structural damage and fibrosis via Nrf2/ARE activation [121]. Furthermore, Tan IIA prevents liver injury via epigenetic activation of Nrf2 and reinforcing antioxidant defense system [122]. Hence, Tan IIA stimulates Nrf2 signaling as a way of recovering redox homeostasis and inhibiting pulmonary fibrosis [123].

In alleviation of DOX-induced cardiotoxicity, Tan IIA increases cell viability and prevents damage-associated morphological alterations in H9C2 cells. In addition, a decrease occurs in generation of ROS levels, while GSH undergoes up-regulation in activity. These protective effects of Tan IIA are mediated by activating Nrf2 signaling and its downstream targets HO-1 and NQO1 [124].

Punicalagin (PUN) is a polyphenol isolated from pomegranate and displays a variety of pharmacological activities, of which antioxidant and anti-inflammatory are the most important [125,126]. It seems that antioxidant activity of PUN is mediated via its impact on Nrf2 signaling pathway. In this way, PUN induces Nrf2/HO-1 axis in protecting DOX-mediated cardiotoxicity. The protective impacts of PUN are abolished via Nrf2 down-regulation. By Nrf2 activation, PUN not only reduces oxidative stress parameters, but also prevents loss of mitochondrial membrane potential, cytochrome C release and apoptosis induction [127]. Experiments discussed in this section demonstrate that phytochemicals can effectively induce Nrf2 signaling in protecting against DOX-mediated toxicity.

Importantly, as natural compounds suffer from poor bioavailability, using nanoparticles for their delivery can promote their therapeutic effects and impact on Nrf2 signaling that are of importance for ameliorating DOX-mediated toxicity. Future studies will shed some light on this aspect.

6. Nrf2 Modulation

MiRNAs are upstream mediators of a variety of molecular pathways due to their role in coordinating detailed biological mechanisms [128–135]. As occurs in different pathological events, miRNA dysregulation leads to alterations in normal cellular events [136,137]. Increasing evidence demonstrates that Nrf2 signaling is under surveillance of miRNAs in different pathological events for regulating response of cells to oxidative stress [138,139]. It is noteworthy that miRNA and Nrf2 interaction is of importance in DOX toxicity. It has been reported that miRNA-140-5p binds to $3'$-untranslated region ($3'$-UTR) to reduce its expression. This leads to a reduction in activity of antioxidant enzymes such as HO-1, NQO1, and GCLM that subsequently, deteriorates DOX-mediated cardiotoxicity [140]. MiRNA-200a is another non-coding RNA that regulates Nrf2 signaling. It appears that miRNA-200a ameliorates diabetes endothelial dysfunction via reducing Keap1 expression and subsequent induction of Nrf2 signaling [141]. Furthermore, miRNA-200a inhibits apoptosis and inflammation in cardiomyocytes by regulating Keap1/Nrf2 signaling in favor of cell protection [142]. In mice exposed to DOX, miRNA-200a enhances Nrf2 expression to improve contractile function, and prevent apoptosis and oxidative stress [143].

The involvement of Nrf2 signaling in organ protection is confirmed by the study of Li and colleagues showing that Nrf2 silencing deteriorates DOX-mediated toxicity [144]. This experiment demonstrated a novel pathway in which Nrf2 follows to alleviate DOX-mediated cardiotoxicity. In this way, Nrf2 affects a mechanism known as autophagy. Primarily, autophagy is considered as a "self-digestion" mechanism that degrades toxic and aged organelles and macromolecules [145,146]. It has been reported that there is a close association between autophagy and oxidative stress in cells, so that autophagy activation can ameliorate oxidative stress [147]. This relationship is of importance in relieving oxidative damage in cells. For instance, autophagy stimulation can improve integrity of intestinal barrier against ROS and oxidative damage [148]. In reducing DOX-mediated cardiac dysfunction, Nrf2 activation can promote levels of light chain-3II (LC-3II) to induce autophagy, leading to amelioration of DOX-mediated cardiotoxicity [144]. Following Nrf2 degradation and inhibition, oxidative stress increases and apoptosis markers such as caspase-3 and caspase-9 undergo up-regulation that mediate toxic effects of DOX on organs of body [149]. An interesting point should be noted that autophagy has also interactions with apoptosis [150–152]. In respect to effect of Nrf2 on autophagy and also, the interaction between autophagy and apoptosis, further studies can evaluate autophagy induction by Nrf2, and its impact on incidence of apoptosis in cells exposed to DOX.

Orosomucoid 1 (ORM1) was first discovered by Tokita and Schmid in a century ago and is an acute phase protein synthesized in liver [153,154]. ORM1 has a variety of functions in cells including modulating immune system, preserving capillary barrier function, and reducing ROS levels [155–157]. Due to its impact of oxidative stress and ROS levels, ORM1 may be capable of regulating Nrf2 signaling. It has been reported that ORM1 overexpression is associated with activation on Nrf2 signaling and its downstream target HO-1, leading to a reduction in oxidative stress and apoptosis (caspase-3 down-regulation) that are of importance in ameliorating DOX-mediated cardiotoxicity [158].

A 3-dimensional model (3D) of cardiac system demonstrates that Nrf2 activation is a positive factor in protecting cells against DOX-mediated cardiotoxicity, further confirming role of Nrf2 in cardioprotection [159]. One of the emerging upstream mediators of Nrf2 signaling is GSK-3β that is a serine/threonine kinase with ubiquitous expression [160,161]. GSK-3β is an inhibitor of Nrf2 signaling and is correlated with development of a variety of pathological events including diabetes [162], aging [163], liver disease [164] and neurological disorders [165–167]. There is a reverse relationship between Nrf2 signaling and GSK-3β in cells exposed to DOX, so that GSK-3β down-regulation provides condition for Nrf2 activation and reducing DOX-mediated toxicity [168]. It is worth mentioning that chronic exposure to DOX is associated with Nrf2 inhibition that further aggravates organ toxicity [169]. Therefore, a wide variety of signaling networks, both inhibitor and inducer of Nrf2 signaling are involved in regulated DOX-mediated toxicity on organs and understanding their interactions can provide a new insight for designing novel therapeutics (Table 1, Figure 2).

Table 1. Nrf2 signaling as a chemoprotection mechanism.

Toxicity	Signaling Network	Compound	Nrf2 Expression	Outcomes	Refs
Cardiotoxicity	MiRNA-140-5p/Nrf2	–	Down-regulation	Deteriorating DOX-mediated cardiotoxicity Reducing expressions of NQO1 and HO-1 Enhancing oxidative stress level	[140]
Cardiotoxicity Hepatotoxicity Renotoxicity	–	Asiatic acid	Up-regulation	Reducing necrosis, congestion and hyaline degeneration in heart Decreasing leukocyte inflammation, necrosis, apoptosis and fatty change in liver Decreasing necrosis and inflammation in kidney Mediating these protective effects via Nrf2 induction	[98]
Cardiotoxicity	Nrf2/HO-1 Nrf2/NQO1 Nrf2/GCL	Pristimerin	Up-regulation	Increasing expressions of Nrf2 and its downstream targets HO-1, NQO1 and GCL Reducing oxidative stress and fibrosis	[91]
Cardiotoxicity	Nrf2/HO-1 Nrf2/NQO1	Tert-butylhydroquinone	Up-regulation	Ameliorating cardiotoxicity via induction of Nrf2 and its downstream targets	[113]
Cardiotoxicity	Nrf2/HO-1	b-LAPachone	Up-regulation	Triggering nuclear translocation of Nrf2 Enhancing expressions of HO-1 and antioxidant enzymes such as SOD, CAT and GPx	[101]
Cardiotoxicity	Nrf2/HO-1 Nrf2/NQO1	Cardamonin	Up-regulation	Protecting cells against inflammation and oxidative stress Reducing oxidative stress, apoptosis, and inflammation Inducing Nrf2 signaling and its downstream targets HO-1 and NQO1	[105]
Cardiotoxicity	Nrf2/HO-1	Curdione	Up-regulation	Alleviating oxidative stress Preventing ROS overgeneration and mediating mitochondrial dysfunction Triggering Nrf2/HO-1 axis as an antioxidant axis	[102]
Cardiotoxicity	MAPK/Nrf2/ARE	Chitosan oligosaccharide	Up-regulation	Decreasing oxidative stress and apoptosis Stimulating MAPK and subsequent induction of Nrf2/ARE axis Reinforcing antioxidant defense system	[112]

Table 1. Cont.

Toxicity	Signaling Network	Compound	Nrf2 Expression	Outcomes	Refs
Cardiotoxicity	MiRNA-200a/Nrf2	–	Up-regulation	Improving cardiomyocyte contractile function Reducing levels of cardiac troponin I Ameliorating oxidative stress, inflammation and apoptosis Inducing Nrf2 signaling	[143]
Cardiotoxicity	Nrf2/ARE	3,3'-diindolylmethane	Up-regulation	Suppressing apoptosis Improving histopathological profile Enhancing expressions of HO-1, NQO1 and GST Reducing Bax and caspase-3 expression	[114]
Cardiotoxicity	Sirt1/AMPK/Nrf2	Acacetin	Up-regulation	Alleviation of cardiomyopathy Enhancing cell viability Preventing ROS overgeneration Activation of Sirt1/AMPK to induce Nrf2 signaling Triggering cell defense system	[170]
Cardiotoxicity	Nrf2/HO-1	Genistein	Up-regulation	Inducing Nrf2/HO-1 axis Reducing ROS levels by its scavenging feature Reducing lipid peroxidation and DNA damage	[171]
Cardiotoxicity	Nrf2/LC-3II/autophagy	–	Down-regulation	Reducing oxidative stress Activating autophagy as a protective mechanism via LC-3II up-regulation Nrf2 inhibition aggravates DOX-mediated cardiotoxicity via impairing autophagy and enhancing oxidative stress	[144]
Cardiotoxicity	–	p-coumaric acid	Up-regulation	Enhancing cell survival Inhibiting apoptosis and oxidative stress Providing nuclear translocation of Nrf2	[118]
Cardiotoxicity	Nrf2/NQO1	Tanshinone IIA	Up-regulation	Enhancing cell viability and morphological profile Reducing oxidative parameters Up-regulation of NQO1	[124]
Cardiotoxicity	ORM1/Nrf2	–	Up-regulation	ORM1 is correlated with a decrease in oxidative stress and apoptosis Up-regulation of Nrf2 and its downstream target HO-1	[158]
Testicular toxicity	–	–	Down-regulation	Inducing apoptosis and oxidative stress in testis Reducing Nrf2 expression	[149]
Nephrotoxicity	–	Thymoquinone	Up-regulation	Reducing malondialdehyde and lipid peroxidation levels Enhancing SOD and GST levels Preventing necrosis and oxidative stress Activation of Nrf2 and improving antioxidant defense system	[119]

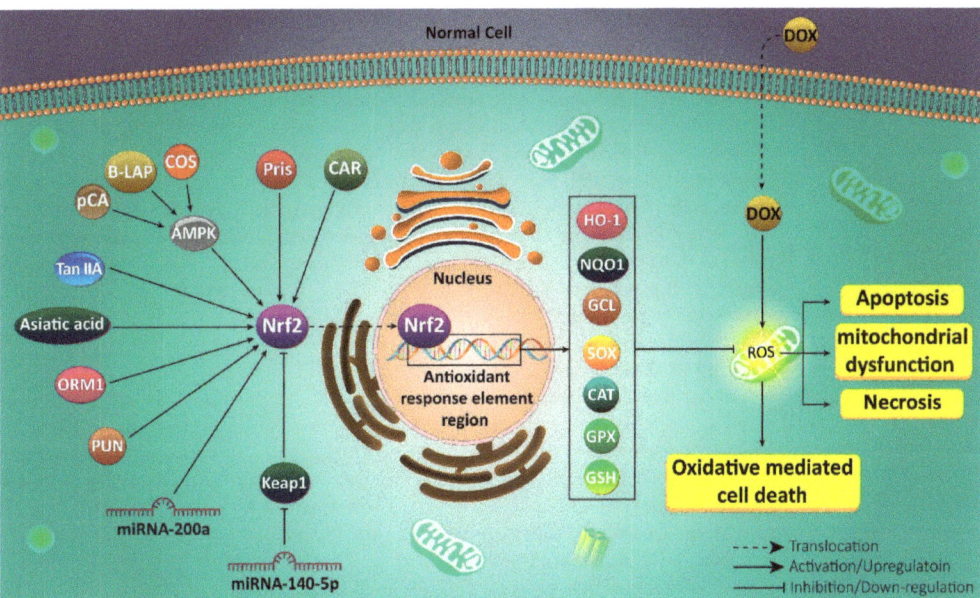

Figure 2. Targeting Nrf2 signaling pathway in chemoprotection. Regulation of Nrf2 signaling by upstream mediators and protective compounds in decreasing adverse effects of doxorubicin. Apoptosis, mitochondrial dysfunction, necrosis and cell death are prevented upon Nrf2 activation.

7. Nrf2 in Doxorubicin Resistance

Due to the potential role of Nrf2 signaling in triggering DOX resistance, much attention has been directed towards targeting this pathway in reversing chemoresistance. For this purpose, Singh and colleagues have designed a small molecule inhibitor of Nrf2 signaling, known as ML385 that binds to Neh1 domain of Nrf2 and inhibits its DNA binding. This leads to an increase in anti-tumor activity of DOX against lung cancer cells [172]. Therefore, first strategy can be considered developing a novel inhibitor capable of binding to Nrf2 domain and suppressing its activity and nuclear translocation. The second strategy that has not been tried yet, but can be considered in next experiments, is designing molecules capable of binding to Keap1 and promoting its activity in inhibiting Nrf2. Furthermore, natural products can be utilized in targeting Nrf2 signaling for providing DOX sensitivity. Parthenolide (PN) is a sesquiterpene lactone exclusively found in *Tanacetum parthenium* and is famous due to its inhibitory effect on cancer progression [173–175]. In DOX-resistance breast cancer cells, Nrf2 undergoes up-regulation that mediates increased levels of P-glycoprotein (P-gp), Bcl-2, CAT, SOD and heat shock protein 70 (HSP70). PN administration along with DOX inhibits Nrf2 signaling and its downstream targets to promote ROS generation, leading to reversing DOX resistance [176].

Chrysin is a flavonoid compound that has demonstrated anti-tumor activity against different cancers via regulating molecular pathways. Increasing evidence exhibits that chrysin suppresses cancer progression and proliferation and stimulates apoptosis via down-regulating phosphoinositide 3-kinase (PI3K)/protein kinase B (Akt) axis [177,178]. Furthermore, chrysin diminishes expression level of extracellular-signal regulated kinase (ERK) in disrupting cancer progression [179,180]. In enhancing DOX sensitivity of cancer cells, chrysin affects two distinct pathways including PI3K/Akt/Nrf2 and ERK/Nrf2. In this way, chrysin reduces expression levels of ERK and PI3K/Akt to suppress Nrf2 signaling, leading to enhanced DOX sensitivity [181]. What is noteworthy is that it seems that PI3K/Nrf2 signaling has association with activity and expression of drug resistance proteins that has been evaluated. Vialenin P (VP) can suppress PI3K/Nrf2 signaling to down-regulate multidrug resistance protein 1 (MRP1), leading to enhanced accumulation of DOX in breast cancer cells, and sensitizing them to chemotherapy [182].

Apigenin (APG) is a natural bioflavonoid present in fruits and vegetables and has anti-tumor activity against different cancers. APG administration is of importance in suppressing cisplatin resistance of ovarian cancer cells via apoptosis induction and Mcl-1 down-regulation [183]. In increasing DOX cytotoxicity, APG inhibits DNA repair of breast cancer cells [184]. Furthermore, co-administration of APG with other anti-tumor agents such as sorafenib increases its efficacy in triggering apoptosis and cell cycle arrest in cancer cells [185]. In DOX-resistant hepatocellular carcinoma cells, APG enhances expression of miRNA-101 as a tumor-suppressing factor. Then, up-regulated miRNA-101 reduces Nrf2 expression to promote DOX sensitivity of cancer cells [186].

In addition to miRNAs, PI3K/Akt signaling pathway is affected by APG in suppressing DOX resistance. As it was mentioned, PI3K/Akt induction is in favor of cancer progression and its inhibition can be considered as a promising strategy in cancer therapy [187,188]. It seems that APG down-regulates PI3K/Akt signaling to inhibit Nrf2, leading to increased sensitivity to DOX chemotherapy [189]. These studies demonstrate that how molecular pathways such as Nrf2 with its main role in providing redox balance, can participate in DOX resistance [190]. Consequently, targeting Nrf2, and its upstream and downstream mediators can be considered as ideal strategies in cancer therapy and reversing DOX resistance [191].

Wogonin is a bioactive flavonoid isolated from *Scutellaria baicalensis* with capability of suppressing chemoresistance via down-regulating expression and activity of P-gp [192]. Wogonin functions as an enhancer of ROS levels in inducing cell proliferation inhibition [193]. Wogonin can enhance efficacy of immune system in cancer eradication and promote macrophage M1 polarization [194]. In DOX-resistant breast cancer cells, wogonin suppresses defense system mediated via Nrf2 inhibition and decreasing expressions of HO-1 and NQO1 [195]. Another experiment investigates potential of plant-derived extracts in increasing sensitivity of lung cancer cells to DOX chemotherapy. It has been reported that cinnamomic cortex extract provides Nrf2 down-regulation in promoting DOX sensitivity [196].

Similar to wogonin, luteolin also belongs to flavonoid family. Luteolin acts as a potent anti-cancer agent [197] in suppressing cancer migration and invasion via down-regulating epithelial-to-mesenchymal transition (EMT) and focal adhesion kinase [198,199]. Cancer progression occurs in hypoxic conditions, and luteolin administration is of importance in reducing HIF-1α expression and disrupting hypoxia-mediated cancer progression. Furthermore, luteolin induces apoptosis and autophagy in breast and colon cancer cells [200]. These studies advocate the fact that luteolin administration negatively affects cancer progression, and this agent is advantageous in reversing DOX resistance. In this way, luteolin reduces Nrf2 expression at mRNA level by 34% and is involved in regaining sensitivity of lung cancer cells to DOX chemotherapy [201]. Luteolin can also enhance DOX sensitivity of breast cancer cells. Luteolin dually inhibits Nrf2/HO-1 and Nrf2/MDR1 signaling pathways to remove defense system mechanism in enhancing DOX sensitivity [202].

Consequently, using anti-tumor compounds, as most of them are phytochemicals, is of importance in reversing DOX resistance via Nrf2 down-regulation [203]. However, it should be noted that anti-tumor agents, especially naturally occurring compounds suffer from poor bioavailability [204,205], and using carriers such as nanostructures for their delivery can remarkably promote their potential in down-regulating Nrf2 signaling and enhancing DOX sensitivity of cancer cells.

8. Nrf2, Upstream and Downstream Targets

In the previous section, we demonstrated that both synthesized and natural compounds can be of importance in suppressing DOX resistance via regulating Nrf2 and its downstream targets. In this section, a mechanistic discussion of signaling networks in which Nrf2 is key player and lead to DOX resistance, is provided to provide insights for developing novel therapeutics.

One of the important aspects of Nrf2 signaling is its association with drug transporters. Nrf2 can promote expression of P-gp transporter in enhancing colorectal cancer progression and triggering chemoresistance [206]. Such a relationship is found between Nrf2 and ABCB1 in DOX resistant. In hypoxic conditions, liver cancer cells increase Nrf2 expression to up-regulate activity and expression of ABCB1. Then, intracellular accumulation of DOX decreases in cancer cells that provides their resistance to apoptosis [207]. It has been reported that Nrf2 down-regulation is associated with P-gp inhibition and triggering DOX sensitivity of cancer cells [208]. Targeting Nrf2 is of importance for increasing sensitivity of cancer cells to DOX chemotherapy.

Small interfering RNA (siRNA) is a powerful genetic tool that is extensively applied in targeting molecular pathways and genes responsible for cancer progression. Recent studies have shown that siRNA can be utilized for increasing sensitivity of cancer cells to chemotherapeutic agents such as cisplatin, paclitaxel, docetaxel and so on [209–211]. Similarly, siRNA can be used for mediating DOX sensitivity via targeting Nrf2. Down-regulating Nrf2 expression at mRNA and protein levels is performed by siRNA, and its downstream targets such as HO-1 and NQO1 undergo down-regulation, resulting in ROS overgeneration and enhanced sensitivity to DOX chemotherapy [212]. The interesting point is that in vitro and in vivo experiments have confirmed that Nrf2 overexpression is associated with cancer proliferation, survival and chemoresistance. Abrogation of Nrf2 expression results in an increase in DOX sensitivity via enhancing ROS levels and triggering cancer cell death [213].

Cluster of differentiation 44 (CD44) is a glycoprotein and a receptor for extracellular matrix (ECM) components such as hyaluronic acid (HA). This cell-surface glycoprotein is a cancer stem cell (CSC) marker and can undergo alternative splicing and post-transcriptional modification. CD44 overexpression is an obvious finding in cancer cells and mediates their malignancy [214,215]. It has been reported that CD44 can trigger drug resistance of breast cancer stem cells. CD44 enhances p62 expression to induce Nrf2 and DOX resistance [216]. This is maybe due to increased malignancy of cancer cells, so that Keap1 down-regulation and subsequent Nrf2 induction provide conditions for cancer growth [217]. CSCs that are resistant to DOX chemotherapy, demonstrate simultaneous up-regulation of Nrf2 and ABCB1 [218]. As it was mentioned earlier, Nrf2 stimulates DOX resistance via enhancing activity and expression of drug transporters. Therefore, up-regulation of Nrf2 and ABCB1 in CSCs may have associations that should be considered in further experiments.

MRTF-A is a co-activator of serum response factor (SRF) that functions as a tumor-promoting factor in increasing proliferation, and metastasis as well as triggering drug resistance [219]. MRTF-A can cooperate with signal transducer and activator of transcription 3 (STAT3) in inducing BRSM1 hypermethylation and increasing breast cancer invasion [220]. In mediating DOX resistance, MRTF-A generates a complex containing SRF attached to CarG on promoter region of Nrf2 to stimulate its expression and reduce sensitivity of cancer cells to apoptosis [221].

Sometimes, interaction between enzymes and their product can direct conditions towards developing chemoresistance. Such association is obvious in lysophosphatidate (LPA) that is generated by autotaxin (ATX). Primarily, LPA is involved in repairing tissues by inducing proliferation, migration, angiogenesis and other important biological mechanisms. These impacts are of importance in improving pathological conditions such as arthritis, pulmonary fibrosis and inflammatory bowel disease [222–226]. However, it has been reported that LPA and ATX can induce cancer progression and LPA up-regulation is correlated with development of colon cancer and hepatitis [227–229]. In DOX-resistant breast cancer cells, LPA enhances stabilization of Nrf2 to up-regulate its expression, resulting in activation of antioxidant parameters and drug transporters that are vital for inducing DOX resistance [230]. Table 2 provides a summary of molecular pathways involved in

DOX resistance, and anti-tumor agents capable of regulating Nrf2 signaling in suppressing DOX resistance (Table 2, Figure 3).

Table 2. Activation/suppression of Nrf2 signaling and its association with DOX resistance/sensitivity.

Cancer Type	Signaling Network	Compound/Agent	Nrf2 Expression	Remarks	Refs
Breast cancer	P62/Nrf2	–	Up-regulation	Reducing oxidative stress Mediating DOX resistance Promoting colony formation and migration capacities Improving cancer stem cell features	[216]
Breast cancer	Cul3/Nrf2	–	Down-regulation	Association of Cul3 with Nrf2 depletion Inducing oxidative stress Increasing DOX sensitivity	[231]
Breast cancer	PI3K/Nrf2/MRP1	Vielanin P	Down-regulation	Inhibiting PI3K/Nrf2 axis Suppressing MRP1 expression Promoting DOX sensitivity	[182]
Breast cancer	Nrf2/HSP70	Parthenolide	Down-regulation	Reducing expressions of Nrf2 and HSP70 Enhancing DOX sensitivity of breast cancer cells	[176]
Breast cancer	Nrf2/HO-1 Nrf2/MDR1	Luteolin	Down-regulation	Enhancing number of cancer cells undergoing cell death Increasing cytotoxicity of DOX Down-regulation of Nrf2 and subsequent inhibition of its downstream targets HO-1 and MDR1	[202]
Breast cancer	Nrf2/HO-1 Nrf2/NQO1	Wogonin	Down-regulation	Impairing cellular defense systemNrf2 signaling inhibition Down-regulation of HO-1 and NQO1 Increasing DOX cytotoxicity towards cancer cells	[195]
Breast cancer	HER2/Nrf2	–	Up-regulation	Conferring drug resistance Enhancing activities of antioxidant enzymes such as GSTA2, GSTP1 and HO-1	[232]
Breast cancer	Nrf2/p62	Pseudomonas aeruginosa mannose-sensitive hemagglutinin	Down-regulation	Inhibiting Nrf2 signaling and its downstream target p62 Increasing DOX sensitivity Impairing cancer growth	[190]
Hepatocellular carcinoma	MiRNA-101/Nrf2	Apigenin	Down-regulation	Enhancing miRNA-101 expression Inhibiting Nrf2 signaling by binding to 3$'$-UTR Enhancing DOX sensitivity	[186]
Hepatocellular carcinoma	PI3K/Akt/Nrf2	Apigenin	Down-regulation	Reducing mRNA and protein levels of Nrf2 via PI3K/Akt inhibition Reducing cell proliferation Inducing apoptosis Promoting DOX sensitivity	[189]
Liver cancer	Nrf2/ABCB1	–	Up-regulation	Nrf2 overexpression occurs in hypoxic conditions Reducing apoptosis and DNA damage Inducing DOX resistance ABCB1 up-regulation	[207]
Different cancers	MRTF-A/Nrf2	–	Up-regulation	Reducing apoptosis Triggering DOX resistance	[221]
Different cancers	–	–	Down-regulation	SiRNA is a powerful in Nrf2 down-regulation Inhibiting activities of ABCC3, ABCC4 and ABCG2 Enhancing DOX sensitivity	[212]
Different cancers	PI3K/Akt/Nrf2 ERK/Nrf2	Chrysin	Down-regulation	Suppressing PI3K/Akt/Nrf2 and ERK/Nrf2 signaling pathwaysNrf2 down-regulation and inhibiting its downstream targets HO-1 Enhancing DOX sensitivity	[181]

Table 2. Cont.

Cancer Type	Signaling Network	Compound/Agent	Nrf2 Expression	Remarks	Refs
Ovarian cancer	ALDH/Nrf2	All-trans retinoic acid	Down-regulation	Promoting cancer stem features Enhancing colony formation capacity Mediating DOX resistance Suppressing ALDH/Nrf2 signaling by retinoic acid in reducing DOX resistance	[191]
Ovarian cancer	-	-	Up-regulation	Overexpression of Nrf2 in DOX-resistant cancer cells Reducing tumor growth following Nrf2 down-regulation	[233]
Ovarian cancer	-	-	Up-regulation	Obtaining DOX resistance via Nrf2 signaling and reducing cell death	[234]
Ovarian cancer	Nrf2/miRNA-206/c-MET/EGFR	-	Up-regulation	Reducing miRNA-206 expression Inducing expressions of c-MET and EGFR expressions Triggering DOX resistance	[235]
Colorectal cancer	Nrf2/P-gp	-	Up-regulation	Enhancing P-gp expressions Reducing cell death Inducing DOX resistance	[208]
Lung cancer	-	ML385	Down-regulation	ML385 functions as an inhibitor of Nrf2 signaling Promoting DOX sensitivity	[172]
Myeloid leukemia	Nrf2/HO-1 Nrf2/NQO1	Tritolide	Down-regulation	Enhancing drug sensitivity Apoptosis induction Suppressing Nrf2 and its downstream targets	[203]

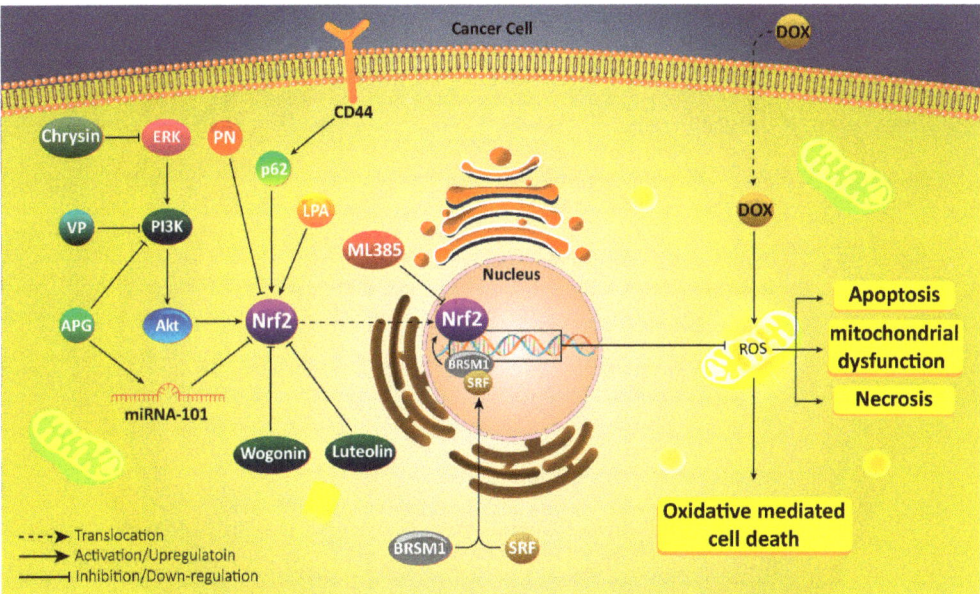

Figure 3. Nrf2 signaling in mediating DOX resistance of cancer cells. Suppressing Nrf2 signaling as a pro-survival pathway is associated with induction of apoptosis and necrosis in cancer cells, and their sensitivity to chemotherapy.

9. Room for Drug Discovery

In treatment of cancer patients, DOX is considered as a first option and is mostly preferred to surgery, as an invasive strategy. However, resistance to this well-known chemotherapeutic agent has resulted in failure in treatment of cancer patients. Nrf2 is involved in DOX resistance, and after chemotherapy, compounds activating Nrf2 signaling can be applied. As it was mentioned earlier in the main text, most of the anti-tumor compounds for providing DOX sensitivity are phytochemicals. For synthesizing new small molecule inhibitors of Nrf2 signaling, much attention should be directed towards Nrf2 and Keap1 structures. Furthermore, new chemically synthesized anti-tumor agents can also inhibit nuclear translocation of Nrf2 by binding to it and providing ubiquitination and degradation. After DOX chemotherapy, the story is completely different and if a protective agent wants to be synthesized, it should be capable of binding to Nrf2 and mediating its nuclear translocation or suppressing Keap1 activity.

10. Conclusions and Remarks

In the present review, two important aspects of Nrf2 signaling including chemoprotection and chemoresistance were discussed in view of DOX. Each section was divided into two parts describing involved molecular pathways and role of anti-tumor and protective compounds in targeting Nrf2 signaling during DOX chemotherapy. It is noteworthy that most of the compounds targeting Nrf2 signaling are phytochemicals. In the case of protecting against adverse effects of DOX, protective compounds induce Nrf2 signaling and its downstream targets such as HO-1 and NQO1 in reinforcing antioxidant defense systems and supporting against oxidative damage, while anti-tumor compounds inhibit Nrf2 signaling in promoting ROS levels and oxidative damage, resulting in cell death in cancer cells.

These statements clearly demonstrate the dual role of Nrf2 signaling in cancer chemotherapy. In fact, the aim is determining factor for stimulating or suppressing Nrf2 signaling. The notion should be considered that chemoprotection should be performed after DOX chemotherapy, since inducing Nrf2 signaling is associated with DOX resistance. Therefore, Nrf2 inhibition should be conducted during DOX chemotherapy and Nrf2 induction after this period to prevent or ameliorate its side effects on major organs of the body. The interesting point is that Nrf2 signaling can promote stem cell population in providing DOX resistance. Hence, by targeting Nrf2 signaling, both cancer cells and CSCs are affected that are of importance in effective DOX chemotherapy.

To date, most of the studies have focused on using compounds for targeting Nrf2 signaling in chemoprotection and reversing chemoresistance. However, more progress can be performed using nanoparticles for delivery of these anti-tumor agents. Nanocarriers can significantly promote intracellular accumulation of anti-tumor agents in cancer cells and enhance their efficiency in Nrf2 inhibition and providing DOX sensitivity. Furthermore, the ability of compounds to protect during DOX chemotherapy can be improved using nanocarriers. Another important aspect is using genetic tools in targeting Nrf2 signaling. As it was mentioned, siRNA system has been applied for affecting Nrf2 signaling. Other techniques such as CRISPR/Cas9 system can also be used, and furthermore, more studies are needed to elucidate potential of siRNA for using in DOX sensitivity. Similar to compounds, nanoarchitectures can promote efficiency of genetic tools in gene silencing that should be considered in future experiments.

Author Contributions: M.A., H.K. and A.P.K. conceptualized the review, collate articles and performed critical revision of the manuscript. S.M., A.Z. (Amirhossein Zabolian), F.H., H.S., N.A., S.H., M.V.F. and K.H. contributed to preparing draft manuscript. A.Z. (Ali Zarrabi) performed software works. All authors have read and agreed to the published version of the manuscript.

Funding: This work was supported by grants from Singapore Ministry of Education [T2EP30120-0042], the National Research Foundation Singapore and the Singapore Ministry of Education under its Research Centre's of Excellence initiative to Cancer Science Institute of Singapore, National University of Singapore to A.P.K.

Conflicts of Interest: The authors declare no conflict of interest.

Abbreviations

DOX	Doxorubicin
ROS	reactive oxygen species
TFAM	mitochondrial transcription factor A
AMPK	AMP-activated protein kinase
VASH2	vasohibin2
SpK1	sphingosine kinase 1
HIF-1α	hypoxia inducible factor-1α
ncRNAs	non-coding RNAs
lncRNAs	long non-coding RNAs
miRNAs	microRNAs
GI	gastrointestinal
MMP-2	matrix metalloproteinase-2
Nrf2	nuclear factor erythroid 2-related factor 2
Keap1	kelch-like ECH-associated protein 1
Cul3	cullin3
GSK-3β	glycogen synthase-kinase 3β
βTrCP	β transducing repeat containing E3 ubiquitin-protein ligase
HO-1	heme oxygenase-1
NQO1	NAD(p)H dehydrogenase quinone 1
ARE	antioxidant response elemento
PPARγ	peroxisome proliferator-activated receptor gama
MDA	malondialdehyde
SOD	superoxide dismutase
CAT	catálase
GSH	glutathione
Pris	pristimerin
AA	Asiatic acid
B-LAP	β-LAPachone
CAR	cardamonin
COS	chitosan oligosaccharide
pCA	p-coumaric acid
LPS	lipopolysaccharide
Tan IIA	tanshinone IIA
PUN	punicalagin
3′-UTR	3′-untranslated region
LC-3II	light chain-3II
ORM1	orosomucoid 1
3D	3-dimensional
PN	parthenolide
P-gp	P-glycoprotein
HSP70	heat shock protein 70
PI3K	phosphatidylinositide 3-kinase
Akt	protein kinase-B
ERK	extracellular signal-regulated kinase
VP	vialenin P
MRP1	multidrug resistance protein 1
APG	apigenin
EMT	epithelial-to-mesenchymal transition
siRNA	small interfering RNA
CD44	cluster of differentiation 44
ECM	extracellular matrix
CSC	cancer stem cell
SRF	serum response factor
STAT3	signal transducer and activator of transcription 3
LPA	lisophosphatidate
ATX	autotaxin

References

1. Prathumsap, N.; Shinlapawittayatorn, K.; Chattipakorn, S.C.; Chattipakorn, N. Effects of doxorubicin on the heart: From molecular mechanisms to intervention strategies. *Eur. J. Pharmacol.* **2020**, *866*, 172818. [CrossRef]
2. Denard, B.; Lee, C.; Ye, J. Doxorubicin blocks proliferation of cancer cells through proteolytic activation of CREB3L1. *elife* **2012**, *1*, e00090. [CrossRef]
3. Lu, M.; Xie, K.; Lu, X.; Lu, L.; Shi, Y.; Tang, Y. Notoginsenoside R1 counteracts mesenchymal stem cell-evoked oncogenesis and doxorubicin resistance in osteosarcoma cells by blocking IL-6 secretion-induced JAK2/STAT3 signaling. *Investig. New Drugs* **2020**. [CrossRef]
4. Ghandhariyoun, N.; Jaafari, M.R.; Nikoofal-Sahlabadi, S.; Taghdisi, S.M.; Moosavian, S.A. Reducing Doxorubicin resistance in breast cancer by liposomal FOXM1 aptamer: In vitro and in vivo. *Life Sci.* **2020**, *262*, 118520. [CrossRef] [PubMed]
5. Ashrafizadeh, M.; Zarrabi, A.; Hashemi, F.; Zabolian, A.; Saleki, H.; Bagherian, M.; Azami, N.; Bejandi, A.K.; Hushmandi, K.; Ang, H.L.; et al. Polychemotherapy with Curcumin and Doxorubicin via Biological Nanoplatforms: Enhancing Antitumor Activity. *Pharmaceutics* **2020**, *12*, 1084. [CrossRef]
6. Poh, H.M.; Chiou, Y.S.; Chong, Q.Y.; Chen, R.M.; Rangappa, K.S.; Ma, L.; Zhu, T.; Kumar, A.P.; Pandey, V.; Lee, S.C.; et al. Inhibition of TFF3 Enhances Sensitivity-and Overcomes Acquired Resistance-to Doxorubicin in Estrogen Receptor-Positive Mammary Carcinoma. *Cancers* **2019**, *11*, 1528. [CrossRef] [PubMed]
7. Yang, L.; Li, D.; Tang, P.; Zuo, Y. Curcumin increases the sensitivity of K562/DOX cells to doxorubicin by targeting S100 calcium-binding protein A8 and P-glycoprotein. *Oncol. Lett.* **2020**, *19*, 83–92. [CrossRef]
8. Xinyong, C.; Zhiyi, Z.; Lang, H.; Peng, Y.; Xiaocheng, W.; Ping, Z.; Liang, S. The role of toll-like receptors in myocardial toxicity induced by doxorubicin. *Immunol. Lett.* **2020**, *217*, 56–64. [CrossRef]
9. Wei, T.; Xiaojun, X.; Peilong, C. Magnoflorine improves sensitivity to doxorubicin (DOX) of breast cancer cells via inducing apoptosis and autophagy through AKT/mTOR and p38 signaling pathways. *Biomed. Pharmacother.* **2020**, *121*, 109139. [CrossRef]
10. Abd-Rabou, A.A.; Ahmed, H.H.; Shalby, A.B. Selenium Overcomes Doxorubicin Resistance in Their Nano-platforms Against Breast and Colon Cancers. *Biol. Trace Elem. Res.* **2020**, *193*, 377–389. [CrossRef]
11. Zhu, Y.; Xu, J.; Hu, W.; Wang, F.; Zhou, Y.; Xu, W.; Gong, W.; Shao, L. TFAM depletion overcomes hepatocellular carcinoma resistance to doxorubicin and sorafenib through AMPK activation and mitochondrial dysfunction. *Gene* **2020**, *753*, 144807. [CrossRef]
12. Tan, X.; Liao, Z.; Zou, S.; Ma, L.; Wang, A. VASH2 Promotes Cell Proliferation and Resistance to Doxorubicin in Non-Small Cell Lung Cancer via AKT Signaling. *Oncol. Res.* **2020**, *28*, 3–11. [CrossRef]
13. Tanaka, I.; Chakraborty, A.; Saulnier, O.; Benoit-Pilven, C.; Vacher, S.; Labiod, D.; Lam, E.W.F.; Bièche, I.; Delattre, O.; Pouzoulet, F.; et al. ZRANB2 and SYF2-mediated splicing programs converging on ECT2 are involved in breast cancer cell resistance to doxorubicin. *Nucleic Acids Res.* **2020**, *48*, 2676–2693. [CrossRef]
14. Datta, A.; Loo, S.Y.; Huang, B.; Wong, L.; Tan, S.S.; Tan, T.Z.; Lee, S.C.; Thiery, J.P.; Lim, Y.C.; Yong, W.P.; et al. SPHK1 regulates proliferation and survival responses in triple-negative breast cancer. *Oncotarget* **2014**, *5*, 5920–5933. [CrossRef]
15. Ma, Z.; Wang, L.Z.; Cheng, J.T.; Lam, W.S.T.; Ma, X.; Xiang, X.; Wong, A.L.; Goh, B.C.; Gong, Q.; Sethi, G.; et al. Targeting HIF-1-mediated Metastasis for Cancer Therapy. *Antioxid. Redox Signal.* **2020**. [CrossRef]
16. Ren, X.; Su, C. Sphingosine kinase 1 contributes to doxorubicin resistance and glycolysis in osteosarcoma. *Mol. Med. Rep.* **2020**, *22*, 2183–2190. [CrossRef]
17. Wu, H.; Gu, J.; Zhou, D.; Cheng, W.; Wang, Y.; Wang, Q.; Wang, X. LINC00160 mediated paclitaxel-And doxorubicin-resistance in breast cancer cells by regulating TFF3 via transcription factor C/EBPβ. *J. Cell. Mol. Med.* **2020**, *24*, 8589–8602. [CrossRef]
18. Wang, B.; Xu, L.; Zhang, J.; Cheng, X.; Xu, Q.; Wang, J.; Mao, F. LncRNA NORAD accelerates the progression and doxorubicin resistance of neuroblastoma through up-regulating HDAC8 via sponging miR-144-3p. *Biomed. Pharmacother.* **2020**, *129*, 110268. [CrossRef]
19. Ong, M.S.; Cai, W.; Yuan, Y.; Leong, H.C.; Tan, T.Z.; Mohammad, A.; You, M.L.; Arfuso, F.; Goh, B.C.; Warrier, S.; et al. 'Lnc'-ing Wnt in female reproductive cancers: Therapeutic potential of long non-coding RNAs in Wnt signalling. *Br. J. Pharmacol.* **2017**, *174*, 4684–4700. [CrossRef]
20. Mishra, S.; Verma, S.S.; Rai, V.; Awasthee, N.; Chava, S.; Hui, K.M.; Kumar, A.P.; Challagundla, K.B.; Sethi, G.; Gupta, S.C. Long non-coding RNAs are emerging targets of phytochemicals for cancer and other chronic diseases. *Cell. Mol. Life Sci.* **2019**, *76*, 1947–1966. [CrossRef]
21. Ashrafizadeh, M.; Zarrabi, A.; Hushmandi, K.; Kalantari, M.; Mohammadinejad, R.; Javaheri, T.; Sethi, G. Association of the Epithelial-Mesenchymal Transition (EMT) with Cisplatin Resistance. *Int. J. Mol. Sci.* **2020**, *21*, 4002. [CrossRef]
22. Li, Y.; Li, X.; Lu, Y.; Chaurasiya, B.; Mi, G.; Shi, D.; Chen, D.; Webster, T.J.; Tu, J.; Shen, Y. Co-delivery of Poria cocos extract and doxorubicin as an 'all-in-one' nanocarrier to combat breast cancer multidrug resistance during chemotherapy. *Nanomedicine* **2020**, *23*, 102095. [CrossRef] [PubMed]
23. Pfister, C.; Gravis, G.; Fléchon, A.; Soulié, M.; Guy, L.; Laguerre, B.; Mottet, N.; Joly, F.; Allory, Y.; Harter, V.; et al. Randomized Phase III Trial of Dose-dense Methotrexate, Vinblastine, Doxorubicin, and Cisplatin, or Gemcitabine and Cisplatin as Perioperative Chemotherapy for Patients with Muscle-invasive Bladder Cancer. Analysis of the GETUG/AFU V05 VESPER Trial Secondary Endpoints: Chemotherapy Toxicity and Pathological Responses. *Eur. Urol.* **2020**. [CrossRef]

24. Gadisa, D.A.; Assefa, M.; Wang, S.H.; Yimer, G. Toxicity profile of Doxorubicin-Cyclophosphamide and Doxorubicin-Cyclophosphamide followed by Paclitaxel regimen and its associated factors among women with breast cancer in Ethiopia: A prospective cohort study. *J. Oncol. Pharm. Pract.* **2020**, *26*, 1912–1920. [CrossRef]
25. Harahap, Y.; Ardiningsih, P.; Corintias Winarti, A.; Purwanto, D.J. Analysis of the Doxorubicin and Doxorubicinol in the Plasma of Breast Cancer Patients for Monitoring the Toxicity of Doxorubicin. *Drug Des. Dev. Ther.* **2020**, *14*, 3469–3475. [CrossRef]
26. Li, X.Q.; Liu, Y.K.; Yi, J.; Dong, J.S.; Zhang, P.P.; Wan, L.; Li, K. MicroRNA-143 Increases Oxidative Stress and Myocardial Cell Apoptosis in a Mouse Model of Doxorubicin-Induced Cardiac Toxicity. *Med. Sci. Monit.* **2020**, *26*, e920394. [CrossRef]
27. Chan, B.Y.H.; Roczkowsky, A.; Cho, W.J.; Poirier, M.; Sergi, C.; Keschrumrus, V.; Churko, J.M.; Granzier, H.; Schulz, R. MMP inhibitors attenuate doxorubicin cardiotoxicity by preventing intracellular and extracellular matrix remodeling. *Cardiovasc. Res.* **2020**. [CrossRef]
28. Boratto, F.A.; Franco, M.S.; Barros, A.L.B.; Cassali, G.D.; Malachias, A.; Ferreira, L.A.M.; Leite, E.A. Alpha-tocopheryl succinate improves encapsulation, pH-sensitivity, antitumor activity and reduces toxicity of doxorubicin-loaded liposomes. *Eur. J. Pharm. Sci.* **2020**, *144*, 105205. [CrossRef]
29. Khan, T.H.; Ganaie, M.A.; Alharthy, K.M.; Madkhali, H.; Jan, B.L.; Sheikh, I.A. Naringenin prevents doxorubicin-induced toxicity in kidney tissues by regulating the oxidative and inflammatory insult in Wistar rats. *Arch. Physiol. Biochem.* **2020**, *126*, 300–307. [CrossRef]
30. Oh, J.; Lee, B.S.; Lim, G.; Lim, H.; Lee, C.J.; Park, S.; Lee, S.H.; Chung, J.H.; Kang, S.M. Atorvastatin protects cardiomyocyte from doxorubicin toxicity by modulating survivin expression through FOXO1 inhibition. *J. Mol. Cell. Cardiol.* **2020**, *138*, 244–255. [CrossRef]
31. Uruno, A.; Matsumaru, D.; Ryoke, R.; Saito, R.; Kadoguchi, S.; Saigusa, D.; Saito, T.; Saido, T.C.; Kawashima, R.; Yamamoto, M. Nrf2 Suppresses Oxidative Stress and Inflammation in App Knock-In Alzheimer's Disease Model Mice. *Mol. Cell. Biol.* **2020**, *40*. [CrossRef]
32. Zhou, Y.; Wang, K.; Zhou, Y.; Li, T.; Yang, M.; Wang, R.; Chen, Y.; Cao, M.; Hu, R. HEATR1 deficiency promotes pancreatic cancer proliferation and gemcitabine resistance by up-regulating Nrf2 signaling. *Redox Biol.* **2020**, *29*, 101390. [CrossRef]
33. Hassanein, E.H.; Sayed, A.M.; Hussein, O.E.; Mahmoud, A.M. Coumarins as Modulators of the Keap1/Nrf2/ARE Signaling Pathway. *Oxidative Med. Cell. Longev.* **2020**, *2020*, 1675957. [CrossRef]
34. Rosa, P.L.; Bertini, E.S.; Piemonte, F. The NRF2 Signaling Network Defines Clinical Biomarkers and Therapeutic Opportunity in Friedreich's Ataxia. *Int. J. Mol. Sci.* **2020**, *21*, 916. [CrossRef]
35. Kohandel, Z.; Farkhondeh, T.; Aschner, M.; Samarghandian, S. Nrf2 a molecular therapeutic target for Astaxanthin. *Biomed. Pharmacother.* **2021**, *137*, 111374. [CrossRef]
36. Uddin, M.S.; Al Mamun, A.; Jakaria, M.; Thangapandiyan, S.; Ahmad, J.; Rahman, M.A.; Mathew, B.; Abdel-Daim, M.M.; Aleya, L. Emerging promise of sulforaphane-mediated Nrf2 signaling cascade against neurological disorders. *Sci. Total Environ.* **2020**, *707*, 135624. [CrossRef]
37. Raghunath, A.; Sundarraj, K.; Arfuso, F.; Sethi, G.; Perumal, E. Dysregulation of Nrf2 in Hepatocellular Carcinoma: Role in Cancer Progression and Chemoresistance. *Cancers* **2018**, *10*, 481. [CrossRef]
38. Kirtonia, A.; Sethi, G.; Garg, M. The multifaceted role of reactive oxygen species in tumorigenesis. *Cell. Mol. Life Sci.* **2020**, *77*, 4459–4483. [CrossRef]
39. Anandhan, A.; Dodson, M.; Schmidlin, C.J.; Liu, P.; Zhang, D.D. Breakdown of an Ironclad Defense System: The Critical Role of NRF2 in Mediating Ferroptosis. *Cell. Chem. Biol.* **2020**, *27*, 436–447. [CrossRef]
40. Taguchi, K.; Yamamoto, M. The KEAP1-NRF2 System as a Molecular Target of Cancer Treatment. *Cancers* **2020**, *13*, 46. [CrossRef] [PubMed]
41. Farkhondeh, T.; Folgado, S.L.; Pourbagher-Shahri, A.M.; Ashrafizadeh, M.; Samarghandian, S. The therapeutic effect of resveratrol: Focusing on the Nrf2 signaling pathway. *Biomed. Pharmacother.* **2020**, *127*, 110234. [CrossRef]
42. Samarghandian, S.; Pourbagher-Shahri, A.M.; Ashrafizadeh, M.; Khan, H.; Forouzanfar, F.; Aramjoo, H.; Farkhondeh, T. A pivotal role of the nrf2 signaling pathway in spinal cord injury: A prospective therapeutics study. *CNS Neurol. Disord. Drug Targets Former. Curr. Drug Targets-CNS Neurol. Disord.* **2020**, *19*, 207–219. [CrossRef]
43. Ahmadi, Z.; Ashrafizadeh, M. Melatonin as a potential modulator of Nrf2. *Fundam. Clin. Pharmacol.* **2020**, *34*, 11–19. [CrossRef]
44. Ashrafizadeh, M.; Fekri, H.S.; Ahmadi, Z.; Farkhondeh, T.; Samarghandian, S. Therapeutic and biological activities of berberine: The involvement of Nrf2 signaling pathway. *J. Cell. Biochem.* **2020**, *121*, 1575–1585. [CrossRef]
45. Itoh, K.; Wakabayashi, N.; Katoh, Y.; Ishii, T.; Igarashi, K.; Engel, J.D.; Yamamoto, M. Keap1 represses nuclear activation of antioxidant responsive elements by Nrf2 through binding to the amino-terminal Neh2 domain. *Genes Dev.* **1999**, *13*, 76–86. [CrossRef]
46. Kobayashi, A.; Kang, M.I.; Okawa, H.; Ohtsuji, M.; Zenke, Y.; Chiba, T.; Igarashi, K.; Yamamoto, M. Oxidative stress sensor Keap1 functions as an adaptor for Cul3-based E3 ligase to regulate proteasomal degradation of Nrf2. *Mol. Cell. Biol.* **2004**, *24*, 7130–7139. [CrossRef]
47. Eggler, A.L.; Liu, G.; Pezzuto, J.M.; van Breemen, R.B.; Mesecar, A.D. Modifying specific cysteines of the electrophile-sensing human Keap1 protein is insufficient to disrupt binding to the Nrf2 domain Neh2. *Proc. Natl. Acad. Sci. USA* **2005**, *102*, 10070–10075. [CrossRef]

48. Shaw, P.; Chattopadhyay, A. Nrf2-ARE signaling in cellular protection: Mechanism of action and the regulatory mechanisms. *J. Cell. Physiol.* **2020**, *235*, 3119–3130. [CrossRef]
49. Cuadrado, A. Structural and functional characterization of Nrf2 degradation by glycogen synthase kinase 3/β-TrCP. *Free Radic. Biol. Med.* **2015**, *88*, 147–157. [CrossRef]
50. Venugopal, R.; Jaiswal, A.K. Nrf2 and Nrf1 in association with Jun proteins regulate antioxidant response element-mediated expression and coordinated induction of genes encoding detoxifying enzymes. *Oncogene* **1998**, *17*, 3145–3156. [CrossRef]
51. Saeedi, B.J.; Liu, K.H.; Owens, J.A.; Hunter-Chang, S.; Camacho, M.C.; Eboka, R.U.; Chandrasekharan, B.; Baker, N.F.; Darby, T.M.; Robinson, B.S.; et al. Gut-Resident Lactobacilli Activate Hepatic Nrf2 and Protect Against Oxidative Liver Injury. *Cell. Metab.* **2020**, *31*, 956–968.e955. [CrossRef] [PubMed]
52. Yu, J.; Wang, W.N.; Matei, N.; Li, X.; Pang, J.W.; Mo, J.; Chen, S.P.; Tang, J.P.; Yan, M.; Zhang, J.H. Ezetimibe Attenuates Oxidative Stress and Neuroinflammation via the AMPK/Nrf2/TXNIP Pathway after MCAO in Rats. *Oxidative Med. Cell. Longev.* **2020**, *2020*, 4717258. [CrossRef] [PubMed]
53. Alcaraz, M.J.; Ferrándiz, M.L. Relevance of Nrf2 and heme oxygenase-1 in articular diseases. *Free Radic. Biol. Med.* **2020**, *157*, 83–93. [CrossRef]
54. Kasai, S.; Shimizu, S.; Tatara, Y.; Mimura, J.; Itoh, K. Regulation of Nrf2 by Mitochondrial Reactive Oxygen Species in Physiology and Pathology. *Biomolecules* **2020**, *10*, 320. [CrossRef]
55. Ahn, K.S.; Sethi, G.; Jain, A.K.; Jaiswal, A.K.; Aggarwal, B.B. Genetic deletion of NAD(P)H:quinone oxidoreductase 1 abrogates activation of nuclear factor-kappaB, IkappaBalpha kinase, c-Jun N-terminal kinase, Akt, p38, and p44/42 mitogen-activated protein kinases and potentiates apoptosis. *.J. Biol. Chem.* **2006**, *281*, 19798–19808. [CrossRef]
56. Soares, M.P.; Seldon, M.P.; Gregoire, I.P.; Vassilevskaia, T.; Berberat, P.O.; Yu, J.; Tsui, T.Y.; Bach, F.H. Heme oxygenase-1 modulates the expression of adhesion molecules associated with endothelial cell activation. *J. Immunol.* **2004**, *172*, 3553–3563. [CrossRef]
57. Li, F.; Shanmugam, M.K.; Chen, L.; Chatterjee, S.; Basha, J.; Kumar, A.P.; Kundu, T.K.; Sethi, G. Garcinol, a polyisoprenylated benzophenone modulates multiple proinflammatory signaling cascades leading to the suppression of growth and survival of head and neck carcinoma. *Cancer Prev. Res.* **2013**, *6*, 843–854. [CrossRef]
58. Shanmugam, M.K.; Ong, T.H.; Kumar, A.P.; Lun, C.K.; Ho, P.C.; Wong, P.T.; Hui, K.M.; Sethi, G. Ursolic acid inhibits the initiation, progression of prostate cancer and prolongs the survival of TRAMP mice by modulating pro-inflammatory pathways. *PLoS ONE* **2012**, *7*, e32476. [CrossRef] [PubMed]
59. Pan, H.; Wang, H.; Wang, X.; Zhu, L.; Mao, L. The absence of Nrf2 enhances NF-κB-dependent inflammation following scratch injury in mouse primary cultured astrocytes. *Mediat. Inflamm.* **2012**, *2012*, 217580. [CrossRef]
60. Abd El-Twab, S.M.; Hussein, O.E.; Hozayen, W.G.; Bin-Jumah, M.; Mahmoud, A.M. Chicoric acid prevents methotrexate-induced kidney injury by suppressing NF-κB/NLRP3 inflammasome activation and up-regulating Nrf2/ARE/HO-1 signaling. *Inflamm. Res.* **2019**, *68*, 511–523. [CrossRef]
61. Mahmoud, A.M.; Hussein, O.E.; Abd El-Twab, S.M.; Hozayen, W.G. Ferulic acid protects against methotrexate nephrotoxicity via activation of Nrf2/ARE/HO-1 signaling and PPARγ, and suppression of NF-κB/NLRP3 inflammasome axis. *Food Funct.* **2019**, *10*, 4593–4607. [CrossRef]
62. Aladaileh, S.H.; Abukhalil, M.H.; Saghir, S.A.M.; Hanieh, H.; Alfwuaires, M.A.; Almaiman, A.A.; Bin-Jumah, M.; Mahmoud, A.M. Galangin Activates Nrf2 Signaling and Attenuates Oxidative Damage, Inflammation, and Apoptosis in a Rat Model of Cyclophosphamide-Induced Hepatotoxicity. *Biomolecules* **2019**, *9*, 346. [CrossRef]
63. HAS, A.L.; Alotaibi, M.F.; Bin-Jumah, M.; Elgebaly, H.; Mahmoud, A.M. Olea europaea leaf extract up-regulates Nrf2/ARE/HO-1 signaling and attenuates cyclophosphamide-induced oxidative stress, inflammation and apoptosis in rat kidney. *Biomed. Pharmacother.* **2019**, *111*, 676–685. [CrossRef]
64. Ranneh, Y.; Akim, A.M.; Hamid, H.A.; Khazaai, H.; Fadel, A.; Mahmoud, A.M. Stingless bee honey protects against lipopolysaccharide induced-chronic subclinical systemic inflammation and oxidative stress by modulating Nrf2, NF-κB and p38 MAPK. *Nutr. Metab.* **2019**, *16*, 15. [CrossRef]
65. Mahmoud, A.M.; Germoush, M.O.; Al-Anazi, K.M.; Mahmoud, A.H.; Farah, M.A.; Allam, A.A. Commiphora molmol protects against methotrexate-induced nephrotoxicity by up-regulating Nrf2/ARE/HO-1 signaling. *Biomed. Pharmacother.* **2018**, *106*, 499–509. [CrossRef]
66. Manu, K.A.; Shanmugam, M.K.; Li, F.; Chen, L.; Siveen, K.S.; Ahn, K.S.; Kumar, A.P.; Sethi, G. Simvastatin sensitizes human gastric cancer xenograft in nude mice to capecitabine by suppressing nuclear factor-kappa B-regulated gene products. *J. Mol. Med.* **2014**, *92*, 267–276. [CrossRef]
67. Dai, X.; Ahn, K.S.; Wang, L.Z.; Kim, C.; Deivasigamni, A.; Arfuso, F.; Um, J.Y.; Kumar, A.P.; Chang, Y.C.; Kumar, D.; et al. Ascochlorin Enhances the Sensitivity of Doxorubicin Leading to the Reversal of Epithelial-to-Mesenchymal Transition in Hepatocellular Carcinoma. *Mol. Cancer Ther.* **2016**, *15*, 2966–2976. [CrossRef]
68. Manu, K.A.; Shanmugam, M.K.; Ramachandran, L.; Li, F.; Siveen, K.S.; Chinnathambi, A.; Zayed, M.E.; Alharbi, S.A.; Arfuso, F.; Kumar, A.P.; et al. Isorhamnetin augments the anti-tumor effect of capecitabine through the negative regulation of NF-κB signaling cascade in gastric cancer. *Cancer lett.* **2015**, *363*, 28–36. [CrossRef]
69. Pinto, V.; Bergantim, R.; Caires, H.R.; Seca, H.; Guimarães, J.E.; Vasconcelos, M.H. Multiple Myeloma: Available Therapies and Causes of Drug Resistance. *Cancers* **2020**, *12*, 407. [CrossRef]

70. Wei, L.; Sun, J.; Zhang, N.; Zheng, Y.; Wang, X.; Lv, L.; Liu, J.; Xu, Y.; Shen, Y.; Yang, M. Noncoding RNAs in gastric cancer: Implications for drug resistance. *Mol. Cancer* **2020**, *19*, 62. [CrossRef]
71. Zhou, Y.Q.; Liu, D.Q.; Chen, S.P.; Chen, N.; Sun, J.; Wang, X.M.; Cao, F.; Tian, Y.K.; Ye, D.W. Nrf2 activation ameliorates mechanical allodynia in paclitaxel-induced neuropathic pain. *Acta Pharmacol. Sin.* **2020**, *41*, 1041–1048. [CrossRef]
72. Zhou, Y.Q.; Liu, D.Q.; Chen, S.P.; Chen, N.; Sun, J.; Wang, X.M.; Li, D.Y.; Tian, Y.K.; Ye, D.W. PPARγ activation mitigates mechanical allodynia in paclitaxel-induced neuropathic pain via induction of Nrf2/HO-1 signaling pathway. *Biomed. Pharmacother.* **2020**, *129*, 110356. [CrossRef]
73. Mohamed, M.E.; Abduldaium, Y.S.; Younis, N.S. Ameliorative Effect of Linalool in Cisplatin-Induced Nephrotoxicity: The Role of HMGB1/TLR4/NF-κB and Nrf2/HO1 Pathways. *Biomolecules* **2020**, *10*, 1488. [CrossRef] [PubMed]
74. Abdel-Wahab, B.A.; Alkahtani, S.A.; Elagab, E.A.M. Tadalafil alleviates cisplatin-induced reproductive toxicity through the activation of the Nrf2/HO-1 pathway and the inhibition of oxidative stress and apoptosis in male rats. *Reprod. Toxicol.* **2020**, *96*, 165–174. [CrossRef] [PubMed]
75. Azouz, A.A.; Abdel-Nassir Abdel-Razek, E.; Abo-Youssef, A.M. Amlodipine alleviates cisplatin-induced nephrotoxicity in rats through gamma-glutamyl transpeptidase (GGT) enzyme inhibition, associated with regulation of Nrf2/HO-1, MAPK/NF-κB, and Bax/Bcl-2 signaling. *Saudi Pharm. J.* **2020**, *28*, 1317–1325. [CrossRef]
76. Lu, Y.; Wu, S.; Xiang, B.; Li, L.; Lin, Y. Curcumin Attenuates Oxaliplatin-Induced Liver Injury and Oxidative Stress by Activating the Nrf2 Pathway. *Drug Des. Dev. Ther.* **2020**, *14*, 73–85. [CrossRef] [PubMed]
77. Fang, Y.; Ye, J.; Zhao, B.; Sun, J.; Gu, N.; Chen, X.; Ren, L.; Chen, J.; Cai, X.; Zhang, W.; et al. Formononetin ameliorates oxaliplatin-induced peripheral neuropathy via the KEAP1-NRF2-GSTP1 axis. *Redox Biol.* **2020**, *36*, 101677. [CrossRef]
78. Yu, Y.P.; Cai, L.C.; Wang, X.Y.; Cheng, S.Y.; Zhang, D.M.; Jian, W.G.; Wang, T.D.; Yang, J.K.; Yang, K.B.; Zhang, C. BMP8A promotes survival and drug resistance via Nrf2/TRIM24 signaling pathway in clear cell renal cell carcinoma. *Cancer Sci.* **2020**, *111*, 1555–1566. [CrossRef]
79. Leung, H.W.; Lau, E.Y.T.; Leung, C.O.N.; Lei, M.M.L.; Mok, E.H.K.; Ma, V.W.S.; Cho, W.C.S.; Ng, I.O.L.; Yun, J.P.; Cai, S.H.; et al. NRF2/SHH signaling cascade promotes tumor-initiating cell lineage and drug resistance in hepatocellular carcinoma. *Cancer Lett.* **2020**, *476*, 48–56. [CrossRef]
80. Jiang, G.; Liang, X.; Huang, Y.; Lan, Z.; Zhang, Z.; Su, Z.; Fang, Z.; Lai, Y.; Yao, W.; Liu, T.; et al. p62 promotes proliferation, apoptosis-resistance and invasion of prostate cancer cells through the Keap1/Nrf2/ARE axis. *Oncol. Rep.* **2020**, *43*, 1547–1557. [CrossRef] [PubMed]
81. Mukhopadhyay, S.; Goswami, D.; Adiseshaiah, P.P.; Burgan, W.; Yi, M.; Guerin, T.M.; Kozlov, S.V.; Nissley, D.V.; McCormick, F. Undermining Glutaminolysis Bolsters Chemotherapy While NRF2 Promotes Chemoresistance in KRAS-Driven Pancreatic Cancers. *Cancer Res.* **2020**, *80*, 1630–1643. [CrossRef]
82. Escoll, M.; Lastra, D.; Pajares, M.; Robledinos-Antón, N.; Rojo, A.I.; Fernández-Ginés, R.; Mendiola, M.; Martínez-Marín, V.; Esteban, I.; López-Larrubia, P.; et al. Transcription factor NRF2 uses the Hippo pathway effector TAZ to induce tumorigenesis in glioblastomas. *Redox Biol.* **2020**, *30*, 101425. [CrossRef]
83. Cucci, M.A.; Grattarola, M.; Dianzani, C.; Damia, G.; Ricci, F.; Roetto, A.; Trotta, F.; Barrera, G.; Pizzimenti, S. Ailanthone increases oxidative stress in CDDP-resistant ovarian and bladder cancer cells by inhibiting of Nrf2 and YAP expression through a post-translational mechanism. *Free Radic. Biol. Med.* **2020**, *150*, 125–135. [CrossRef]
84. Fouzder, C.; Mukhuty, A.; Kundu, R. Kaempferol inhibits Nrf2 signalling pathway via downregulation of Nrf2 mRNA and induces apoptosis in NSCLC cells. *Arch. Biochem. Biophys.* **2020**, *697*, 108700. [CrossRef] [PubMed]
85. Ma, C.S.; Lv, Q.M.; Zhang, K.R.; Tang, Y.B.; Zhang, Y.F.; Shen, Y.; Lei, H.M.; Zhu, L. NRF2-GPX4/SOD2 axis imparts resistance to EGFR-tyrosine kinase inhibitors in non-small-cell lung cancer cells. *Acta Pharmacol. Sin.* **2020**. [CrossRef]
86. Jiang, C.; Luo, P.; Li, X.; Liu, P.; Li, Y.; Xu, J. Nrf2/ARE is a key pathway for curcumin-mediated protection of TMJ chondrocytes from oxidative stress and inflammation. *Cell Stress Chaperones* **2020**, *25*, 395–406. [CrossRef]
87. Rasheed, M.S.U.; Tripathi, M.K.; Patel, D.K.; Singh, M.P. Resveratrol Regulates Nrf2-Mediated Expression of Antioxidant and Xenobiotic Metabolizing Enzymes in Pesticides-Induced Parkinsonism. *Protein Pept. Lett.* **2020**, *27*, 1038–1045. [CrossRef] [PubMed]
88. Yu, X.; Li, Y.; Mu, X. Effect of Quercetin on PC12 Alzheimer's Disease Cell Model Induced by Aβ (25-35) and Its Mechanism Based on Sirtuin1/Nrf2/HO-1 Pathway. *Biomed. Res. Int.* **2020**, *2020*, 8210578. [CrossRef]
89. Costa, P.M.; Ferreira, P.M.; Bolzani Vda, S.; Furlan, M.; de Freitas Formenton Macedo Dos Santos, V.A.; Corsino, J.; de Moraes, M.O.; Costa-Lotufo, L.V.; Montenegro, R.C.; Pessoa, C. Antiproliferative activity of pristimerin isolated from Maytenus ilicifolia (Celastraceae) in human HL-60 cells. *Toxicol. In Vitro* **2008**, *22*, 854–863. [CrossRef]
90. Tong, L.; Nanjundaiah, S.M.; Venkatesha, S.H.; Astry, B.; Yu, H.; Moudgil, K.D. Pristimerin, a naturally occurring triterpenoid, protects against autoimmune arthritis by modulating the cellular and soluble immune mediators of inflammation and tissue damage. *Clin. Immunol.* **2014**, *155*, 220–230. [CrossRef]
91. El-Agamy, D.S.; El-Harbi, K.M.; Khoshhal, S.; Ahmed, N.; Elkablawy, M.A.; Shaaban, A.A.; Abo-Haded, H.M. Pristimerin protects against doxorubicin-induced cardiotoxicity and fibrosis through modulation of Nrf2 and MAPK/NF-kB signaling pathways. *Cancer Manag. Res.* **2019**, *11*, 47–61. [CrossRef] [PubMed]
92. Aktaş, I.; Özmen, Ö.; Tutun, H.; Yalçın, A.; Türk, A. Artemisinin attenuates doxorubicin induced cardiotoxicity and hepatotoxicity in rats. *Biotech. Histochem.* **2020**, *95*, 121–128. [CrossRef] [PubMed]

93. Prospero, A.G.; Fidelis-de-Oliveira, P.; Soares, G.A.; Miranda, M.F.; Pinto, L.A.; Dos Santos, D.C.; Silva, V.D.S.; Zufelato, N.; Bakuzis, A.F.; Miranda, J.R. AC biosusceptometry and magnetic nanoparticles to assess doxorubicin-induced kidney injury in rats. *Nanomedicine* **2020**, *15*, 511–525. [CrossRef]
94. Oh, S.-K.; Rha, C.; Kadir, A.; Ng, T. Use of Asiatic Acid or Asiaticoside for Treatment of Cancer. U.S. Patent Application No. 10/362,720, 20 May 2004.
95. Han, Y.; Jiang, Y.; Li, Y.; Wang, M.; Fan, T.; Liu, M.; Ke, Q.; Xu, H.; Yi, Z. An aligned porous electrospun fibrous scaffold with embedded asiatic acid for accelerating diabetic wound healing. *J. Mater. Chem. B* **2019**, *7*, 6125–6138. [CrossRef]
96. Hu, W.Y.; Li, X.X.; Diao, Y.F.; Qi, J.J.; Wang, D.L.; Zhang, J.B.; Sun, B.X.; Liang, S. Asiatic acid protects oocytes against in vitro aging-induced deterioration and improves subsequent embryonic development in pigs. *Aging* **2020**, *12*. [CrossRef]
97. Lian, G.Y.; Wang, Q.M.; Tang, P.M.; Zhou, S.; Huang, X.R.; Lan, H.Y. Combination of Asiatic Acid and Naringenin Modulates NK Cell Anti-cancer Immunity by Rebalancing Smad3/Smad7 Signaling. *Mol. Ther.* **2018**, *26*, 2255–2266. [CrossRef] [PubMed]
98. Kamble, S.M.; Patil, C.R. Asiatic Acid Ameliorates Doxorubicin-Induced Cardiac and Hepato-Renal Toxicities with Nrf2 Transcriptional Factor Activation in Rats. *Cardiovasc. Toxicol.* **2018**, *18*, 131–141. [CrossRef]
99. Song, C.; Heping, H.; Shen, Y.; Jin, S.; Li, D.; Zhang, A.; Ren, X.; Wang, K.; Zhang, L.; Wang, J.; et al. AMPK/p38/Nrf2 activation as a protective feedback to restrain oxidative stress and inflammation in microglia stimulated with sodium fluoride. *Chemosphere* **2020**, *244*, 125495. [CrossRef]
100. Lee, E.H.; Baek, S.Y.; Park, J.Y.; Kim, Y.W. Rifampicin activates AMPK and alleviates oxidative stress in the liver as mediated with Nrf2 signaling. *Chem. Biol. Interact.* **2020**, *315*, 108889. [CrossRef]
101. Nazari Soltan Ahmad, S.; Sanajou, D.; Kalantary-Charvadeh, A.; Hosseini, V.; Roshangar, L.; Khojastehfard, M.; Haiaty, S.; Mesgari-Abbasi, M. β-LAPachone ameliorates doxorubicin-induced cardiotoxicity via regulating autophagy and Nrf2 signalling pathways in mice. *Basic Clin. Pharmacol. Toxicol.* **2020**, *126*, 364–373. [CrossRef]
102. Wu, Z.; Zai, W.; Chen, W.; Han, Y.; Jin, X.; Liu, H. Curdione Ameliorated Doxorubicin-Induced Cardiotoxicity Through Suppressing Oxidative Stress and Activating Nrf2/HO-1 Pathway. *J. Cardiovasc. Pharmacol.* **2019**, *74*, 118–127. [CrossRef]
103. Yoo, O.K.; Choi, W.J.; Keum, Y.S. Cardamonin Inhibits Oxazolone-Induced Atopic Dermatitis by the Induction of NRF2 and the Inhibition of Th2 Cytokine Production. *Antioxidants* **2020**, *9*, 834. [CrossRef] [PubMed]
104. Tan, Y.; Wan, H.H.; Sun, M.M.; Zhang, W.J.; Dong, M.; Ge, W.; Ren, J.; Peng, H. Cardamonin protects against lipopolysaccharide-induced myocardial contractile dysfunction in mice through Nrf2-regulated mechanism. *Acta Pharmacol. Sin.* **2020**. [CrossRef]
105. Qi, W.; Boliang, W.; Xiaoxi, T.; Guoqiang, F.; Jianbo, X.; Gang, W. Cardamonin protects against doxorubicin-induced cardiotoxicity in mice by restraining oxidative stress and inflammation associated with Nrf2 signaling. *Biomed. Pharmacother.* **2020**, *122*, 109547. [CrossRef] [PubMed]
106. Wang, W.; Meng, Q.; Li, Q.; Liu, J.; Zhou, M.; Jin, Z.; Zhao, K. Chitosan derivatives and their application in biomedicine. *Int. J. Mol. Sci.* **2020**, *21*, 487. [CrossRef]
107. Li, Y.; Liu, H.; Xu, Q.-S.; Du, Y.-G.; Xu, J. Chitosan oligosaccharides block LPS-induced O-GlcNAcylation of NF-κB and endothelial inflammatory response. *Carbohydr. Polym.* **2014**, *99*, 568–578. [CrossRef] [PubMed]
108. Fernandes, J.C.; Sereno, J.; Garrido, P.; Parada, B.; Cunha, M.F.; Reis, F.; Pintado, M.E.; Santos-Silva, A. Inhibition of bladder tumor growth by chitooligosaccharides in an experimental carcinogenesis model. *Marine Drugs* **2012**, *10*, 2661–2675. [CrossRef]
109. Muanprasat, C.; Chatsudthipong, V. Chitosan oligosaccharide: Biological activities and potential therapeutic applications. *Pharmacol. Ther.* **2017**, *170*, 80–97. [CrossRef]
110. Zou, P.; Yang, X.; Wang, J.; Li, Y.; Yu, H.; Zhang, Y.; Liu, G. Advances in characterisation and biological activities of chitosan and chitosan oligosaccharides. *Food Chem.* **2016**, *190*, 1174–1181. [CrossRef]
111. Fang, I.-M.; Yang, C.-M.; Yang, C.-H. Chitosan oligosaccharides prevented retinal ischemia and reperfusion injury via reduced oxidative stress and inflammation in rats. *Exp. Eye Res.* **2015**, *130*, 38–50. [CrossRef]
112. Zhang, Y.; Ahmad, K.A.; Khan, F.U.; Yan, S.; Ihsan, A.U.; Ding, Q. Chitosan oligosaccharides prevent doxorubicin-induced oxidative stress and cardiac apoptosis through activating p38 and JNK MAPK mediated Nrf2/ARE pathway. *Chem. Biol. Interact.* **2019**, *305*, 54–65. [CrossRef]
113. Wang, L.F.; Su, S.W.; Wang, L.; Zhang, G.Q.; Zhang, R.; Niu, Y.J.; Guo, Y.S.; Li, C.Y.; Jiang, W.B.; Liu, Y.; et al. Tert-butylhydroquinone ameliorates doxorubicin-induced cardiotoxicity by activating Nrf2 and inducing the expression of its target genes. *Am. J. Transl. Res.* **2015**, *7*, 1724–1735.
114. Hajra, S.; Basu, A.; Singha Roy, S.; Patra, A.R.; Bhattacharya, S. Attenuation of doxorubicin-induced cardiotoxicity and genotoxicity by an indole-based natural compound 3,3′-diindolylmethane (DIM) through activation of Nrf2/ARE signaling pathways and inhibiting apoptosis. *Free Radic. Res.* **2017**, *51*, 812–827. [CrossRef]
115. Kanski, J.; Aksenova, M.; Stoyanova, A.; Butterfield, D.A. Ferulic acid antioxidant protection against hydroxyl and peroxyl radical oxidation in synaptosomal and neuronal cell culture systems in vitro: Structure-activity studies. *J. Nutr. Biochem.* **2002**, *13*, 273–281. [CrossRef]
116. Kheiry, M.; Dianat, M.; Badavi, M.; Mard, S.A.; Bayati, V. p-Coumaric Acid Attenuates Lipopolysaccharide-Induced Lung Inflammation in Rats by Scavenging ROS Production: An In Vivo and In Vitro Study. *Inflammation* **2019**, *42*, 1939–1950. [CrossRef] [PubMed]

117. Chen, J.J.; Deng, J.S.; Huang, C.C.; Li, P.Y.; Liang, Y.C.; Chou, C.Y.; Huang, G.J. p-Coumaric-Acid-Containing Adenostemma lavenia Ameliorates Acute Lung Injury by Activating AMPK/Nrf2/HO-1 Signaling and Improving the Anti-oxidant Response. Am. J. Chin. Med. **2019**, 47, 1483–1506. [CrossRef] [PubMed]
118. Sunitha, M.C.; Dhanyakrishnan, R.; PrakashKumar, B.; Nevin, K.G. p-Coumaric acid mediated protection of H9c2 cells from Doxorubicin-induced cardiotoxicity: Involvement of augmented Nrf2 and autophagy. Biomed. Pharmacother. **2018**, 102, 823–832. [CrossRef]
119. Elsherbiny, N.M.; El-Sherbiny, M. Thymoquinone attenuates Doxorubicin-induced nephrotoxicity in rats: Role of Nrf2 and NOX4. Chem. Biol. Interact. **2014**, 223, 102–108. [CrossRef] [PubMed]
120. Xu, S.; Liu, P. Tanshinone II-A: New perspectives for old remedies. Expert Opin. Ther. Pat. **2013**, 23, 149–153. [CrossRef] [PubMed]
121. Feng, F.; Cheng, P.; Zhang, H.; Li, N.; Qi, Y.; Wang, H.; Wang, Y.; Wang, W. The Protective Role of Tanshinone IIA in Silicosis Rat Model via TGF-β1/Smad Signaling Suppression, NOX4 Inhibition and Nrf2/ARE Signaling Activation. Drug Des. Dev. Ther. **2019**, 13, 4275–4290. [CrossRef]
122. Yang, Y.; Liu, L.; Zhang, X.; Jiang, X.; Wang, L. Tanshinone IIA prevents rifampicin-induced liver injury by regulating BSEP/NTCP expression via epigenetic activation of NRF2. Liver Int. **2020**, 40, 141–154. [CrossRef]
123. An, L.; Peng, L.Y.; Sun, N.Y.; Yang, Y.L.; Zhang, X.W.; Li, B.; Liu, B.L.; Li, P.; Chen, J. Tanshinone IIA Activates Nuclear Factor-Erythroid 2-Related Factor 2 to Restrain Pulmonary Fibrosis via Regulation of Redox Homeostasis and Glutaminolysis. Antioxid. Redox Signal. **2019**, 30, 1831–1848. [CrossRef] [PubMed]
124. Guo, Z.; Yan, M.; Chen, L.; Fang, P.; Li, Z.; Wan, Z.; Cao, S.; Hou, Z.; Wei, S.; Li, W.; et al. Nrf2-dependent antioxidant response mediated the protective effect of tanshinone IIA on doxorubicin-induced cardiotoxicity. Exp. Ther. Med. **2018**, 16, 3333–3344. [CrossRef] [PubMed]
125. Feng, X.; Yang, Q.; Wang, C.; Tong, W.; Xu, W. Punicalagin Exerts Protective Effects against Ankylosing Spondylitis by Regulating NF-κB-TH17/JAK2/STAT3 Signaling and Oxidative Stress. Biomed. Res. Int. **2020**, 2020, 4918239. [CrossRef]
126. Wang, W.; Bai, J.; Zhang, W.; Ge, G.; Wang, Q.; Liang, X.; Li, N.; Gu, Y.; Li, M.; Xu, W.; et al. Protective Effects of Punicalagin on Osteoporosis by Inhibiting Osteoclastogenesis and Inflammation via the NF-κB and MAPK Pathways. Front. Pharmacol. **2020**, 11, 696. [CrossRef] [PubMed]
127. Ye, M.; Zhang, L.; Yan, Y.; Lin, H. Punicalagin protects H9c2 cardiomyocytes from doxorubicin-induced toxicity through activation of Nrf2/HO-1 signaling. Biosci. Rep. **2019**, 39. [CrossRef]
128. Arnold, J.; Engelmann, J.C.; Schneider, N.; Bosserhoff, A.K.; Kuphal, S. miR-488-5p and its role in melanoma. Exp. Mol. Pathol. **2020**, 112, 104348. [CrossRef]
129. Kolenda, T.; Guglas, K.; Kopczyńska, M.; Sobocińska, J.; Teresiak, A.; Bliźniak, R.; Lamperska, K. Good or not good: Role of miR-18a in cancer biology. Rep. Pract. Oncol. Radiother. **2020**, 25, 808–819. [CrossRef]
130. Ashrafizadeh, M.; Hushmandi, K.; Hashemi, M.; Akbari, M.E.; Kubatka, P.; Raei, M.; Koklesova, L.; Shahinozzaman, M.; Mohammadinejad, R.; Najafi, M.; et al. Role of microRNA/Epithelial-to-Mesenchymal Transition Axis in the Metastasis of Bladder Cancer. Biomolecules **2020**, 10, 1159. [CrossRef]
131. Aggarwal, V.; Tuli, H.S.; Varol, A.; Thakral, F.; Yerer, M.B.; Sak, K.; Varol, M.; Jain, A.; Khan, M.A.; Sethi, G. Role of Reactive Oxygen Species in Cancer Progression: Molecular Mechanisms and Recent Advancements. Biomolecules **2019**, 9, 735. [CrossRef] [PubMed]
132. Dastmalchi, N.; Hosseinpourfeizi, M.A.; Khojasteh, S.M.B.; Baradaran, B.; Safaralizadeh, R. Tumor suppressive activity of miR-424-5p in breast cancer cells through targeting PD-L1 and modulating PTEN/PI3K/AKT/mTOR signaling pathway. Life Sci. **2020**, 259, 118239. [CrossRef] [PubMed]
133. Aslan, C.; Maralbashi, S.; Kahroba, H.; Asadi, M.; Soltani-Zangbar, M.S.; Javadian, M.; Shanehbandi, D.; Baradaran, B.; Darabi, M.; Kazemi, T. Docosahexaenoic acid (DHA) inhibits pro-angiogenic effects of breast cancer cells via down-regulating cellular and exosomal expression of angiogenic genes and microRNAs. Life Sci. **2020**, 258, 118094. [CrossRef]
134. Khalili, N.; Nouri-Vaskeh, M.; Hasanpour Segherlou, Z.; Baghbanzadeh, A.; Halimi, M.; Rezaee, H.; Baradaran, B. Diagnostic, prognostic, and therapeutic significance of miR-139-5p in cancers. Life Sci. **2020**, 256, 117865. [CrossRef]
135. Azarbarzin, S.; Hosseinpour-Feizi, M.A.; Banan Khojasteh, S.M.; Baradaran, B.; Safaralizadeh, R. MicroRNA -383-5p restrains the proliferation and migration of breast cancer cells and promotes apoptosis via inhibition of PD-L1. Life Sci. **2021**, 267, 118939. [CrossRef] [PubMed]
136. Godínez-Rubí, M.; Ortuño-Sahagún, D. miR-615 Fine-Tunes Growth and Development and Has a Role in Cancer and in Neural Repair. Cells **2020**, 9, 1566. [CrossRef]
137. Ferrari, E.; Gandellini, P. Unveiling the ups and downs of miR-205 in physiology and cancer: Transcriptional and post-transcriptional mechanisms. Cell Death Dis. **2020**, 11, 980. [CrossRef]
138. Mu, Z.; Zhang, H.; Lei, P. Piceatannol inhibits pyroptosis and suppresses oxLDL-induced lipid storage in macrophages by regulating miR-200a/Nrf2/GSDMD axis. Biosci. Rep. **2020**, 40. [CrossRef] [PubMed]
139. Wang, X.; Ye, L.; Zhang, K.; Gao, L.; Xiao, J.; Zhang, Y. Upregulation of microRNA-200a in bone marrow mesenchymal stem cells enhances the repair of spinal cord injury in rats by reducing oxidative stress and regulating Keap1/Nrf2 pathway. Artif. Organs **2020**, 44, 744–752. [CrossRef]
140. Zhao, L.; Qi, Y.; Xu, L.; Tao, X.; Han, X.; Yin, L.; Peng, J. MicroRNA-140-5p aggravates doxorubicin-induced cardiotoxicity by promoting myocardial oxidative stress via targeting Nrf2 and Sirt2. Redox Biol. **2018**, 15, 284–296. [CrossRef]

141. Jiang, Z.; Wu, J.; Ma, F.; Jiang, J.; Xu, L.; Du, L.; Huang, W.; Wang, Z.; Jia, Y.; Lu, L.; et al. MicroRNA-200a improves diabetic endothelial dysfunction by targeting KEAP1/NRF2. *J. Endocrinol.* **2020**, *245*, 129–140. [CrossRef]
142. Ma, Y.; Pan, C.; Tang, X.; Zhang, M.; Shi, H.; Wang, T.; Zhang, Y. MicroRNA-200a represses myocardial infarction-related cell death and inflammation by targeting the Keap1/Nrf2 and β-catenin pathways. *Hellenic. J. Cardiol.* **2020**. [CrossRef] [PubMed]
143. Hu, X.; Liu, H.; Wang, Z.; Hu, Z.; Li, L. miR-200a Attenuated Doxorubicin-Induced Cardiotoxicity through Upregulation of Nrf2 in Mice. *Oxidative Med. Cell. Longev.* **2019**, *2019*, 1512326. [CrossRef] [PubMed]
144. Li, S.; Wang, W.; Niu, T.; Wang, H.; Li, B.; Shao, L.; Lai, Y.; Li, H.; Janicki, J.S.; Wang, X.L.; et al. Nrf2 deficiency exaggerates doxorubicin-induced cardiotoxicity and cardiac dysfunction. *Oxidative Med. Cell. Longev.* **2014**, *2014*, 748524. [CrossRef] [PubMed]
145. Singh, S.S.; Vats, S.; Chia, A.Y.; Tan, T.Z.; Deng, S.; Ong, M.S.; Arfuso, F.; Yap, C.T.; Goh, B.C.; Sethi, G.; et al. Dual role of autophagy in hallmarks of cancer. *Oncogene* **2018**, *37*, 1142–1158. [CrossRef]
146. Patra, S.; Mishra, S.R.; Behera, B.P.; Mahapatra, K.K.; Panigrahi, D.P.; Bhol, C.S.; Praharaj, P.P.; Sethi, G.; Patra, S.K.; Bhutia, S.K. Autophagy-modulating phytochemicals in cancer therapeutics: Current evidences and future perspectives. *Semin. Cancer Biol.* **2020**. [CrossRef]
147. Ren, H.; Shao, Y.; Wu, C.; Ma, X.; Lv, C.; Wang, Q. Metformin alleviates oxidative stress and enhances autophagy in diabetic kidney disease via AMPK/SIRT1-FoxO1 pathway. *Mol. Cell. Endocrinol.* **2020**, *500*, 110628. [CrossRef]
148. Liang, D.; Zhuo, Y.; Guo, Z.; He, L.; Wang, X.; He, Y.; Li, L.; Dai, H. SIRT1/PGC-1 pathway activation triggers autophagy/mitophagy and attenuates oxidative damage in intestinal epithelial cells. *Biochimie* **2020**, *170*, 10–20. [CrossRef]
149. Renu, K.; Valsala Gopalakrishnan, A. Deciphering the molecular mechanism during doxorubicin-mediated oxidative stress, apoptosis through Nrf2 and PGC-1α in a rat testicular milieu. *Reprod. Biol.* **2019**, *19*, 22–37. [CrossRef]
150. Zhou, B.; Liu, J.; Kang, R.; Klionsky, D.J.; Kroemer, G.; Tang, D. Ferroptosis is a type of autophagy-dependent cell death. *Semin. Cancer Biol.* **2020**, *66*, 89–100. [CrossRef]
151. Liu, Q.; Zhao, M.; Chen, W.; Xu, K.; Huang, F.; Qu, J.; Xu, Z.; Wang, X.; Wang, Y.; Zhu, Y.; et al. Mainstream cigarette smoke induces autophagy and promotes apoptosis in oral mucosal epithelial cells. *Arch. Oral Biol.* **2020**, *111*, 104646. [CrossRef]
152. Deng, S.; Shanmugam, M.K.; Kumar, A.P.; Yap, C.T.; Sethi, G.; Bishayee, A. Targeting autophagy using natural compounds for cancer prevention and therapy. *Cancer* **2019**, *125*, 1228–1246. [CrossRef] [PubMed]
153. Chihara, D.; Westin, J.R.; Oki, Y.; Ahmed, M.A.; Do, B.; Fayad, L.E.; Hagemeister, F.B.; Romaguera, J.E.; Fanale, M.A.; Lee, H.J.; et al. Management strategies and outcomes for very elderly patients with diffuse large B-cell lymphoma. *Cancer* **2016**, *122*, 3145–3151. [CrossRef] [PubMed]
154. McGuckin, M.M.; Giesy, S.L.; Davis, A.N.; Abyeta, M.A.; Horst, E.A.; Saed Samii, S.; Zang, Y.; Butler, W.R.; Baumgard, L.H.; McFadden, J.W.; et al. The acute phase protein orosomucoid 1 is upregulated in early lactation but does not trigger appetite-suppressing STAT3 signaling via the leptin receptor. *J. Dairy Sci.* **2020**, *103*, 4765–4776. [CrossRef] [PubMed]
155. Fandiño-Vaquero, R.; Fernández-Trasancos, Á.; Alvarez, E.; Ahmad, S.; Batista-Oliveira, A.L.; Adrio, B.; Fernández, A.L.; González-Juanatey, J.R.; Eiras, S. Orosomucoid secretion levels by epicardial adipose tissue as possible indicator of endothelial dysfunction in diabetes mellitus or inflammation in coronary artery disease. *Atherosclerosis* **2014**, *235*, 281–288. [CrossRef]
156. Ren, F.; Chen, Y.; Wang, Y.; Yan, Y.; Zhao, J.; Ding, M.; Zhang, J.; Jiang, Y.; Zhai, Y.; Duan, Z. Comparative serum proteomic analysis of patients with acute-on-chronic liver failure: Alpha-1-acid glycoprotein maybe a candidate marker for prognosis of hepatitis B virus infection. *J. Viral. Hepat.* **2010**, *17*, 816–824. [CrossRef]
157. Zhu, H.Z.; Zhou, W.J.; Wan, Y.F.; Ge, K.; Lu, J.; Jia, C.K. Downregulation of orosomucoid 2 acts as a prognostic factor associated with cancer-promoting pathways in liver cancer. *World J. Gastroenterol.* **2020**, *26*, 804–817. [CrossRef]
158. Cheng, X.; Liu, D.; Xing, R.; Song, H.; Tian, X.; Yan, C.; Han, Y. Orosomucoid 1 Attenuates Doxorubicin-Induced Oxidative Stress and Apoptosis in Cardiomyocytes via Nrf2 Signaling. *Biomed. Res. Int.* **2020**, *2020*, 5923572. [CrossRef]
159. Tomlinson, L.; Lu, Z.Q.; Bentley, R.A.; Colley, H.E.; Murdoch, C.; Webb, S.D.; Cross, M.J.; Copple, I.M.; Sharma, P. Attenuation of doxorubicin-induced cardiotoxicity in a human in vitro cardiac model by the induction of the NRF-2 pathway. *Biomed. Pharmacother.* **2019**, *112*, 108637. [CrossRef]
160. Wang, H.; Brown, J.; Martin, M. Glycogen synthase kinase 3: A point of convergence for the host inflammatory response. *Cytokine* **2011**, *53*, 130–140. [CrossRef]
161. Cohen, P.; Frame, S. The renaissance of GSK3. *Nat. Rev. Mol. Cell. Biol.* **2001**, *2*, 769–776. [CrossRef]
162. Bitar, M.S.; Al-Mulla, F. A defect in Nrf2 signaling constitutes a mechanism for cellular stress hypersensitivity in a genetic rat model of type 2 diabetes. *Am. J. Physiol. Endocrinol. Metab.* **2011**, *301*, E1119–E1129. [CrossRef]
163. Tomobe, K.; Shinozuka, T.; Kuroiwa, M.; Nomura, Y. Age-related changes of Nrf2 and phosphorylated GSK-3β in a mouse model of accelerated aging (SAMP8). *Arch. Gerontol. Geriatr.* **2012**, *54*, e1–e7. [CrossRef] [PubMed]
164. Jiang, Y.; Bao, H.; Ge, Y.; Tang, W.; Cheng, D.; Luo, K.; Gong, G.; Gong, R. Therapeutic targeting of GSK3β enhances the Nrf2 antioxidant response and confers hepatic cytoprotection in hepatitis C. *Gut* **2015**, *64*, 168–179. [CrossRef] [PubMed]
165. Rojo, A.I.; Rada, P.; Egea, J.; Rosa, A.O.; López, M.G.; Cuadrado, A. Functional interference between glycogen synthase kinase-3 beta and the transcription factor Nrf2 in protection against kainate-induced hippocampal cell death. *Mol. Cell. Neurosci.* **2008**, *39*, 125–132. [CrossRef] [PubMed]
166. Espada, S.; Rojo, A.I.; Salinas, M.; Cuadrado, A. The muscarinic M1 receptor activates Nrf2 through a signaling cascade that involves protein kinase C and inhibition of GSK-3beta: Connecting neurotransmission with neuroprotection. *J. Neurochem.* **2009**, *110*, 1107–1119. [CrossRef] [PubMed]

167. Correa, F.; Mallard, C.; Nilsson, M.; Sandberg, M. Activated microglia decrease histone acetylation and Nrf2-inducible antioxidant defence in astrocytes: Restoring effects of inhibitors of HDACs, p38 MAPK and GSK3β. *Neurobiol. Dis.* **2011**, *44*, 142–151. [CrossRef]
168. Zhou, S.; Wang, P.; Qiao, Y.; Ge, Y.; Wang, Y.; Quan, S.; Yao, R.; Zhuang, S.; Wang, L.J.; Du, Y.; et al. Genetic and Pharmacologic Targeting of Glycogen Synthase Kinase 3β Reinforces the Nrf2 Antioxidant Defense against Podocytopathy. *J. Am. Soc. Nephrol.* **2016**, *27*, 2289–2308. [CrossRef]
169. Nordgren, K.K.S.; Wallace, K.B. Disruption of the Keap1/Nrf2-Antioxidant Response System After Chronic Doxorubicin Exposure In Vivo. *Cardiovasc. Toxicol.* **2020**, *20*, 557–570. [CrossRef]
170. Wu, W.Y.; Cui, Y.K.; Hong, Y.X.; Li, Y.D.; Wu, Y.; Li, G.; Li, G.R.; Wang, Y. Doxorubicin cardiomyopathy is ameliorated by acacetin via Sirt1-mediated activation of AMPK/Nrf2 signal molecules. *J. Cell. Mol. Med.* **2020**, *24*, 12141–12153. [CrossRef]
171. Chen, M.; Samuel, V.P.; Wu, Y.; Dang, M.; Lin, Y.; Sriramaneni, R.; Sah, S.K.; Chinnaboina, G.K.; Zhang, G. Nrf2/HO-1 Mediated Protective Activity of Genistein Against Doxorubicin-Induced Cardiac Toxicity. *J. Environ. Pathol. Toxicol. Oncol.* **2019**, *38*, 143–152. [CrossRef]
172. Singh, A.; Venkannagari, S.; Oh, K.H.; Zhang, Y.Q.; Rohde, J.M.; Liu, L.; Nimmagadda, S.; Sudini, K.; Brimacombe, K.R.; Gajghate, S.; et al. Small Molecule Inhibitor of NRF2 Selectively Intervenes Therapeutic Resistance in KEAP1-Deficient NSCLC Tumors. *ACS Chem. Biol.* **2016**, *11*, 3214–3225. [CrossRef]
173. Li, X.; Kong, L.; Yang, Q.; Duan, A.; Ju, X.; Cai, B.; Chen, L.; An, T.; Li, Y. Parthenolide inhibits ubiquitin-specific peptidase 7 (USP7), Wnt signaling, and colorectal cancer cell growth. *J. Biol. Chem.* **2020**, *295*, 3576–3589. [CrossRef] [PubMed]
174. Sztiller-Sikorska, M.; Czyz, M. Parthenolide as Cooperating Agent for Anti-Cancer Treatment of Various Malignancies. *Pharmaceuticals* **2020**, *13*, 194. [CrossRef]
175. Jin, X.; Yang, Q.; Cai, N.; Zhang, Z. A cocktail of betulinic acid, parthenolide, honokiol and ginsenoside Rh2 in liposome systems for lung cancer treatment. *Nanomedicine* **2020**, *15*, 41–54. [CrossRef] [PubMed]
176. Carlisi, D.; De Blasio, A.; Drago-Ferrante, R.; Di Fiore, R.; Buttitta, G.; Morreale, M.; Scerri, C.; Vento, R.; Tesoriere, G. Parthenolide prevents resistance of MDA-MB231 cells to doxorubicin and mitoxantrone: The role of Nrf2. *Cell Death Discov.* **2017**, *3*, 17078. [CrossRef] [PubMed]
177. Yang, B.; Huang, J.; Xiang, T.; Yin, X.; Luo, X.; Huang, J.; Luo, F.; Li, H.; Li, H.; Ren, G. Chrysin inhibits metastatic potential of human triple-negative breast cancer cells by modulating matrix metalloproteinase-10, epithelial to mesenchymal transition, and PI3K/Akt signaling pathway. *J. Appl. Toxicol.* **2014**, *34*, 105–112. [CrossRef] [PubMed]
178. Woo, K.J.; Jeong, Y.J.; Park, J.W.; Kwon, T.K. Chrysin-induced apoptosis is mediated through caspase activation and Akt inactivation in U937 leukemia cells. *Biochem. Biophys. Res. Commun.* **2004**, *325*, 1215–1222. [CrossRef]
179. Wang, J.; Wang, H.; Sun, K.; Wang, X.; Pan, H.; Zhu, J.; Ji, X.; Li, X. Chrysin suppresses proliferation, migration, and invasion in glioblastoma cell lines via mediating the ERK/Nrf2 signaling pathway. *Drug Des. Dev. Ther.* **2018**, *12*, 721–733. [CrossRef]
180. Xia, Y.; Lian, S.; Khoi, P.N.; Yoon, H.J.; Joo, Y.E.; Chay, K.O.; Kim, K.K.; Do Jung, Y. Chrysin inhibits tumor promoter-induced MMP-9 expression by blocking AP-1 via suppression of ERK and JNK pathways in gastric cancer cells. *PLoS ONE* **2015**, *10*, e0124007. [CrossRef]
181. Gao, A.M.; Ke, Z.P.; Shi, F.; Sun, G.C.; Chen, H. Chrysin enhances sensitivity of BEL-7402/ADM cells to doxorubicin by suppressing PI3K/Akt/Nrf2 and ERK/Nrf2 pathway. *Chem. Biol. Interact.* **2013**, *206*, 100–108. [CrossRef]
182. Gao, H.L.; Xia, Y.Z.; Zhang, Y.L.; Yang, L.; Kong, L.Y. Vielanin P enhances the cytotoxicity of doxorubicin via the inhibition of PI3K/Nrf2-stimulated MRP1 expression in MCF-7 and K562 DOX-resistant cell lines. *Phytomedicine* **2019**, *58*, 152885. [CrossRef] [PubMed]
183. Qi, Y.; Ding, Z.; Yao, Y.; Ren, F.; Yin, M.; Yang, S.; Chen, A. Apigenin induces apoptosis and counteracts cisplatin-induced chemoresistance via Mcl-1 in ovarian cancer cells. *Exp. Ther. Med.* **2020**, *20*, 1329–1336. [CrossRef]
184. Korga-Plewko, A.; Michalczyk, M.; Adamczuk, G.; Humeniuk, E.; Ostrowska-Lesko, M.; Jozefczyk, A.; Iwan, M.; Wojcik, M.; Dudka, J. Apigenin and Hesperidin Downregulate DNA Repair Genes in MCF-7 Breast Cancer Cells and Augment Doxorubicin Toxicity. *Molecules* **2020**, *25*, 4421. [CrossRef] [PubMed]
185. Şirin, N.; Elmas, L.; Seçme, M.; Dodurga, Y. Investigation of possible effects of apigenin, sorafenib and combined applications on apoptosis and cell cycle in hepatocellular cancer cells. *Gene* **2020**, *737*, 144428. [CrossRef]
186. Gao, A.M.; Zhang, X.Y.; Ke, Z.P. Apigenin sensitizes BEL-7402/ADM cells to doxorubicin through inhibiting miR-101/Nrf2 pathway. *Oncotarget* **2017**, *8*, 82085–82091. [CrossRef] [PubMed]
187. Mohan, C.D.; Srinivasa, V.; Rangappa, S.; Mervin, L.; Mohan, S.; Paricharak, S.; Baday, S.; Li, F.; Shanmugam, M.K.; Chinnathambi, A.; et al. Trisubstituted-Imidazoles Induce Apoptosis in Human Breast Cancer Cells by Targeting the Oncogenic PI3K/Akt/mTOR Signaling Pathway. *PLoS ONE* **2016**, *11*, e0153155. [CrossRef] [PubMed]
188. Ong, P.S.; Wang, L.Z.; Dai, X.; Tseng, S.H.; Loo, S.J.; Sethi, G. Judicious Toggling of mTOR Activity to Combat Insulin Resistance and Cancer: Current Evidence and Perspectives. *Front. Pharmacol.* **2016**, *7*, 395. [CrossRef] [PubMed]
189. Gao, A.M.; Ke, Z.P.; Wang, J.N.; Yang, J.Y.; Chen, S.Y.; Chen, H. Apigenin sensitizes doxorubicin-resistant hepatocellular carcinoma BEL-7402/ADM cells to doxorubicin via inhibiting PI3K/Akt/Nrf2 pathway. *Carcinogenesis* **2013**, *34*, 1806–1814. [CrossRef]
190. Wei, Y.; Liu, D.; Jin, X.; Gao, P.; Wang, Q.; Zhang, J.; Zhang, N. PA-MSHA inhibits the growth of doxorubicin-resistant MCF-7/ADR human breast cancer cells by downregulating Nrf2/p62. *Cancer Med.* **2016**, *5*, 3520–3531. [CrossRef]

191. Kim, D.; Choi, B.H.; Ryoo, I.G.; Kwak, M.K. High NRF2 level mediates cancer stem cell-like properties of aldehyde dehydrogenase (ALDH)-high ovarian cancer cells: Inhibitory role of all-trans retinoic acid in ALDH/NRF2 signaling. *Cell Death Dis.* **2018**, *9*, 896. [CrossRef]
192. Yang, H.Y.; Zhao, L.; Yang, Z.; Zhao, Q.; Qiang, L.; Ha, J.; Li, Z.Y.; You, Q.D.; Guo, Q.L. Oroxylin a reverses multi-drug resistance of human hepatoma BEL7402/5⁻FU cells via downregulation of P⁻glycoprotein expression by inhibiting NF-κB signaling pathway. *Mol. Carcinog.* **2012**, *51*, 185–195. [CrossRef] [PubMed]
193. Koh, H.; Sun, H.N.; Xing, Z.; Liu, R.; Chandimali, N.; Kwon, T.; Lee, D.S. Wogonin Influences Osteosarcoma Stem Cell Stemness Through ROS-dependent Signaling. *In Vivo* **2020**, *34*, 1077–1084. [CrossRef] [PubMed]
194. Yang, D.; Guo, Q.; Liang, Y.; Zhao, Y.; Tian, X.; Ye, Y.; Tian, J.; Wu, T.; Lu, N. Wogonin induces cellular senescence in breast cancer via suppressing TXNRD2 expression. *Arch. Toxicol.* **2020**, *94*, 3433–3447. [CrossRef] [PubMed]
195. Zhong, Y.; Zhang, F.; Sun, Z.; Zhou, W.; Li, Z.Y.; You, Q.D.; Guo, Q.L.; Hu, R. Drug resistance associates with activation of Nrf2 in MCF-7/DOX cells, and wogonin reverses it by down-regulating Nrf2-mediated cellular defense response. *Mol. Carcinog.* **2013**, *52*, 824–834. [CrossRef]
196. Ohnuma, T.; Matsumoto, T.; Itoi, A.; Kawana, A.; Nishiyama, T.; Ogura, K.; Hiratsuka, A. Enhanced sensitivity of A549 cells to the cytotoxic action of anticancer drugs via suppression of Nrf2 by procyanidins from Cinnamomi Cortex extract. *Biochem. Biophys. Res. Commun.* **2011**, *413*, 623–629. [CrossRef]
197. Selvi, R.B.; Swaminathan, A.; Chatterjee, S.; Shanmugam, M.K.; Li, F.; Ramakrishnan, G.B.; Siveen, K.S.; Chinnathambi, A.; Zayed, M.E.; Alharbi, S.A.; et al. Inhibition of p300 lysine acetyltransferase activity by luteolin reduces tumor growth in head and neck squamous cell carcinoma (HNSCC) xenograft mouse model. *Oncotarget* **2015**, *6*, 43806–43818. [CrossRef]
198. Masraksa, W.; Tanasawet, S.; Hutamekalin, P.; Wongtawatchai, T.; Sukketsiri, W. Luteolin attenuates migration and invasion of lung cancer cells via suppressing focal adhesion kinase and non-receptor tyrosine kinase signaling pathway. *Nutr. Res. Pract.* **2020**, *14*, 127–133. [CrossRef]
199. Cao, D.; Zhu, G.Y.; Lu, Y.; Yang, A.; Chen, D.; Huang, H.J.; Peng, S.X.; Chen, L.W.; Li, Y.W. Luteolin suppresses epithelial-mesenchymal transition and migration of triple-negative breast cancer cells by inhibiting YAP/TAZ activity. *Biomed. Pharmacother.* **2020**, *129*, 110462. [CrossRef] [PubMed]
200. Monti, E.; Marras, E.; Prini, P.; Gariboldi, M.B. Luteolin impairs hypoxia adaptation and progression in human breast and colon cancer cells. *Eur. J. Pharmacol.* **2020**, *881*, 173210. [CrossRef]
201. Tang, X.; Wang, H.; Fan, L.; Wu, X.; Xin, A.; Ren, H.; Wang, X.J. Luteolin inhibits Nrf2 leading to negative regulation of the Nrf2/ARE pathway and sensitization of human lung carcinoma A549 cells to therapeutic drugs. *Free Radic. Biol. Med.* **2011**, *50*, 1599–1609. [CrossRef]
202. Sabzichi, M.; Hamishehkar, H.; Ramezani, F.; Sharifi, S.; Tabasinezhad, M.; Pirouzpanah, M.; Ghanbari, P.; Samadi, N. Luteolin-loaded phytosomes sensitize human breast carcinoma MDA-MB 231 cells to doxorubicin by suppressing Nrf2 mediated signalling. *Asian Pac. J. Cancer Prev.* **2014**, *15*, 5311–5316. [CrossRef]
203. Chen, F.; Liu, Y.; Wang, S.; Guo, X.; Shi, P.; Wang, W.; Xu, B. Triptolide, a Chinese herbal extract, enhances drug sensitivity of resistant myeloid leukemia cell lines through downregulation of HIF-1α and Nrf2. *Pharmacogenomics* **2013**, *14*, 1305–1317. [CrossRef] [PubMed]
204. Shanmugam, M.K.; Warrier, S.; Kumar, A.P.; Sethi, G.; Arfuso, F. Potential Role of Natural Compounds as Anti-Angiogenic Agents in Cancer. *Curr. Vasc. Pharmacol.* **2017**, *15*, 503–519. [CrossRef]
205. Kashyap, D.; Tuli, H.S.; Yerer, M.B.; Sharma, A.; Sak, K.; Srivastava, S.; Pandey, A.; Garg, V.K.; Sethi, G.; Bishayee, A. Natural product-based nanoformulations for cancer therapy: Opportunities and challenges. *Semin. Cancer Biol.* **2019**. [CrossRef]
206. Sadeghi, M.R.; Jeddi, F.; Soozangar, N.; Somi, M.H.; Shirmohamadi, M.; Khaze, V.; Samadi, N. Nrf2/P-glycoprotein axis is associated with clinicopathological characteristics in colorectal cancer. *Biomed. Pharmacother.* **2018**, *104*, 458–464. [CrossRef] [PubMed]
207. Xia, X.; Wang, Q.; Ye, T.; Liu, Y.; Liu, D.; Song, S.; Zheng, C. NRF2/ABCB1-mediated efflux and PARP1-mediated dampening of DNA damage contribute to doxorubicin resistance in chronic hypoxic HepG2 cells. *Fundam. Clin. Pharmacol.* **2020**, *34*, 41–50. [CrossRef]
208. Ryoo, I.G.; Kim, G.; Choi, B.H.; Lee, S.H.; Kwak, M.K. Involvement of NRF2 Signaling in Doxorubicin Resistance of Cancer Stem Cell-Enriched Colonospheres. *Biomol. Ther.* **2016**, *24*, 482–488. [CrossRef] [PubMed]
209. Yang, J.; Zhang, Q.; Liu, Y.; Zhang, X.; Shan, W.; Ye, S.; Zhou, X.; Ge, Y.; Wang, X.; Ren, L. Nanoparticle-based co-delivery of siRNA and paclitaxel for dual-targeting of glioblastoma. *Nanomedicine* **2020**, *15*, 1391–1409. [CrossRef] [PubMed]
210. Wu, B.; Yuan, Y.; Han, X.; Wang, Q.; Shang, H.; Liang, X.; Jing, H.; Cheng, W. Structure of LINC00511-siRNA-conjugated nanobubbles and improvement of cisplatin sensitivity on triple negative breast cancer. *FASEB J.* **2020**, *34*, 9713–9726. [CrossRef] [PubMed]
211. Chen, J.; Wu, Z.; Ding, W.; Xiao, C.; Zhang, Y.; Gao, S.; Gao, Y.; Cai, W. SREBP1 siRNA enhance the docetaxel effect based on a bone-cancer dual-targeting biomimetic nanosystem against bone metastatic castration-resistant prostate cancer. *Theranostics* **2020**, *10*, 1619–1632. [CrossRef] [PubMed]
212. Li, P.C.; Tu, M.J.; Ho, P.Y.; Jilek, J.L.; Duan, Z.; Zhang, Q.Y.; Yu, A.X.; Yu, A.M. Bioengineered NRF2-siRNA Is Effective to Interfere with NRF2 Pathways and Improve Chemosensitivity of Human Cancer Cells. *Drug Metab. Dispos.* **2018**, *46*, 2–10. [CrossRef]

213. Shao, J.; Glorieux, C.; Liao, J.; Chen, P.; Lu, W.; Liang, Z.; Wen, S.; Hu, Y.; Huang, P. Impact of Nrf2 on tumour growth and drug sensitivity in oncogenic K-ras-transformed cells in vitro and in vivo. *Free Radic. Res.* **2018**, *52*, 661–671. [CrossRef]
214. Yan, Y.; Zuo, X.; Wei, D. Concise Review: Emerging Role of CD44 in Cancer Stem Cells: A Promising Biomarker and Therapeutic Target. *Stem. Cells Transl. Med.* **2015**, *4*, 1033–1043. [CrossRef]
215. Zöller, M. CD44: Can a cancer-initiating cell profit from an abundantly expressed molecule? *Nat. Rev. Cancer* **2011**, *11*, 254–267. [CrossRef] [PubMed]
216. Ryoo, I.G.; Choi, B.H.; Ku, S.K.; Kwak, M.K. High CD44 expression mediates p62-associated NFE2L2/NRF2 activation in breast cancer stem cell-like cells: Implications for cancer stem cell resistance. *Redox Biol.* **2018**, *17*, 246–258. [CrossRef] [PubMed]
217. Probst, B.L.; McCauley, L.; Trevino, I.; Wigley, W.C.; Ferguson, D.A. Cancer Cell Growth Is Differentially Affected by Constitutive Activation of NRF2 by KEAP1 Deletion and Pharmacological Activation of NRF2 by the Synthetic Triterpenoid, RTA 405. *PLoS ONE* **2015**, *10*, e0135257. [CrossRef]
218. Goto, S.; Kawabata, T.; Li, T.S. Enhanced Expression of ABCB1 and Nrf2 in CD133-Positive Cancer Stem Cells Associates with Doxorubicin Resistance. *Stem. Cells Int.* **2020**, *2020*, 8868849. [CrossRef]
219. Song, Z.; Liu, Z.; Sun, J.; Sun, F.L.; Li, C.Z.; Sun, J.Z.; Xu, L.Y. The MRTF-A/B function as oncogenes in pancreatic cancer. *Oncol. Rep.* **2016**, *35*, 127–138. [CrossRef] [PubMed]
220. Xing, W.J.; Liao, X.H.; Wang, N.; Zhao, D.W.; Zheng, L.; Zheng, D.L.; Dong, J.; Zhang, T.C. MRTF-A and STAT3 promote MDA-MB-231 cell migration via hypermethylating BRSM1. *IUBMB Life* **2015**, *67*, 202–217. [CrossRef]
221. Xu, Y.; Luo, Y.; Wang, Z.Y.; Li, X.; Zheng, P.; Zhang, T.C. MRTF-A can activate Nrf2 to increase the resistance to doxorubicin. *Oncotarget* **2017**, *8*, 8436–8446. [CrossRef]
222. Brindley, D.N.; Lin, F.-T.; Tigyi, G.J. Role of the autotaxin–lysophosphatidate axis in cancer resistance to chemotherapy and radiotherapy. *Biochim. Biophys. Acta BBA Mol. Cell Biol. Lipids* **2013**, *1831*, 74–85. [CrossRef] [PubMed]
223. Kehlen, A.; Lauterbach, R.; Santos, A.; Thiele, K.; Kabisch, U.; Weber, E.; Riemann, D.; Langner, J. IL-1β-and IL-4-induced down-regulation of autotaxin mRNA and PC-1 in fibroblast-like synoviocytes of patients with rheumatoid arthritis (RA). *Clin. Exp. Immunol.* **2001**, *123*, 147–154. [CrossRef] [PubMed]
224. Nikitopoulou, I.; Oikonomou, N.; Karouzakis, E.; Sevastou, I.; Nikolaidou-Katsaridou, N.; Zhao, Z.; Mersinias, V.; Armaka, M.; Xu, Y.; Masu, M. Autotaxin expression from synovial fibroblasts is essential for the pathogenesis of modeled arthritis. *J. Exp. Med.* **2012**, *209*, 925–933. [CrossRef]
225. Tager, A.M.; LaCamera, P.; Shea, B.S.; Campanella, G.S.; Selman, M.; Zhao, Z.; Polosukhin, V.; Wain, J.; Karimi-Shah, B.A.; Kim, N.D. The lysophosphatidic acid receptor LPA 1 links pulmonary fibrosis to lung injury by mediating fibroblast recruitment and vascular leak. *Nat. Med.* **2008**, *14*, 45–54. [CrossRef] [PubMed]
226. Hozumi, H.; Hokari, R.; Kurihara, C.; Narimatsu, K.; Sato, H.; Sato, S.; Ueda, T.; Higashiyama, M.; Okada, Y.; Watanabe, C. Involvement of autotaxin/lysophospholipase D expression in intestinal vessels in aggravation of intestinal damage through lymphocyte migration. *Lab. Investig.* **2013**, *93*, 508–519. [CrossRef] [PubMed]
227. Euer, N.; Schwirzke, M.; Evtimova, V.; Burtscher, H.; Jarsch, M.; Tarin, D.; Weidle, U.H. Identification of genes associated with metastasis of mammary carcinoma in metastatic versus non-metastatic cell lines. *Anticancer Res.* **2002**, *22*, 733–740. [PubMed]
228. Lin, S.; Wang, D.; Iyer, S.; Ghaleb, A.M.; Shim, H.; Yang, V.W.; Chun, J.; Yun, C.C. The absence of LPA2 attenuates tumor formation in an experimental model of colitis-associated cancer. *Gastroenterology* **2009**, *136*, 1711–1720. [CrossRef]
229. Cooper, A.B.; Wu, J.; Lu, D.; Maluccio, M.A. Is autotaxin (ENPP2) the link between hepatitis C and hepatocellular cancer? *J. Gastrointest. Surg.* **2007**, *11*, 1628–1634; discussion 1634–1625. [CrossRef] [PubMed]
230. Venkatraman, G.; Benesch, M.G.; Tang, X.; Dewald, J.; McMullen, T.P.; Brindley, D.N. Lysophosphatidate signaling stabilizes Nrf2 and increases the expression of genes involved in drug resistance and oxidative stress responses: Implications for cancer treatment. *FASEB J.* **2015**, *29*, 772–785. [CrossRef]
231. Loignon, M.; Miao, W.; Hu, L.; Bier, A.; Bismar, T.A.; Scrivens, P.J.; Mann, K.; Basik, M.; Bouchard, A.; Fiset, P.O.; et al. Cul3 overexpression depletes Nrf2 in breast cancer and is associated with sensitivity to carcinogens, to oxidative stress, and to chemotherapy. *Mol. Cancer Ther.* **2009**, *8*, 2432–2440. [CrossRef]
232. Kang, H.J.; Yi, Y.W.; Hong, Y.B.; Kim, H.J.; Jang, Y.J.; Seong, Y.S.; Bae, I. HER2 confers drug resistance of human breast cancer cells through activation of NRF2 by direct interaction. *Sci. Rep.* **2014**, *4*, 7201. [CrossRef] [PubMed]
233. Manandhar, S.; Lee, S.; Kwak, M.K. Effect of stable inhibition of NRF2 on doxorubicin sensitivity in human ovarian carcinoma OV90 cells. *Arch. Pharm. Res.* **2010**, *33*, 717–726. [CrossRef]
234. Shim, G.S.; Manandhar, S.; Shin, D.H.; Kim, T.H.; Kwak, M.K. Acquisition of doxorubicin resistance in ovarian carcinoma cells accompanies activation of the NRF2 pathway. *Free Radic. Biol. Med.* **2009**, *47*, 1619–1631. [CrossRef] [PubMed]
235. Choi, B.H.; Ryu, D.Y.; Ryoo, I.G.; Kwak, M.K. NFE2L2/NRF2 silencing-inducible miR-206 targets c-MET/EGFR and suppresses BCRP/ABCG2 in cancer cells. *Oncotarget* **2017**, *8*, 107188–107205. [CrossRef] [PubMed]

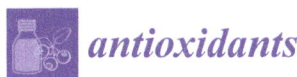

Article

Impact of the APE1 Redox Function Inhibitor E3330 in Non-Small Cell Lung Cancer Cells Exposed to Cisplatin: Increased Cytotoxicity and Impairment of Cell Migration and Invasion

Rita Manguinhas [1], Ana S. Fernandes [2], João G. Costa [2], Nuno Saraiva [2], Sérgio P. Camões [1], Nuno Gil [3], Rafael Rosell [4,5], Matilde Castro [1], Joana P. Miranda [1] and Nuno G. Oliveira [1,*]

[1] Research Institute for Medicines (iMed.ULisboa), Faculty of Pharmacy, Universidade de Lisboa, Av. Professor Gama Pinto, 1649-003 Lisboa, Portugal; rmanguinhas@campus.ul.pt (R.M.); sergiocamoes@campus.ul.pt (S.P.C.); mcastro@ff.ulisboa.pt (M.C.); jmiranda@ff.ulisboa.pt (J.P.M.)

[2] Research Center for Biosciences & Health Technologies (CBIOS), Universidade Lusófona de Humanidades e Tecnologias, Campo Grande 376, 1749-024 Lisboa, Portugal; ana.fernandes@ulusofona.pt (A.S.F.); jgcosta@ulusofona.pt (J.G.C.); nuno.saraiva@ulusofona.pt (N.S.)

[3] Lung Cancer Unit, Champalimaud Centre for the Unknown, Av. Brasília, 1400-038 Lisboa, Portugal; nuno.gil@fundacaochampalimaud.pt

[4] Laboratory of Cellular and Molecular Biology, Institute for Health Science Research Germans Trias i Pujol (IGTP), Campus Can Ruti, Ctra de Can Ruti, Camí de les Escoles, s/n, 08916 Badalona, Barcelona, Spain; rrosell@iconcologia.net

[5] Internal Medicine Department, Universitat Autónoma de Barcelona, Campus de la UAB, Plaça Cívica, 08193 Bellaterra, Barcelona, Spain

* Correspondence: ngoliveira@ff.ulisboa.pt

Received: 12 May 2020; Accepted: 22 June 2020; Published: 24 June 2020

Abstract: Elevated expression levels of the apurinic/apyrimidinic endonuclease 1 (APE1) have been correlated with the more aggressive phenotypes and poor prognosis of non-small cell lung cancer (NSCLC). This study aimed to assess the impact of the inhibition of the redox function of APE1 with E3330 either alone or in combination with cisplatin in NSCLC cells. For this purpose, complementary endpoints focusing on cell viability, apoptosis, cell cycle distribution, and migration/invasion were studied. Cisplatin decreased the viability of H1975 cells in a time- and concentration-dependent manner, with IC$_{50}$ values of 9.6 µM for crystal violet assay and 15.9 µM for 3-(4,5-Dimethylthiazol-2-yl)-5-(3-carboxymethoxyphenyl)-2-(4-sulfophenyl)-2H-tetrazolium (MTS) assay. E3330 was clearly cytotoxic for concentrations above 30 µM. The co-incubation of E3330 and cisplatin significantly decreased cell viability compared to cisplatin alone. Regarding cell cycle distribution, cisplatin led to an increase in sub-G1, whereas the co-treatment with E3330 did not change this profile, which was then confirmed in terms of % apoptotic cells. In addition, the combination of E3330 and cisplatin at low concentrations decreased collective and chemotactic migration, and also chemoinvasion, by reducing these capabilities up to 20%. Overall, these results point to E3330 as a promising compound to boost cisplatin therapy that warrants further investigation in NSCLC.

Keywords: non-small cell lung cancer; cisplatin; apurinic/apyrimidinic endonuclease 1; E3330; cytotoxicity; apoptosis; migration; invasion

---

1. Introduction

Worldwide, lung cancer (LC) is the first cause of cancer-related deaths and the most diagnosed type of cancer for men and women combined. In the US, LC is by far the main cause of death by cancer [1,2]. Non-small cell lung cancer (NSCLC) accounts for the majority of all lung cancer cases and has a low survival rate due to metastasis progression [3]. The most common chemotherapy regimens used in this type of cancer comprise the platinum-based drug cisplatin (Figure 1A), which exerts its effect by cross-linking DNA, inhibiting its replication and transcription, resulting in cell death [4,5]. Even though cisplatin is associated with slightly better survival rates, it is still associated with inherited and acquired resistance to therapy, making it inactive against some tumor types [6]. Indeed, cisplatin resistance is one of the major limitations to its clinical use [4]. Nevertheless, the mechanisms responsible for the resistance of tumor cells are not yet completely understood. For this reason, a number of possible mechanisms for cisplatin resistance were proposed, including reduced intracellular accumulation of cisplatin; enhanced drug inactivation by metallothionein and glutathione; altered expression of oncogenes and regulatory proteins; and increased repair activity of DNA damage [5]. The mechanistic findings on nicotine-induced cisplatin chemoresistance [7,8] should also be mentioned in the context of lung cancer in tobacco smokers. Moreover, both nicotine [9] and cigarette smoking [10] have been associated with oxidative stress.

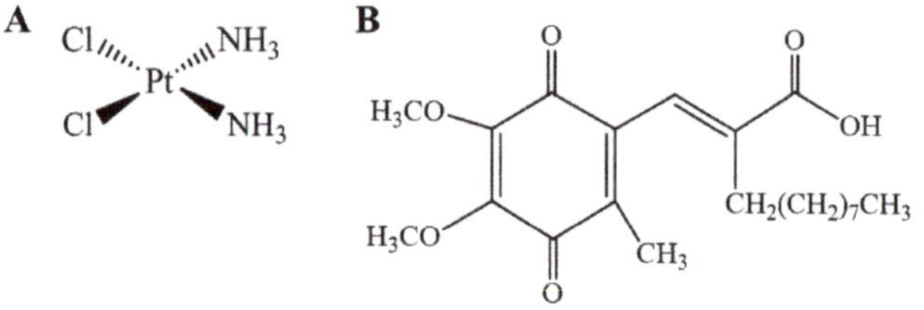

Figure 1. Chemical structure of cisplatin (**A**) and (2E)-2-[(4,5-dimethoxy-2-methyl-3,6-dioxo-1,4-cyclohexadien-1-yl)methylene] undecanoic acid (E3330) (**B**).

The human apurinic/apyrimidinic endonuclease 1 (APE1) is an essential enzyme with two key functions, i.e., repairing DNA damage through the base excision repair (BER) pathway and also a redox signaling protein, modulating the activation of several transcription factors related to cell survival, proliferation, migration/invasion, inflammation, angiogenesis and metastases formation [11–13]. Several transcription factors have been related to APE1's redox activity, particularly the nuclear factor-κB (NF-κB), activator protein 1 (AP-1), early growth response protein-1 (Egr-1), hypoxia-inducible factor 1α (HIF-1α), p53, signal transducer and activator of transcription 3 (STAT3), and Nuclear factor (erythroid-derived 2)-like 2 (Nrf-2) [12,14–20]. In addition, upon oxidative stress, APE1 is known to control the intracellular redox state via the inhibition of reactive oxygen species (ROS) production or by binding with transcription factors (such as p53, HIF-1α, and Nrf-2), promoting an antioxidant response [21–23]. Furthermore, multiple studies have demonstrated that APE1 is overexpressed in numerous types of cancer, such as NSCLC. Increased expression is also associated with more aggressive tumor phenotypes and poor prognosis [13,18,24]. For these reasons, APE1 has gained increasing attention as an emerging druggable target in cancer therapy. A study by Wang et al. [24] suggested that APE1 could be a promising target for the combination of cisplatin-based chemotherapy in NCSLC patients, since its total inhibition using siRNA enhanced sensitivity to cisplatin activity in A549 cells by enabling a synergistic relationship. Other complementary studies also demonstrated that the increased chemoresistance to cisplatin treatment could be related to APE1 overexpression up-regulating transcription factors related to cell survival, such as NF-κB and AP-1, and adaptive response to apoptotic stimulation [25–27]. All this evidence reinforces that APE1 plays a vital role as an upstream effector in cancer progression and reducing its expression levels could help with cisplatin therapy efficiency.

The quinone derivative (2E)-2-[(4,5-dimethoxy-2-methyl-3,6-dioxo-1,4-cyclohexadien-1-yl) methylene] undecanoic acid (E3330 or APX3330, Figure 1B) has been described as a direct and highly specific inhibitor of APE1 redox function, being the first to be identified [28]. For this reason, it has been tested to reduce growth-promoting, inflammatory and anti-apoptotic activities in cells, as well as tumor invasion and metastatic disease in different types of cancer [12,13,28,29]. Its therapeutic potential has been addressed in several cancer-cell-based studies, with interesting results including those from a previous study from our group with human breast cancer cells [13]. A study with prostate cancer also demonstrated important results by reducing cancer cell proliferation and inducing cell cycle arrest upon selective inhibition of the reduction-oxidation function with E3330 [30]. In pancreatic cancer, E3330 was able to impair tumor growth and blocked the activity of NF-κB, AP-1, and HIF-1α [31]. Furthermore, E3330 therapeutic efficacy has been shown to reduce the activity of the transcriptional activators, described previously, regulated by the APE1 redox activity [14–17]. As a result, E3330 has been evaluated in phase I clinical trials in patients with advanced solid tumors [29].

In this context, the present work aimed to assess the impact of APE1's redox function inhibition by E3330 in NSCLC cells in vitro and if this active compound could improve the efficacy of cisplatin administration by enabling a synergistic effect. This evaluation was performed for the first time in the context of NSCLC by integrating multiple endpoints related to cell viability, cell cycle progression, apoptosis, and cell migration and invasion.

2. Materials and Methods

2.1. Chemicals

RPMI-1640 with L-glutamine was purchased from Biowest (Nuaillé, France). Cisplatin, E3330, penicillin-streptomycin solution (10,000 units/mL of penicillin; 10 mg/mL of streptomycin), crystal violet (CV), sodium bicarbonate, extracellular matrix (ECM) gel and dimethylsulfoxide (DMSO) were purchased from Sigma-Aldrich (Madrid, Spain). Sodium pyruvate was purchased from Lonza (Basel, Switzerland) and trypsin (0.25%), and fetal bovine serum (FBS) from Gibco (Eugene, OR, USA). Ethanol absolute, propidium iodide (PI), ethylenediaminetetraacetic acid (EDTA), and acetic acid were obtained from Merck (Darmstadt, Germany). HEPES and D-Glucose were purchased from AppliChem (Darmstadt, Germany). CellTiter 96® Aqueous MTS (3-(4,5-Dimethylthiazol-2-yl)-5-(3-carboxymethoxyphenyl)-2-(4-sulfophenyl)-2H-tetrazolium) was acquired from Promega (Madison, WI, USA) and the Alexa Fluor 488® Annexin V/PI Kit was acquired from Molecular Probes (Eugene, OR, USA).

A 25 mM stock solution of E3330 was prepared in DMSO, aliquoted, and stored at −20 °C. Working solutions were freshly diluted in complete cell culture medium so that, in each final solution, the DMSO concentration was kept at 0.2% (v/v). Cisplatin was dissolved in saline (0.9% NaCl) at a concentration of 2 mM, aliquoted, and stored at −20 °C. In all cell-based assays, vehicle-treated controls were also included, in which H1975 cells were exposed to the respective solvents, i.e., DMSO (final concentration of 0.2% (v/v)) or saline.

2.2. Cell Culture

The human NSCLC cell line H1975 was purchased from the American Type Culture Collection (ATCC, Manassas, VA, USA). This cell line was established in July 1988, originated from lung adenocarcinoma (NSCLC) and the tissue donor was a non-smoker female. H1975 cells were cultured in monolayer in RPMI-1640 medium with L-glutamine supplemented with 10 mM HEPES, 2.5 g/L D-glucose, 1 mM Sodium pyruvate, 1.5 g/L Sodium bicarbonate, 10% FBS and 1% Pen/Strep (complete cell culture medium) and were maintained at 37 °C, under a humidified atmosphere containing 5% CO_2 in air.

2.3. Crystal Violet (CV) Staining Assay

The cytotoxicity of cisplatin/E3330 alone or in combination, in H1975 cells, was evaluated according to a previously described CV staining protocol [13]. Cells were seeded for 24 h at a density of approximately 3×10^3 cells/well in 200 μL of complete culture medium in 96-well plates. After the 24 h period, culture medium was changed and the cells were incubated with a range of cisplatin (1–50 μM) or E3330 (5–50 µM) concentrations, for another 72 h (and also 48 h for cisplatin), in order to assess concentration-response profiles. For combinatory assays, cells were pre-incubated with E3330 (30 µM) for 3 h and then simultaneously exposed to E3330 and different concentrations of cisplatin (5–20 µM) for 72 h. After the incubation periods, H1975 cells were washed with phosphate-buffered saline (PBS) to remove non-adherent cells (non-viable cells). The adherent cells were then fixed with ice-cold 96% ethanol for 10 min and stained with 0.1% crystal violet in 10% ethanol for 5 min. After rinsing with tap water, the stained cells were dissolved in 200 µL of 96% ethanol with 1% acetic acid. Absorbance was measured at 595 nm (OD595) using a SPECTROstar OMEGA microplate reader (BMG Labtech, Offenburg, Germany). Absorbance values presented by vehicle-treated control cells (untreated cells) corresponded to 100% of cell viability. Three to five independent experiments were carried out and six replicates were used for each condition in each independent experiment. The IC_{50} was calculated based on the concentration–response curve using GraphPad Prism® 7.0 (GraphPad Software, Inc., La Jolla, CA, USA).

2.4. MTS Reduction Assay

The MTS reduction assay was carried out as a confirmatory assay of cell viability by applying the same experimental conditions as in the CV assay and following an already described protocol [13]. Briefly, after treatment with the compounds and removal of the incubation medium, cells were washed with PBS, followed by the addition of 100 µL of fresh complete growth medium plus 20 µL of MTS substrate prepared from the CellTiter 96® Aqueous MTS, according to the manufacturer's instructions. Cells were incubated for 2 h with the MTS reagent and the results were measured in terms of absorbance at 490 nm and 690 nm (reference wavelength) using a SPECTROstar OMEGA microplate reader (BMG Labtech, Offenburg, Germany). Absorbance values presented by vehicle-treated control cells corresponded to 100% of cell viability. Three to four independent experiments were carried out and three replicates were used for each condition in each independent experiment. The IC_{50} was also calculated based on the concentration–response curve using GraphPad Prism® 7.0 (GraphPad Software, Inc., La Jolla, CA, USA).

2.5. Cell DNA Content Analysis

Cell DNA content analysis by flow cytometry was performed in order to evaluate the effect of the combination of both compounds in cell cycle distribution. This procedure was carried out according to previously described protocols [32,33]. Briefly, 6×10^4 cells/well were seeded in 6-well plates and cultured for 21 h. Afterwards, cells were incubated with E3330 (30 µM) for 3 h. The culture medium was then changed and both cisplatin (20 µM) and E3330 (30 µM) were added to the cells and incubated for an additional 72-h period. Cells were harvested using 5 mM EDTA in PBS at 37 °C, washed with cold PBS and fixed with chilled 80% ethanol. Cells were stained with PI (10 µg/mL) and simultaneously treated with RNase A (20 µg/mL) for 15–20 min. PI staining was analyzed using a FACSCalibur flow cytometer (Becton Dickinson, San Jose, CA, USA). Data acquisition and analysis were performed using CellQuest® software (Becton Dickinson, San Jose, CA, USA) and FlowJo® (Tree Star Inc., San Carlos, CA, USA), respectively. Three independent experiments were performed.

2.6. Apoptosis Assay

The percentage of apoptotic cells was measured using the flow cytometry dead cell apoptosis kit with Alexa® Fluor 488 Annexin V and PI according to the manufacturers' instructions (Molecular Probes, Eugene, OR, USA). Roughly, 9×10^4 cells were seeded in 6-well plates and grown for 21 h at 37 °C in complete growth medium. After the 21 h period, E3330 (30 µM) was added to the cells for 3 h (pre-incubation). The culture medium was then renewed and both cisplatin (20 µM) and E3330 (30 µM) were added to the cells and incubated for further 72 h. Afterwards, the cells were detached with 5 mM EDTA in PBS at 37 °C and washed with cold PBS. Cells were then stained with PI and Alexa Fluor® 488 annexin V according to the manufacturer's instructions and analysed using a FACSCalibur flow cytometer (Becton Dickinson, San Jose, CA, USA). Three independent experiments were performed. Data acquisition and analysis were performed using CellQuest® software (Becton Dickinson, San Jose, CA, USA) and FlowJo® (Tree Star Inc., San Carlos, CA, USA), respectively.

2.7. Selection of Cisplatin and E3330 Concentrations for the Migration/Invasion Assays

To select non-toxic concentrations of both compounds for the migration and invasion assays, CV and MTS assays were performed as described previously, but using medium with a low serum content instead. This step is of utmost importance to avoid misleading conclusions in migration assays due to cytotoxic effects. Taking this into account, 8×10^3 cells/well were seeded in 96-well plates in complete culture medium containing 10% FBS for 24 h. After the 24 h period, the complete cell culture medium was replaced by culture medium containing 2% FBS and cells were then incubated with a range of low concentrations of cisplatin (0.1–5 µM) or E3330 (10–30 µM) for another 24 h. The CV and MTS assays were subsequently performed and non-toxic concentrations of both E3330 and cisplatin were selected for the following assays. Three to seven independent experiments were performed, each one comprising three (MTS) or six (CV) replicates.

2.8. In Vitro Wound-Healing Assay

For the evaluation of collective cell migration, an in vitro wound-healing assay was performed according to a previously described method [34,35]. H1975 cells were seeded in 24-well plates at a density of approximately 5.5×10^4 cells/well and incubated for 21 h in complete cell culture medium. E3330 was then added to the well at a concentration of 10 µM and incubated for 3 h. Afterwards, the cell culture medium was removed, and a scratch was performed using a 200 µL sterile pipette tip on the cell monolayer. Cells were then washed twice with warm PBS, in order to remove cellular debris, and were left to migrate in cell culture medium containing 2% FBS in the presence of cisplatin (1 µM) and E3330 (10 µM) for further 20 h. Wound closure was evaluated using a Motic AE2000 Inverted Phase Contrast Microscope (Motic, Barcelona, Spain) and pictures of the same areas were captured using a magnification of 40× with a camera Moticam 2500 (Motic, Barcelona, Spain). The scratch width was measured with Motic Images plus v2.0 software (Motic, Barcelona, Spain) at 0, 8, and 20 h after the scratch was performed. The percentage of cell migration was measured in relation to the initial distance between the wound edges. At each time-point, two pictures of the scratch were taken for each condition. Three independent experiments were performed.

2.9. Chemotaxis and Chemoinvasion Assays

As a single-cell migration evaluation, a chemotactic migration assay was performed by adopting a protocol already described by Flórido et al. [36] and Fernandes et al. [34]. Briefly, 3×10^4 cells/well were seeded in cell culture medium containing 2% FBS on the top of a transwell insert with transparent polyethylene terephthalate (PET) membranes containing 8 µm pores (BD Falcon, Bedford, MA, USA) inside 24-well plates. Complete cell culture medium was added to the lower chamber, containing 10% FBS as the chemoattractant. Right after seeding, E3330 (10 µM) alone was added to both chambers and incubated for 3 h. After this 3 h period, cisplatin (1 µM) was also added to both chambers and cells were allowed to migrate through the membrane for another 16 h. Subsequently, non-migrating cells were carefully removed from the upper chamber with a cotton swab and migrating cells (bottom of each membrane) were fixed with cold 96% ethanol for 10 min and then stained with 0.1% crystal violet in 10% ethanol for 15 min. The inserts were thoroughly rinsed using tap water and were allowed to dry for at least 24 h. Five randomly selected fields were photographed for each condition, using a Moticam 2500 (Motic, Barcelona, Spain) placed on a Motic AE2000 Inverted Phase Contrast Microscope (Motic, Barcelona, Spain) with an amplification of 100×. For each picture, migrated cells were manually counted using the software Motic Images plus v3.0 (Motic, Barcelona, Spain). The counted cells were expressed as percentages of vehicle-treated control cells and three independent experiments were performed.

A procedure similar to the abovementioned chemotactic migration assay was carried out for the evaluation of chemoinvasion. The difference between the two setups was the addition of 75 μL of ECM gel (1:25 dilution in serum-free medium) in order to coat the porous membranes of the transwell inserts. The initial seeding density was also adapted to 1.5×10^4 cells/well. The analysis of the results was performed similarly to the abovementioned chemotactic migration assay, and five independent experiments were performed.

3. Results

3.1. Cytotoxicity Profile of Cisplatin in H1975 Cells

In order to determine the impact of cisplatin treatment in H1975 cells viability, a concentration-response profile was established, resorting to CV staining and MTS reduction assays. In the CV staining assay, after 48 and 72 h of cisplatin exposure (Figure 2A), the viability of H1975 cells decreased in a time- and concentration-dependent manner (1–50 μM). Additionally, The MTS reduction assay (Figure 2B) was performed as a mechanistically complementary method and the concentration–response curves showed similar cytotoxicity profiles. The IC_{50} values for the CV assay were 27.5 and 9.6 μM for 48 and 72 h, respectively. In addition, the IC_{50} value calculated for the MTS assay at 72 h was 15.9 μM, in the same range, although slightly higher. Cisplatin was demonstrated to be toxic at low concentrations for a 72 h incubation period, starting to compromise cell viability at 1 μM and dramatically decreasing it at 50 μM, for both MTS and CV assays. Considering these results, the cisplatin concentrations of 5, 10, and 20 μM were selected for the subsequent combinatory assays, since they represent different levels of cytotoxicity, comprising the range of IC_{50} values calculated as well as concentrations slightly above and below this parameter.

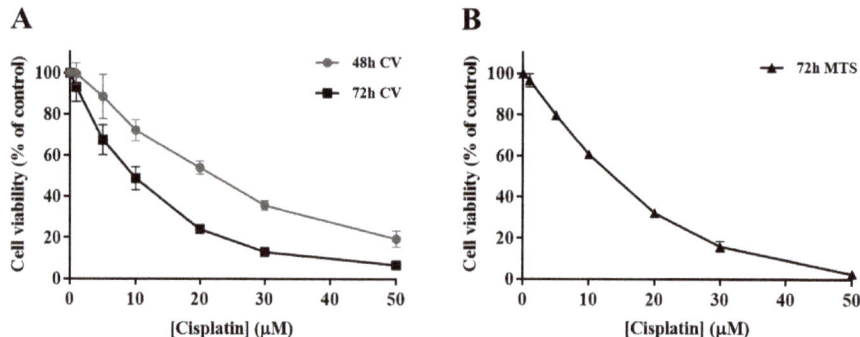

Figure 2. Cytotoxic effects of cisplatin (1–50 μM) in H1975 cells. The viability of cells treated with cisplatin for 48 h and 72 h was assessed by crystal violet (CV) staining assay (**A**) and for 72 h by MTS reduction assay (**B**). Values represent mean ± SD (n = 3–4) and are expressed as percentages of the vehicle-treated control cells.

3.2. Impact of E3330 in the Viability of H1975 Cells

The effect of E3330 was evaluated by exposing H1975 cells during 72 h to a range of concentrations from 5 to 50 μM. Both CV and MTS assays revealed that E3330 was not considerably toxic at low concentrations (Figure 3A,B, respectively). Both assays demonstrated a similar concentration–response curve for E3330. Nevertheless, E3330 at 50 μM showed decreased cell viability in about 45% with the CV assay whereas, with the MTS assay, the decrease was lower, approximately 30%. A similar trend in the differences between these two methods was also observed in the previous cisplatin assays, reflecting the inherent sensitivities of these two mechanistically distinct endpoints. Since the range of E3330 concentrations applied for these experimental conditions did not lead to a 50% loss in cell viability, it was not possible to calculate the IC_{50} values for H1975 cells. The concentration of 30 μM was chosen for the combinatory assays since it was the higher concentration of E3330 tested that displayed a relatively low impact on cell viability.

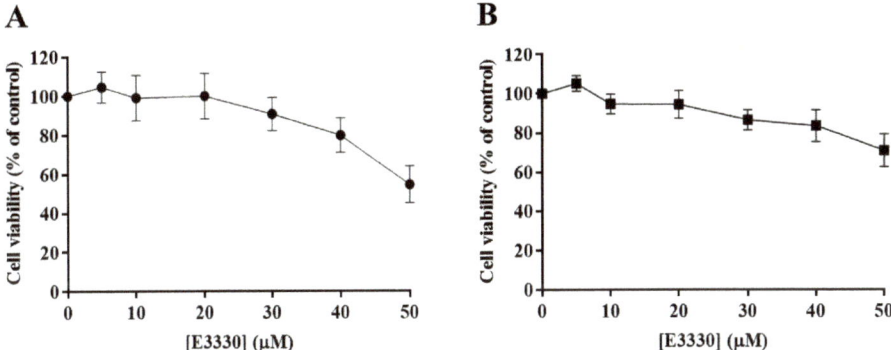

Figure 3. Evaluation of E3330 (5–50 µM) cytotoxicity in H1975 cells. The cell viability of E3330-exposed cells (72 h) was evaluated by CV staining (**A**) and MTS reduction (**B**) assays. Values represent mean ± SD ($n = 3$) and are expressed as percentages of the vehicle-treated control cells.

3.3. The Combination of E3330 and Cisplatin Displays a Synergistic Effect in Cell Viability

With the purpose of evaluating if E3330 enhanced cisplatin treatment in NSCLC, H1975 cells were co-incubated with these two compounds and the effects were evaluated using the CV staining assay and validated with the MTS reduction assay. In the CV assay, E3330 (30 µM) demonstrated a slight decrease in cell viability of around 11% ($p < 0.01$) when compared to the vehicle-treated control cells (Figure 4A). In the MTS assay, this decrease was lower and not statistically significant (Figure 4B). All the concentrations of cisplatin (5, 10, and 20 µM) tested in the CV assay revealed an impairment in cell viability that was clearly intensified when the APE1 redox inhibitor E3330 was co-incubated. This significant combined effect was also confirmed in the MTS assay. In this case, the cells were treated with 20 µM of cisplatin and 30 µM of E3330. In absolute percentage values, the decreases in cell viability observed for 5, 10 and 20 µM of cisplatin, in the presence of E3330, were 18.5% ($p < 0.05$), 22.8% ($p < 0.05$) and 12.4% ($p < 0.01$), respectively, for the CV assay, and 17.1% ($p < 0.05$) for the MTS assay. Considering the relative decreases in cell viability observed, the concentration of E3330 at 30 µM reduced in 36% and 78% the cell viability of 20 µM cisplatin-treated cells for the CV and MTS assays, respectively. As such, this combination was selected for further cell cycle distribution studies. Altogether, these results suggest that for all the concentrations and endpoints tested, a synergistic effect was present.

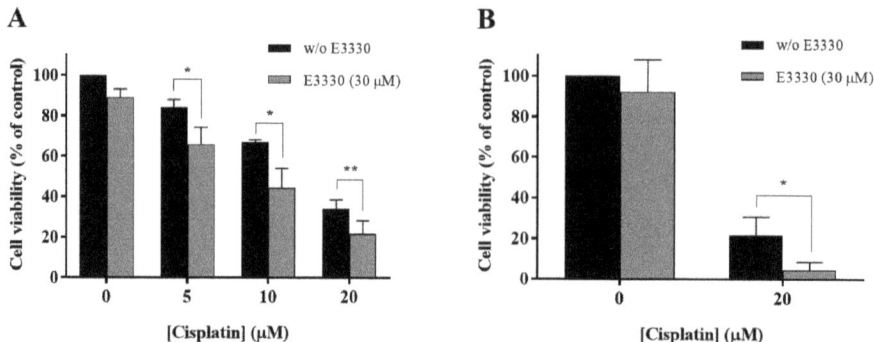

Figure 4. Impact of E3330 on the viability of H1975 cells treated with cisplatin. Cells were pre-incubated with E3330 (30 µM) for 3 h and then simultaneously exposed to E3330 and cisplatin (5–20 µM) for 72 h. The effects in terms of cell viability were evaluated using the CV staining assay (**A**) and MTS reduction assay (**B**). Values represent mean ± SD (n = 3–5) and are expressed as percentages relative to vehicle-treated control cells. * $p < 0.05$ and ** $p < 0.01$ relative to respective cisplatin-treated cells (Student's t-test).

3.4. Effect of the Combination of E3330 and Cisplatin in Cell Cycle Distribution and Cell Death

Since cytotoxicity is frequently accompanied by cell cycle arrest and/or cell death, the impact of E3330 and cisplatin combination in H1975 cells was evaluated by cell DNA content using PI staining for flow cytometry (Figure 5A,B). As expected, the exposure to cisplatin (20 µM, 72 h) alone substantially increased (around five-fold) the sub-G1 population and lead to a decrease in the G0/G1 population when compared to vehicle-treated control cells. E3330 (30 µM, 72 h) did not significantly modify the cell cycle distribution of vehicle-treated or cisplatin-treated cells. In fact, the cell cycle distribution of cisplatin alone or cisplatin with E3330 remained similar. G2/M population maintained unaltered for all the conditions tested.

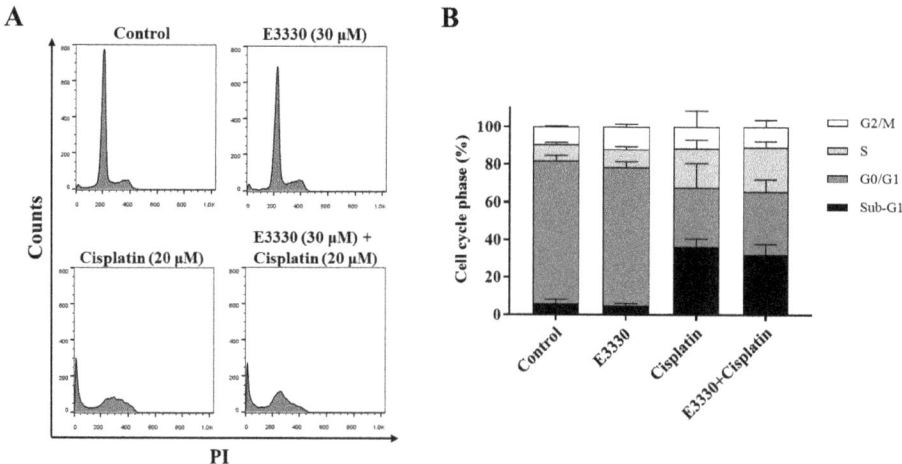

Figure 5. *Cont.*

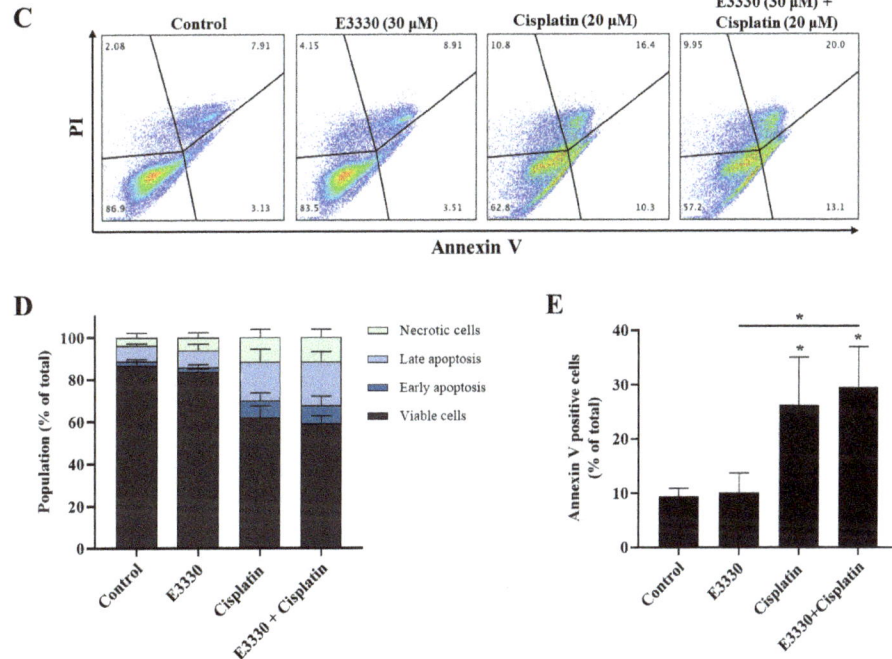

Figure 5. Cell cycle progression and apoptosis of H1975 cells treated with E3330 and/or cisplatin. Cells were pre-incubated with E3330 (30 µM) for 3 h and then cisplatin (20 µM) was added for co-incubation for further 72 h. After this exposure period, cell DNA content analysis with PI staining was performed by flow cytometry. (**A**) Representative flow cytometry histograms. (**B**) Sub-G1, G0/G1, S, and G2/M populations' summary results. The percentage of apoptotic cells was determined by PI and Annexin V staining after the same incubation profile as in the cell DNA content analysis. (**C**) Representative flow cytometry dot-plots. (**D**) Percentage of viable cells, cells undergoing early and late apoptosis, and necrotic cells summary results. (**E**) Summary results demonstrate the percentage of apoptotic cells (Annexin V positive cells). Values represent mean ± SD (n = 3), * $p < 0.05$ (one-way ANOVA with Tukey's test).

The induction of apoptosis was analyzed by flow cytometry after staining with Annexin V-FITC and PI (Figure 5C–E). Representative graphs obtained by flow cytometry are displayed in Figure 5C. Incubation with cisplatin (20 µM, 72 h) alone led to a ~3-fold increase in the % of apoptotic cells when compared to vehicle-treated cells (Figure 5E; ~26% vs 9%, respectively), which is in line with the observed increase in the sub-G1 population. Moreover, although the exposure to E3330 did not significantly alter the % of apoptotic cells in cisplatin-treated cultures, a small trend towards a synergistic effect was observed (Figure 5E).

3.5. E3330 in Combination with Cisplatin Reduces Both Collective and Chemotactic Cell Migration

Considering an impairment in cell viability would interfere with possible results in cell migration and invasion processes, it was necessary to ascertain that non-toxic concentrations of E3330 and cisplatin were used. As such, the H1975 cells were exposed to a range of low concentrations of either cisplatin (0.1–5 µM) or E3330 (10–30 µM) for 24 h in order to select the conditions of migration/invasion assays. Accordingly, in these experiments, a complete culture medium with 2% FBS was used. The effect of cisplatin was assessed using the CV assay (Figure 6A). Cell viability was not markedly affected up to 2.5 µM (~10% reduction). At a concentration of 5 µM, this decrease reached around 17%. As for E3330, cell viability started to be affected at the concentration of 20 µM with a reduction of 12% in the CV assay (Figure 6B), although in the MTS assay this concentration level was not cytotoxic (Figure 6C). Overall, considering both assays and compounds, we decided to select the representative non-cytotoxic concentrations of 1 µM for cisplatin and 10 µM for E3330 for the migration and invasion assays.

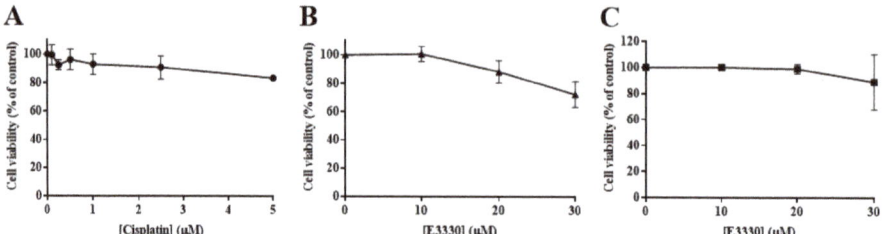

Figure 6. Viability of H1975 cells exposed to low concentrations of cisplatin or E3330 in culture medium with 2% FBS. (**A**) Effect of cisplatin (0.1–5 µM; 24 h) on cell viability, in the presence of 2% FBS, evaluated by the CV assay. Effect of E3330 (10–30 µM; 24 h) on cell viability in the presence of 2% FBS evaluated by both CV (**B**) and MTS assays (**C**). Values for cell viability represent mean ± SD (n = 4–7) and are expressed as percentages relative to vehicle-treated control cells.

Metastases development comprises multiple biological mechanisms, including an increase in cell motility. For this reason, after the selection of non-cytotoxic concentrations of both E3330 and cisplatin, the migration capacity of H1975 cells was evaluated by resorting to two mechanistically different methods. Firstly, collective cell migration was assessed with the wound-healing assay as an evaluation of the cells' movement across a horizontal surface with the conservation of functional cell–cell junctions (Figure 7A). Both E3330 and cisplatin alone did not demonstrate an effect on wound closure. Importantly, their combination significantly reduced this closure in about 20% ($p < 0.05$) when compared to vehicle-treated control cells. This decrease was also statistically significant when comparing the combination of both compounds with cisplatin-treated cells ($p < 0.01$). Microphotographs were also taken at a timepoint of 8 h of co-incubation, already revealing a slight impairment for the combinatory condition (data not shown).

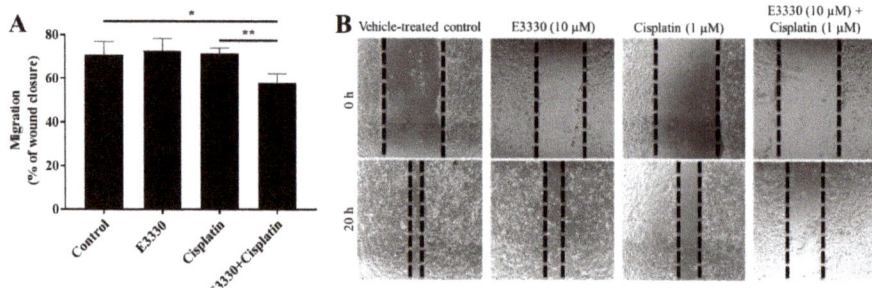

Figure 7. *Cont.*

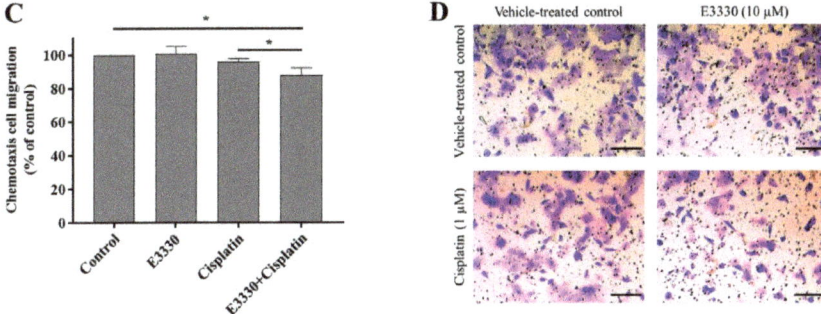

Figure 7. E3330 effect on collective and chemotactic migration of H1975 cells exposed to cisplatin. Collective cell migration was evaluated by the wound-healing assay (**A**) and chemotaxis was measured using a transwell assay (**C**). Representative microscopy images of the wound-healing assay (40×, **B**) and the chemotaxis assay (migrating cells stained with crystal violet—100×, **D**). Scale bars = 200 µm. Values for the wound-healing assay represent mean ± SD ($n = 3$) and are expressed as percentage of wound closure, calculated relative to the initial width; * $p < 0.05$ and ** $p < 0.01$ (Student's t-test). Values for the chemotaxis assay represent mean ± SD ($n = 3$) and are expressed as percentages relative to vehicle-treated control cells; * $p < 0.05$ (Student's t-test).

For the determination of chemotactic individual cell migration, the transwell assay was performed (Figure 7C) as a measurement of the ability of single cells to directionally respond to a chemoattractant gradient. In this assay, E3330 and cisplatin alone also did not influence chemotactic migration, but again their combination reduced this type of migration in approximately 12% ($p < 0.05$) when compared to vehicle-treated control cells. The decrease observed was also statistically significant when compared to cisplatin-treated H1975 cells ($p < 0.05$). Representative images of the wound-healing assay and the chemotaxis migration assay are presented in Figure 7B,D, respectively.

3.6. The Combination of E3330 and Cisplatin Decreases Invasion of H1975 Cells

For the progression of cancer and metastases formation, cancerous cells located in the primary tumor need to be able to invade through the extracellular matrix and consequently migrate throughout blood circulation and/or lymphatic vessels and attach to a distant site in response to a stimulus. Considering these processes, the effect of E3330 on the invasion of cisplatin-treated H1975 cells was evaluated by the transwell chemoinvasion assay (Figure 8A). Since the proteolytic degradation of basement membranes is essential for invasion processes and subsequent metastasis formation, this assay was performed under the same conditions as the chemotaxis migration assay but with the incorporation of an ECM gel. Similar to the results from the migration assays, both E3330 and cisplatin alone did not induce a significant effect in terms of cell invasiveness. However, when both compounds were combined, there was a statistically significant decrease of approximately 17% ($p < 0.01$) in chemoinvasion when compared to vehicle-treated control cells. This decrease was also statistically significant when comparing the combination of compounds with cisplatin-treated H1975 cells ($p < 0.05$). Representative images of the chemoinvasion assay are presented in Figure 8B.

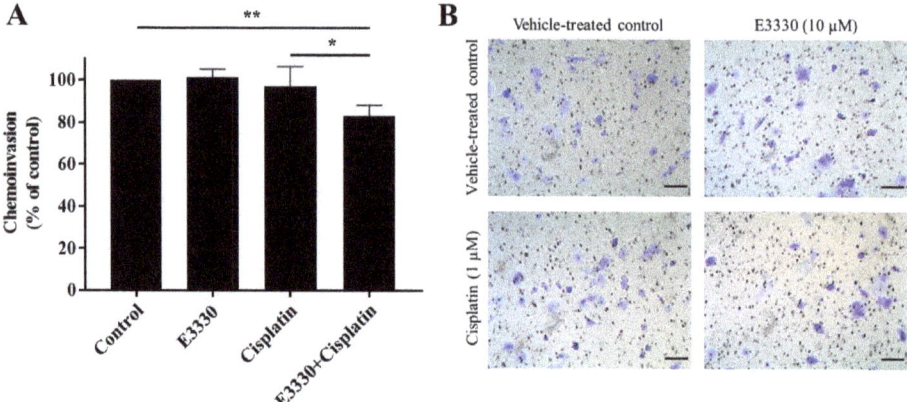

Figure 8. Effect of E3330 on the invasiveness of cisplatin-treated H1975 cells. (**A**) Transwell chemoinvasion was assessed after a pre-incubation period of 3 h with E3330 and a subsequent period of 16 h with both compounds. Values represent mean ± SD (n = 5) and are expressed as percentages relative to vehicle-treated control cells; * p < 0.05 and ** p < 0.01 (Student's t-test). (**B**) Representative microscopy images of invading cells stained with crystal violet (100×). Scale bars = 100 µm.

4. Discussion

As aforementioned, NSCLC is the most frequent lung cancer sub-type, presenting low survival rates due to metastasis progression, which is often resistant to platinum-based chemotherapy. The usefulness of genetics to predict the response of cisplatin was reviewed by Karachaliou et al. [37]. Rosell et al. [38] also recently highlighted the novel molecular targets for the treatment of NSCLC, identifying different prognostic markers. In fact, there are important molecular markers that should be considered in NSCLC. For instance, HIF-1α was reported as a prognostic factor for lung cancer patients [39]. In the scope of the present study, and as described in the Introduction Section, the elevated expression levels of APE1 have also been correlated with more aggressive phenotypes and poor prognosis of NSCLC patients.

APE1, besides being a key DNA repair enzyme, also works as a redox signaling protein, modulating the activation of several transcription factors related to cancer progression and metastasis formation. For this reason, the aim of the present work was to address in vitro the impact of a novel therapeutic strategy based on targeting APE1 redox function in NSCLC in order to increase the efficacy of platinum-based chemotherapy and reduce its possible resistance. This innovative approach constitutes the first report on the effect of E3330 alone or in combination with cisplatin in NSCLC cells using complementary endpoints. The representative cell model chosen for this purpose is the H1975 human lung adenocarcinoma cell line that was established from a non-smoker patient and possesses a mutation in the gene that confers resistance to EGFR inhibitors [40]. It is considered as a highly invasive cell line used as an adequate tool in preclinical studies towards the discovery of novel drugs for NSCLC and also in xenograft models [41].

According to two complementary cell viability assays, cisplatin displayed a concentration- and time-dependent cytotoxic effect with IC_{50} values ranging from approximately 10 to 16 µM for 72 h, being more than two-fold higher for a shorter incubation period of 48 h. Considering the results available in the literature, the effect of cisplatin in H1975 cells viability herein obtained is comparable to those described by other authors using different methodologies such as sulforhodamine B assay (IC_{50} = 8.31 µM [27]) and MTT (3-(4,5-dimethylthiazol-2-yl)-2,5-diphenyltetrazolium bromide) assay (IC_{50} = 6.71 µM [42] and IC_{50} = 11 µM [43]) for the same 72 h incubation period. As for 48 h of cisplatin incubation in the same cell line, our results differ from the study of Zhao et al. [44] that found an IC_{50} value of 3 µM using the MTT assay. In contrast, Sun et al. [45] with the Cell Counting kit-8 assay, obtained an IC_{50} value of around 30 µM for H1975 cells, which was comparable to our results. It is known that cell viability for similar cisplatin concentrations varies among different cell lines, even for cells originating from the same NSCLC cancer subtype, due to various reasons including acquired cisplatin resistance. For example, A549 cells appear to be more sensitive to cisplatin incubation (72 h) than the H1975 cells as shown by Wang et al. (IC_{50} = 1.54 µM [24]), Deben et al. (IC_{50} = 4.12 µM [27]) and Wang et al. (IC_{50} = 5.7 µM [43]). In contrast, H1993 is a NSCLC cell line more resistant to cisplatin, with an IC_{50} value of 19.58 µM [46]. In this sense, the choice for H1975 cells was considered here in view of its average sensitivity to cisplatin effects.

In the present work, E3330 did not induce significant cytotoxicity at low concentrations in H1975 cells. However, this compound has demonstrated a significant impact on different cancer cell lines. At the same incubation period, and with an MTT assay, E3330 was demonstrated to be more cytotoxic to ovarian cancer cell lines with IC_{50} values of 33 µM and 37 µM in Hey-C2 and SKOC-3X cell lines, respectively [47]. In the case of prostatic cancer, McIlwain et al. [30] presented the following IC_{50} values for a five day incubation period with E3330: PC-3, 54.7 µM; C4-2, 89.5 µM, and LNCaP, 71.9 µM. As for pancreatic cancer, E3330 cytotoxicity was demonstrated to fluctuate between different cell lines by presenting an IC_{50} of 50 µM for PANC1 cells [48] and causing only 20% loss of cell viability at the same concentration in Pa03C cells [19]. However, this compound has only been tested in a NSCLC cell line (A549) with a concentration of 25 µM for 72 h, resulting in less than 5% loss in cell viability [49], which was similar to the results obtained in the present work. Based on these results, it can be concluded that E3330 is not considerably cytotoxic to H1975 cells at concentrations up to 30-40 µM, displaying only a clear cytotoxic effect at 50 µM. Interestingly, the blood levels found in clinical trials varied between 50 and 150 µM [30], higher than the range of E3330 concentrations that were effective in the combinatory experiments with cisplatin described in the present study.

Importantly, when both drugs were combined in the CV and MTS assays, a significant decrease in cell viability was revealed. Since cytotoxicity is frequently accompanied by cell cycle arrest and apoptosis induction, we aimed to explore this synergistic relationship between E3330 and cisplatin in terms of cell cycle distribution. However, the addition of E3330 did not alter the profile of H1975 cisplatin-treated cells. Moreover, E3330 per se did not have an impact on the cell cycle distribution. This could be a consequence of its low cytotoxic potential (Figure 3). Similar results were also observed in representative cell lines of pancreatic cancer (PANC1 [48]) and breast cancer (MDA-MB-231 [13]). The cytotoxicity of cisplatin is mediated through the induction of apoptosis and cell cycle arrest resulting from its interaction with DNA [5]. It has been demonstrated that cisplatin can affect the Gl-S checkpoint, when the cell is entering the S-phase, or the G2/M checkpoint, after DNA replication [50,51]. For example, in a study with A549 cells, it was demonstrated that an incubation with 11 µM of cisplatin for 24 h increased the G2/M phase population (cell cycle arrest) and a decrease in G0/G1 population [52]. This impact is also observed in our results. Considering the results achieved in the cytotoxicity assays, the evaluation of apoptosis was also performed. As expected, the incubation of cisplatin alone induced a high increase in the number of apoptotic cells. However, E3330 did not significantly increase the apoptosis induced in cisplatin-treated cells. Taking this into consideration, other cell mechanisms could be involved in promoting the loss of cell viability when E3330 and cisplatin are combined.

The ability of cells to migrate and invade surrounding tissues is essential for the development of metastases, and APE1's redox function has been shown to modulate several transcription factors and signaling pathways related to these mechanisms [11,12]. Since E3330 inhibits this redox function, the combination of this compound with cisplatin was evaluated on these processes by assessing two mechanistically different migration endpoints and performing the reference chemoinvasion assay. E3330 and cisplatin alone did not interfere with both migration and invasion endpoints tested. However, when these compounds were combined, both collective and chemotactic cell migration, and also chemoinvasion, were reduced in levels up to 20%, this being also a relevant finding of the present study. It should be noted that higher concentrations of E3330 would likely lead to more pronounced results. However, the use of high concentrations of a given anti-migratory drug may enclose cytotoxicity, thus precluding the accurate assessment of migration. In addition, Nyland et al. demonstrated that in order to have redox inhibition by E3330, in ovarian Hey-C2 cells, a concentration of 10 µM was sufficient [53]. The use of E3330 potential to interfere with migration has been evaluated by other authors in different cancer models. For instance, E3330 impaired migration in pancreatic cancer cells [48] and retinal endothelial cells [54]. A previous study from our group using breast cancer cells (MDA-MB-231) also demonstrated a significant decrease in collective cell migration but not in chemotaxis [13]. Additionally, E3330 promoted a significant decrease in chemoinvasion when combined with docetaxel, a standard chemotherapeutic drug for breast cancer.

Overall, it is clear that the combination of E3330 and cisplatin is able to sensitize NSCLC cells, promoting a better response in terms of cytotoxicity and cell migration and invasion. A previous study by Li et al. showed that NF-κB expression is linked to chemoresistance in NSCLC cells (H460 cells), and consequent inhibition of this transcription factor enhances the sensitivity of these cells to cisplatin [55]. Furthermore, NF-κB, and also AP-1, have been associated with several downstream mechanisms related to cell migration and invasion such as matrix metalloproteinases (MMPs) and the hyaluronan cell-surface receptor CD44 activity. E3330 was able to suppress CD44 expression in pancreatic cancer cells, promoting a direct consequence for cell migration [48]. Besides, overexpression of this receptor has been correlated with occurrence and migration of NSCLC [56]. MMPs have also been established as key players in mechanisms of tumor invasion and metastasis formation by ECM degradation and are regulated by AP-1 and NF-κB, being MMP-9 strongly regulated by the latter [57,58]. In addition, this MMP has been found to be upregulated in NSCLC [59].

Altogether, the blocked transcription factors and subsequent downstream effectors may be responsible for the abovementioned effects in cytotoxicity and the reduction in migration and invasion upon treatment with both compounds. In this sense, the evaluation of the role of transcriptional factors constitutes a further step of this work in order to elucidate the mechanisms involved. This study should be performed in a holistic manner, focusing on a set of putative key targets (e.g., AP-1, Nrf2, NF-κB, HIF-1α). In accordance, it should be also pertinent to perform experiments to gain insights on other unknown transcriptional targets, resorting to RNA sequencing by Next Generation Sequencing (NGS) followed by protein expression confirmation. The inclusion of in vivo animal data is also anticipated after further elucidation of the putative mechanisms. There are several NSCLC rodent models available, including patient-derived xenografts, which can be adequate to study the combination of cisplatin (i.v.) with E3330 orally administered. Finally, it should be emphasized that E3330 has been tested in cancer clinical trials for solid tumors (oral administration, twice a day). In view of this, the collection of in vitro and in vivo data will be determinant to support the potential clinical use of this drug in combination with standard platinum-based therapy in NSCLC.

5. Conclusions

The work developed herein enabled us to evaluate the impact of the APE1 redox inhibitor E3330 in H1975 cells treated with cisplatin by characterizing the cytotoxicity, cell cycle distribution, apoptosis, and migration and invasion processes. Overall, the results pointed to E3330 as a promising compound to boost cisplatin therapy that warrants further investigation in NSCLC. The results highlight that additional studies should be performed to elucidate the underlying mechanisms involved, such as verifying the expression of transcription factors under APE1 redox function which are also related to cell migration and invasion.

Author Contributions: Conceptualization, N.G.O.; formal analysis, R.M., A.S.F., J.G.C. and N.S.; funding acquisition, A.S.F., R.R., J.P.M. and N.G.O.; investigation, R.M., J.G.C. and N.S.; methodology, R.M., A.S.F., J.G.C., N.S. and S.P.C.; resources, A.S.F., M.C., J.P.M. and N.G.O.; software, R.M., J.G.C. and N.S.; supervision, N.G.O.; validation, A.S.F., N.S. and N.G.O.; writing—original draft, R.M. and N.G.O.; writing—review & editing, A.S.F., J.G.C., S.P.C., N.G., R.R., M.C., J.P.M. and N.G.O. All authors have read and agreed to the published version of the manuscript.

Funding: This research was funded by Fundação para a Ciência e a Tecnologia (FCT) through grants UID/DTP/04138/2019 to iMed.ULisboa; UID/DTP/04567/2019 to CBIOS; PD/BD/114280/2016 to S.P.C.; TUBITAK/003/2014 and PTDC/MED-TOX/29183/2017. R.R. reports grants from La Caixa Foundation and from the Spanish Association Against Cancer (PROYE18012ROSE). Research developed with funding from Universidade Lusófona/ILIND (Grant Programme FIPID 2019/2020).

Acknowledgments: The authors acknowledge Jordi Berenguer for the technical assistance related to the selection of NSCLC cells.

Conflicts of Interest: The authors declare no conflict of interest.

References

1. Bray, F.; Ferlay, J.; Soerjomataram, I.; Siegel, R.L.; Torre, L.A.; Jemal, A. Global cancer statistics 2018: GLOBOCAN estimates of incidence and mortality worldwide for 36 cancers in 185 countries. *CA Cancer J. Clin.* **2018**, *68*, 394–424. [CrossRef] [PubMed]
2. Siegel, R.L.; Miller, K.D.; Jemal, A. Cancer statistics, 2019. *CA Cancer J. Clin.* **2019**, *69*, 7–34. [CrossRef]
3. Zappa, C.; Mousa, S.A. Non-small cell lung cancer: Current treatment and future advances. *Transl. Lung Cancer Res.* **2016**, *5*, 288–300. [CrossRef]
4. Rocha, C.R.R.; Silva, M.M.; Quinet, A.; Cabral-Neto, J.B.; Menck, C.F.M. DNA repair pathways and cisplatin resistance: An intimate relationship. *Clinics* **2018**, *73*, e478s. [CrossRef] [PubMed]
5. Wang, G.; Reed, E.; Li, Q.Q. Molecular basis of cellular response to cisplatin chemotherapy in non-small cell lung cancer (Review). *Oncol. Rep.* **2004**, *12*, 955–965. [CrossRef] [PubMed]
6. Rajeswaran, A.; Trojan, A.; Burnand, B.; Giannelli, M. Efficacy and side effects of cisplatin- and carboplatin-based doublet chemotherapeutic regimens versus non-platinum-based doublet chemotherapeutic regimens as first line treatment of metastatic non-small cell lung carcinoma: A systematic review of randomi. *Lung Cancer* **2008**, *59*, 1–11. [CrossRef] [PubMed]
7. Zhang, J.; Kamdar, O.; Le, W.; Rosen, G.D.; Upadhyay, D. Nicotine induces resistance to chemotherapy by modulating mitochondrial signaling in lung cancer. *Am. J. Respir. Cell Mol. Biol.* **2009**, *40*, 135–146. [CrossRef]
8. Nishioka, T.; Luo, L.Y.; Shen, L.; He, H.; Mariyannis, A.; Dai, W.; Chen, C. Nicotine increases the resistance of lung cancer cells to cisplatin through enhancing Bcl-2 stability. *Br. J. Cancer* **2014**, *110*, 1785–1792. [CrossRef]
9. Zhang, Q.; Ganapathy, S.; Avraham, H.; Nishioka, T.; Chen, C. Nicotine exposure potentiates lung tumorigenesis by perturbing cellular surveillance. *Br. J. Cancer* **2020**, *122*, 904–911. [CrossRef]
10. Goldkorn, T.; Filosto, S.; Chung, S. Lung injury and lung cancer caused by cigarette smoke-induced oxidative stress: Molecular mechanisms and therapeutic opportunities involving the ceramide-generating machinery and epidermal growth factor receptor. *Antioxid. Redox Signal.* **2014**, *21*, 2149–2174. [CrossRef]
11. Tell, G.; Fantini, D.; Quadrifoglio, F. Understanding different functions of mammalian AP endonuclease (APE1) as a promising tool for cancer treatment. *Cell. Mol. Life Sci.* **2010**, *67*, 3589–3608. [CrossRef] [PubMed]
12. Kelley, M.R.; Georgiadis, M.M.; Fishel, M.L. APE1/Ref-1 Role in Redox Signaling: Translational Applications of Targeting the Redox Function of the DNA Repair/Redox Protein APE1/Ref-1. *Curr. Mol. Pharmacol.* **2012**, *5*, 36–53. [CrossRef] [PubMed]
13. Guerreiro, P.S.; Corvacho, E.; Costa, J.G.; Saraiva, N.; Fernandes, A.S.; Castro, M.; Miranda, J.P.; Oliveira, N.G. The APE1 redox inhibitor E3330 reduces collective cell migration of human breast cancer cells and decreases chemoinvasion and colony formation when combined with docetaxel. *Chem. Biol. Drug Des.* **2017**, *90*, 561–571. [CrossRef] [PubMed]
14. Logsdon, D.P.; Grimard, M.; Luo, M.; Shahda, S.; Jiang, Y.; Tong, Y.; Yu, Z.; Zyromski, N.; Schipani, E.; Carta, F.; et al. Regulation of HIF1α under Hypoxia by APE1/Ref-1 Impacts CA9 Expression: Dual Targeting in Patient-Derived 3D Pancreatic Cancer Models. *Mol. Cancer Ther.* **2016**, *15*, 2722–2732. [CrossRef]
15. Cardoso, A.A.; Jiang, Y.; Luo, M.; Reed, A.M.; Shahda, S.; He, Y.; Maitra, A.; Kelley, M.R.; Fishel, M.L. APE1/Ref-1 Regulates STAT3 Transcriptional Activity and APE1/Ref-1-STAT3 Dual-Targeting Effectively Inhibits Pancreatic Cancer Cell Survival. *PLoS ONE* **2012**, *7*, e47462. [CrossRef]
16. Cesaratto, L.; Codarin, E.; Vascotto, C.; Leonardi, A.; Kelley, M.R.; Tiribelli, C.; Tell, G. Specific Inhibition of the Redox Activity of Ape1/Ref-1 by E3330 Blocks Tnf-A-Induced Activation of Il-8 Production in Liver Cancer Cell Lines. *PLoS ONE* **2013**, *8*, e70909. [CrossRef]
17. Biswas, A.; Khanna, S.; Roy, S.; Pan, X.; Sen, C.K.; Gordillo, G.M. Endothelial cell tumor growth is ape/ref-1 dependent. *Am. J. Physiol. Cell Physiol.* **2015**, *309*, C296–C307. [CrossRef]

18. Jiang, Y.; Zhou, S.; Sandusky, G.E.; Kelley, M.R.; Fishel, M.L. Reduced Expression of DNA Repair and Redox Signaling Protein APE1/Ref-1 Impairs Human Pancreatic Cancer Cell Survival, Proliferation, and Cell Cycle Progression. *Cancer Investig.* **2010**, *28*, 885–895. [CrossRef]
19. Fishel, M.L.; Wu, X.; Devlin, C.M.; Logsdon, D.P.; Jiang, Y.; Luo, M.; He, Y.; Yu, Z.; Tong, Y.; Lipking, K.P.; et al. Apurinic/apyrimidinic endonuclease/redox factor-1 (APE1/Ref-1) redox function negatively regulates NRF2. *J. Biol. Chem.* **2015**, *290*, 3057–3068. [CrossRef]
20. Lando, D.; Pongratz, I.; Poellinger, L.; Whitelaw, M.L. A redox mechanism controls differential DNA binding activities of hypoxia-inducible factor (HIF) 1α and the HIF-like factor. *J. Biol. Chem.* **2000**, *275*, 4618–4627. [CrossRef]
21. Shan, J.L.; He, H.T.; Li, M.X.; Zhu, J.W.; Cheng, Y.; Hu, N.; Wang, G.; Wang, D.; Yang, X.Q.; He, Y.; et al. APE1 promotes antioxidant capacity by regulating Nrf-2 function through a redox-dependent mechanism. *Free Radic. Biol. Med.* **2015**, *78*, 11–22. [CrossRef] [PubMed]
22. Yoo, D.G.; Song, Y.J.; Cho, E.J.; Lee, S.K.; Park, J.B.; Yu, J.H.; Lim, S.P.; Kim, J.M.; Jeon, B.H. Alteration of APE1/ref-1 expression in non-small cell lung cancer: The implications of impaired extracellular superoxide dismutase and catalase antioxidant systems. *Lung Cancer* **2008**, *60*, 277–284. [CrossRef] [PubMed]
23. Tell, G.; Quadrifoglio, F.; Tiribelli, C.; Kelley, M.R. The many functions of APE1/Ref-1: Not only a DNA repair enzyme. *Antioxid. Redox Signal.* **2009**, *11*, 601–619. [CrossRef] [PubMed]
24. Wang, D.; Xiang, D.B.; Yang, X.Q.; Chen, L.S.; Li, M.X.; Zhong, Z.Y.; Zhang, Y.S. APE1 overexpression is associated with cisplatin resistance in non-small cell lung cancer and targeted inhibition of APE1 enhances the activity of cisplatin in A549 cells. *Lung Cancer* **2009**, *66*, 298–304. [CrossRef]
25. Pacifico, F.; Mauro, C.; Barone, C.; Crescenzi, E.; Mellone, S.; Monaco, M.; Chiappetta, G.; Terrazzano, G.; Liguoro, D.; Vito, P.; et al. Oncogenic and anti-apoptotic activity of NF-κB in human thyroid carcinomas. *J. Biol. Chem.* **2004**, *279*, 54610–54619. [CrossRef]
26. Yeh, P.Y.; Chuang, S.E.; Yeh, K.H.; Song, Y.C.; Ea, C.K.; Cheng, A.L. Increase of the resistance of human cervical carcinoma cells to cisplatin by inhibition of the MEK to ERK signaling pathway partly via enhancement of anticancer drug-induced NFκB activation. *Biochem. Pharmacol.* **2002**, *63*, 1423–1430. [CrossRef]
27. Deben, C.; Deschoolmeester, V.; De Waele, J.; Jacobs, J.; Van Den Bossche, J.; Wouters, A.; Peeters, M.; Rolfo, C.; Smits, E.; Lardon, F.; et al. Hypoxia-induced cisplatin resistance in non-small cell lung cancer cells is mediated by HIF-1α and mutant p53 and can be overcome by induction of oxidative stress. *Cancers* **2018**, *10*, 126. [CrossRef]
28. Shimizu, N.; Sugimoto, K.; Tang, J.; Nishi, T.; Sato, I.; Hiramoto, M.; Aizawa, S.; Hatakeyama, M.; Ohba, R.; Hatori, H.; et al. High-performance affinity beads for identifying drug receptors. *Nat. Biotechnol.* **2000**, *18*, 877–881. [CrossRef]
29. Shah, F.; Logsdon, D.; Messmann, R.A.; Fehrenbacher, J.C.; Fishel, M.L.; Kelley, M.R. Exploiting the Ref-1-APE1 node in cancer signaling and other diseases: From bench to clinic. *NPJ Precis. Oncol.* **2017**, *1*, 1–19. [CrossRef]
30. McIlwain, D.W.; Fishel, M.L.; Boos, A.; Kelley, M.R.; Jerde, T.J. APE1/Ref-1 redox-specific inhibition decreases survivin protein levels and induces cell cycle arrest in prostate cancer cells. *Oncotarget* **2018**, *9*, 10962–10977. [CrossRef]
31. Fishel, M.L.; Jiang, Y.; Rajeshkumar, N.V.; Scandura, G.; Sinn, A.L.; He, Y.; Shen, C.; Jones, D.R.; Pollok, K.E.; Ivan, M.; et al. Impact of APE1/Ref-1 Redox Inhibition on Pancreatic Tumor Growth. *Mol. Cancer Ther.* **2012**, *10*, 1698–1708. [CrossRef] [PubMed]
32. Costa, J.G.; Saraiva, N.; Guerreiro, P.S.; Louro, H.; Silva, M.J.; Miranda, J.P.; Castro, M.; Batinic-Haberle, I.; Fernandes, A.S.; Oliveira, N.G. Ochratoxin A-induced cytotoxicity, genotoxicity and reactive oxygen species in kidney cells: An integrative approach of complementary endpoints. *Food Chem. Toxicol.* **2016**, *87*, 65–76. [CrossRef] [PubMed]
33. Costa, J.G.; Saraiva, N.; Batinic-Haberle, I.; Castro, M.; Oliveira, N.G.; Fernandes, A.S. The SOD mimic MnTnHex-2-PyP5+ reduces the viability and migration of 786-O human renal cancer cells. *Antioxidants* **2019**, *8*, 490. [CrossRef] [PubMed]
34. Fernandes, A.S.; Flórido, A.; Saraiva, N.; Cerqueira, S.; Ramalhete, S.; Cipriano, M.; Cabral, M.F.; Miranda, J.P.; Castro, M.; Costa, J.; et al. Role of the Copper(II) Complex Cu[15]pyN5 in Intracellular ROS and Breast Cancer Cell Motility and Invasion. *Chem. Biol. Drug Des.* **2015**, *86*, 578–588. [CrossRef] [PubMed]

35. Costa, J.G.; Keser, V.; Jackson, C.; Saraiva, N.; Guerreiro, Í.; Almeida, N.; Camões, S.P.; Manguinhas, R.; Castro, M.; Miranda, J.P.; et al. A multiple endpoint approach reveals potential in vitro anticancer properties of thymoquinone in human renal carcinoma cells. *Food Chem. Toxicol.* **2020**, *136*, 111076. [CrossRef] [PubMed]
36. Flórido, A.; Saraiva, N.; Cerqueira, S.; Almeida, N.; Parsons, M.; Batinic-Haberle, I.; Miranda, J.P.; Costa, J.G.; Carrara, G.; Castro, M.; et al. The manganese(III) porphyrin MnTnHex-2-PyP5+ modulates intracellular ROS and breast cancer cell migration: Impact on doxorubicin-treated cells. *Redox Biol.* **2019**, *20*, 367–378. [CrossRef]
37. Karachaliou, N.; Moreno, M.D.L.L.G.; Sosa, A.E.; Santarpia, M.; Lazzari, C.; Capote, A.R.; Massuti, B.; Rosell, R. Using genetics to predict patient response to platinum-based chemotherapy. *Expert Rev. Precis. Med. Drug Dev.* **2017**, *2*, 21–32. [CrossRef]
38. Rosell, R.; Karachaliou, N.; Arrieta, O. Novel molecular targets for the treatment of lung cancer. *Curr. Opin. Oncol.* **2020**, *32*, 37–43. [CrossRef]
39. Wang, Q.; Hu, D.F.; Rui, Y.; Jiang, A.B.; Liu, Z.L.; Huang, L.N. Prognosis value of HIF-1α expression in patients with non-small cell lung cancer. *Gene* **2014**, *541*, 69–74. [CrossRef]
40. Okabe, T.; Okamoto, I.; Tamura, K.; Terashima, M.; Yoshida, T.; Satoh, T.; Takada, M.; Fukuoka, M.; Nakagawa, K. Differential constitutive activation of the epidermal growth factor receptor in non-small cell lung cancer cells bearing EGFR gene mutation and amplification. *Cancer Res.* **2007**, *67*, 2046–2053. [CrossRef]
41. Umelo, I.A.; De Wever, O.; Kronenberger, P.; Noor, A.; Teugels, E.; Chen, G.; Bracke, M.; De Grève, J. Combined inhibition of rho-associated protein kinase and EGFR suppresses the invasive phenotype in EGFR-dependent lung cancer cells. *Lung Cancer* **2015**, *90*, 167–174. [CrossRef]
42. Chen, X.; Yang, Y.; Katz, S.I. Dexamethasone pretreatment impairs the thymidylate synthase inhibition mediated flare in thymidine salvage pathway activity in non-small cell lung cancer. *PLoS ONE* **2018**, *13*, e0202384. [CrossRef] [PubMed]
43. Wang, M.C.; Liang, X.; Liu, Z.Y.; Cui, J.; Liu, Y.; Jing, L.; Jiang, L.L.; Ma, J.Q.; Han, L.L.; Guo, Q.Q.; et al. In vitro synergistic antitumor efficacy of sequentially combined chemotherapy/icotinib in non-small cell lung cancer cell lines. *Oncol. Rep.* **2015**, *33*, 239–249. [CrossRef] [PubMed]
44. Zhao, M.; Xu, P.; Liu, Z.; Zhen, Y.; Chen, Y.; Liu, Y.; Fu, Q.; Deng, X.; Liang, Z.; Li, Y.; et al. Dual roles of miR-374a by modulated c-Jun respectively targets CCND1-inducing PI3K/AKT signal and PTEN-suppressing Wnt/β-catenin signaling in non-small-cell lung cancer article. *Cell Death Dis.* **2018**, *9*, 1–17. [CrossRef] [PubMed]
45. Sun, Y.; Miao, H.; Ma, S.; Zhang, L.; You, C.; Tang, F.; Yang, C.; Tian, X.; Wang, F.; Luo, Y.; et al. FePt-Cys nanoparticles induce ROS-dependent cell toxicity, and enhance chemo-radiation sensitivity of NSCLC cells in vivo and in vitro. *Cancer Lett.* **2018**, *418*, 27–40. [CrossRef] [PubMed]
46. Baker, A.F.; Hanke, N.T.; Sands, B.J.; Carbajal, L.; Anderl, J.L.; Garland, L.L. Carfilzomib demonstrates broad anti-tumor activity in pre-clinical non-small cell and small cell lung cancer models. *J. Exp. Clin. Cancer Res.* **2014**, *33*, 1–12. [CrossRef]
47. Luo, M.; Delaplane, S.; Jiang, A.; Reed, A.; He, Y.; Fishel, M.; Nyland, R.L.; Borch, R.F.; Qiao, X.; Georgiadis, M.M.; et al. Role of the multifunctional DNA repair and redox signaling protein Ape1/Ref-1 in cancer and endothelial cells: Small-molecule inhibition of the redox function of Ape1. *Antioxid. Redox Signal.* **2008**, *10*, 1853–1867. [CrossRef]
48. Zou, G.-M.; Maitra, A. Small-molecule inhibitor of the AP endonuclease 1/REF-1 E3330 inhibits pancreatic cancer cell growth and migration. *Mol. Cancer Ther.* **2008**, *7*, 2012–2021. [CrossRef]
49. Singh-Gupta, V.; Joiner, M.C.; Runyan, L.; Yunker, C.K.; Sarkar, F.H.; Miller, S.; Gadgeel, S.M.; Konski, A.A.; Hillman, G.G. Soy isoflavones augment radiation effect by inhibiting APE1/ref-1 DNA repair activity in non-small cell lung cancer. *J. Thorac. Oncol.* **2011**, *6*, 688–698. [CrossRef] [PubMed]
50. Shapiro, G.I.; Edwards, C.D.; Ewen, M.E.; Rollins, B.J. p16INK4A Participates in a G1 Arrest Checkpoint in Response to DNA Damage. *Mol. Cell. Biol.* **1998**, *18*, 378–387. [CrossRef] [PubMed]
51. Sorenson, C.M.; Barry, M.A.; Eastman, A. Analysis of events associated with cell cycle arrest at G2 phase and cell death induced by cisplatin. *J. Natl. Cancer Inst.* **1990**, *82*, 749–755. [CrossRef] [PubMed]
52. Sarin, N.; Engel, F.; Kalayda, G.V.; Mannewitz, M.; Cinatl, J.; Rothweiler, F.; Michaelis, M.; Saafan, H.; Ritter, C.A.; Jaehde, U.; et al. Cisplatin resistance in non-small cell lung cancer cells is associated with an abrogation of cisplatin-induced G2/M cell cycle arrest. *PLoS ONE* **2017**, *12*, e0181081. [CrossRef] [PubMed]

53. Nyland, R.L.; Luo, M.; Kelley, M.R.; Borch, R.F. Design and Synthesis of Novel Quinone Inhibitors Targeted to the Redox Function of Apurinic/Apyrimidinic Endonuclease 1/Redox Enhancing Factor-1 (Ape1/Ref-1). *J. Med. Chem.* **2010**, *53*, 1200–1210. [CrossRef]
54. Jiang, A.; Gao, H.; Kelley, M.R.; Qiao, X. Inhibition of APE1/Ref-1 Redox Activity with APX3330 Blocks Retinal Angiogenesis in vitro and in vivo. *Vis. Res.* **2011**, *51*, 93–100. [CrossRef] [PubMed]
55. Li, Y.; Ahmed, F.; Ali, S.; Philip, P.A.; Kucuk, O.; Sarkar, F.H. Inactivation of Nuclear Factor kB by Soy Isoflavone Genistein Contributes to Increased Apoptosis Induced by Chemotherapeutic Agents in Human Cancer Cells. *Cancer Res.* **2005**, *65*, 6934–6942. [CrossRef] [PubMed]
56. Li, G.; Gao, Y.; Cui, Y.; Zhang, T.; Cui, R.; Jiang, Y.; Shi, J. Overexpression of CD44 is associated with the occurrence and migration of non-small cell lung cancer. *Mol. Med. Rep.* **2016**, *14*, 3159–3167. [CrossRef] [PubMed]
57. Bauvois, B. New facets of matrix metalloproteinases MMP-2 and MMP-9 as cell surface transducers: Outside-in signaling and relationship to tumor progression. *Biochim. Biophys. Acta* **2012**, *1825*, 29–36. [CrossRef]
58. Yan, C.; Boyd, D.D. Regulation of matrix metalloproteinase gene expression. *J. Cell. Physiol.* **2007**, *211*, 19–26. [CrossRef]
59. El-badrawy, M.K.; Yousef, A.M.; Shaalan, D.; Elsamanoudy, A.Z. Matrix Metalloproteinase-9 Expression in Lung Cancer Patients and Its Relation to Serum MMP-9 Activity, Pathologic Type, and Prognosis. *J. Bronchol. Interv. Pulmonol.* **2014**, *21*, 327–334. [CrossRef] [PubMed]

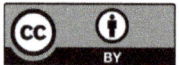

© 2020 by the authors. Licensee MDPI, Basel, Switzerland. This article is an open access article distributed under the terms and conditions of the Creative Commons Attribution (CC BY) license (http://creativecommons.org/licenses/by/4.0/).

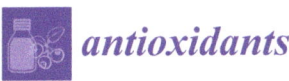

Review

LOXL2 Inhibitors and Breast Cancer Progression

Sandra Ferreira [1], Nuno Saraiva [1], Patrícia Rijo [1,2] and Ana S. Fernandes [1,*]

[1] CBIOS, Universidade Lusófona's Research Center for Biosciences & Health Technologies, Campo Grande 376, 1749-024 Lisbon, Portugal; sandra.ferreira@ulusofona.pt (S.F.); nuno.saraiva@ulusofona.pt (N.S.); patricia.rijo@ulusofona.pt (P.R.)

[2] Instituto de Investigação do Medicamento (iMed.ULisboa), Faculdade de Farmácia, Universidade de Lisboa, 1649-003 Lisboa, Portugal

* Correspondence: ana.fernandes@ulusofona.pt; Tel.: +351-217-515-500 (ext. 627)

Abstract: LOX (lysyl oxidase) and lysyl oxidase like-1–4 (LOXL 1–4) are amine oxidases, which catalyze cross-linking reactions of elastin and collagen in the connective tissue. These amine oxidases also allow the cross-link of collagen and elastin in the extracellular matrix of tumors, facilitating the process of cell migration and the formation of metastases. LOXL2 is of particular interest in cancer biology as it is highly expressed in some tumors. This protein also promotes oncogenic transformation and affects the proliferation of breast cancer cells. LOX and LOXL2 inhibition have thus been suggested as a promising strategy to prevent metastasis and invasion of breast cancer. BAPN (β-aminopropionitrile) was the first compound described as a LOX inhibitor and was obtained from a natural source. However, novel synthetic compounds that act as LOX/LOXL2 selective inhibitors or as dual LOX/LOX-L inhibitors have been recently developed. In this review, we describe LOX enzymes and their role in promoting cancer development and metastases, with a special focus on LOXL2 and breast cancer progression. Moreover, the recent advances in the development of LOXL2 inhibitors are also addressed. Overall, this work contextualizes and explores the importance of LOXL2 inhibition as a promising novel complementary and effective therapeutic approach for breast cancer treatment.

Keywords: BAPN; breast cancer; cell invasion; EMT; lysyl-oxidase; lysyl-oxidase like 2; metastases; inhibitors

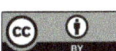

1. Introduction

LOX (lysyl oxidase or protein lysine 6-oxidase) and lysyl oxidase like-1 through 4 (LOXL1–LOXL4) are copper-dependent amine oxidases that covalently cross-link collagen and elastin in the extracellular matrix (ECM) [1,2]. These enzymes are expressed in various tissues and organs, such as skin, aorta, heart, lung, liver, cartilage, kidney, stomach, small intestine, colon, retina, ovary, testis, and brain [3]. LOX/LOXL proteins have been implicated in the pathogenesis of various diseases, including cancer. Therefore, inhibitors of these enzymes have been developed for therapeutic purposes. In this work, the impact of LOX/LOXL enzymes in cancer progression and the state of the art of the development of inhibitors are reviewed.

2. Historical Perspective

The discovery of LOX enzymes was initially associated with the toxic effects described for the inhibitor β-aminopropionitrile (BAPN; Figure 1). Reports on BAPN can be found in the literature since the 1950s [4]. BAPN is a potent irreversible inhibitor of LOX enzymes that severely disrupts cross-linkage of collagen and elastin [5]. This natural compound was originally found in sweet peas, *Lathyrus odoratus* L. The ingestion of seeds or food products of these genus spp. is associated with toxic effects, namely with lathyrism. This condition is characterized by skeletal and tissue deformities, growth malformations, and vascular alterations that result from connective tissue disruption, especially by inhibition of collagen and elastin cross-linking [5]. Hippocrates was the first to describe the deleterious effect of lathyrism, which caused paralysis of the legs after the consumption of certain species of peas. In 1883, the phenomenon of lathyrism was described by Louis Astier. Since then, several researchers have described the consequences of the ingestion of certain plants on connective tissue disorders, especially on collagen and elastin cross-linking [5].

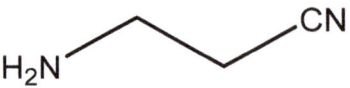

Figure 1. Chemical structure of β-aminopropionitrile (BAPN).

In the late 1960s, LOX enzymes were identified while studying the role of collagen and elastin cross-link associated with bone loss [6,7]. Pinnell and Martin, 1968 [7] detected an enzyme that converts peptide-bound lysine to allysine in embryonic chick bone. The authors demonstrated that the enzyme was inhibited by the lathyrogen BAPN. This compound showed in vitro and in vivo inhibition of collagen and elastin cross-linking by blocking the lysine-to-allysine conversion. The authors concluded that this enzymatic inactivation promoted the primary lesion of lathyrism. It was the first time that the enzyme responsible for converting lysyl residues to allysyl residues was identified [7,8]. Although LOX is known since the late 1960s, the 3D crystalline structure of human lysyl oxidase-like 2 (Figure 2A) was only obtained in 2018 [9].

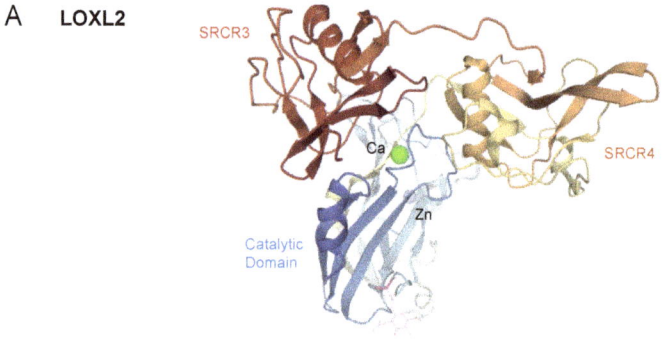

	LOX	LOXL1	LOXL2	LOXL3	LOXL4
	417 aa	574 aa	774 aa	753 aa	756 aa
C-terminal	copper binding motif, LTQ residues, CRL domain				
N-terminal	Pro-domains		SRCR domains		

Figure 2. Structure of LOX proteins. (A) Crystal structure of human LOXL2 in a precursor state obtained by Zhang et al. (2018) [9]. The SRCR domains 3 and 4 are colored in red and orange, respectively; the catalytic domain is colored in blue. The glycosyl groups at Asn-644 are shown. Zinc and calcium ions are represented as purple, blue and green spheres, respectively. Image was prepared with PDB (PDBID 5ZE3) [10]. (B) Schematic representation of the structure and homology of human LOX isoenzymes. Due to similarities in the domain arrangement, LOX and LOXL1 represent one LOX subfamily, whereas LOXL2-4 constitute another LOX subfamily.

3. LOX Enzymes

The mammalian lysyl oxidase family of proteins is encoded by five genes: *LOX, LOXL1, LOXL2, LOXL3,* and *LOXL4*. These genes encode proteins with the conserved C-terminal region that includes a copper binding site, lysine tyrosylquinone (LTQ) cofactor residues, and a cytokine receptor-like (CRL) domain [1,11]. The diverse N-terminal pro-peptide regions determine the classification into two subfamilies consisting of LOX and LOXL1, and LOXL2–LOXL4. The prodomains in LOX and LOXL1 enable their secretion as pro-enzymes, which are then activated extracellularly in a process that involves proteolytic cleavage. LOXL2, LOXL3, and LOXL4 contain four scavenger receptor cysteine-rich domains (SRCR) that are thought to be involved in protein-protein interactions. (Figure 2B) [1,11]. Xu et al., 2013 [12] have demonstrated that recombinant human LOXL2 secreted from *Drosophila* Schneider 2 cells is N-glycosylated. N-linked glycans at Asn-455 and Asn-644 are essential for proper protein folding, stability, and secretion.

The catalytic domain of LOX enzymes harbors a copper-binding motif and a functional quinone group, which has been identified as lysyl tyrosylquinone (LTQ; Figure 3). This quinone cofactor is generated through posttranslational cross-linkage between specific lysine and tyrosine residues. Copper is essential for LTQ generation, as previously demonstrated by Zhang et al. (2018) [9]. In fact, copper is involved in oxygen electron transfer to facilitate oxidative deamination of peptidyl lysyl to internally catalyze the formation of the quinone cofactor (Figure 3) [9].

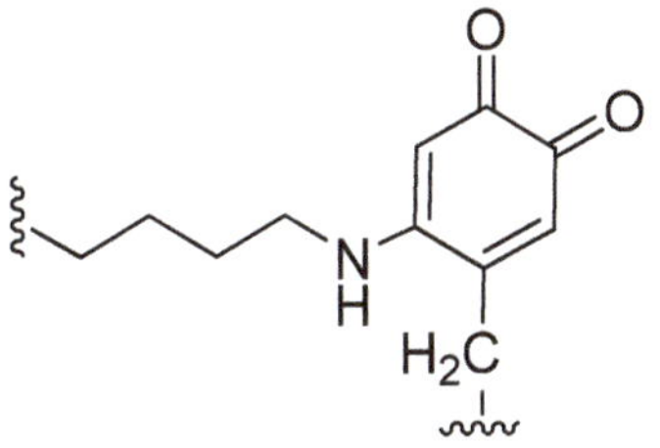

Figure 3. Lysine tyrosylquinone (LTQ).

Lysyl oxidases catalyze the extracellular oxidative deamination of lysine residues in elastin and of lysine and hydroxylysine in collagen precursors, generating highly reactive aldehydes. These aldehydes further react in their microenvironment, to form higher-order cross-linkages that are essential for the formation and repair of ECM fiber networks and the development of connective tissues [13,14]. Despite its higher affinity for collagen, these proteins also catalyze the deamination of other monoamines, diamines and lysine-rich proteins [15]. In the primary structure of LOX enzymes, there are also binding domains for cytokines [2,13]. Despite the extracellular proteolytic cleavage leading to the enzymatic activation of LOX proteins, they may also be active inside the cell. For example, LOXL2 can modulate intracellular events, such as epithelial to mesenchymal transition (EMT) [16], as described below.

Among the different LOX enzymes, this review gives particular emphasis to the human LOXL2 (hLOXL2) due to the importance of this particular isoform to breast cancer progression.

4. LOX and Disease

The human LOX proteins are expressed in several different tissues and organs [1,3]. Although their specific functions and substrate preferences in vivo remain to be elucidated, these proteins may play different roles. These might include regulating gene transcription, and controlling cell proliferation and motility [16,17]. Given the determinant role of LOX in the formation, maintenance, and functional properties of ECM and connective tissues, the expression dysregulation of these enzymes is associated with the onset and progression of multiple pathologies affecting connective tissue. These include fibrotic processes, cancer, and neurodegenerative and cardiovascular diseases [11,18,19]. The decreased expression of LOX can lead to diseases such as myocardial ischemia [20], cutis laxa [21], and Menkes syndrome [22], while its overexpression can be associated with atherosclerosis [23], pulmonary fibrosis [6], and cancer progression [11].

5. LOXL2 and Cancer

Several members of the LOX family have been implicated in cancer development. However, data published so far does not exclude opposite effects for these enzymes as stimulators or suppressors of tumor promotion/progression (reviewed in [24]). Different protein isoforms, their intra and extracellular locations, the proteolytic cleavage status in the case of LOX and LOXL1, and other cellular events contribute to these different outcomes in cancer. The tumor suppression activity has been mostly associated with the LOX propeptide (LOX-PP) that is generated by the cleavage of the secreted pro-LOX by procollagen-C-proteinase (reviewed in [24]). LOXL2-4 do not generate this type of propeptide.

Solid tumors are characterized by unregulated growth, generating hypoxic conditions. LOX expression is upregulated under hypoxic conditions [25] and contributes to the induction of EMT, i.e., cells undergo biochemical, molecular, and morphological modifications, which give them a greater capacity to migrate, invade, and resist apoptosis [26].

In breast, nasopharynx, gastric, pancreatic, pulmonary, renal, lung, ovarian, and thyroid cancers, lysyl oxidase and collagen were found to influence the architecture of the ECM, creating a favorable microenvironment for tumor development and progression [26,27]. Leeming et al., 2019 [28] found that healthy humans presented serum LOXL2 enzyme levels of $\approx$46.8 ng/mL. In patients with breast, colorectal, lung, ovarian, and pancreatic cancer, the levels of LOXL2 in serum were significantly elevated, varying between 49 ng/mL and 84 ng/mL. Regarding patients with breast cancer, serum LOXL2 levels were elevated by 218% compared to healthy controls [28]. A study from Janyasupab et al. (2016) [29] measured LOXL2 levels in human serum, plasma, and urine. The researchers found differential LOXL2 concentrations in patients with breast cancer ($\approx$ 2.7 μM in blood; $\approx$ 40 μM in urine), when compared to the cancer-free individuals ($\approx$ 0.6 μM in blood; $\approx$ 25 μM in urine).

High LOX and LOXL2 expression is considered a risk factor for the early occurrence of metastases, mostly due to their ability to stimulate tumor cell migration and invasion [26,30]. The secretion of this enzyme not only by tumor cells, but also by stromal cells, may also play a role in the evolution of metastases [31]. The mechanisms by which LOXL2 promotes metastases and invasion are still not fully characterized, but both extra- and intracellularly localized LOXL2 seem to be implicated in cancer progression [32], as depicted in Figure 4.

ECM collagen cross-linking by extracellular LOXL2 is mediated by the aforementioned deamination of lysine residues and increases ECM stiffness. This process can promote tumor cell invasion and progression by modulating integrin activity and focal adhesions assembly and signaling [31].

LOXL2 also plays a role in angiogenesis. LOXL2 is involved in endothelial cell proliferation and migration, as well as in vessel formation, by influencing the deposition of collagen in the vascular microenvironment [33]. The involvement in angiogenesis stimulation is dependent on both LOXL2 non-enzymatic and enzymatic activities. The organization of endothelial cells into tubes depends on LOXL2 expression levels. However, the equilibrium of the basement membrane structures and vessels requires enzymatic activity [34]. LOXL2 is also a vital prolymphangiogenic molecule and affects the function of lymphatic endothelial cells (LEC), both in vitro and in vivo [35]. The lymphangiogenesis process is critical for breast cancer malignancy and is associated with reduced survival of breast cancer patients [35].

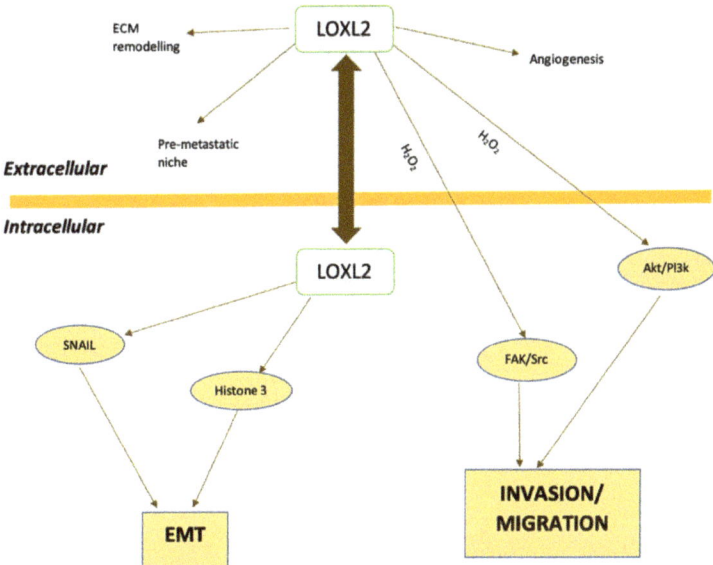

Figure 4. Intracellular and extracellular pathways involving LOXL2 in cancer metastasis-related processes. Akt, protein kinase B; EMT, epithelial–mesenchymal transition; FAK, focal adhesion kinase; PI3k, phosphoinositide 3-kinases; SNAIL, zinc finger protein; Src, proto-oncogene tyrosine-protein kinase Src. Adapted from [31,32].

The upregulation of LOX under hypoxic conditions is also involved in the recruitment of inflammatory stromal cells and bone marrow-derived cells at sites distant to the primary tumor, aiding the formation of the premetastatic niche [31]. Transgenic mouse models of PyMT-induced breast cancer were used to explore the role of LOXL2 in driving breast cancer metastases [36]. Using these models, the researchers demonstrated that LOXL2 action, together with elevated levels of SNAIL1 and expression of several cytokines, promoted the pre-metastatic niche formation [36].

In addition to the extracellular mechanisms described so far, intracellular LOX is also implicated in tumor progression. Intracellular LOXL2 prevents the degradation of SNAIL1. The stabilization of this transcriptional repressor results in the down-regulation of E-cadherin (CDH1), an adhesion receptor crucial in EMT and consequentially in the regulation of metastases formation [31]. LOXL2 deaminates unmethylated and trimethylated lysine 4 in histone H3 (H3K4me3) through an amino-oxidase reaction, releasing the amino group and converting K4 into an allysine (H3K4ox) [37]. This modification is also linked to the repression of the E-cadherin gene and heterochromatin transcription and to the deregulation of EMT [37,38].

Mechanistic studies carried out by Moreno-Bueno et al. (2011) [39] have demonstrated that LOXL2 is involved on the transcriptional downregulation of the proteins lethal giant larvae 2 (Lgl2) and claudin1, and disorganization of cell polarity and tight junctions, thus maintaining the mesenchymal phenotype of basal-like carcinoma cells.

LOXL2 also contributes positively to the activation of the focal adhesion kinase (FAK) signaling pathway and participates in the assembly of focal adhesion complexes. During the oxidation reaction catalyzed by lysyl oxidases, hydrogen peroxide is generated as a by-product. Hydrogen peroxide accumulation induces the upregulation of Src phosphorylation in the Src kinase/focal adhesion kinase pathway (FAK/Src), which can contribute to the pro-invasive effects of LOXL2. The produced H_2O_2 also stimulates the PI3K/Akt pathway [30,40]. In addition to these signaling pathways, other H_2O_2-mediated mechanisms could be implicated in LOX effects since these reactive oxygen species have been shown to modulate other cancer progression-related events in different experimental models [41–43].

LOXL2 is overexpressed in some cancers, thus contributing to poor prognosis and a higher risk of distant metastases. This overexpression was previously described in breast cancer (detailed in the next section), as well as in non-small cell lung cancer (NSCLC) [44], hepatocellular carcinoma (HCC) [26], oral squamous cell carcinoma (OSCC) [27], colorectal cancer, pancreatic cancer, esophageal squamous cell carcinoma, head and neck squamous cell carcinomas, gastric cancer and renal carcinoma [32]. Table 1 summarizes some examples of the consequences of altered LOXL2 expression described in experimental models or in patients with these cancers.

Table 1. The impact of LOXL2 in different types of cancer.

Cancer Type	Effect Observed
Lung cancer (NSCLC)	High cytoplasmatic LOXL2 associated with (↑) size of tumor and (↓) overall survival.
Oral squamous cell carcinoma (OSCC)	LOXL2 has been shown to be a marker of poor survival.
Hepatocellular carcinoma (HCC)	LOXL2 promotes proliferation, migration, and invasion of HCC cells. LOXL2 is overexpressed in HCC patients and is positively correlated with tumor grade, metastasis, vasculogenic mimicry formation, and poor survival.
Colorectal cancer	LOXL2 was upregulated in SW480 cells, which presented high migratory potential. Patients with high LOXL2 expression had a significantly increased rate of distant metastases and decreased survival.
Pancreatic cancer	LOXL2 is upregulated in human pancreatic cancer showing a sevenfold increase comparing with healthy human tissue. Silencing LOXL2 renders cells sensitive to chemotherapy.
Esophageal squamous cell carcinoma (ESCC)	LOXL2 plays a key role in the invasion of ESCC cell lines, through the disruption of cytoskeletal components. Patients with decreased levels of nuclear LOXL2 and increased cytoplasmic LOXL2 levels had lower survival rates. Increased LOXL2 expression drives tumor cell invasion and is associated with poor prognosis.
Head and neck squamous cell carcinomas	LOXL2 knock down cells had an upregulation of epidermal differentiation genes. LOXL2 and SNAIL knockdown reduced invasion in a mouse carcinogenesis model.
Gastric cancer	Significant reduction in the survival rate of gastric cancer patients positive for LOXL2 in both stromal and cancer cells.
Clear cell renal carcinoma (ccRCC)	LOXL2 siRNA knockdown significantly inhibited cell growth, migration, and invasion of ccRCC cell lines. Elevated LOXL2 expression correlated with the pathologic stages of ccRCC patients.

LOXL2—lysyl oxidase-like 2; NSCLC—non-small-cell lung carcinoma; SW480—colon cancer cell lines; SNAIL—zinc finger protein. Table 1 constructed with data collected from references [11,32,44–47].

6. LOXL2 and Breast Cancer

A bioinformatics study, aimed at identifying potential prognostic marker genes associated with breast cancer progression, identified and validated eight candidates [48]. One of those genes was LOXL2, that was particularly relevant in the luminal subtype.

Kirschmann et al. (2002) [49] studied the expression of LOX and LOXL1-4 in the human breast cancer cell line MDA-MB-231, a highly invasive/metastatic cell line. Their results suggested that LOX and LOXL2 had the strongest association with an invasive/metastatic phenotype. In vitro tests using LOXL2-silenced cell lines of invasive ductal carcinoma (BT549 and MDA-MB-231) showed that down-regulation of this protein induces a process similar to the mesenchymal-epithelial transition and thus to a decrease in cell migration and invasion [50].

Normal breast tissue has lower levels of LOXL2 expression and this protein is found in the stroma and luminal layer of epithelial cells. Conversely, breast cancer tissues show increased LOXL2 expression, located intracellularly in the cytoplasm and cell nuclei, and extracellularly in the ECM [39,51]. Immunohistochemical studies demonstrated that approximately 60% of basal breast carcinomas have increased intracellular LOXL2 with perinuclear distribution, associated with mRNA overexpression [39]. In addition, there is an increase in LOX expression in metastatic tissues compared with primary tumors [31]. Using immunohistochemistry, Ahn et al. (2013) [50] demonstrated that LOXL2 is an independent prognostic marker of metastatic disease and death in patients with breast cancer. In addition, LOXL2 is an independent prognostic factor for overall survival (OS) and metastasis-free survival (MFS) in breast cancer (hazard ratio of 2.27 and 2.10, respectively) [50].

A retrospective study found that patients with ER-negative tumors expressing high levels of LOXL2 mRNA have a poorer prognosis [52]. This study also showed that LOXL2 expression significantly correlated with decreased overall survival and metastasis-free survival [52].

Triple-negative breast cancer (TNBC) is strongly related with metastatic disease and represents 15% of breast cancer cases [53]. Previous studies have found that the expression of both LOX [53] and LOXL2 [50] is increased in TNBC patients. These proteins are thus possible targets for systemic therapy of TNBC. In addition, the inhibition of LOXL2 has been proposed as a strategy to sensitize TNBC cells to conventional therapy [37].

Barker et al. (2011) [52] demonstrated that the inhibition of LOXL2 by genetic, chemical, or antibody-mediated tools leads to a decrease in metastases in in vivo models [52]. The authors attributed this finding to the LOXL2-dependent promotion of invasion by regulating the expression and activity of the proteins metallopeptidase inhibitor 1 (TIMP1) and matrix metalloproteinase 9 (MMP9). LOXL2 inhibition did not alter the expression of other LOX-like proteins, suggesting that these enzymes do not compensate for each other [52].

Previous studies have concluded that LOXL2 pro-metastatic action is intrinsic to breast tumor cells and mostly independent of the extracellular action of this protein on the ECM. Therefore, the possible therapeutic strategies for inhibiting LOXL2 in breast cancer will be more efficient if intracellular LOXL2 is blocked [36].

Considering the therapeutic potential of blocking LOXL2 in cancer treatment, several inhibitors of this protein have been developed. The next sections summarize the state of the art of the discovery of LOXL2 inhibitors.

7. LOX Inhibitors

7.1. β-Aminopropionitrile (BAPN)

As mentioned in Section 2, BAPN was the first LOX inhibitor to be identified. BAPN inhibits intramolecular and intermolecular covalent cross-linking of collagen and elastin connective tissue proteins [6]. In fact, BAPN is described as a potent and irreversible non-specific LOX inhibitor, which also has an affinity for other amine oxidases [54].

LOX inhibitory activity of BAPN was evaluated in an assay developed in rats [55]. The authors found that doses of BAPN ranging from 1 to 40 mg per 100 g bw were efficient in inhibiting LOX activity from 6 and up to 48 h. They also studied the kinetics of both BAPN and its major metabolite, the cyanoacetic acid (CAA), in the same model. After a single intraperitoneal dose, most of the BAPN was excreted unchanged in the urine, while the rest was metabolized slowly in CAA [55].

Tang et al. (1983) [56] suggested a possible mechanism for the interaction between BAPN and LOX. By using BAPN with isotopically labeled carbons, the authors found that this molecule covalently binds to LOX to equivalent extents and in parallel with the development of inactivation, without the elimination of nitrile moiety. The copper of the enzyme is not altered upon interaction with BAPN, and BAPN is not processed to a free aldehyde product. The suggested inhibition mechanism involves the formation of a covalent bond between an enzyme nucleophile and a ketenimine formed from BAPN.

This LOX inhibitor has shown anticancer properties in several in vitro and in vivo models of different cancer types. For example, Yang et al. (2013) [57] demonstrated that BAPN (500 µM) blocked the hypoxia-induced invasion and migration capabilities of cervical cancer cells. Zhao et al. (2019) [58] have shown that the inhibition of LOX by BAPN in BGC-823 gastric cancer cells inhibits the expression and activity of matrix metalloproteinases 2 and 9.

Regarding the effects of BAPN in breast cancer, Cohen et al. (1979) [59] used rats with breast tumors induced by 7,12-dimethylbenzanthracene. The authors found that BAPN inhibited the collagen cross-link and promoted an 82% decrease in tumor formation and a significant reduction in tumor volume. In another experiment, luciferase-expressing breast cancer cells (MDA-MB-231-Luc2) were injected in mice to explore the effects of BAPN in invasion to other organs [60]. The results show that BAPN reduced the appearance of metastases. The number of metastases was decreased by 44%, and 27%, when BAPN treatment was initiated the day before or on the same day as the intra-cardiac injection of cancer cells, respectively. However, BAPN showed no effect on the growth of established metastases. The authors concluded that LOX inhibition might be a useful strategy for metastasis prevention [60].

Another potential use of BAPN and LOX inhibitors was suggested by Rachman-Tzemah et al. (2017). Increased LOX activity and expression, fibrillary collagen cross-linking, and focal adhesion signaling observed after breast tumor resection contribute to increasing the risk of lung metastases [61]. LOX pharmacological inhibition using BAPN or an anti-LOX antibody prior to surgical intervention was able to reduce lung metastasis after surgery and increased animal survival in a murine model of breast cancer [61].

Despite the interesting results obtained with BAPN, this molecule lacks suitable sites for chemical modifications [62]. This fact does not facilitate the preclinical optimization. Conversely, novel classes of LOX enzyme inhibitors do not present this drawback, making it an advantage in drug discovery, as described in the subsequent sections.

7.2. Copper Chelators

Cox, Gartland, and Erler (2016) [63] proposed an indirect approach for LOX inhibition, using tetrathiomolybdate (TM). This is a potent copper chelator that targets the catalytic activity of LOX by binding to copper and depleting it. Copper has a significant influence on the functional activity of LOX, although it does not directly interfere with its expression levels. In preclinical studies, tetrathiomolybdate showed antiangiogenic activity, antifibrogenic and anti-inflammatory actions. A recent study found that copper was elevated in fibrotic kidney tissue and such increase promoted LOX activity and extracellular collagen cross-linking [64]. Copper chelation by TM leads to a decrease in activated LOX protein [64].

Another copper chelator initially suggested to be a LOXL2 inhibitor is D-penicillamine (D-pen) [65]. Contrarily to BAPN, D-pen structure has a secondary amine [32]. D-pen drastically inhibits rhLOXL2 activity at a concentration of 10 µM [52]. However, despite some conflicting data regarding its mechanism of action, as a copper chelator, D-pen is considered a non-selective inhibitor of LOXL2 enzyme (reviewed in [32,65]). In an orthotopic breast cancer mouse model, D-pen showed no effect on tumor growth rate. However, mice bearing tumors treated with D-pen displayed fewer lung and liver metastases than untreated mice [52]. Accordingly, in a transgenic breast cancer model, D-pen treatment led to a decreased development of lung metastases when compared to control mice [52].

Despite some encouraging results obtained with TM and D-pen, the chelation of cooper is not selective for LOXL2 or even for enzymes of the LOX family. Since copper ions play a part in several biological processes and are implicated in different enzymatic reactions [66], the use of such chelators will likely disturb other biological functions.

7.3. LOX/LOXL2 Selective Inhibitors

Following the discovery of BAPN, some compounds have been developed with LOX and LOXL2 inhibitory activity and favorable pharmacokinetics parameters. However, targeting LOXs with specific small molecule inhibitors presents a challenge due to the lack of crystalline structures, since only the LOXL2 crystalline structure is available.

The LOXL2 inhibitors PXS-S1A and PXS-S2A are haloallylamine-based molecules (the structures are not disclosed) [67]. PXS-S1A is a first-generation LOX inhibitor that exhibits an identical activity and selectivity when comparing to BAPN. The pIC_{50} values against LOXL2 are 6.8 ± 0.2 for PXS-S1A and 6.4 ± 0.1 for BAPN, and the two compounds also have similar pIC_{50} values when tested against the native human LOX enzyme. PXS-S1A allows for structural modifications that can be introduced to improve the inhibiting potency of LOX/LOXL2, thus leading to significant increases in selectivity. Chemical modifications of PXS-S1A led to the development of PXS-S2A, a potent and specific inhibitor of LOXL2 (pIC_{50} = 8.3 M). The discovery of PXS-S2A established the basis for dissecting the functional role of LOXL2 in the progression of solid tumors such as breast cancer [67]. These two LOX/LOXL2 inhibitors reduced the in vitro 2D and 3D proliferation of the breast cancer cell line MDA-MB-231 in a dose-dependent way [67]. This cell line has a high level of LOXL2 expression. Although authors also describe a significant impairment in 2D and 3D cell motility, the assays were performed under similar conditions to those that lead to a reduction in cell proliferation. Thus, implying that the observed reduction in cell motility may also be partially due to the reduced cell proliferation of cells treated with the compounds. Importantly, the authors observed a clear reduction of in vivo orthotopic MDA-MB-231 primary tumor volume and tumor cell proliferation upon treatment with PXS-S1A and PXS-S2A [67]. All the above-mentioned inhibitory effects were more pronounced for PXS-S1A when compared with PXS-S2A.

Another class of LOXL2 inhibitors is the patented collection of diazabicyclo[3.2.2]nonanes with a des-primary amine group. Compounds of this class were tested in a transgenic mouse breast cancer model and led to a reduction in the formation of lung metastases (reviewed in [32]).

PAT-1251 (Figure 5) was the first small molecule that acts as an irreversible LOXL2 inhibitor to advance to clinical trials (see Section 7.5). This compound is a potent and highly selective oral LOXL2 inhibitor that is based on a benzylamine with 2-substituted pyridine-4-ylmethanamines [65,68].

Epigallocatechin gallate (EGCG) is a trihydroxyphenolic compound that was suggested as a dual inhibitor of LOXL2 and transforming growth factor-β1 (TGFβ1) receptor kinase [69,70]. This compound induces the auto-oxidation of a LOXL2/3–specific lysine (K731) in a time-dependent manner that inhibits LOXL2 irreversibly [69]. ECGC attenuates TGFβ1 signaling and collagen accumulation and was thus suggested as a possible therapeutic approach against fibrotic diseases [69,70].

Besides small molecules, the LOXL2 inhibiting strategies developed so far also include biological drugs. The anti-LOXL2 functional antibody named Simtuzumab is an IgG4 humanized monoclonal antibody, that is a non-competitive inhibitor of extracellular LOXL2 via allosteric inhibition by binding to the fourth SRCR domain. This antibody revealed beneficial effects in various preclinical models of fibrosis and cancer [52,71]. Moreover, Simtuzumab has been evaluated in several clinical trials, as detailed in Section 7.5. While Simtuzumab targets noncatalytic regions of LOXL2, Grossman et al. (2016) [72] developed specific antibodies that targeted the active site of this enzyme. Among those, the antibody clone designated GS341 displayed binding affinity to LOXL2 at the subnanomolar range and prevented the assembly of linear collagen fibers, producing visible variations in fibrillary collagen morphology. The GS341antibody was evaluated in a breast cancer xenograft model using MDA-MB-231 cells into immunocompromised SCID mice. Treatment with GS341 resulted in a decrease in tumor volume and in the number of lung metastases. In addition, the tumor fibrils in the GS341-treated animals were thinner when compared with the vehicle-treated ones [72].

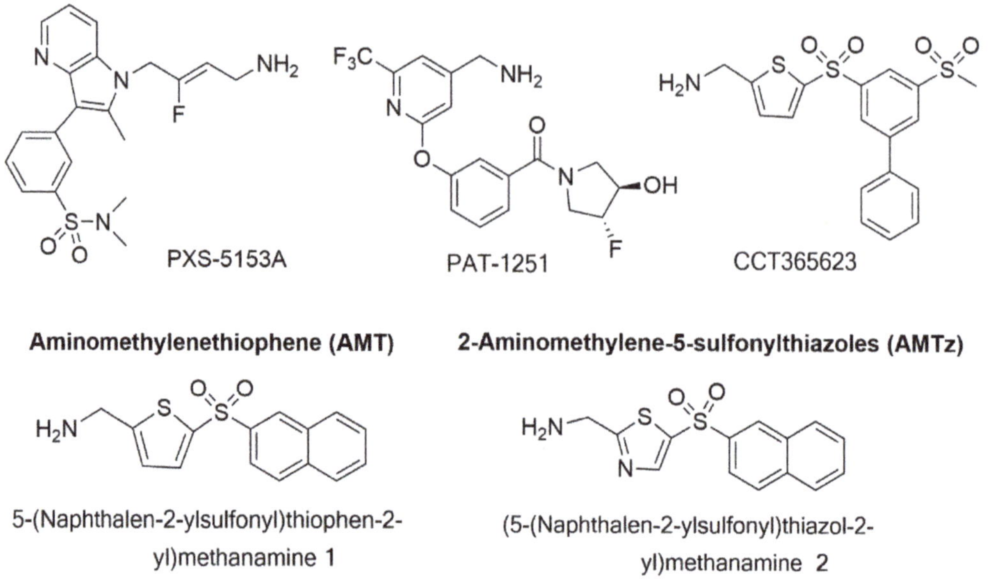

Figure 5. Structures of PXS-5153A; PAT-1251; CCT365623; an aminomethylenethiophene (AMT), 5-(naphthalen-2-ylsulfonyl)thiophen-2-yl)methanamine 1; and a 2-aminomethylene-5-sulponylthiazole (AMTz), (5-(naphthalen-2-ylsulfonyl)thiazol-2-yl)methanamine 2.

7.4. Dual LOX/LOX-L Inhibitors

The small molecule PXS-5153A (Figure 5) demonstrated complete and irreversible enzyme inhibition for LOXL2 and LOXL3, unlike Simtuzumab or PAT-1251 (Figure 5). This innovative molecule is thus a useful tool to better understand the impact of LOXL2/LOXL3 activity in fibrotic diseases [73]. It interacts with the LTQ cofactor in the enzymatic pocket of LOXL2 and LOXL3, and after fluoride elimination, leads to a covalently bound enzyme inhibitor complex [73]. In vitro, PXS-5153A reduced LOXL2-mediated collagen oxidation and cross-linking, in a concentration-dependent manner. This dual LOXL2/LOXL3 inhibitor has shown beneficial effects in models of liver fibrosis and myocardial infarction [73].

Leung et al. (2019) [74] developed an orally bioavailable LOX inhibitor named CCT365623 (Figure 5). This is an aminomethylenethiophene (AMT) based inhibitor, which helped to elucidate the mechanisms by which LOX drives tumor progression. The AMT inhibitors are selective for LOX/LOXL2 and led to a significant reduction in tumor growth and metastases in an in vivo model of transgenic LOX-dependent breast tumor mice [74]. In another study, a substantial reduction of the growth of primary and metastatic tumors of MMT-PyMT breast transgenic model was observed when animals were treated daily by oral gavage with 70 mg kg^{-1} of CCT365623 [75]. This effect was ascribed to the ability of this small molecule to disrupt epidermal growth factor receptor (EGFR) cell surface retention. Thus, demonstrating the potential of this orally delivered inhibitor to reduce breast cancer progression.

Taking AMT compounds as a starting point, several systematic modifications were introduced to a hit molecule identified by high-throughput screen (HTS), leading to submicromolar IC$_{50}$ inhibitors with desirable selectivity and pharmacokinetic properties [62]. The 2,5-substituted thiophene core was replaced with other five-membered heterocyclic rings. However, only a 2-aminomethylene-5-sulfonyl thiazole core maintains activity, where the naphthalenesulfonyl-substituted thiazole 2 showed a LOX inhibition comparable to that of the analogous thiophene compound 1 (Figure 5). For the active thiazole compound 2, a modest increase in potency toward LOXL2 inhibition was observed, rendering this compound equipotent against LOX and LOXL2 isoforms. These important observations allowed the development of 2-aminomethylene-5-sulfonylthiazoles (AMTz) as dual LOX/LOXL2 inhibitors. Overall, the introduction of a thiazole core led to the improvement of the potency toward LOXL2 inhibition via an irreversible binding. These dual inhibitors exhibit good pharmacokinetic properties [62]. An in vivo study was carried out using a spontaneous breast cancer genetically engineered mouse model in order to assess the efficacy of an AMTz compound. A delay in primary tumor development, as well as a significant reduction in tumor growth rate, was observed in treated animals when comparing with controls [62].

Overall, an important motif that has been maintained in the majority of the small molecules successfully developed as LOXL2 inhibitors is a primary amine. This chemical motif competes with lysine in the direct interaction and reaction with the LTQ cofactor in the active site of LOXL2, allowing for specific binding to this enzyme [32].

7.5. Clinical Use of LOX Inhibitors

Specific targeting of LOX enzymes for the treatment of breast cancer and metastases seems to offer a significant promise with reduced risk. In mouse models treated with specific anti-LOX therapies, no adverse effects were observed. However, it remains to be thoroughly explored whether this would pertain to the patient setting [63].

Lysyl oxidase-like 2 inhibitors are already in phase II clinical trials for fibrotic diseases, heart failure, glaucoma, oncological and angiogenic diseases. The antibody Simtuzumab is an IgG4 humanized monoclonal antibody, that acts a non-competitive inhibitor of extracellular LOXL2 via allosteric inhibition by binding to the fourth SRCR domain [76]. This antibody has reached phase II clinical trials for several conditions related with fibrosis, including idiopathic pulmonary fibrosis, primary sclerosing cholangitis, hepatic fibrosis, compensated cirrhosis, and myelofibrosis (a fibrosis-related blood cancer) [32,77,78]. In the field of oncology, phase II clinical trials were also conducted with Simtuzumab in conjunction with gemcitabine for patients with pancreatic cancer [79]. Another phase II clinical trial was done with a combination of Simtuzumab and FOLFIRI (folinic acid, fluorouracil, and irinotecan) in patients with KRAS mutant colorectal cancer [80]. Simtuzumab was generally well tolerated in these clinical trials, with frequencies of adverse effects similar between treatment and control groups [32]. However, the clinical benefits observed were limited and some studies stopped due to lack of efficacy [32,77]. The failure of these clinical trials may be ascribed to the fact that Simtuzumab only targets extracellular LOXL2 [32]. As mentioned above, LOXL2 intracellular mechanisms are critical for cancer progression. Therefore, targeting this enzyme by a small molecule with the ability to block both intra- and extracellular LOXL2 would be a more effective approach to fight cancer progression and metastases.

The orally administered small molecule PAT-1251, currently designated as GB2064, concluded phase I clinical trials in healthy participants [81]. A phase IIa study designed to evaluate its safety, tolerability, pharmacokinetics and pharmacodynamics in participants with myelofibrosis is planned and results are expected by 2022 [82]. PXS-5382A, another orally administered LOXL2 inhibitor, completed a phase I pharmacokinetic study in healthy adult males in 2020 [83]. By the time this review was written, no results were publicly available yet.

The pan-lysyl oxidase inhibitor PXS-5505 demonstrated an excellent safety profile and was well tolerated in healthy male volunteers [84]. An open-label phase I/IIa study is now planned to assess the safety and tolerability of PXS-5505 in patients with primary, postpolycythemia vera or post-essential thrombocythemia myelofibrosis. The results of this study are expected by 2023 [85].

An early phase I clinical trial to evaluate EGCG is currently recruiting participants. The first part of the study will determine the pharmacokinetic profile of orally given EGCG in normal volunteers. In the second part of this study, lung biopsy fragments and urine samples from patients with interstitial lung disease treated with EGCG will be analyzed to assess the specific inhibition of LOXL2 and TGFbeta1 signaling [86].

Copper chelators, namely D-penicilamine and TM, have also been studied in phase I and phase II clinical trials for different diseases, including fibrotic and oncological conditions [87,88]. As far as breast cancer is concerned, a phase II study of TM is currently ongoing in patients with breast cancer at moderate to high risk of recurrence [88]. However, as mentioned in Section 7.2, this approach does not provide a selective LOX inhibition, as multiple pathways will be affected by the chelation of copper.

Despite the different clinical trials focused on LOX inhibitors, clinical data in breast cancer remain essentially inexistent. Small molecule inhibitors are likely to provide better efficacy than the anti-LOXL2 antibodies strategy, as they may target both intra- and extracellular LOXL2. However, their clinical development is at a much earlier stage than the biological approach. In the upcoming years, we expect to obtain more detailed information on the pharmacokinetics and safety profiles of small molecule LOXL2 inhibitors. These data will be determinant for the progress of LOXL2 inhibitors development and may support the design of clinical trials in breast cancer patients.

8. Conclusions

LOX enzymes, and specifically LOXL2, are critical for cancer progression and metastases. The inhibition of this enzyme was suggested as a promising therapeutic strategy for oncological diseases, including breast cancer. Various synthetic compounds have been studied as having LOX enzymes/LOXL2 inhibitory activities and favorable pharmacokinetics parameters. Although the clinical studies focused on this approach are still very scarce, the preclinical data is encouraging. More studies are needed to develop effective inhibitors. Given the importance of LOX enzymes to the formation of conjunctive tissue, its systemic inhibition may have undesirable side effects. Therefore, adequate pharmacokinetics properties, selectivity, and delivery systems are needed. The combination of LOX enzyme inhibitors with standard anticancer treatments is another approach that should be further explored in future studies.

Author Contributions: Conceptualization, A.S.F. and P.R.; investigation, S.F.; writing—original draft preparation, S.F. and P.R.; writing—review and editing, A.S.F. and N.S.; visualization, N.S. and S.F.; supervision, A.S.F.; project administration, A.S.F. and P.R.; funding acquisition, A.S.F. and P.R.; All authors have read and agreed to the published version of the manuscript.

Funding: This work is funded by national funds through FCT-Foundation for Science and Technology, I.P., under the UIDB/04567/2020 and UIDP/04567/2020 projects. Research developed with funding from Universidade Lusófona/ILIND (Grant Programmes FIPID 2019/2020 and ILIND/F+/EI/01/2020).

Conflicts of Interest: The authors declare no conflict of interest. The funders had no role in the design of the study; in the collection, analyses, or interpretation of data; in the writing of the manuscript, or in the decision to publish the results.

References

1. Molnar, J.; Fong, K.; He, Q.; Hayashi, K.; Kim, Y.; Fong, S.; Fogelgren, B.; Szauter, K.M.; Mink, M.; Csiszar, K. Structural and functional diversity of lysyl oxidase and the LOX-like proteins. *Biochim. Biophys. Acta Proteins Proteom.* **2003**, *1647*, 220–224. [CrossRef]
2. Rucker, R.B.; Kosonen, T.; Clegg, M.S.; Mitchell, A.E.; Rucker, B.R.; Uriu-Hare, J.Y.; Keen, C.L. Copper, lysyl oxidase, and extracellular matrix protein cross-linking. *Am. J. Clin. Nutr.* **1998**, *67*, 996S–1002S. [CrossRef]
3. Hayashi, K.; Fong, K.S.K.; Mercier, F.; Boyd, C.D.; Csiszar, K.; Hayashi, M. Comparative immunocytochemical localization of lysyl oxidase (LOX) and the lysyl oxidase-like (LOXL) proteins: Changes in the expression of LOXL during development and growth of mouse tissues. *J. Mol. Histol.* **2004**, *35*, 845–855. [CrossRef]
4. Schilling, E.D.; Strong, F.M. Isolation, Structure and Synthesis of a Lathyrus Factor From L. Odoratus1,2. *J. Am. Chem. Soc.* **1955**, *77*, 2843–2845. [CrossRef]
5. Sherif, H.M. In search of a new therapeutic target for the treatment of genetically triggered thoracic aortic aneurysms and cardiovascular conditions: Insights from human and animal lathyrism. *Interact. Cardiovasc. Thorac. Surg.* **2010**, *11*, 271–276. [CrossRef] [PubMed]

6. Barry-Hamilton, V.; Spangler, R.; Marshall, D.; McCauley, S.A.; Rodriguez, H.M.; Oyasu, M.; Mikels, A.; Vaysberg, M.; Ghermazien, H.; Wai, C.; et al. Allosteric inhibition of lysyl oxidase–like-2 impedes the development of a pathologic microenvironment. *Nat. Med.* **2010**, *16*, 1009–1017. [CrossRef]
7. Pinnell, S.R.; Martin, G.R. The cross-linking of collagen and elastin: Enzymatic conversion of lysine in peptide linkage to alpha-aminoadipic-delta-semialdehyde (allysine) by an extract from bone. *Proc. Natl. Acad. Sci. USA* **1968**, *61*, 708–716. [CrossRef] [PubMed]
8. Blaschko, H. The natural history of amine oxidases. *Rev. Physiol. Biochem. Pharmacol.* **1974**, *70*, 83–148. [CrossRef]
9. Zhang, X.; Wang, Q.; Wu, J.; Wang, J.; Shi, Y.; Liu, M. Crystal structure of human lysyl oxidase-like 2 (hLOXL2) in a precursor state. *Proc. Natl. Acad. Sci. USA* **2018**, *115*, 3828–3833. [CrossRef] [PubMed]
10. Sehnal, D.; Rose, A.S.; Koca, J.; Burley, S.K.; Velankar, S. Mol: Towards a Common Library and Tools for Web Molecular Graphics. In Proceedings of the Molecular Graphics and Visual Analysis of Molecular Data 2018, Brno, Czech Republic, 4 June 2018.
11. Barker, H.E.; Cox, T.R.; Erler, J.T. The rationale for targeting the LOX family in cancer. *Nat. Rev. Cancer* **2012**, *12*, 540–552. [CrossRef]
12. Xu, L.; Go, E.P.; Finney, J.; Moon, H.; Lantz, M.; Rebecchi, K.; Desaire, H.; Mure, M. Post-translational Modifications of Recombinant Human Lysyl Oxidase-like 2 (rhLOXL2) Secreted from Drosophila S2 Cells. *J. Biol. Chem.* **2013**, *288*, 5357–5363. [CrossRef] [PubMed]
13. Kagan, H.M.; Li, W. Lysyl oxidase: Properties, specificity, and biological roles inside and outside of the cell. *J. Cell. Biochem.* **2003**, *88*, 660–672. [CrossRef] [PubMed]
14. Kim, Y.-M.; Kim, E.-C.; Kim, Y. The human lysyl oxidase-like 2 protein functions as an amine oxidase toward collagen and elastin. *Mol. Biol. Rep.* **2010**, *38*, 145–149. [CrossRef]
15. Nagan, N.; Kagan, H. Modulation of lysyl oxidase activity toward peptidyl lysine by vicinal dicarboxylic amino acid residues. Implications for collagen cross-linking. *J. Biol. Chem.* **1994**, *269*, 22366–22371. [CrossRef]
16. Wu, L.; Zhu, Y. The function and mechanisms of action of LOXL2 in cancer (Review). *Int. J. Mol. Med.* **2015**, *36*, 1200–1204. [CrossRef]
17. Yeung, T.; Georges, P.C.; Flanagan, L.A.; Marg, B.; Ortiz, M.; Funaki, M.; Zahir, N.; Ming, W.; Weaver, V.; Janmey, P.A. Effects of substrate stiffness on cell morphology, cytoskeletal structure, and adhesion. *Cell Motil. Cytoskelet.* **2004**, *60*, 24–34. [CrossRef] [PubMed]
18. Kumari, S.; Panda, T.K.; Pradhan, T. Lysyl Oxidase: Its Diversity in Health and Diseases. *Indian J. Clin. Biochem.* **2016**, *32*, 134–141. [CrossRef]
19. Jeong, Y.J.; Park, S.H.; Mun, S.H.; Kwak, S.G.; Lee, S.; Oh, H.K. Association between lysyl oxidase and fibrotic focus in relation with inflammation in breast cancer. *Oncol. Lett.* **2017**, *15*, 2431–2440. [CrossRef]
20. Sibon, I.; Sommer, P.; Lamaziere, J.M.D.; Bonnet, J. Lysyl oxidase deficiency: A new cause of human arterial dissection. *Heart* **2005**, *91*, e33. [CrossRef]
21. Khakoo, A.; Thomas, R.; Trompeter, R.; Duffy, P.; Price, R.; Pope, F.M. Congenital cutis laxa and lysyl oxidase deficiency. *Clin. Genet.* **2008**, *51*, 109–114. [CrossRef]
22. Royce, P.M.; Camakaris, J.; Danks, D.M. Reduced lysyl oxidase activity in skin fibroblasts from patients with Menkes' syndrome. *Biochem. J.* **1980**, *192*, 579–586. [CrossRef] [PubMed]
23. Kagan, H.M.; Raghavan, J.; Hollander, W. Changes in aortic lysyl oxidase activity in diet-induced atherosclerosis in the rabbit. *Arter.* **1981**, *1*, 287–291. [CrossRef] [PubMed]
24. Wang, T.-H.; Hsia, S.-M.; Shieh, T.-M. Lysyl Oxidase and the Tumor Microenvironment. *Int. J. Mol. Sci.* **2016**, *18*, 62. [CrossRef]
25. Wong, C.C.-L.; Gilkes, D.M.; Zhang, H.; Chen, J.; Wei, H.; Chaturvedi, P.; Fraley, S.I.; Khoo, U.-S.; Ng, I.O.-L.; Wirtz, D.; et al. Hypoxia-inducible factor 1 is a master regulator of breast cancer metastatic niche formation. *Proc. Natl. Acad. Sci. USA* **2011**, *108*, 16369–16374. [CrossRef] [PubMed]
26. Umezaki, N.; Nakagawa, S.; Yamashita, Y.; Kitano, Y.; Arima, K.; Miyata, T.; Hiyoshi, Y.; Okabe, H.; Nitta, H.; Hayashi, H.; et al. Lysyl oxidase induces epithelial-mesenchymal transition and predicts intrahepatic metastasis of hepatocellular carcinoma. *Cancer Sci.* **2019**, *110*, 2033–2043. [CrossRef]
27. Yu, M.; Shen, W.; Shi, X.; Wang, Q.; Zhu, L.; Xu, X.; Yu, J.; Liu, L. Upregulated LOX and increased collagen content associated with aggressive clinicopathological features and unfavorable outcome in oral squamous cell carcinoma. *J. Cell. Biochem.* **2019**, *120*, 14348–14359. [CrossRef]
28. Leeming, D.; Willumsen, N.; Sand, J.; Nielsen, S.H.; Dasgupta, B.; Brodmerkel, C.; Curran, M.; Bager, C.; Karsdal, M. A serological marker of the N-terminal neoepitope generated during LOXL2 maturation is elevated in patients with cancer or idiopathic pulmonary fibrosis. *Biochem. Biophys. Rep.* **2019**, *17*, 38–43. [CrossRef]
29. Janyasupab, M.; Lee, Y.-H.; Zhang, Y.; Liu, C.W.; Cai, J.; Popa, A.; Samia, A.C.; Wang, K.W.; Xu, J.; Hu, C.-C.; et al. Detection of Lysyl Oxidase-Like 2 (LOXL2), a Biomarker of Metastasis from Breast Cancers Using Human Blood Samples. *Recent Pat. Biomark.* **2016**, *5*, 93–100. [CrossRef]
30. Levental, K.R.; Yu, H.; Kass, L.; Lakins, J.N.; Egeblad, M.; Erler, J.T.; Fong, S.F.; Csiszar, K.; Giaccia, A.; Weninger, W.; et al. Matrix Crosslinking Forces Tumor Progression by Enhancing Integrin Signaling. *Cell* **2009**, *139*, 891–906. [CrossRef]
31. Cano, A.; Santamaria, P.G.; Moreno-Bueno, G. LOXL2 in epithelial cell plasticity and tumor progression. *Future Oncol.* **2012**, *8*, 1095–1108. [CrossRef]

32. Chopra, V.; Sangarappillai, R.M.; Romero-Canelón, I.; Jones, A.M. Lysyl Oxidase Like-2 (LOXL2): An Emerging Oncology Target. *Adv. Ther.* **2020**, *3*, 1900119. [CrossRef]
33. Bignon, M.; Pichol-Thievend, C.; Hardouin, J.; Malbouyres, M.; Bréchot, N.; Nasciutti, L.; Barret, A.; Teillon, J.; Guillon, E.; Etienne, E.; et al. Lysyl oxidase-like protein-2 regulates sprouting angiogenesis and type IV collagen assembly in the endothelial basement membrane. *Blood* **2011**, *118*, 3979–3989. [CrossRef]
34. De Jong, O.G.; Van Der Waals, L.M.; Kools, F.R.W.; Verhaar, M.C.; Van Balkom, B.W.M. Lysyl oxidase-like 2 is a regulator of angiogenesis through modulation of endothelial-to-mesenchymal transition. *J. Cell. Physiol.* **2018**, *234*, 10260–10269. [CrossRef]
35. Wang, C.; Xu, S.; Tian, Y.; Ju, A.; Hou, Q.; Liu, J.; Fu, Y.; Luo, Y. Lysyl Oxidase-Like Protein 2 Promotes Tumor Lymphangiogenesis and Lymph Node Metastasis in Breast Cancer. *Neoplasia* **2019**, *21*, 413–427. [CrossRef]
36. Salvador, F.; Martin, A.; López-Menéndez, C.; Moreno-Bueno, G.; Santos, V.; Vázquez-Naharro, A.; Santamaria, P.G.; Morales, S.; Dubus, P.R.; Muinelo-Romay, L.; et al. Lysyl Oxidase–like Protein LOXL2 Promotes Lung Metastasis of Breast Cancer. *Cancer Res.* **2017**, *77*, 5846–5859. [CrossRef]
37. Cebrià-Costa, J.P.; Pascual-Reguant, L.; Gonzalez-Perez, A.; Serra-Bardenys, G.; Querol, J.; Cosín, M.; Verde, G.; Cigliano, R.A.; Sanseverino, W.; Segura-Bayona, S.; et al. LOXL2-mediated H3K4 oxidation reduces chromatin accessibility in triple-negative breast cancer cells. *Oncogene* **2020**, *39*, 79–121. [CrossRef]
38. Millanes-Romero, A.; Herranz, N.; Perrera, V.; Iturbide, A.; Loubat-Casanovas, J.; Gil, J.; Jenuwein, T.; De Herreros, A.G.; Peiró, S. Regulation of Heterochromatin Transcription by Snail1/LOXL2 during Epithelial-to-Mesenchymal Transition. *Mol. Cell* **2013**, *52*, 746–757. [CrossRef]
39. Moreno-Bueno, G.; Salvador, F.; Martín, A.; Floristán, A.; Cuevas, E.P.; Santos, V.; Montes, A.; Morales, S.; Castilla, M.A.; Rojo-Sebastián, A.; et al. Lysyl oxidase-like 2 (LOXL2), a new regulator of cell polarity required for metastatic dissemination of basal-like breast carcinomas. *EMBO Mol. Med.* **2011**, *3*, 528–544. [CrossRef]
40. Payne, S.L.; Fogelgren, B.; Hess, A.R.; Seftor, E.A.; Wiley, E.L.; Fong, S.F.; Csiszar, K.; Hendrix, M.J.; Kirschmann, D.A. Lysyl Oxidase Regulates Breast Cancer Cell Migration and Adhesion through a Hydrogen Peroxide–Mediated Mechanism. *Cancer Res.* **2005**, *65*, 11429–11436. [CrossRef]
41. Egea, J.; Fabregat, I.; Frapart, Y.M.; Ghezzi, P.; Görlach, A.; Kietzmann, T.; Kubaichuk, K.; Knaus, U.G.; Lopez, M.G.; Olaso-Gonzalez, G.; et al. European contribution to the study of ROS: A summary of the findings and prospects for the future from the COST action BM1203 (EU-ROS). *Redox Biol.* **2017**, *13*, 94–162. [CrossRef]
42. Flórido, A.; Saraiva, N.; Cerqueira, S.; Almeida, N.; Parsons, M.; Batinic-Haberle, I.; Miranda, J.P.; Costa, J.G.; Carrara, G.; Castro, M.; et al. The manganese(III) porphyrin MnTnHex-2-PyP5+ modulates intracellular ROS and breast cancer cell migration: Impact on doxorubicin-treated cells. *Redox Biol.* **2019**, *20*, 367–378. [CrossRef]
43. Almeida, N.; Carrara, G.; Palmeira, C.M.; Fernandes, A.S.; Parsons, M.; Smith, G.L.; Saraiva, N. Stimulation of cell invasion by the Golgi Ion Channel GAAP/TMBIM4 via an H2O2-Dependent Mechanism. *Redox Biol.* **2020**, *28*, 101361. [CrossRef] [PubMed]
44. Zhan, P.; Lv, X.-J.; Ji, Y.-N.; Xie, H.; Yu, L.-K. Increased lysyl oxidase-like 2 associates with a poor prognosis in non-small cell lung cancer. *Clin. Respir. J.* **2016**, *12*, 712–720. [CrossRef] [PubMed]
45. Wu, L.; Zhang, Y.; Zhu, Y.; Cong, Q.; Xiang, Y.; Fu, L. The effect of LOXL2 in hepatocellular carcinoma. *Mol. Med. Rep.* **2016**, *14*, 1923–1932. [CrossRef] [PubMed]
46. Shao, B.; Zhao, X.; Liu, T.; Zhang, Y.; Sun, R.; Dong, X.; Liu, F.; Zhao, N.; Zhang, D.; Wu, L.; et al. LOXL2 promotes vasculogenic mimicry and tumour aggressiveness in hepatocellular carcinoma. *J. Cell. Mol. Med.* **2019**, *23*, 1363–1374. [CrossRef]
47. Hase, H.; Jingushi, K.; Ueda, Y.; Kitae, K.; Egawa, H.; Ohshio, I.; Kawakami, R.; Kashiwagi, Y.; Tsukada, Y.; Kobayashi, T.; et al. LOXL2 Status Correlates with Tumor Stage and Regulates Integrin Levels to Promote Tumor Progression in ccRCC. *Mol. Cancer Res.* **2014**, *12*, 1807–1817. [CrossRef]
48. Wang, C.C.; Li, C.Y.; Cai, J.-H.; Sheu, P.C.-Y.; Tsai, J.J.; Wu, M.-Y.; Hou, M.-F. Identification of Prognostic Candidate Genes in Breast Cancer by Integrated Bioinformatic Analysis. *J. Clin. Med.* **2019**, *8*, 1160. [CrossRef]
49. Kirschmann, D.A.; Seftor, E.A.; Fong, S.F.T.; Nieva, D.R.C.; Sullivan, C.M.; Edwards, E.M.; Sommer, P.; Csiszar, K.; Hendrix, M.J.C. A molecular role for lysyl oxidase in breast cancer invasion. *Cancer Res.* **2002**, *62*, 4478–4483.
50. Ahn, S.G.; Dong, S.M.; Oshima, A.; Kim, W.H.; Lee, H.M.; Lee, S.A.; Kwon, S.-H.; Lee, J.-H.; Lee, J.M.; Jeong, J.; et al. LOXL2 expression is associated with invasiveness and negatively influences survival in breast cancer patients. *Breast Cancer Res. Treat.* **2013**, *141*, 89–99. [CrossRef]
51. Hollósi, P.; Yakushiji, J.K.; Fong, K.S.; Csiszar, K.; Fong, S.F. Lysyl oxidase-like 2 promotes migration in noninvasive breast cancer cells but not in normal breast epithelial cells. *Int. J. Cancer* **2009**, *125*, 318–327. [CrossRef]
52. Barker, H.E.; Chang, J.; Cox, T.R.; Lang, G.; Bird, D.; Nicolau, M.; Evans, H.R.; Gartland, A.; Erler, J.T. LOXL2-Mediated Matrix Remodeling in Metastasis and Mammary Gland Involution. *Cancer Res.* **2011**, *71*, 1561–1572. [CrossRef]
53. Leo, C.; Cotic, C.; Pomp, V.; Fink, D.; Varga, Z. Overexpression of Lox in triple-negative breast cancer. *Ann. Diagn. Pathol.* **2018**, *34*, 98–102. [CrossRef]
54. Hajdú, I.; Kardos, J.; Major, B.; Fabó, G.; Lőrincz, Z.; Cseh, S.; Dormán, G. Inhibition of the LOX enzyme family members with old and new ligands. Selectivity analysis revisited. *Bioorganic Med. Chem. Lett.* **2018**, *28*, 3113–3118. [CrossRef] [PubMed]
55. Arem, A.J.; Misiorowski, R.; Chvapil, M. Effects of low-dose BAPN on wound healing. *J. Surg. Res.* **1979**, *27*, 228–232. [CrossRef]
56. Tang, S.S.; Trackman, P.C.; Kagan, H.M. Reaction of Aortic Lysyl Oxidase with Beta-Aminopropionitrile. *J. Biol. Chem.* **1983**, *258*, 4331–4338. [CrossRef]

57. Yang, X.; Li, S.; Li, W.; Chen, J.; Xiao, X.; Wang, Y.; Yan, G.; Chen, L. Inactivation of lysyl oxidase by β-aminopropionitrile inhibits hypoxia-induced invasion and migration of cervical cancer cells. *Oncol. Rep.* **2013**, *29*, 541–548. [CrossRef] [PubMed]
58. Zhao, L.; Niu, H.; Liu, Y.; Wang, L.; Zhang, N.; Zhang, G.; Liu, R.; Han, M. LOX inhibition downregulates MMP-2 and MMP-9 in gastric cancer tissues and cells. *J. Cancer* **2019**, *10*, 6481–6490. [CrossRef]
59. Cohen, I.K.; Moncure, C.W.; Witorsch, R.J.; Diegelmann, R.F. Collagen Synthesis in Capsules Surrounding Dimethylbenzanthracene-Induced Rat Breast Tumors and the Effect of Pretreatment with β-Aminopropionitrile. *Cancer Res.* **1979**, *39*, 2923–2927. [PubMed]
60. Bondareva, A.; Downey, C.M.; Ayres, F.; Liu, W.; Boyd, S.K.; Hallgrimsson, B.; Jirik, F.R. The Lysyl Oxidase Inhibitor, β-Aminopropionitrile, Diminishes the Metastatic Colonization Potential of Circulating Breast Cancer Cells. *PLoS ONE* **2009**, *4*, e5620. [CrossRef]
61. Rachman-Tzemah, C.; Zaffryar-Eilot, S.; Grossman, M.; Ribero, D.; Timaner, M.; Mäki, J.M.; Myllyharju, J.; Bertolini, F.; Hershkovitz, D.; Sagi, I.; et al. Blocking Surgically Induced Lysyl Oxidase Activity Reduces the Risk of Lung Metastases. *Cell Rep.* **2017**, *19*, 774–784. [CrossRef]
62. Smithen, D.A.; Leung, L.M.H.; Challinor, M.; Lawrence, R.; Tang, H.; Niculescu-Duvaz, D.; Pearce, S.P.; McLeary, R.; Lopes, F.; Aljarah, M.; et al. 2-Aminomethylene-5-sulfonylthiazole Inhibitors of Lysyl Oxidase (LOX) and LOXL2 Show Significant Efficacy in Delaying Tumor Growth. *J. Med. Chem.* **2019**, *63*, 2308–2324. [CrossRef] [PubMed]
63. Cox, T.R.; Gartland, A.; Erler, J.T. Lysyl Oxidase, a Targetable Secreted Molecule Involved in Cancer Metastasis. *Cancer Res.* **2016**, *76*, 188–192. [CrossRef] [PubMed]
64. Niu, Y.-Y.; Zhang, Y.-Y.; Zhu, Z.; Zhang, X.-Q.; Liu, X.; Zhu, S.-Y.; Song, Y.; Jin, X.; Lindholm, B.; Yu, C. Elevated intracellular copper contributes a unique role to kidney fibrosis by lysyl oxidase mediated matrix crosslinking. *Cell Death Dis.* **2020**, *11*, 1–14. [CrossRef] [PubMed]
65. Setargew, Y.F.; Wyllie, K.; Grant, R.D.; Chitty, J.L.; Cox, T.R. Targeting Lysyl Oxidase Family Mediated Matrix Cross-Linking as an Anti-Stromal Therapy in Solid Tumours. *Cancers* **2021**, *13*, 491. [CrossRef]
66. Fernandes, A.S.; Cabral, M.F.; Costa, J.; Castro, M.; Delgado, R.; Drew, M.G.; Félix, V. Two macrocyclic pentaaza compounds containing pyridine evaluated as novel chelating agents in copper(II) and nickel(II) overload. *J. Inorg. Biochem.* **2011**, *105*, 410–419. [CrossRef]
67. Chang, J.; Lucas, M.C.; Leonte, L.E.; Garcia-Montolio, M.; Singh, L.B.; Findlay, A.D.; Deodhar, M.; Foot, J.S.; Jarolimek, W.; Timpson, P.; et al. Pre-clinical evaluation of small molecule LOXL2 inhibitors in breast cancer. *Oncotarget* **2017**, *8*, 26066–26078. [CrossRef] [PubMed]
68. Rowbottom, M.W.; Bain, G.; Calderon, I.; Lasof, T.; Lonergan, D.; Lai, A.; Huang, F.; Darlington, J.; Prodanovich, P.; Santini, A.M.; et al. Identification of 4-(Aminomethyl)-6-(trifluoromethyl)-2-(phenoxy)pyridine Derivatives as Potent, Selective, and Orally Efficacious Inhibitors of the Copper-Dependent Amine Oxidase, Lysyl Oxidase-Like 2 (LOXL2). *J. Med. Chem.* **2017**, *60*, 4403–4423. [CrossRef] [PubMed]
69. Wei, Y.; Kim, T.J.; Peng, D.H.; Duan, D.; Gibbons, D.L.; Yamauchi, M.; Jackson, J.R.; Le Saux, C.J.; Calhoun, C.; Peters, J.; et al. Fibroblast-specific inhibition of TGF-β1 signaling attenuates lung and tumor fibrosis. *J. Clin. Investig.* **2017**, *127*, 3675–3688. [CrossRef]
70. Wei, Y.; Dong, W.; Jackson, J.; Ho, T.-C.; Le Saux, C.J.; Brumwell, A.; Li, X.; Klesney-Tait, J.; Cohen, M.L.; Wolters, P.J.; et al. Blocking LOXL2 and TGFβ1 signalling induces collagen I turnover in precision-cut lung slices derived from patients with idiopathic pulmonary fibrosis. *Thorax* **2021**. [CrossRef]
71. Ikenaga, N.; Peng, Z.-W.; Vaid, A.K.; Liu, S.B.; Yoshida, S.; Sverdlov, D.Y.; Mikels-Vigdal, A.; Smith, V.; Schuppan, D.; Popov, Y.V. Selective targeting of lysyl oxidase-like 2 (LOXL2) suppresses hepatic fibrosis progression and accelerates its reversal. *Gut* **2017**, *66*, 1697–1708. [CrossRef]
72. Grossman, M.; Ben-Chetrit, N.; Zhuravlev, A.; Afik, R.; Bassat, E.; Solomonov, I.; Yarden, Y.; Sagi, I. Tumor Cell Invasion Can Be Blocked by Modulators of Collagen Fibril Alignment That Control Assembly of the Extracellular Matrix. *Cancer Res.* **2016**, *76*, 4249–4258. [CrossRef] [PubMed]
73. Schilter, H.; Findlay, A.D.; Perryman, L.; Yow, T.T.; Moses, J.; Zahoor, A.; Turner, C.I.; Deodhar, M.; Foot, J.S.; Zhou, W.; et al. The lysyl oxidase like 2/3 enzymatic inhibitor, PXS-5153A, reduces crosslinks and ameliorates fibrosis. *J. Cell. Mol. Med.* **2018**, *23*, 1759–1770. [CrossRef] [PubMed]
74. Leung, L.; Niculescu-Duvaz, D.; Smithen, D.; Lopes, F.; Callens, C.; McLeary, R.; Saturno, G.; Davies, L.; Aljarah, M.; Brown, M.; et al. Anti-metastatic Inhibitors of Lysyl Oxidase (LOX): Design and Structure–Activity Relationships. *J. Med. Chem.* **2019**, *62*, 5863–5884. [CrossRef] [PubMed]
75. Tang, H.; Leung, L.; Saturno, G.; Viros, A.; Smith, D.; Di Leva, G.; Morrison, E.; Niculescu-Duvaz, D.; Lopes, F.; Johnson, L.; et al. Lysyl oxidase drives tumour progression by trapping EGF receptors at the cell surface. *Nat. Commun.* **2017**, *8*, 14909. [CrossRef] [PubMed]
76. Rodriguez, H.M.; Vaysberg, M.; Mikels, A.; McCauley, S.; Velayo, A.C.; Garcia, C.; Smith, V. Modulation of Lysyl Oxidase-like 2 Enzymatic Activity by an Allosteric Antibody Inhibitor. *J. Biol. Chem.* **2010**, *285*, 20964–20974. [CrossRef] [PubMed]
77. Raghu, G.; Brown, K.K.; Collard, H.R.; Cottin, V.; Gibson, K.F.; Kaner, R.J.; Lederer, D.J.; Martinez, F.J.; Noble, P.W.; Song, J.W.; et al. Efficacy of simtuzumab versus placebo in patients with idiopathic pulmonary fibrosis: A randomised, double-blind, controlled, phase 2 trial. *Lancet Respir. Med.* **2017**, *5*, 22–32. [CrossRef]

78. Meissner, E.G.; McLaughlin, M.; Matthews, L.; Gharib, A.M.; Wood, B.J.; Levy, E.; Sinkus, R.; Virtaneva, K.; Sturdevant, D.; Martens, C.; et al. Simtuzumab treatment of advanced liver fibrosis in HIV and HCV-infected adults: Results of a 6-month open-label safety trial. *Liver Int.* **2016**, *36*, 1783–1792. [CrossRef]
79. Benson, A.B.; Wainberg, Z.A.; Hecht, J.R.; Vyushkov, D.; Dong, H.; Bendell, J.; Kudrik, F. A Phase II Randomized, Double-Blind, Placebo-Controlled Study of Simtuzumab or Placebo in Combination with Gemcitabine for the First-Line Treatment of Pancreatic Adenocarcinoma. *Oncologist* **2017**, *22*, 241-e15. [CrossRef]
80. Hecht, J.R.; Benson, A.B.; Vyushkov, D.; Yang, Y.; Bendell, J.; Verma, U. A Phase II, Randomized, Double-Blind, Placebo-Controlled Study of Simtuzumab in Combination with FOLFIRI for the Second-Line Treatment of Metastatic KRAS Mutant Colorectal Adenocarcinoma. *Oncologist* **2017**, *22*, 243-e23. [CrossRef]
81. PharmAkea, Inc. A Phase 1, Randomised, Placebo-Controlled, Ascending Single and Multiple Dose Safety, Tolerability, Pharmacokinetic and Food Effect Study of PAT-1251 in Healthy Adult Subjects; Clinical Trial Registration NCT02852551. 2016. Available online: clinicaltrials.gov (accessed on 25 January 2021).
82. Galecto Biotech, A.B. An Open-Label, Phase IIa Study of the Safety, Tolerability, Pharmacokinetics and Pharmacodynamics of Oral GB2064 (a LOXL2 Inhibitor) in Participants with Myelofibrosis (MF); Clinical Trial Registration NCT04679870. 2021. Available online: clinicaltrials.gov (accessed on 10 February 2021).
83. Pharmaxis. A Two-Part Pharmacokinetic Study of PXS-5382A in Healthy Adult Males; Clinical Trial Registration NCT04183517. 2020. Available online: clinicaltrials.gov (accessed on 10 February 2021).
84. How, J.; Liu, Y.; Story, J.L.; Neuberg, S.D.S.; Ravid, D.K.; Jarolimek, W.; Charlton, B.; Hobbs, G.S. Evaluation of a Pan-Lysyl Oxidase Inhibitor, Pxs-5505, in Myelofibrosis: A Phase I, Randomized, Placebo Controlled Double Blind Study in Healthy Adults. *Blood* **2020**, *136*, 16. [CrossRef]
85. Pharmaxis. A Phase 1/2a Study to Evaluate Safety, Pharmacokinetic and Pharmacodynamic Dose Escalation and Expansion Study of PXS-5505 in Patients With Primary, Postpolycythemia Vera or Post-Essential Thrombocythemia Myelofibrosis; Clinical Trial Registration NCT04676529. 2020. Available online: clinicaltrials.gov (accessed on 10 February 2021).
86. University of California. Fibroblast Specific Inhibition of LOXL2 and TGFbeta1 Signaling in Patients with Pulmonary Fibrosis. Clinical Trial Registration NCT03928847. 2021. Available online: clinicaltrials.gov (accessed on 8 February 2021).
87. Sidney Kimmel Comprehensive Cancer Center at Johns Hopkins. Phase II Study of Penicillamine and Reduction of Copper for Angiosuppressive Therapy of Adults with Newly Diagnosed Glioblastoma; Clinical Trial Registration NCT00003751. 2012. Available online: clinicaltrials.gov (accessed on 8 February 2021).
88. Memorial Sloan Kettering Cancer Center. A Phase II Study of Tetrathiomolybdate (TM) in Patients with Breast Cancer at Moderate to High Risk of Recurrence; Clinical Trial Registration NCT00195091. 2020. Available online: clinicaltrials.gov (accessed on 11 February 2021).

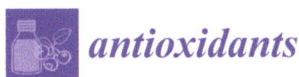

Article

Withanolide C Inhibits Proliferation of Breast Cancer Cells via Oxidative Stress-Mediated Apoptosis and DNA Damage

Tzu-Jung Yu [1,2], Jen-Yang Tang [3,4], Li-Ching Lin [5,6,7], Wan-Ju Lien [8], Yuan-Bin Cheng [2,9], Fang-Rong Chang [2], Fu Ou-Yang [1,*] and Hsueh-Wei Chang [2,10,11,12,*]

1. Division of Breast Surgery and Department of Surgery, Kaohsiung Medical University Hospital, Kaohsiung 80708, Taiwan; u107500035@kmu.edu.tw
2. Graduate Institute of Natural Products, Kaohsiung Medical University, Kaohsiung 80708, Taiwan; jmb@kmu.edu.tw (Y.-B.C.); aaronfrc@kmu.edu.tw (F.-R.C.)
3. Department of Radiation Oncology, Faculty of Medicine, College of Medicine, Kaohsiung Medical University, Kaohsiung 80708, Taiwan; reyata@kmu.edu.tw
4. Department of Radiation Oncology, Kaohsiung Medical University Hospital, Kaohsiung 80708, Taiwan
5. Department of Radiation Oncology, Chi-Mei Foundation Medical Center, Tainan 71004, Taiwan; 8508a6@mail.chimei.org.tw
6. School of Medicine, Taipei Medical University, Taipei 11031, Taiwan
7. Chung Hwa University Medical Technology, Tainan 71703, Taiwan
8. Department of Biomedical Science and Environmental Biology, Ph.D Program in Life Sciences, College of Life Sciences, Kaohsiung Medical University, Kaohsiung 80708, Taiwan; u106023002@kmu.edu.tw
9. Department of Marine Biotechnology and Resources, National Sun Yat-sen University, Kaohsiung 80424, Taiwan
10. Center for Cancer Research, Kaohsiung Medical University, Kaohsiung 80708, Taiwan
11. Cancer Center, Kaohsiung Medical University Hospital, Kaohsiung 80708, Taiwan
12. Institute of Medical Science and Technology, National Sun Yat-sen University, Kaohsiung 80424, Taiwan
* Correspondence: swfuon@kmu.edu.tw or kmufrank@gmail.com (F.O.-Y.); changhw@kmu.edu.tw (H.-W.C.); Tel.: +886-7-312-1101 (ext. 8105) (F.O.-Y.); +886-7-312-1101 (ext. 2691) (H.-W.C.)

Received: 21 July 2020; Accepted: 14 September 2020; Published: 16 September 2020

Abstract: Some withanolides, particularly the family of steroidal lactones, show anticancer effects, but this is rarely reported for withanolide C (WHC)—especially anti-breast cancer effects. The subject of this study is to evaluate the ability of WHC to regulate the proliferation of breast cancer cells, using both time and concentration in treatment with WHC. In terms of ATP depletion, WHC induced more antiproliferation to three breast cancer cell lines, SKBR3, MCF7, and MDA-MB-231, than to normal breast M10 cell lines. SKBR3 and MCF7 cells showing higher sensitivity to WHC were used to explore the antiproliferation mechanism. Flow cytometric apoptosis analyses showed that subG1 phase and annexin V population were increased in breast cancer cells after WHC treatment. Western blotting showed that cleaved forms of the apoptotic proteins poly (ADP-ribose) polymerase (c-PARP) and cleaved caspase 3 (c-Cas 3) were increased in breast cancer cells. Flow cytometric oxidative stress analyses showed that WHC triggered reactive oxygen species (ROS) and mitochondrial superoxide (MitoSOX) production as well as glutathione depletion. In contrast, normal breast M10 cells showed lower levels of ROS and annexin V expression than breast cancer cells. Flow cytometric DNA damage analyses showed that WHC triggered γH2AX and 8-oxo-2′-deoxyguanosine (8-oxodG) expression in breast cancer cells. Moreover, N-acetylcysteine (NAC) pretreatment reverted oxidative stress-mediated ATP depletion, apoptosis, and DNA damage. Therefore, WHC kills breast cancer cells depending on oxidative stress-associated mechanisms.

Keywords: withanolide; breast cancer; apoptosis; oxidative stress; DNA damage

1. Introduction

Withanolide is a general name for at least 300 natural C-28 steroidal lactones [1,2]. Several kinds of withanolides are reported to have anticancer effects [3]. For example, withaferin A has anticancer effects on oral [4], colon [5], and breast [6] cancer cells. 4β-hydroxywithanolide [7] and withanone [8] caused selective killing against oral and breast cancer cells, respectively. Withanolide E had anticancer effects against renal cancer cells [9].

Accumulating evidence shows that a series of withanolides induce apoptosis of several cancer cells through oxidative stress. For example, withaferin A induces reactive oxygen species (ROS)-mediated apoptosis in oral [4], head and neck [10], and melanoma [11] cancer cells. Similarly, 4β-hydroxywithanolide induces ROS leading to apoptosis of oral cancer cells [7]. However, the mechanisms of anticancer action of other withanolides have not been fully explored as of yet. Further screening of other withanolide candidates for their antiproliferative potency is warranted.

Breast cancer is the most common cancer type in women worldwide. Breast cancer exhibits complex and heterogeneous characters with three typical clinical subtypes, such as hormone receptor (HR) positive, human epidermal growth factor receptor 2 (HER2) positive, and triple-negative breast cancer (TNBC). Breast cancer was also considered to have five molecular classification subtypes, including luminal A, luminal B, HER2, basal, and Claudin-low, with different combinations of positive and negative for HER2, HR, and estrogen receptor (ER) [12]. Different clinical subtypes of breast cancer show different responses to different treatments. Among these breast cancer subtypes, TNBC is the most difficult subtype for treatment due to the lack of HR, HER2, and ER overexpression. In addition to target therapy, chemotherapy provides an alternative mainstay for treatment of all subtypes of breast cancer cells. Clinical drugs were used for breast cancer therapy but they generally caused side effects to normal tissues. Therefore, new drug development for breast cancer therapy continues to be required.

Among the many withanolides, we noted that withanolide C (WHC), one of the active compounds isolated from the solanacean plant *Physalis peruviana*, was rarely investigated. Although WHC was shown to have anticancer potency in 2009, only IC_{50} values in a MTT study of liver (HepG2 and Hep3B), lung (A549) and breast (MDA-MB-231 and MCF7) cancer cells [13] were investigated as yet. The detailed anticancer mechanisms and antiproliferation effect of WHC on other cancer cells have not been yet explored. Therefore, the aim of the present study was to investigate its antiproliferation function and the mechanisms involved in WHC-treated breast cancer cell responses.

2. Materials and Methods

2.1. Cell Culture

SKBR3, MCF7, and MDA-MB-231 were the three cell lines for human breast cancer, obtained from the American Tissue Culture Collection (ATCC, Manassas, VA, USA). M10 is a normal human breast cell line, obtained from the Bioresource Collection and Research Center (BCRC; HsinChu, Taiwan). SKBR3, MCF7, and MDA-MB-231 cells are HER2+, luminal A, and Claudin-low subtypes of breast cancer cell lines exhibiting metastasis ability, respectively [14,15]. Dulbecco's Modified Eagle Medium (DMEM)/F12 (3:2 mixture) with 10% bovine serum (Gibco, Grand Island, NE, USA), antibiotics, and glutamine were used for culturing the SKBR3, MCF7, and MDA-MB-231 cells. Alpha medium with 10% fetal bovine serum (Gibco) and common antibiotics (penicillin and streptomycin) were used for the M10 cells. The cells were cultured in a humidified atmosphere 5% CO_2 at 37 °C.

2.2. ATP and MTS Assays

Double checking of the proliferation status was performed by both ATP and MTS assays. The cell viability in terms of cellular ATP content was measured by ATP-lite assay kit (PerkinElmer Life Sciences, Boston, MA, USA) [16]. The cell viability in terms of mitochondrial metabolic activity was measured by a colorimetric MTS assay (Promega Corporation, Madison, WI, USA) [17].

2.3. Drug Information

This purification of the WHC was performed as follows. The plant materials of *Physalis peruviana* were collected in Tainan county, in September 2017. The species was identified by Dr. Yuan-Bin Cheng and a voucher specimen (PPR-18) was deposited in the Graduate Institute of Natural Products, Kaohsiung Medical University. The air-dried roots of *P. peruviana* (20.0 kg) were extracted with MeOH (15 L) thrice to yield a crude extract. This extract was partitioned between water and EtOAc to get the EtOAc portion (45.2 g). The later portion was further partitioned between hexanes and 75% MeOH$_{aq}$ to gain a terpene-enriched portion (26.8 g). This portion was subjected to a silica gel flash column stepwise eluting with hexanes/EtOAc/MeOH to furnish eight fractions. Fraction 5 (20.3 g) was separated by another silica gel column stepwise elution with methylene chloride and MeOH to provide six subfractions. Subfraction 5-3 (9.0 g) was purified by reverse phase column stepwise elution with MeOH and H$_2$O to yield eight fractions. Fraction 5-3-4 (3.4 g) was isolated by silica gel open column stepwise elution with hexane and acetone to give a subfraction 5-3-4-1 (587.3 mg). Subfraction 5-3-4-1 was purified by reversed phase high performance liquid chromatography (RP-HPLC) (C$_{18}$ column, 62% MeOH, isocratic) to produce WHC (40.0 mg).

N-acetylcysteine (NAC) (Sigma-Aldrich, St. Louis, MO, USA) was used as an inhibitor for oxidative stress [18,19]. The pretreatment condition for the NAC used in the cells was 10 mM for 1 h. Cisplatin (Selleckchem, Houston, TX, USA) was used as a positive control for treatment to breast cancer cells and normal breast cells. WHC, NAC, and cisplatin were dissolved in dimethyl sulfoxide (DMSO), double-distilled water, and phosphate-buffered saline (PBS) for drug treatments. For the control treatment, cells were cultured with a low concentration of a DMSO-containing medium, where all treatments (control, NAC, WHC, and NAC/WHC) had the same DMSO concentrations in the same experiments, as indicated.

2.4. Antibody Information

For Western blotting, the primary antibodies were specifically recognized of the cleaved forms of poly (ADP-ribose) polymerase (c-PARP) (Asp214) (D64E10), caspase 3 (c-Cas 3) (Asp175) (5A1E) (1:1000 dilution), and mAb-β-actin (control) (1:5000 dilution), which were obtained from Cell Signalling Technology Inc. (Danvers, MA, USA) and Sigma-Aldrich [20]. For flow cytometry, the primary antibodies for p-Histone H2A.X (Ser 139) (γH2AX) and the 8-OHdG antibody (E-8) Fluorescein isothiocyanate (FITC), as well as the Alexa 488-conjugated secondary antibody for the γH2AX primary antibody, were obtained from the Santa Cruz Biotechnology (Santa Cruz, CA, USA) and Cell Signalling Technology Inc.

2.5. Cell Cycle Assay

Cellular DNA contents were stained with 7-aminoactinomycin D (7AAD) (Biotium Inc., Hayward, CA, USA) (1 µg/mL, 30 min, 37 °C) as described previously [4]. A flow cytometer (Guava® easyCyte™; Luminex, TX, USA) and FlowJo software (Becton-Dickinson; Franklin Lakes, NJ, USA) were used for cell cycle determination.

2.6. Annexin V/7AAD Assay

An Annexin V/7AAD dual staining kit (Strong Biotech Corp., Taipei, Taiwan) was chosen for apoptosis detection as previously described [17] and analyses were conducted using a BD Accuri C6 flow cytometer. Annexin V (10 μg/mL) and 7AAD (1 μg/mL) were used for dual staining at 37 °C for 30 min.

2.7. ROS and Glutathione (GSH) Assays

Cellular ROS was probed with 2′,7′-dichlorodihydrofluorescein diacetate (H_2DCF-DA) (Sigma-Aldrich) (10 μM, 30 min, 37 °C) as previously described [21] and analyzed using a BD Accuri C6 flow cytometer. Cellular GSH was probed with CellTracker Green 5-chloromethylfluorescein (CMFDA) (Thermo Fisher Scientific, Carlsbad, CA, USA) (0.1 μM, 30 min, 37 °C) as previously described [22] and analyzed using a flow cytometer (Guava® easyCyte™) and FlowJo software (Becton-Dickinson).

2.8. Mitochondrial Superoxide (MitoSOX) Assay

MitoSOX was probed with MitoSOX™ Red (Thermo Fisher Scientific, Carlsbad, CA, USA) (50 nM, 30 min, 37 °C) and analyzed using a BD Accuri C6 flow cytometer as previously described [23].

2.9. γH2AX Assay

The primary antibody against γH2AX (1:500 dilution, 4 °C, 1 h) and its coupled Alexa 488-conjugated secondary antibody, as well as 7AAD (5 μg/mL, 30 min, 37 °C), were used [24]. An analysis was subsequently performed using a flow cytometer (Guava® easyCyte™) and FlowJo software (Becton-Dickinson) as previously described.

2.10. 8-Oxo-2′-Deoxyguanosine (8-oxodG) Assay

Cells were probed with the antibody 8-OHdG (E-8) FITC (1:10000 dilution, 4 °C, 1 h) to detect an oxidative DNA damage marker (8-oxodG) [25]. An analysis was subsequently performed using a BD Accuri C6 flow cytometer as previously described.

2.11. Statistics

Significance for multiple comparison was determined by analysis of variance (ANOVA) coupled with Tukey's HSD Post-Hoc Tests using JMP® 12 software. For the purposes of multiple comparisons, data columns were marked with small letters. When data columns were without overlapping letters, there were significant differences between them.

3. Results

3.1. WHC Inhibits Proliferation of Breast Cancer and Normal Cells Involving ROS

In terms of the ATP assay, at 48 h, WHC had decreased the cell viability of the three subtypes of breast cancer (SKBR3, MCF7 and MDA-MB-231) cells more than normal breast (M10) cells (Figure 1A, left). Accordingly, WHC exhibited higher antiproliferation of breast cancer cells than normal breast cells. For the sake of higher sensitivity to WHC, SKBR3 and MCF7 cells were chosen for other experiments to explore its antiproliferation mechanism in breast cancer cells. In terms of the MTS assay, at 48 h, WHC at 1 μM had decreased the cell viability of two subtypes of breast cancer (SKBR3 and MCF7) cells more than normal breast (M10) cells (Figure 1A, right), i.e., 66.6% and 43.0% vs. 83.4%, respectively.

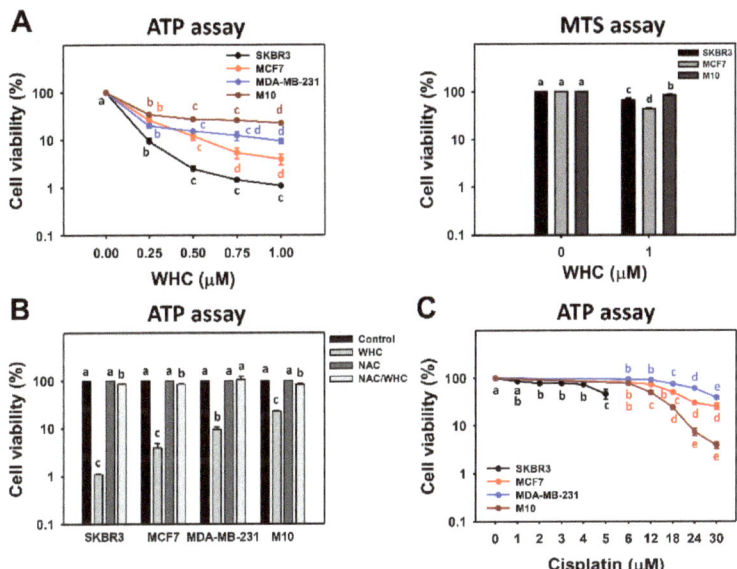

Figure 1. Withanolide C (WHC) inhibited the cell viabilities of breast cancer and normal breast cells differentially. Cell viabilities were determined by ATP assays. (**A**) ATP and MTS assays for determining cell viability after WHC treatment. For the ATP assay, breast cancer (SKBR3, MCF7 and MDA-MB-231) cells and breast normal (M10) cells were exposed to 0 (0.1% DMSO only), 0.25, 0.5, 0.75, and 1 µM of WHC for 48 h. For the MTS assay, breast cancer (SKBR3 and MCF7) cells and M10 cells were exposed to 0 (0.1% DMSO only) and 1 µM of WHC for 48 h. WHC also dissolved in the same concentration of DMSO. (**B**) N-acetylcysteine (NAC) pretreatment reversed WHC-induced ATP changes. Following pretreatment with NAC (10 mM for 1 h), cells were treated with the control and 1 µM of WHC for 48 h, i.e., NAC/WHC. (**C**) ATP assay for determining cell viability after cisplatin treatment for 48 h. Data are means ± SDs (n = 3). Results marked without overlapping letters show significant differences ($p < 0.05$ to 0.0001).

There was a pretreatment with NAC to examine the effect of ROS on the antiproliferation function of WHC. The cell viabilities of breast cancer and normal cells after the WHC time course treatment were recovered to control by NAC pretreatment (Figure 1B). For comparison, the clinical drug cisplatin was used as a positive control to breast cancer cells and normal breast cells (Figure 1C). The drug sensitivity of WHC was higher than cisplatin for breast cancer cells. The cytotoxicity of WHC was lower than cisplatin for normal breast (M10) cells.

3.2. WHC Disturbs Cell Cycle Progression of Breast Cancer Cells

The dose and time course changes of cell cycle progression in breast cancer cells were determined by 7AAD flow cytometry (Figure 2A,C). WHC showed dose- and time-dependent increases in subG1 populations, decreases in G1 population, and increases in G2/M population in breast cancer (SKBR3 and MCF7) cells (Figure 2B,D).

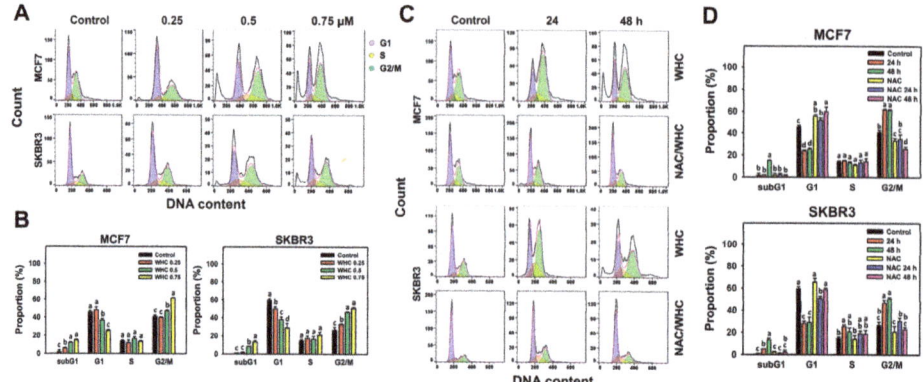

Figure 2. WHC disturbed cell cycle progression of breast cancer cells. (**A,B**) Cell cycle profiles and statistics for dose effects of WHC. Breast cancer (MCF7 and SKBR3) cells were treated with WHC (control (0.075% DMSO), 0.25, 0.5, and 0.75 µM, respectively) for 48 h. (**C,D**) NAC pretreatments reversed the WHC induced cell cycle disturbance. Following pretreatments with NAC (10 mM for 1 h), cells were treated with the control (0.075% DMSO) and 0.75 µM of WHC for 0, 24, and 48 h, i.e., NAC/WHC. Data are means ± SDs ($n = 3$). Results marked without overlapping letters show significant differences ($p < 0.05$ to 0.0001).

NAC pretreatment was used to examine the effects of pm the WHC function of cell cycle disturbance. Cell cycle disturbance of breast cancer cells after the WHC time course treatment was recovered by NAC pretreatment (Figure 2D).

3.3. WHC Differentially Induces Apoptosis (Annexin V/7AAD) of Breast Cancer and Normal Cells

The dose and time course changes of annexin V/7AAD in breast cancer and normal breast cells were determined by flow cytometry (Figure 3A,C). The WHC treatment showed dose- and time-dependent increases in the apoptotic (annexin V) population of breast cancer (SKBR3 and MCF7) cells (Figure 3B,D), which was higher than that of normal breast (M10) cells (Figure 3B). The apoptosis changes were further confirmed by performing Western blotting. c-PAPR and c-Cas 3 were overexpressed in the breast cancer (SKBR3 and MCF7) cells (Figure 3E).

NAC pretreatment was used to examine the effects of ROS on apoptosis (annexin V) caused by WHC. Increasing apoptosis (annexin V) populations of breast cancer cells after the WHC time course treatment were recovered by NAC pretreatment (Figure 3D). Moreover, WHC-induced c-PAPR overexpression in breast cancer cells was suppressed by NAC pretreatment (Figure 3E). Similarly, WHC induced another apoptotic protein c-Cas 3 overexpression in breast cancer cells which was suppressed by NAC pretreatment.

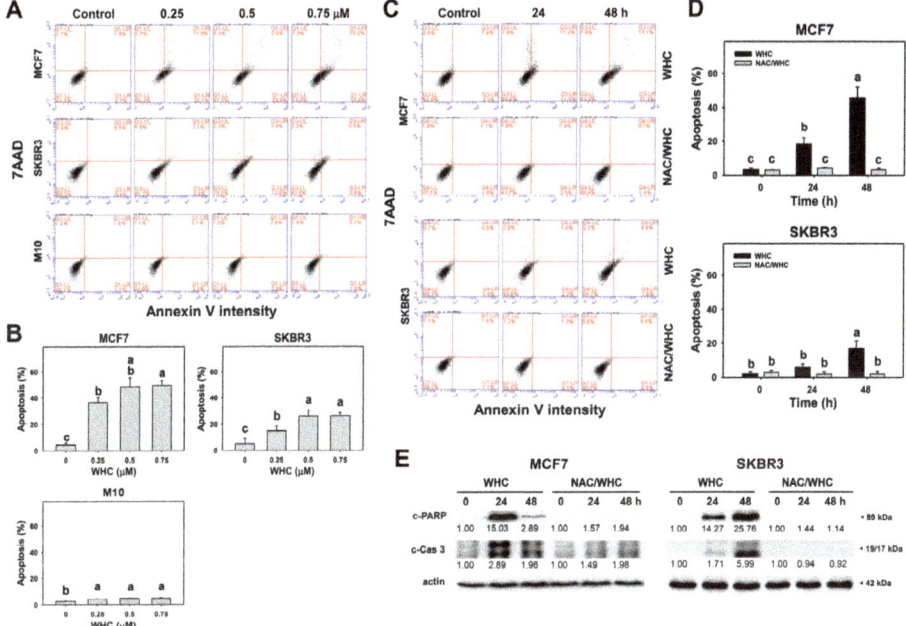

Figure 3. WHC induced apoptosis (annexin V/7AAD) differentially in breast cancer and normal breast cells. (**A,B**) Annexin V/7AAD profiles and statistics for dose effect of WHC. Breast cancer (MCF7 and SKBR3) cells and normal breast (M10) cells were treated with WHC (control (0.075% DMSO), 0.25, 0.5, and 0.75 µM) for 48 h. Annexin V (+) (%) was counted for the apoptosis (%). (**C,D**) NAC pretreatments reversed the WHC-induced apoptosis. Following pretreatments with NAC (10 mM for 1 h), cells were treated with control (0.075% DMSO) and 0.75 µM of WHC for 0, 24, and 48 h, i.e., NAC/WHC. Data are means ± SDs (n = 3). Results marked without overlapping letters showed significant differences (p < 0.05 to 0.001). (**E**) Apoptosis Western blotting of WHC. Cleaved PARP (c-PARP) and c-Cas 3 expressions were quantified referring to β-actin expression.

3.4. WHC Differentially Induced ROS Generation and GSH Depletion of Breast Cancer and Normal Cells

The dose and time course changes of ROS generation in breast cancer and normal breast cells were determined by flow cytometry (Figure 4A,C). The WHC treatment showed dose- and time-dependent increases in the ROS (+) population in breast cancer (SKBR3 and MCF7) cells (Figure 4B,D), which was higher than that of normal breast (M10) cells (Figure 4B).

NAC pretreatment was used to examine the ROS function of WHC. Increasing ROS (+) populations of breast cancer cells after the WHC time course treatment were recovered by NAC pretreatment (Figure 4D). Moreover, the time course changes of the GSH content in breast cancer cells were determined by flow cytometry (Figure 4E). The WHC treatment showed decreases in the GSH (+) population in breast cancer (SKBR3 and MCF7) cells over time compared to the control (Figure 4F).

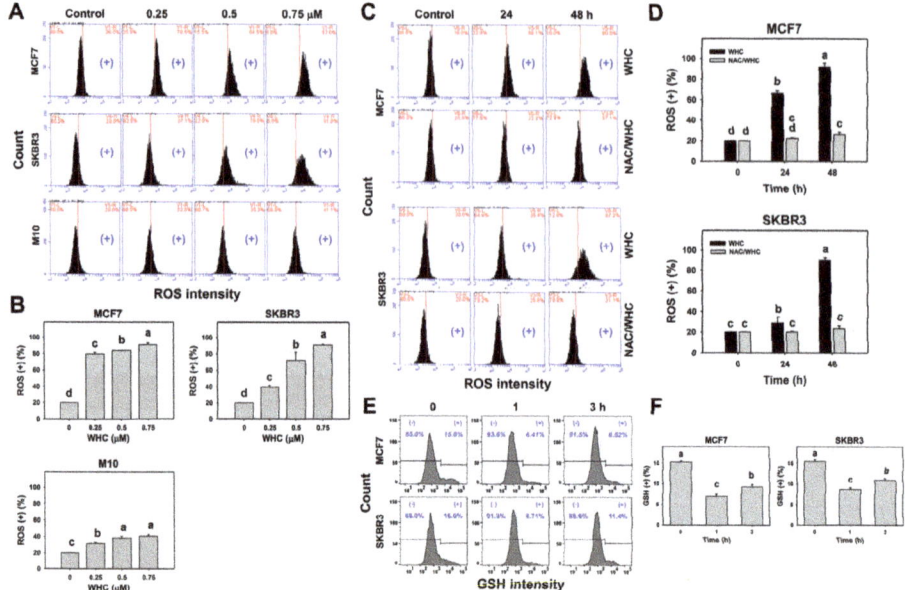

Figure 4. WHC differentially induced reactive oxygen species (ROS) generation among breast cancer and normal breast cells. (**A,B**) ROS profiles and statistics for dose effects to WHC. Breast cancer (MCF7 and SKBR3) cells and normal breast (M10) cells were treated with WHC (control (0.075% DMSO), 0.25, 0.5, and 0.75 µM) for 48 h. (+) located at the right side of each profile is counted for ROS (+) (%). (**C,D**) NAC pretreatment reversed the WHC induced ROS generation. Following pretreatments with NAC (10 mM for 1 h), cells were treated with control (0.075% DMSO) and 0.75 µM of WHC for 0, 24, and 48 h, i.e., NAC/WHC. (**E,F**) GSH profiles and statistics for time course changes to WHC. Breast cancer MCF7 and SKBR3 cells were treated with WHC (control (0.075% DMSO) and 0.75 µM) for 0, 1, and 3 h. (+) located at right side of each profile is counted for GSH (+) (%). Data, means ± SDs ($n = 3$). Results marked without overlapping letters show significant differences ($p < 0.05$ to 0.0001).

3.5. WHC Overexpresses MitoSOX in Breast Cancer Cells

The dose and time course changes of MitoSOX generation in breast cancer cells were determined by flow cytometry (Figure 5A,C). WHC showed dose- and time-dependent increases for MitoSOX (+) population in breast cancer (SKBR3 and MCF7) cells (Figure 5B,D).

NAC pretreatment was used to examine the effect of ROS on WHC-induced MitoSOX generation. Increasing MitoSOX (+) populations of breast cancer cells after the WHC time course treatment were recovered by NAC pretreatment (Figure 5D).

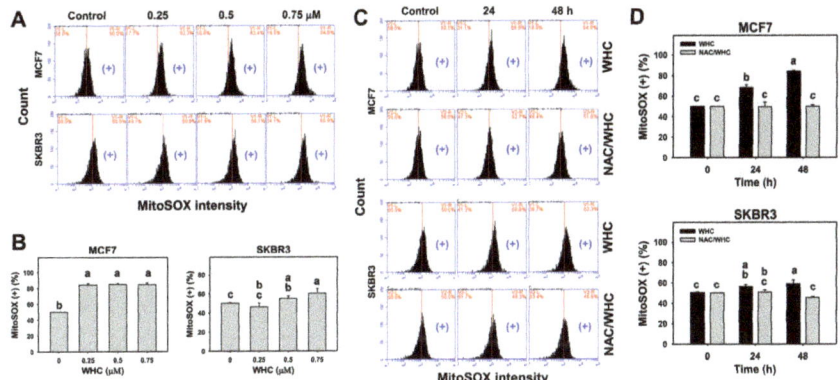

Figure 5. WHC differentially induces MitoSOX generation of breast cancer cells. (**A,B**) MitoSOX profiles and statistics for dose effects on WHC. Breast cancer MCF7 and SKBR3 cells and normal breast (M10) cells were treated with WHC (control (0.075% DMSO), 0.25, 0.5, and 0.75 µM) for 48 h. (+) located on the right side of each profile was counted for MitoSOX (+) (%). (**C,D**) NAC pretreatments reversed the WHC-induced MitoSOX generation. Following pretreatments with NAC (10 mM for 1 h), cells were treated with the control (0.075% DMSO) and 0.75 µM of WHC for 0, 24, and 48 h, i.e., NAC/WHC. Data are means ± SDs (n = 3). Results marked without overlapping letters show significant differences (p < 0.05 to 0.01).

3.6. WHC Overexpresses γH2AX in Breast Cancer Cells

The dose and time course changes of γH2AX expression in breast cancer cells were determined by flow cytometry (Figure 6A,C). WHC showed dose- and time-dependent increases in γH2AX (+) populations in breast cancer (SKBR3 and MCF7) cells (Figure 6B,D).

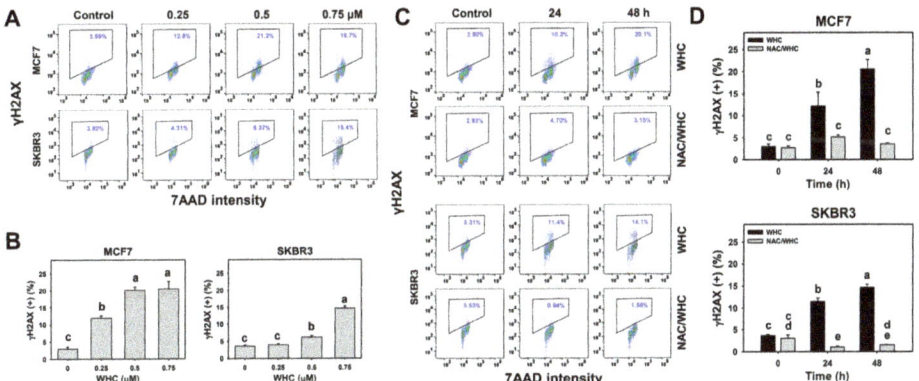

Figure 6. WHC differentially induced DNA double strand break (DSB) damage (γH2AX) of breast cancer cells. (**A,B**) γH2AX profiles and statistics for dose effects on WHC. Breast cancer (MCF7 and SKBR3) cells were treated with WHC (control (0.075% DMSO), 0.25, 0.5, and 0.75 µM) for 48 h. Box region of each profile is counted for γH2AX (+) (%). (**C,D**) NAC pretreatments reversed the WHC induced γH2AX generation. Following pretreatments with NAC (10 mM for 1 h), cells were treated with control (0.075% DMSO) and 0.75 µM of WHC for 0, 24, and 48 h, i.e., NAC/WHC. Data are means ± SDs (n = 3). Results marked without overlapping letters show significant differences (p < 0.005 to 0.0001).

NAC pretreatment was used to examine the effect of ROS on WHC-induced γH2AX expression. Increasing γH2AX (+) populations of breast cancer cells after WHC time course treatment were recovered by NAC pretreatment (Figure 6D).

3.7. WHC Overexpresses 8-OxodG in Breast Cancer Cells

The dose and time course changes of 8-oxodG expression in breast cancer cells were determined by flow cytometry (Figure 7A,C). WHC treatment showed dose- and time-dependent increases in 8-oxodG (+) populations in breast cancer (SKBR3 and MCF7) cells (Figure 7B,D).

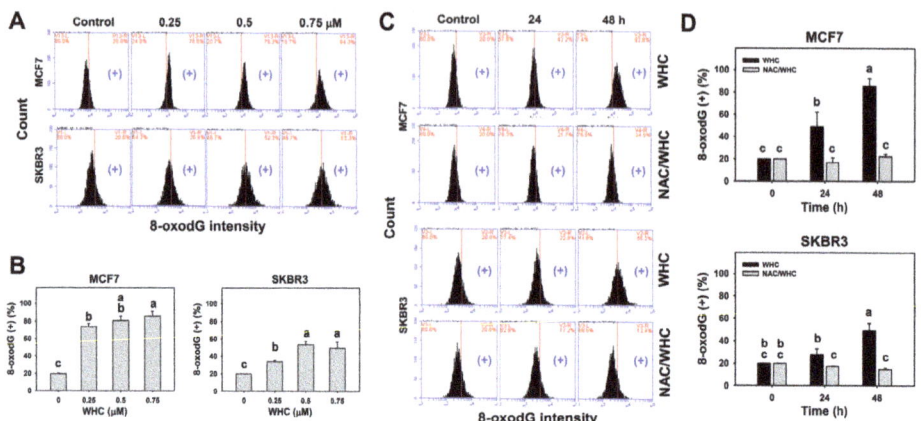

Figure 7. WHC differentially induced oxidative DNA damage (8-oxodG) of breast cancer cells. (**A,B**) 8-oxodG profiles and statistics for dose effects of WHC. Breast cancer (MCF7 and SKBR3) cells were treated with WHC (control (0.075% DMSO), 0.25, 0.5, and 0.75 µM) for 48 h. (+) located on the right side of each profile is counted for 8-oxodG (+) (%). (**C,D**) NAC pretreatments reversed the WHC induced 8-oxodG generation. Following pretreatments with NAC (10 mM for 1 h), cells were treated with control (0.075% DMSO) and 0.75 µM of WHC for 0, 24, and 48 h, i.e., NAC/WHC. Data are means ± SDs ($n = 3$). Results marked without overlapping letters show significant differences ($p < 0.05$ to 0.0001).

NAC pretreatment was used to examine the effect of ROS on WHC-induced 8-oxodG expression. Increasing 8-oxodG (+) populations of breast cancer cells after the WHC time course treatment were recovered by NAC pretreatment (Figure 7D).

4. Discussion

4.1. Withanolides Show Antiproliferative Potential for Cancer Cells

A number of withanolides showed antiproliferative activity against human breast cancer cell lines [26]. For example, the IC_{50} values for withanolide E (WHE) in a 72 h MTT study of breast cancer (MDA-MB-231 and MCF7) cells were 0.97 and 4.03 µM, respectively [13]. The IC_{50} values for withaferin A (WFA) after a 24 h MTS study of oral cancer (Ca9-22 and CAL 27) cells were 3 and 2 µM, respectively. However, WHC was not included in those study.

Recently, WHC cytotoxicity results were reported, i.e., the IC_{50} values for WHC in a 72 h MTT study of liver (HepG2 and Hep3B), lung (A549), and breast (MDA-MB-231 and MCF7) cancer cells were 0.13, 0.11, 1.24, 0.52, and 1.53 µM, respectively [13]. However, only cytotoxic IC_{50} values were reported, without addressing the detailed mechanisms.

In the current study, we found that the IC$_{50}$ values for WHC in a 48 h ATP study of breast cancer (SKBR3, MCF7, and MDA-MB-231) cells and normal breast (M10) cells were 0.134, 0.172, 0.159, and 0.191 µM, respectively (Figure 1A, left). However, different kinds of assays are helpful for double checking cell proliferation. The proliferation statuses based on MTS and ATP assays were compared. In the 48 h MTS assay, normal breast cells (M10) showed higher viability than other breast cancer cells (MCF7 and SKBR3) (Figure 1A, right). The IC$_{50}$ value for WHC in the 48 h MTS study of breast cancer (MCF7) cells was 0.89 µM. These results supported the concept that the luminescent ATP assay is more sensitive than the colorimetric MTS tetrazolium assay [27,28]. Moreover, this shows that WHC selectively kills breast cancer cells and is less harmful to normal breast cells.

In comparison, the IC$_{50}$ values for cisplatin in the 48 h MTS study of breast cancer (SKBR3 and MCF7) cells were 12.37 and 34.83 µM, respectively [22]. In the 48 h ATP study, the IC$_{50}$ values for cisplatin for breast cancer cells (SKBR3, MCF7, and MDA-MB-231) and normal breast cells (M10) were 4.9, 17.9, 26.9, and 12.0 µM, respectively (Figure 1C). This shows that cisplatin non-selectively kills more normal breast (M10) cells than breast cancer (MCF7 and MDA-MB-231) cells. Therefore, WHC has a higher drug sensitivity and selectivity to antiproliferation of breast cancer cells than cisplatin. We further suggest using a xenograft assay of breast cancer cell lines to examine the anticancer effect of WHC in an animal model (e.g., zebrafish embryo, mouse) in vivo in the future.

4.2. WHC Exhibits Higher ATP Depletion for Breast Cancer Cells than Normal Breast Cells

ATP production is the main function of mitochondria. ATP depletion may occur coupled with MitoSOX production. For example, manoalide inhibits ATP production in 3D cultures and induces MitoSOX production [17]. Accordingly, ATP depletion reflects mitochondrial impairment. Moreover, mitochondrial damage induced by proteasome inhibition also overproduces MitoSOX, subsequently triggering cytosolic oxidation and leading to cell death [29]. Consistently, we found that WHC induced ATP depletion (Figure 1) and MitoSOX (Figure 5) and ROS generation (Figure 4) in breast cancer cells (SKBR3 and MCF7).

Since ATP depletion and MitoSOX generation are related to mitochondrial dysfunction, WHC may regulate other mitochondrial functions. For example, mitochondrial fitness [30] is regulated by mitochondrial dynamic changes, such as mitochondrial fusion and fission. Detailed investigation of the mitochondrial fitness of breast cancer cells after WHC treatments would further increase our understanding.

4.3. WHC Exhibiting Antioxidant Property May Contribute to Its Antiproliferation Ability to Breast Cancer Cells

Although some structures were not identified, such as WHC, 13 of 15 constituents of *Withania somnifera* root extract showed 2,2-Diphenyl-1-picrylhydrazyl (DPPH) scavenging effects, suggesting that most constituents of *W. somnifera* show an antioxidant ability [31]. Similarly, in our preliminary result, we found that WHC showed DPPH scavenging activity (Supplementary Figure S1), suggesting that WHC is an antioxidant agent. It is known that antioxidants perform dual functions for regulating cellular oxidative stress in a dose-dependent manner [32]. Under a high dose of an antioxidant, oxidative stress is induced. This concept may partly explain how WHC exhibiting an antioxidant property may induce oxidative stress which inhibits proliferation of breast cancer cells.

4.4. WHC Induces Differential Oxidative Stress and Apoptosis in Breast Cancer Cells

Generally, cancer cells show higher ROS levels than normal cells [33]. In chemotherapy, oxidative stress-modulating anticancer drugs commonly produce higher oxidative stress levels in cancer cells than in normal cells. Consequently, the drugs generate oxidative stress that is beyond ROS tolerance thresholds in cancer cells and inhibit cancer cell proliferation. In contrast, drug-generated oxidative stress in normal cells is less than their ROS tolerance threshold and is tolerated by normal cells. As a consequence, drug-generated oxidative stress selectively kills cancer cells [8,34–37]. This is partly attributed to the fact that oxidative stress can induce early apoptosis [38] by triggering mitochondrial dysfunction [39,40]. For example, withanone demonstrated selective killing and apoptosis against breast cancer cells [8]. Similarly, WHC induced more ATP depletion, ROS generation, and apoptosis (annexin V) in breast cancer cells (SKBR3 and MCF7) than in normal breast cells (Figure 1, Figure 3, and Figure 4), showing a selective killing potential to breast cancer cells.

Moreover, redox homeostasis is unbalanced when the antioxidant system is suppressed, resulting in oxidative stress overexpression after WHC treatment. This rational is further supported by our finding that GSH depletion was induced by WHC in breast cancer cells. Since oxidative stress is a kind of systemic cellular response, central metabolism/signaling pathways are likely involved here. For example, ROS may enhance glycolysis [41]. The TP53-inducible regulator of glycolysis and apoptosis (TIGAR) promotes the pentose phosphate pathway (PPP) [37] to generate the reduced form of nicotinamide adenine dinucleotide phosphate (NADPH) and prevent oxidative stress. Therefore, it warrants further investigation to explore the role of central metabolism/signaling pathways, such as glycolysis and PPP, in WHC-treated breast cancer cells in the future.

4.5. WHC Triggers DNA Damage in Breast Cancer Cells

Oxidative stress at a cytotoxic level is able to induce DNA damage [17,19,42,43]. Consistently, we found that WHC induced oxidative stress, such ROS and MitoSOX, and, therefore, was prone to lead to γH2AX DNA double strand breaks and 8-oxodG oxidative DNA damage in breast cancer cells (SKBR3 and MCF7) (Figures 6 and 7).

4.6. NAC Reverts WHC-Induced Oxidative Stress Associated Changes in Breast Cancer Cells

All WHC-induced oxidative stress-associated changes were suppressed by NAC pretreatment. This holds for ATP depletion, cell cycle arrest, apoptosis, ROS/MitoSOX generation, and γH2AX/8-oxodG DNA damage. These results suggest that WHC-induced antiproliferation of breast cancer cells is oxidative stress-dependent.

5. Conclusions

A series of withanolides have been reported to exhibit antiproliferation potential against several types of cancer cells. However, the anticancer effect of WHC was rarely evaluated, especially on breast cancer cells. In the current study, the antiproliferation effect of WHC on breast cancer cells was confirmed. Detailed mechanisms of breast cancer cell antiproliferation were explored. The mechanisms were confirmed to depend on oxidative stress by NAC pretreatment experiments. Therefore, WHC showing antiproliferation effects represents a potential natural anticancer product against breast cancer cells by generating oxidative stress-mediated cell cycle changes, apoptosis, and DNA damage.

Supplementary Materials: The following are available online at http://www.mdpi.com/2076-3921/9/9/873/s1, Figure S1: The DPPH radical scavenging activity of WHC.

Author Contributions: Conceptualization, H.-W.C. and F.O.-Y.; Data curation, T.-J.Y.; Formal analysis, T.-J.Y. and W.-J.L.; Methodology, J.-Y.T., L.-C.L., F.-R.C., Y.-B.C.; Supervision, F.O.-Y. and H.-W.C.; Writing—original draft, T.-J.Y. and H.-W.C.; Writing—review and editing, F.O.-Y. and H.-W.C. All authors have read and agreed to the published version of the manuscript.

Funding: This work was partly supported by funds from the Ministry of Science and Technology (MOST 108-2320-B-037-015-MY3, MOST 108-2314-B-037-080, MOST 109-2314-B-037-018), the National Sun Yat-sen University-Kaohsiung Medical University (KMU) Joint Research Project (#NSYSUKMU 109-I002), the Chimei-KMU joint project (109CM-KMU-007), the Kaohsiung Medical University Hospital (KMUH104-4R20), the Kaohsiung Medical University Research Center (KMU-TC108A04), and the Health and Welfare Surcharge of Tobacco Products, the Ministry of Health and Welfare, Taiwan, China (MOHW 109-TDU-B-212-134016). The authors thank our colleague Hans-Uwe Dahms for editing the manuscript.

Conflicts of Interest: The authors declare that there are no conflicts of interest among them.

References

1. Chen, L.X.; He, H.; Qiu, F. Natural withanolides: An overview. *Nat. Prod. Rep.* **2011**, *28*, 705–740. [CrossRef] [PubMed]
2. Huang, M.; He, J.X.; Hu, H.X.; Zhang, K.; Wang, X.N.; Zhao, B.B.; Lou, H.X.; Ren, D.M.; Shen, T. Withanolides from the genus *Physalis*: A review on their phytochemical and pharmacological aspects. *J. Pharm. Pharmacol.* **2020**, *72*, 649–669. [CrossRef] [PubMed]
3. Samadi, A.K. Chapter three—Potential anticancer properties and mechanisms of action of withanolides. In *The Enzymes*; Bathaie, S.Z., Tamanoi, F., Eds.; Academic Press: Cambridge, MA, USA, 2015; Volume 37, pp. 73–94.
4. Chang, H.W.; Li, R.N.; Wang, H.R.; Liu, J.R.; Tang, J.Y.; Huang, H.W.; Chan, Y.H.; Yen, C.Y. Withaferin A induces oxidative stress-mediated apoptosis and DNA damage in oral cancer cells. *Front. Physiol.* **2017**, *8*, 634. [CrossRef] [PubMed]
5. Xia, S.; Miao, Y.; Liu, S. Withaferin A induces apoptosis by ROS-dependent mitochondrial dysfunction in human colorectal cancer cells. *Biochem. Biophys. Res. Commun.* **2018**, *503*, 2363–2369. [CrossRef] [PubMed]
6. Royston, K.J.; Paul, B.; Nozell, S.; Rajbhandari, R.; Tollefsbol, T.O. Withaferin A and sulforaphane regulate breast cancer cell cycle progression through epigenetic mechanisms. *Exp. Cell Res.* **2018**, *368*, 67–74. [CrossRef] [PubMed]
7. Chiu, C.C.; Haung, J.W.; Chang, F.R.; Huang, K.J.; Huang, H.M.; Huang, H.W.; Chou, C.K.; Wu, Y.C.; Chang, H.W. Golden berry-derived 4beta-hydroxywithanolide E for selectively killing oral cancer cells by generating ROS, DNA damage, and apoptotic pathways. *PLoS ONE* **2013**, *8*, e64739. [CrossRef]
8. Widodo, N.; Priyandoko, D.; Shah, N.; Wadhwa, R.; Kaul, S.C. Selective killing of cancer cells by Ashwagandha leaf extract and its component Withanone involves ROS signaling. *PLoS ONE* **2010**, *5*, e13536. [CrossRef]
9. Henrich, C.J.; Brooks, A.D.; Erickson, K.L.; Thomas, C.L.; Bokesch, H.R.; Tewary, P.; Thompson, C.R.; Pompei, R.J.; Gustafson, K.R.; McMahon, J.B.; et al. Withanolide E sensitizes renal carcinoma cells to TRAIL-induced apoptosis by increasing cFLIP degradation. *Cell Death Dis.* **2015**, *6*, e1666. [CrossRef]
10. Park, J.W.; Min, K.J.; Kim, D.E.; Kwon, T.K. Withaferin A induces apoptosis through the generation of thiol oxidation in human head and neck cancer cells. *Int. J. Mol. Med.* **2015**, *35*, 247–252. [CrossRef]
11. Mayola, E.; Gallerne, C.; Esposti, D.D.; Martel, C.; Pervaiz, S.; Larue, L.; Debuire, B.; Lemoine, A.; Brenner, C.; Lemaire, C. Withaferin A induces apoptosis in human melanoma cells through generation of reactive oxygen species and down-regulation of Bcl-2. *Apoptosis* **2011**, *16*, 1014–1027. [CrossRef]
12. Holliday, D.L.; Speirs, V. Choosing the right cell line for breast cancer research. *Breast Cancer Res.* **2011**, *13*, 215. [CrossRef] [PubMed]
13. Lan, Y.H.; Chang, F.R.; Pan, M.J.; Wu, C.C.; Wu, S.J.; Chen, S.L.; Wang, S.S.; Wu, M.J.; Wu, Y.C. New cytotoxic withanolides from *Physalis peruviana*. *Food Chem.* **2009**, *116*, 462–469. [CrossRef]
14. Li, Y.; Li, W.; Ying, Z.; Tian, H.; Zhu, X.; Li, J.; Li, M. Metastatic heterogeneity of breast cancer cells is associated with expression of a heterogeneous TGFβ-activating miR424–503 gene cluster. *Cancer Res.* **2014**, *74*, 6107–6118. [CrossRef] [PubMed]
15. Gomez-Cuadrado, L.; Tracey, N.; Ma, R.; Qian, B.; Brunton, V.G. Mouse models of metastasis: Progress and prospects. *Dis. Model Mech.* **2017**, *10*, 1061–1074. [CrossRef] [PubMed]
16. Chen, C.Y.; Yen, C.Y.; Wang, H.R.; Yang, H.P.; Tang, J.Y.; Huang, H.W.; Hsu, S.H.; Chang, H.W. Tenuifolide B from *Cinnamomum tenuifolium* stem selectively inhibits proliferation of oral cancer cells via apoptosis, ROS generation, mitochondrial depolarization, and DNA damage. *Toxins* **2016**, *8*, 319. [CrossRef]
17. Wang, H.R.; Tang, J.Y.; Wang, Y.Y.; Farooqi, A.A.; Yen, C.Y.; Yuan, S.F.; Huang, H.W.; Chang, H.W. Manoalide preferentially provides antiproliferation of oral cancer cells by oxidative stress-mediated apoptosis and DNA damage. *Cancers* **2019**, *11*, 1303. [CrossRef]
18. Huang, C.H.; Yeh, J.M.; Chan, W.H. Hazardous impacts of silver nanoparticles on mouse oocyte maturation and fertilization and fetal development through induction of apoptotic processes. *Environ. Toxicol.* **2018**, *33*, 1039–1049. [CrossRef]
19. Wang, T.S.; Lin, C.P.; Chen, Y.P.; Chao, M.R.; Li, C.C.; Liu, K.L. CYP450-mediated mitochondrial ROS production involved in arecoline N-oxide-induced oxidative damage in liver cell lines. *Environ. Toxicol.* **2018**, *33*, 1029–1038. [CrossRef] [PubMed]

20. Yu, C.; Chen, J.; Huang, L. A study on the antitumour effect of total flavonoids from *Pteris multifida* Poir in H22 tumour-bearing mice. *Afr. J. Tradit. Complement. Altern. Med.* **2013**, *10*, 459–463. [CrossRef] [PubMed]
21. Yen, C.Y.; Chiu, C.C.; Haung, R.W.; Yeh, C.C.; Huang, K.J.; Chang, K.F.; Hseu, Y.C.; Chang, F.R.; Chang, H.W.; Wu, Y.C. Antiproliferative effects of goniothalamin on Ca9-22 oral cancer cells through apoptosis, DNA damage and ROS induction. *Mutat. Res.* **2012**, *747*, 253–258. [CrossRef]
22. Ou-Yang, F.; Tsai, I.H.; Tang, J.Y.; Yen, C.Y.; Cheng, Y.B.; Farooqi, A.A.; Chen, S.R.; Yu, S.Y.; Kao, J.K.; Chang, H.W. Antiproliferation for breast cancer cells by ethyl acetate extract of *Nepenthes thorellii* x (*ventricosa* x *maxima*). *Int. J. Mol. Sci.* **2019**, *20*, 3238. [CrossRef] [PubMed]
23. Chang, Y.T.; Huang, C.Y.; Tang, J.Y.; Liaw, C.C.; Li, R.N.; Liu, J.R.; Sheu, J.H.; Chang, H.W. Reactive oxygen species mediate soft corals-derived sinuleptolide-induced antiproliferation and DNA damage in oral cancer cells. *Onco Targets Ther.* **2017**, *10*, 3289–3297. [CrossRef] [PubMed]
24. Tang, J.Y.; Peng, S.Y.; Cheng, Y.B.; Wang, C.L.; Farooqi, A.A.; Yu, T.J.; Hou, M.F.; Wang, S.C.; Yen, C.H.; Chan, L.P.; et al. Ethyl acetate extract of *Nepenthes adrianii* x *clipeata* induces antiproliferation, apoptosis, and DNA damage against oral cancer cells through oxidative stress. *Environ. Toxicol.* **2019**, *34*, 891–901. [CrossRef]
25. Tang, J.Y.; Huang, H.W.; Wang, H.R.; Chan, Y.C.; Haung, J.W.; Shu, C.W.; Wu, Y.C.; Chang, H.W. 4beta-Hydroxywithanolide E selectively induces oxidative DNA damage for selective killing of oral cancer cells. *Environ. Toxicol.* **2018**, *33*, 295–304. [CrossRef]
26. Machin, R.P.; Veleiro, A.S.; Nicotra, V.E.; Oberti, J.C.; Padrón, J.M. Antiproliferative activity of withanolides against human breast cancer cell lines. *J. Nat. Prod.* **2010**, *73*, 966–968. [CrossRef] [PubMed]
27. Riss, T.L.; Moravec, R.A.; Niles, A.L.; Duellman, S.; Benink, H.A.; Worzella, T.J.; Minor, L. Cell viability assays. In *Assay Guidance Manual*; Markossian, S., Sittampalam, G.S., Grossman, A., Brimacombe, K., Arkin, M., Auld, D., Austin, C.P., Baell, J., Caaveiro, J.M.M., Chung, T.D.Y., Eds.; Bethesda: Rockville, MD, USA, 2004.
28. Ozturk, S.; Erkisa, M.; Oran, S.; Ulukaya, E.; Celikler, S.; Ari, F. Lichens exerts an anti-proliferative effect on human breast and lung cancer cells through induction of apoptosis. *Drug Chem Toxicol* **2019**, 1–9. [CrossRef] [PubMed]
29. Maharjan, S.; Oku, M.; Tsuda, M.; Hoseki, J.; Sakai, Y. Mitochondrial impairment triggers cytosolic oxidative stress and cell death following proteasome inhibition. *Sci. Rep.* **2014**, *4*, 5896. [CrossRef]
30. Rossman, M.J.; Gioscia-Ryan, R.A.; Clayton, Z.S.; Murphy, M.P.; Seals, D.R. Targeting mitochondrial fitness as a strategy for healthy vascular aging. *Clin. Sci.* **2020**, *134*, 1491–1519. [CrossRef]
31. Devkar, S.T.; Jagtap, S.D.; Katyare, S.S.; Hegde, M.V. Estimation of antioxidant potential of individual components present in complex mixture of *Withania somnifera* (Ashwagandha) root fraction by thin-layer chromatography-2,2-diphenyl-1-picrylhdrazyl method. *JPC J Planar Chromatogr. Mod. TLC* **2014**, *27*, 157–161. [CrossRef]
32. Bouayed, J.; Bohn, T. Exogenous antioxidants–Double-edged swords in cellular redox state: Health beneficial effects at physiologic doses versus deleterious effects at high doses. *Oxid. Med. Cell. Longev.* **2010**, *3*, 228–237. [CrossRef]
33. Trachootham, D.; Alexandre, J.; Huang, P. Targeting cancer cells by ROS-mediated mechanisms: A radical therapeutic approach? *Nat. Rev. Drug Discov.* **2009**, *8*, 579–591. [CrossRef] [PubMed]
34. Lee, J.C.; Hou, M.F.; Huang, H.W.; Chang, F.R.; Yeh, C.C.; Tang, J.Y.; Chang, H.W. Marine algal natural products with anti-oxidative, anti-inflammatory, and anti-cancer properties. *Cancer Cell Int.* **2013**, *13*, 55. [CrossRef] [PubMed]
35. Sun, Y.; St Clair, D.K.; Xu, Y.; Crooks, P.A.; Clair, W.H.S. A NADPH oxidase-dependent redox signaling pathway mediates the selective radiosensitization effect of parthenolide in prostate cancer cells. *Cancer Res.* **2010**, *70*, 2880–2890. [CrossRef]
36. Suzuki-Karasaki, Y.; Suzuki-Karasaki, M.; Uchida, M.; Ochiai, T. Depolarization controls TRAIL-sensitization and tumor-selective killing of cancer cells: Crosstalk with ROS. *Front. Oncol.* **2014**, *4*, 128. [CrossRef]
37. Tang, J.Y.; Ou-Yang, F.; Hou, M.F.; Huang, H.W.; Wang, H.R.; Li, K.T.; Fayyaz, S.; Shu, C.W.; Chang, H.W. Oxidative stress-modulating drugs have preferential anticancer effects—Involving the regulation of apoptosis, DNA damage, endoplasmic reticulum stress, autophagy, metabolism, and migration. *Semin. Cancer Biol.* **2019**, *58*, 109–117. [CrossRef] [PubMed]

38. Samhan-Arias, A.K.; Martin-Romero, F.J.; Gutierrez-Merino, C. Kaempferol blocks oxidative stress in cerebellar granule cells and reveals a key role for reactive oxygen species production at the plasma membrane in the commitment to apoptosis. *Free Radic. Biol. Med.* **2004**, *37*, 48–61. [CrossRef]
39. Oh, S.H.; Lim, S.C. A rapid and transient ROS generation by cadmium triggers apoptosis via caspase-dependent pathway in HepG2 cells and this is inhibited through N-acetylcysteine-mediated catalase upregulation. *Toxicol. Appl. Pharmacol.* **2006**, *212*, 212–223. [CrossRef]
40. Li, J.J.; Tang, Q.; Li, Y.; Hu, B.R.; Ming, Z.Y.; Fu, Q.; Qian, J.Q.; Xiang, J.Z. Role of oxidative stress in the apoptosis of hepatocellular carcinoma induced by combination of arsenic trioxide and ascorbic acid. *Acta Pharmacol. Sin.* **2006**, *27*, 1078–1084. [CrossRef]
41. Ghanbari Movahed, Z.; Rastegari-Pouyani, M.; Mohammadi, M.H.; Mansouri, K. Cancer cells change their glucose metabolism to overcome increased ROS: One step from cancer cell to cancer stem cell? *Biomed. Pharmacother.* **2019**, *112*, 108690. [CrossRef]
42. Wu, C.F.; Lee, M.G.; El-Shazly, M.; Lai, K.H.; Ke, S.C.; Su, C.W.; Shih, S.P.; Sung, P.J.; Hong, M.C.; Wen, Z.H.; et al. Isoaaptamine induces T-47D cells apoptosis and autophagy via oxidative stress. *Mar. Drugs* **2018**, *16*, 18. [CrossRef]
43. Hung, J.H.; Chen, C.Y.; Omar, H.A.; Huang, K.Y.; Tsao, C.C.; Chiu, C.C.; Chen, Y.L.; Chen, P.H.; Teng, Y.N. Reactive oxygen species mediate Terbufos-induced apoptosis in mouse testicular cell lines via the modulation of cell cycle and pro-apoptotic proteins. *Environ. Toxicol.* **2016**, *31*, 1888–1898. [CrossRef] [PubMed]

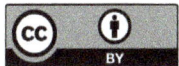

© 2020 by the authors. Licensee MDPI, Basel, Switzerland. This article is an open access article distributed under the terms and conditions of the Creative Commons Attribution (CC BY) license (http://creativecommons.org/licenses/by/4.0/).

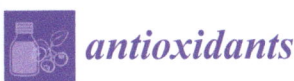

Article

Unique Cellular and Biochemical Features of Human Mitochondrial Peroxiredoxin 3 Establish the Molecular Basis for Its Specific Reaction with Thiostrepton

Kimberly J. Nelson [1,†], Terri Messier [2,†], Stephanie Milczarek [2], Alexis Saaman [2], Stacie Beuschel [2], Uma Gandhi [1], Nicholas Heintz [2], Terrence L. Smalley, Jr. [1], W. Todd Lowther [1,3,*] and Brian Cunniff [2,*]

[1] Center for Structural Biology, Department of Biochemistry, Wake Forest School of Medicine, Medical Center Blvd., Winston-Salem, NC 27157, USA; kjnelson@wakehealth.edu (K.J.N.); ugandhi@wakehealth.edu (U.G.); tsmalley@wakehealth.edu (T.L.S.J.)
[2] Department of Pathology and Laboratory Medicine, University of Vermont Cancer Center, Larner College of Medicine, University of Vermont, 149 Beaumont Ave., Burlington, VT 05405, USA; Terri.Messier@med.uvm.edu (T.M.); stephanie.milczarek@med.uvm.edu (S.M.); alexis.saaman@gmail.com (A.S.); grnmtntarheel@gmail.com (S.B.); nicholas.heintz@med.uvm.edu (N.H.)
[3] Wake Forest Baptist Comprehensive Cancer Center, Medical Center Blvd., Winston-Salem, NC 27157, USA
* Correspondence: tlowther@wakehealth.edu (W.T.L.); bcunniff@uvm.edu (B.C.); Tel.: +336-716-7420 (W.T.L.); +802-656-2188 (B.C.)
† These authors contributed equally to this work.

Abstract: A central hallmark of tumorigenesis is metabolic alterations that increase mitochondrial reactive oxygen species (mROS). In response, cancer cells upregulate their antioxidant capacity and redox-responsive signaling pathways. A promising chemotherapeutic approach is to increase ROS to levels incompatible with tumor cell survival. Mitochondrial peroxiredoxin 3 (PRX3) plays a significant role in detoxifying hydrogen peroxide (H_2O_2). PRX3 is a molecular target of thiostrepton (TS), a natural product and FDA-approved antibiotic. TS inactivates PRX3 by covalently adducting its two catalytic cysteine residues and crosslinking the homodimer. Using cellular models of malignant mesothelioma, we show here that PRX3 expression and mROS levels in cells correlate with sensitivity to TS and that TS reacts selectively with PRX3 relative to other PRX isoforms. Using recombinant PRXs 1–5, we demonstrate that TS preferentially reacts with a reduced thiolate in the PRX3 dimer at mitochondrial pH. We also show that partially oxidized PRX3 fully dissociates to dimers, while partially oxidized PRX1 and PRX2 remain largely decameric. The ability of TS to react with engineered dimers of PRX1 and PRX2 at mitochondrial pH, but inefficiently with wild-type decameric protein at cytoplasmic pH, supports a novel mechanism of action and explains the specificity of TS for PRX3. Thus, the unique structure and propensity of PRX3 to form dimers contribute to its increased sensitivity to TS-mediated inactivation, making PRX3 a promising target for prooxidant cancer therapy.

Keywords: mitochondrial reactive oxygen species; peroxiredoxin 3; pro-oxidant therapy; thiostrepton

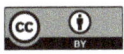

1. Introduction

Thiostrepton (TS) is an FDA-approved, thiazole antibiotic produced by Streptomycetes. A recent study reported by Corsello et al. tested the ability of 4518 drugs from the Drug Repurposing Hub at the Broad Institute to kill 578 cancer cells lines [1]. TS showed significant efficacy in 403 tumor cells lines. Thus, TS was highlighted as "a drug of greatest interest for mechanistic follow-up." Importantly, previous work from our groups identified peroxiredoxin 3 (PRX3) as a key molecular target of TS [2,3]. Our data demonstrated that TS irreversibly crosslinks PRX3 through its active site Cys residues to form inactive covalent dimers, leading to increased mROS levels, reduced FOXM1 expression and anti-tumor activity in both in vitro and in vivo malignant mesothelioma (MM) tumor models.

PRX3 like all other PRXs share a common first step in catalysis in which the peroxidatic cysteine residue attacks a molecule of hydroperoxide to form a Cys sulfenic acid intermediate (Cys-S$_P$OH) (Figure 1) [4]. This intermediate then reacts with the resolving Cys residue (Cys-S$_R$). For the PRXs 1–4 (called the typical 2-Cys or PRX1 class), the disulfide bond formed is intermolecular across the subunit interface of the head-to-tail homodimer. Reduction of the disulfide-bonded dimers is catalyzed by thioredoxin 1 (TRX1) in the cytosol and thioredoxin 2 (TRX2) in the mitochondria [5].

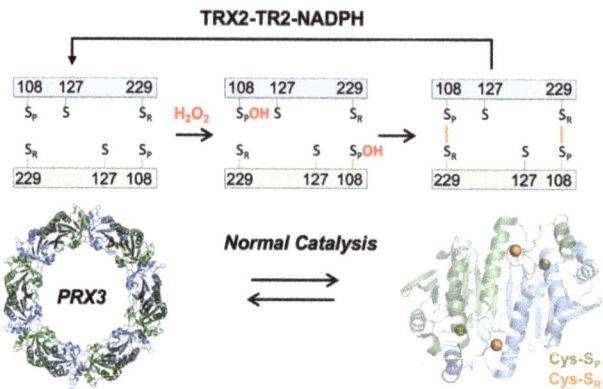

Figure 1. Catalytic cycle of PRX3. Hydrogen peroxide reacts with the peroxidatic Cys residue (Cys108-S$_P$) to form a Cys-sulfenic acid intermediate (Cys108-S$_P$OH). The resolving Cys residue (Cys229-S$_R$) then reacts to form a disulfide. Disulfide bond formation facilitates collapse of the dodecamer to form 6 dimers; reduction of the disulfide by the thioredoxin 2-thioredoxin reductase 2-NADPH (TRX2-TR2-NADPH) reducing system shifts the equilibrium back toward dodecamer. Note that each active site can form a disulfide bond in the absence of TS. In the presence of TS, the data herein supports the formation of an asymmetric dimer with 1 disulfide and 1 TS-mediated crosslink.

Despite the mechanistic and primary sequence similarity, the 2-Cys mechanistic class members differ in: (i) their oligomeric state (e.g., PRX3 is active as a dodecamer, while PRX2 is a decamer), (ii) the thioredoxin-thioredoxin reductase (TRX-TR) system used, (iii) their specificity for hydroperoxide substrates, (iv) disulfide bond formation and reduction rates, (v) susceptibility to hyperoxidation, and (vi) subcellular distribution [4,6–9]. PRX1 and PRX2 reside in the cytoplasm. PRX3 is exclusively expressed in the mitochondrial matrix, and PRX4 is expressed in the endoplasmic reticulum. In contrast, PRX5 contains both mitochondrial and peroxisomal targeting sequences and belongs to a different class of PRXs, where the resolving Cys residue is in the same subunit and an intramolecular disulfide bond is formed during catalysis [4,10]. Because of the high degree of similarity between the PRX active sites and the different roles for these proteins in the cell, the identification of selective PRX inhibitors is both highly challenging and critical to the development of PRX-based therapeutics.

In this study, we demonstrated that TS cytotoxicity is correlated with expression levels of PRX3 and mitochondrial ROS (mROS) levels using a panel of normal mesothelial and patient-derived malignant mesothelioma (MM) cell lines. This activity is not dependent upon the mitochondrial membrane potential. Western blot analysis of PRXs 1–5 shows that only the formation of the PRX3-TS adduct is potentiated by gentian violet (GV), but this reaction does depend upon the mitochondrial membrane potential. Detailed biochemical studies with purified PRXs 1–5 support the observed cellular specificity. In particular, the higher pH of the mitochondrial compartment and the unique oligomeric state dynamics and redox properties of PRX3 make it the most sensitive to TS adduction. Since PRX3 is overexpressed in most cancers, targeting PRX3 with a specific inhibitor represents a significant therapeutic opportunity.

2. Materials and Methods

2.1. Reagents and Chemicals

Thiostrepton (Millipore, Burlington, MA, USA), Gentian Violet (Sigma, St. Louis, MO, USA), 2-[2-[4-(trifluoromethoxy)phenyl]hydrazinylidene]-propanedinitrile (FCCP, Sigma), S-Methyl Methanethiosulfonate (MMTS, TCI Chemicals, Portland, OR, USA), Bovine Serum Albumin (BSA, GOLDBIO, St. Louis, MO, USA), TCEP (Fisher, Waltham, MA, USA), DTT (Fisher) Optima HPLC grade water (Fisher), hydrogen peroxide (Honeywell, Charlotte, NC, USA), NADPH (Roche, Basel, Switzerland), IPTG (Fisher), glucose 6-phosphate dehydrogenase (Alfa Aesar, Haverhill, MA, USA), glucose 6-phosphate (ACROS Organics, Morris Plains, NJ, USA), BioGel P6 Resin (BioRad, Hercules, CA, USA).

2.2. Cells and Cell Culture

Primary and immortalized mesothelial cells and malignant mesothelioma cells were cultured as previously described [2,3]. The STR profiles are of human origin, analysis was performed in the Vermont Integrative Genomics Resource DNA Facility and was supported by University of Vermont Cancer Center, Lake Champlain Cancer Research Organization, and the UVM Larner College of Medicine. The STR profiles matched previously annotated DNA fingerprints [3].

2.3. Immunoblotting

Cells were plated in 6 well plates at a density of 200,000 cells per well. After 24 h, cells were treated with indicated compounds as described in the text. Cell lysates were harvested at indicated time points using RIPA buffer (50 mM Tris-HCl, 150 mM NaCl, 1 mM EDTA, 1% NP-40, 0.25% Sodium deoxycholate, 0.1% sodium dodecyl sulfate, in deionized (DI) water) for reducing samples to be analyzed by reducing SDS-PAGE. For samples to be analyzed by non-reducing SDS-PAGE, cells were incubated in 100 mM S-Methyl Methanethiosulfonate (MMTS, TCI), to prevent artifactual oxidation of reduced cysteines, diluted in warm PBS for 20 min followed by lysis with RIPA buffer containing 100 mM MMTS. Protein concentrations were determined via Bradford Assay (ThermoScientific, Rockford, IL, USA). Lysates (15 μg protein/well) were resolved by SDS-PAGE under reducing conditions (Dithiothreitol (DTT) was omitted for non-reducing gels) on 4–12% gradient Bis-Tris Midi gel (Invitrogen, Carlsbad, CA, USA) at constant 200 V for 50 m. The gel was transferred to a PVDF membrane at constant 1A for 50 min, blocked with 5% BSA diluted in 1× Tris-buffered saline with 1% Tween-20 (TBS-T) for a minimum of one h, and incubated with appropriate primary antibody (Table S1) at indicated dilution in 5% BSA TBS-T at 4 °C overnight. The membrane was washed with 1× TBS-T for 1 h, incubated with appropriate secondary antibody at indicated dilution for 1 h, and washed again with 1× TBS-T for 1 h. Membranes were incubated with ECL Reagent (ThermoScientific, Rockford, IL, USA) and visualized using a GE Amersham Imager chemiluminescent detection system. Blots were washed with 1× TBS-T and re-probed with loading control antibody to verify equal protein loading. Densitometry was performed using ImageJ (NIH).

2.4. Cell Viability Assays

Cell Lines were plated in 96-well plates (Corning, Kennebunk, ME, USA) at a density of 2500 cells per well. The following day, cells were treated with test compounds diluted in complete media followed by incubation for 48 h. Post-incubation cells were washed with PBS (Corning Cellgro, Manassas, VA, USA), fixed with 3.0% formaldehyde (Fisher BioReagents, Fair Lawn, NJ, USA) in PBS, and stained for 30 min with 0.1% crystal violet (Acros Organics, Fair Lawn, NJ, USA) in water. Crystal violet stain was removed, and plates were washed with H_2O and allowed to dry. To quantify cell viability, plates were imaged using the Lionheart Plate reader (BioTek Instruments, Winooski, VT, USA) and/or analyzed by absorbance at 540 nm (crystal violet dye dissolved in 100% methanol) using the Synergy HTX plate reader (BioTek Instruments, Winooski, VT, USA). To determine the effective cytotoxic concentration (EC_{50}) of test compounds the data were plotted using a 4-parameter non-linear regression model using GraphPad Prism7 software (GraphPad Software, San Diego, CA, USA).

2.5. Agilent Seahorse XF Cell Mito Stress Test Assay

A total of 6000 cells of each cell line were plated in 80 µL complete media into individual wells of a XF96 cell culture microplate excluding cells from 4 corner control wells (5 technical replicates per assay). The following day, cells were treated with test compounds diluted in complete media followed by incubation for indicated time. Post-incubation cells were washed 2× with warm, sterile filtered Seahorse XF RPMI media supplemented with 1 mM pyruvate, 2 mM glutamine, and 10 mM glucose at pH 7.4. 80 µL of supplemented Seahorse XF RPMI assay media was added back to each well. Cells were allowed to equilibrate for 1 h in a 37 °C CO_2 free humidified incubator before loading into a XFe96 extracellular flux analyzer temperature adjusted to 37 °C (Seahorse Bioscience, Billerica, MA, USA). Sensor cartridges were equilibrated with XF calibrant for 24 h before loading with inhibitors. Inhibitor concentrations were titrated to determine optimal drug concentrations to establish bioenergetic profiles (data not shown), final well concentrations used were 1.0 µM oligomycin, 1.0 µM carbonyl cyanide-4 (trifluoromethoxy) phenylhydrazone (FCCP), and 0.5 µM rotenone and antimycin A. Oxygen and proton concentrations were measured every 8.5 min for 1 h and 35 min, inhibitors (oligomycin, FCCP, rotenone/antimycin A, respectively) to measure mitochondrial bioenergetics were added to the plates through the microinjection ports at the indicated time points. Oxygen consumption rates (OCR) and spare reserve capacity (difference between maximal and basal OCR) are shown. Cells were imaged using the Lionheart FX Automated Microscope (BioTek Instruments, Winooski, VT, USA) to confirm cell adherence before and after assay.

2.6. MitoSOX Red Detection of Mitochondrial ROS

Indicated cell lines were loaded with 5 µM MitoSOX Red (Invitrogen, Carlsbad, CA, USA), diluted in DMSO, in tissue culture medium for 30 min. Cells were washed with Hanks buffered salt solution with calcium and magnesium (HBSS) and incubated with 1% BSA in HBSS. MitoSOX Red fluorescence was collected at 593 nm following excitation with the RFP filter cube (ex 531-nm) using the Lionheart Plate reader (BioTek Instruments, Winooski, VT, USA). Cell number was counted and used to normalize MitoSOX Red signal to cell number. Primary mesothelial cells immediately lifted from the plate when incubated with MitoSOX Red and therefore were not amenable to this procedure.

2.7. Expression and Purification of Recombinant Proteins

Wild-type human PRX1, PRX1 C83E, and wild-type PRX2 were expressed without a tag from the pET17b vector and purified as previously described [2]. Untagged wild-type PRX3 (residues 62–256) was expressed in C41 (DE3) cells from the PTYB21 expression vector with an N-terminal Intein fusion and purified as previously described [9]. The engineered dimer of PRX3 with and without the resolving Cys (PRX3-S139E/A142E and PRX3-S139E/A142E/C229S) as well as the engineered dimer of PRX2 (PRX2-T82E) were purified from BL21 Gold (DE3) *Escherichia coli* cells with a non-cleavable N-terminal His-tag from the pET15b vector, as previously described [2]. *E. coli* thioredoxin 2 (Trx2, the trxC gene product) was expressed and purified as previously described [11]. For all purifications, HisPur Cobalt affinity resin (Thermo Scientific, Waltham, MA, USA) was used. PRX fractions were pooled, concentrated, flash-frozen with liquid nitrogen, and stored at −80 °C until use. All proteins were stored in a buffer without dithiothreitol (DTT) except for the PRX3 C229S variant. Wild-type PRX3 was oxidized to disulfide by 1.5 equivalents H_2O_2 prior to storage.

E. coli thioredoxin reductase (eTR) was expressed from the pET15pp vector [12]. BL21 Gold (DE3) cells containing the TrxR construct were grown at 37 °C in 2 12 L fermenters until the OD_{600} = 0.8 and induced with 0.5 mM isopropyl 1-thio-β-D-galactopyranoside at 18 °C for 18–20 h. The cells were lysed in 100 ml of Affinity buffer (20 mM HEPES, pH 7.9,

500 mM KCl) supplemented with 1–2 mg FAD, 10% glycerol, 0.1% Triton X-100, 0.1 mM PMSF and 0.1 mM benzamidine using an Emulsiflex C5 homogenizer (Avestin, Inc, Ottawa, ON, Canada). After centrifugation, proteins were purified from the supernatant by affinity chromatography using HisPur cobalt affinity resin (Thermo Scientific). The N-terminal His tag was cleaved by adding 1 mg HRV-3C protease for every 15 mg of protein and allowing the cleavage to proceed overnight at 4 °C during dialysis into buffer containing 20 mM HEPES, 100 mM NaCl, pH 7.5. The fractions containing the protein of interest were further purified by Q-Sepharose FF and Superdex 200 columns (both GE Healthcare). The final storage buffer was 25 mM Hepes pH 7.5, 100 mM NaCl.

The human PRDX4 gene (residues 84–271) was codon optimized for expression in E. coli by GenScript and subcloned into the pET15pp vector. The resultant protein contained a non-cleavable, N-terminal His-tag. The engineered PRX4 dimer (T155E) was generated by Genscript from the same vector. His-tagged PRX4 and PRX4-T155E were purified as described above for eTR except that the buffers were not supplemented with FAD and no protease was added. The mature form of recombinant human PRX5 protein containing a non-cleavable N-terminal 6X His-tag was expressed and purified as previously described [13].

2.8. In Vitro Turnover Assays with TS and PRX

Reactions comparing wild-type PRXs 1–5 and engineered PRX dimers contained 100 µM PRX, 5 µM E. coli TRX2, 0.5 µM E. coli TR, and a NADPH regenerating system composed of 3.2 mM glucose 6-phosphate, 3.2 U/ml glucose 6-phosphate dehydrogenase and 0.4 mM NADPH. Samples were incubated at 37 °C with either 0.25 mM TS or an equivalent volume of DMSO (<1%). To determine the pH dependence of TS, the engineered dimers of PRX1s 1–3 were diluted to 100 µM with 5 mM TCEP in BPCDN buffer at various pH values. BPCDN buffer contains 20 mM phosphate (pK_{a2} = 7.2), 20 mM boric acid (pK_a = 9.0), 20 mM sodium citrate (pK_{a2} = 5.2), 0.2 mM diethylenetriamine pentaacetate (DTPA), and 200 mM sodium chloride and allows for a single buffer solution to be used across pH values ranging from 4.2–10 [14]. Assay components were pulsed with successive additions of 50 µM H_2O_2 to induce turnover of PRX3 and incubated at 37 °C for 10–15 min between H_2O_2 additions. Reactions were stopped by the addition of 5× SDS loading buffer containing 100 mM DTT, heated to 100 °C for 10 min, and proteins were separated by 12% SDS-PAGE and stained for total protein using GelCode Blue (Life Technologies, Carlsbad, CA, USA). The intensity of the non-reducible PRX dimer was divided by the summed intensity of all PRX bands within each lane. Results are presented as mean values ± SD from a minimum of three independent replicates. Data were analyzed by two-way ANOVA with a Tukey HSD post-hoc correction using GraphPad Prism version 7.04.

2.9. Reaction of TS with PRX3-SH vs. PRX3-SOH

The PRX3 EE C229S variant was reduced for 10–20 min at ambient temperature with 20 mM DTT. The sample was then passed through a Bio-Gel P6 spin column equilibrated in 50 mM Tris, pH 8.0 to remove excess DTT. To prevent spontaneous oxidation of the reduced protein, all buffers for this experiment were made using HPLC-grade water. To test the reduced sample, PRX3-EE-C229S was diluted to a final concentration of 20 µM and incubated for 90 min at 37 °C with either 200 µM TS, 20 mM dimedone, or an equivalent amount of DMSO. To test the sulfenic acid form of the protein, 20 µM reduced PRX3-EE-C229S was treated with 30 µM H2O2 for 3 min prior to the addition of DMSO, dimedone, or TS. Samples were stored at −20 °C overnight, and 10 µL of each sampler was passed through a 100 µL BioGel P6 column equilibrated in 25 mM ammonium acetate in HPLC water. Samples were analyzed on a Bruker Autoflex MALDI-TOF mass spectrometer in positive ion and linear acquisition mode using a matrix containing 20 mg/mL sinapic acid, 50% acetonitrile, and 0.1% formic acid in water.

2.10. SEC-MALS Analysis to Measure PRX Size Distribution

Approximate molecular weights of PRX proteins were determined using size exclusion chromatography coupled with multiangle light scattering (SEC-MALS) analysis. SEC-MALS buffers were made in HPLC water and contained 50 mM HEPES, pH 7.5 and 100 mM NaCl. PRXs were diluted into SEC-MALS buffer prior to resolution on a TSK Gel 4000 SW gel filtration column (8 μm particle size, 7.8 × 30 cm, Tosoh Biosciences, Tokyo, Japan). Chromatographic separation was performed over 35 min at a flow rate of 0.5 mL/min, monitoring elution spectrophotometrically at A_{280} and MALS using a HELIOS II detector (Wyatt Technology). Molecular weights were estimated for prominent peaks (determined from the A_{280} traces) from MALS data using Astra 6 software (Wyatt Technology, Goletta, CA, USA).

To measure the oligomeric state of reduced and oxidized PRXs at pH 7.0, 7.5, or 8.0 PRX proteins were diluted to 2 mg/mL (90–93 μM) in SEC-MALS buffer to a final volume of 0.12 mL at the indicated pH values. Reduced samples included 10 mM DTT and oxidized samples included 1.2 equivalents of H_2O_2. Chromatographic separation was performed on 100 μL (0.2 μg) PRX protein in the absence of reducing agents.

To measure the oligomeric state of PRX with sub-stoichiometric amounts of disulfide formation (Figure S6), wild-type, untagged PRX3 or PRX2 were reduced with 20 mM DTT for 10–20 min at RT. Samples were then passed through a 1 mL BioGel P6 spin column to remove excess DTT and to exchange into SEC-MALS buffer pH 7.4 (PRX2) or pH 8.0 (PRX3). PRXs were diluted to 100 μM in 120 μL SEC-MALS buffer and 24 μL of a 5 × stock of peroxide was added to obtain the desired final concentration of H_2O_2. PRX2 (100 μM) was titrated with final peroxide concentrations of: 0 (reduced), 20 μM (2/10 equivalents), 40 μM (4/10 equivalents), 60 μM (6/10 equivalents), 80 μM (8/10 equivalents), or 100 μM (1 equivalence) H_2O_2. PRX3 (93 μM) was titrated with final peroxide concentrations of: 0 (reduced), 15.5 μM (2/12 equivalents), 31 μM (4/12 equivalents), 46.0 μM (6/12 equivalents), 62 μM (8/12 equivalents), 77.5 μM (10/12 equivalents), or 93 μM (1 equivalence) H_2O_2.

3. Results

3.1. PRX3 Expression and Mitochondrial ROS Levels Correlate with Sensitivity to Thiostrepton

Aggressive tumors rely on increased antioxidant expression for survival under otherwise inhospitable redox conditions [15,16]. To determine if there was differential sensitivity to TS, we profiled a panel of primary mesothelial, normal immortalized mesothelial and MM cell lines using cell-viability assays. The concentration of TS required to kill 50, 90 and 99% (EC_{50}, EC_{90}, EC_{99}) of cells was calculated from dose-response curves (Figure 2A,B and Figure S1A). Primary and immortalized non-tumorigenic mesothelial cells were moderately sensitive to TS with EC_{50} values between ~2.8–4.7 μM. Tumorigenic MM cell lines, representative of both pleural and peritoneal disease from sarcomatoid and biphasic histologic subtypes, were more sensitive to TS compared to normal cell lines, with EC_{50} values of ~0.9–2.4 μM TS. EC_{99} values extrapolated from survival curves show MM cell lines are on average ~10 × more sensitive to TS than normal mesothelial cells at their respective EC_{99} concentrations (Figure S1A).

We next examined PRX3 protein expression levels in normal and MM cell lines by immunoblotting (Figure S1B). PRX3 protein expression is elevated in most MM cell lines compared to normal mesothelial cells (Figure 2C). We compared TS sensitivity (EC_{50}) to PRX3 protein expression levels and identified a linear relationship between the two variables (Figure 2D). The slope of the line comparing TS sensitivity and PRX3 expression was significantly non-zero ($p = 0.025$). The levels of mROS in normal and MM cell lines were also determined by staining their mitochondria with MitoSOX Red, a redox-sensitive fluorescent dye (most reactive with superoxide). The fluorescence intensity of this dye was also significantly increased in the majority of MM cell lines as compared to LP9 normal mesothelial cells (Figure 2E), indicating higher mROS levels in MM tumor cell lines. We compared TS sensitivity (EC_{50}) to MitoSOX Red fluorescence intensity and identified a linear relationship between the two variables (Figure 2F). The slope of the line comparing the levels of mROS and sensitivity to TS was significantly non-zero ($p = 0.028$). In addition, mitochondrial bioenergetics in normal and MM cell lines was evaluated using Seahorse Extracellular Flux analysis (Figure S1C). The spare reserve capacity of mitochondria in MM cells was significantly lower when compared to normal mesothelial cells (Figure S1D). Interestingly, this readout of the ability to respond to bioenergetic stress did not significantly correlate with TS sensitivity. Altogether, these data provide evidence that elevated PRX3 protein expression and increased mitochondrial oxidant levels in MM cell lines correlate with sensitivity to TS.

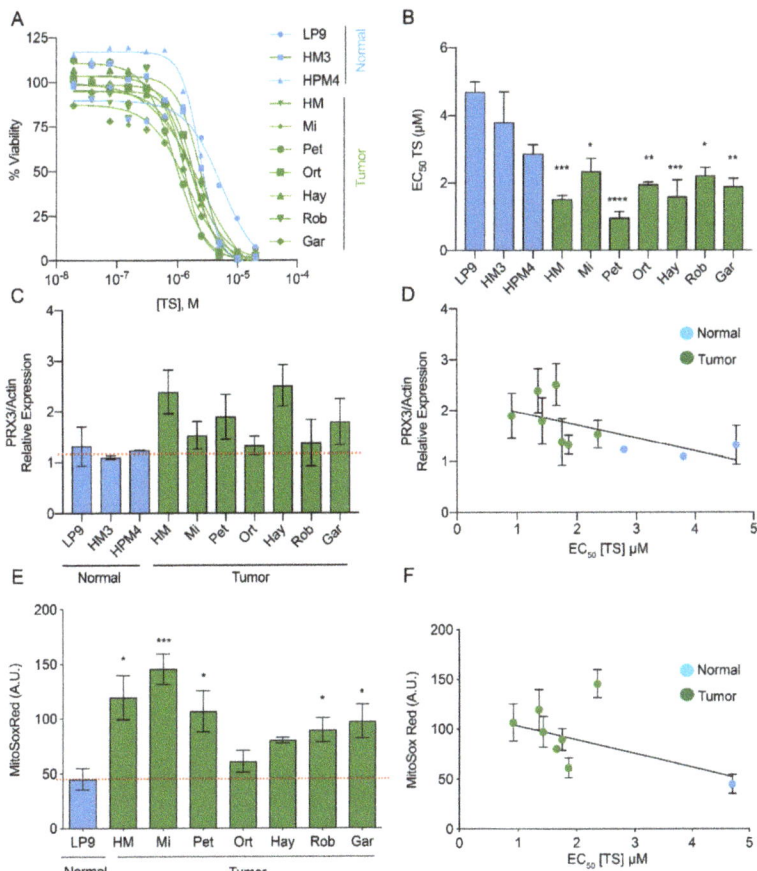

Figure 2. Mitochondrial ROS levels and PRX3 expression correlates with sensitivity to thiostrepton. (**A**) Dose-response curves of normal and MM tumor cell lines to thiostrepton (TS). (**B**) EC_{50} values for TS in normal and MM cell lines (* $p < 0.05$, ** $p < 0.01$, *** $p < 0.001$, **** $p < 0.0001$, $n = 4$ biological replicates). (**C**) Relative PRX3 protein expression levels in MM tumor and normal cells (normalized to actin; See Figure S1 for representative Western blot). Red dotted line for reference to mean expression of PRX3 in normal cell lines ($n = 2$ replicates, ±SEM). (**D**) Relationship between PRX3 expression and EC_{50} values for TS in normal and MM tumor cells ($p = 0.025$, $n = 2$). (**E**) MitoSOX Red levels in normal and MM tumor cell lines (* $p < 0.05$, *** $p < 0.001$, $n = 4$). Red dotted line for reference to mean MitoSOX Red levels in normal cells (Of note, primary mesothelial cells were not amenable to analysis using MitoSOX Red). (**F**) Relationship between MitoSOX Red levels and EC_{50} values for TS in normal and MM tumor cells (* $p = 0.028$, $n = 4$).

3.2. In Vitro (Cellular) Specificity of TS for Mitochondrial PRX3

TS induces the formation of an irreversible PRX3-TS-PRX3 protein species, in vitro and in vivo, that migrates at ~45 kDa on reducing SDS-PAGE gels, the expected molecular weight of PRX3 dimers (Figure 3A) [2]. The TS-mediated PRX crosslink persists despite the treatment of samples with 10 mM DTT in SDS buffer prior to separation by SDS-PAGE electrophoresis, indicating that the covalent TS complex is highly stable once formed. To determine whether TS was able to crosslink other typical 2-Cys PRXs in cells, MM cells were treated with 2.5 or 5 μM TS for 24 h and cell lysates were collected. We immunoblotted the cell lysates with antibodies specific for cytosolic PRX1 and PRX2, mitochondrial PRX3 and the endoplasmic reticulum (ER) localized isoform PRX4. TS induced the formation of a dose-dependent, non-reducible PRX3 dimer in MM cells (Figure 3A,B). In contrast, TS induced non-significant modifications to cytosolic PRXs 1 and 2 and had no observable effect on PRX4. These data provide evidence that TS preferentially reacts with mitochondrial PRX3 and has minimal reactivity with cytosolic or ER resident PRXs in MM cells.

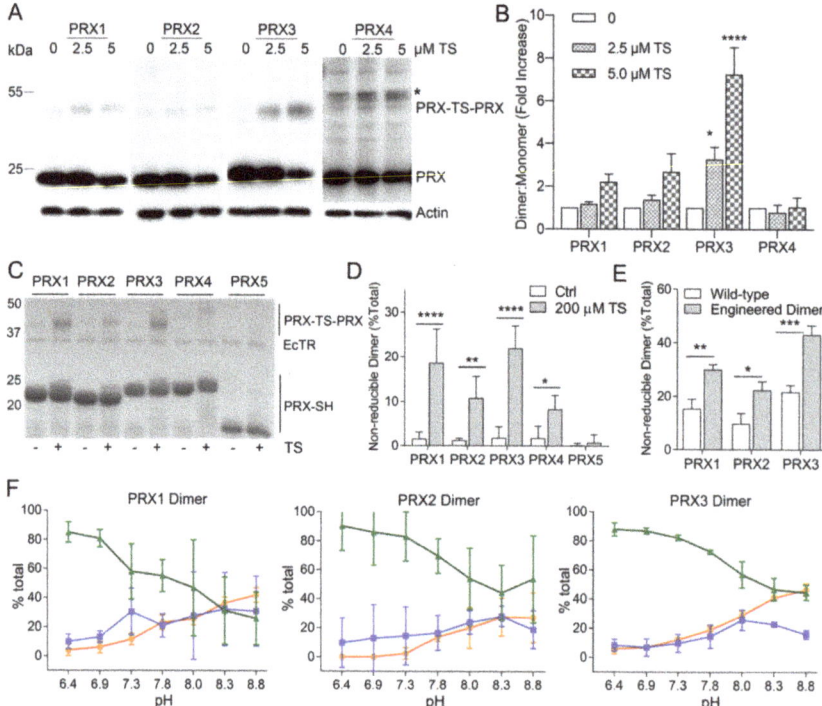

Figure 3. Specificity of TS for cellular and recombinant mitochondrial PRX3. (**A**) Western blots of PRXs 1–4 from MM tumor cells (HM cell line) incubated with indicated concentrations of TS for 24 h. Lysates were run on reducing SDS-PAGE gels (* = PRX-TS-PRX indicated the TS-mediated, cross-linked dimer, * = non-specific band in PRX4 sample). (**B**) Quantification of PRXs 1–4 covalent crosslink by TS in MM tumor cells ($n = 3$). Significance is shown relative to no TS control for each PRX. (**C**) Human PRXs 1–5 (100 μM) were cycled at 37 °C at pH 8 in the presence or absence of 50 μM TS, 5 μM E. coli TRX2, 0.5 μM E. coli TR, a NADPH regenerating system, and 6 successive additions of 50 μM H_2O_2 and run on a reducing SDS-PAGE gel. PRX4 was purified with an N-terminal His tag. PRXs 1–3 & 5 were untagged. (**D**) Quantification of the TS crosslink (dimer:total PRX ratio) for wild-type PRXs 1–5 (mean values ± SD, $n = 3$). (**E**) Quantification of TS crosslink for wild-type proteins and their dimeric variants (mean values ± SD, n = 3). WT and engineered dimers of PRXs 1–3 were untagged. (**F**) pH-dependence of TS adduct formation for the untagged, engineered dimers of PRX1, PRX2, and PRX3. The amount of reduced protein monomer (green), TS monomer adduct (blue) and TS crosslinked dimer (orange) were determined by SDS-PAGE in triplicate, see Methods for details. * p-value < 0.05, ** p-value < 0.005, *** p-value < 0.0005, and **** p-value < 0.0001.

3.3. Specificity of TS for Recombinant PRX3

Although TS exhibits a clear preference for PRX3 in cells, it is not known whether this specificity arises from innate differences in the structure and reactivity of PRX3 compared to other PRX proteins. We tested the ability of TS to form crosslinks between recombinant human PRXs 1–5. Importantly, PRXs 1–3 did not contain any extra residues or affinity tags, since the inclusion of tags can influence the oligomerization and kinetics of typical 2-Cys PRXs [17,18]. Because changes in pH are known to perturb the equilibrium between dimer and decamer/dodecamer, the protonation state of the peroxidatic and resolving Cys residues, and the activity of the E. coli TRX/TR system, our initial assays were all performed at pH 8.0 [2]. Multiple cycles of enzymatic turnover were accomplished by the addition of NADPH and six subsequent additions of 50 µM hydrogen peroxide (See Methods for details). The formation of a TS-induced crosslink was visualized by the appearance of a non-reducible dimer on a reducing SDS-PAGE gel (Figure 3C). PRXs 1–3 all showed the appearance of some cross-linked dimer (12–23%, Figure 3D) in the presence of TS. In contrast, no significant TS crosslink was observed for PRX4. PRX5 belongs to a different class of PRXs but is of interest because it does reside in the mitochondria [10]. Because the disulfide in human PRX5 is intramolecular, a TS crosslink would be expected to increase the size of the monomer rather than induce the formation of a non-reducible dimer. No TS adduct was observed for PRX5 by either gel electrophoresis or mass spectrometry (Figure 3C and Figure S2). It is important to reiterate here that these experiments were performed at pH 8.0, which mimics the mitochondrial environment. Thus, the PRX isoforms (PRXs 1, 2 and 4) that normally function in a lower pH environment may behave differently when tested under conditions that mimic their normal environment, as demonstrated in the experiments below.

3.4. Thiostrepton Preferentially Adducts Dimeric PRX Species

In solution, PRXs 1–4 proteins exist in an equilibrium between dimers and higher order oligomers that include decamers (PRXs 1, 2, and 4) and dodecamers (PRX3). This equilibrium is influenced by numerous conditions including protein concentration, ionic strength, post-translational modifications, redox state and pH [4]. In particular, the dodecamer of oxidized PRX3 is less stable and dissociates into dimers [6]. Therefore, we tested whether PRX1 and PRX2 would become more reactive to TS, if present in the dimeric form. Previous published results from our groups and others have shown that the introduction of one or two negatively charged residues into the dimer-dimer interface disrupts decamer/dodecamer formation [19–22]. The resulting PRX1 C83E, PRX2 T82E, and PRX3 S139E/A142E variants are exclusively dimeric independent of oxidation state and under the conditions used in the studies herein (Figure S3). At pH 8.0, all the engineered dimer variants formed TS-crosslinks more efficiently than the wild-type proteins (Figure 3E).

3.5. TS Adducts PRX Dimers Only at Mitochondrial pH

Performing in vitro experiments at pH 8 is only relevant for mitochondrial PRX3, where pH values range between 7.5 and 8.2; the pH of the cytosol is significantly lower (7.0–7.2) [23]. To determine whether the pH differences between the subcellular compartments contribute to the observed selectivity of TS in vivo, TS reactivity with human PRXs 1–3 were evaluated across a range of pH values (Figure S4). For these experiments, we used TCEP as an alternative reducing system because it is able to efficiently reduce disulfides across a broad pH range [24], unlike the TRX-TR system [25]. TS was more reactive with WT PRXs 1–3 at the higher pH values (5–15% PRX-TS-PRX adduct) found in the mitochondria compared to the lower pH values found in the cytosol (2–5% PRX-TS-PRX adduct, Figure S4). To decouple the pH dependence in reactivity with TS from the pH dependence of the dimer-oligomer equilibrium between the proteins, we evaluated the TS reactivity with the engineered dimers of PRXs 1–3 across the same range of pH values (Figure 3F). The dimeric versions of PRX1, PRX2, and PRX3 were all more reactive at higher pH values (20–50% PRX-TS-PRX adduct at pH 8 vs. 0–7% at pH 7). Thus, the data support that the pH differences between the mitochondria and the cytosol are likely to contribute to the intracellular specificity of TS for PRX3. We have also shown that the dimeric form of PRXs is the species that most readily reacts with TS.

3.6. TS Reacts with the Reduced Cys Thiolate in PRX3, but Not the Sulfenic Acid Intermediate

We have reported that TS adduction by PRX3 requires both the peroxidatic (Cys108) and resolving (Cys229) cysteines, and that the crosslinked adduct accumulates over time with multiple rounds of enzymatic turnover [2]. Both the reduced cysteine thiolate and the cysteine sulfenic acid intermediate in PRX proteins (Figure 1) are nucleophilic and form a covalent complex with electrophilic thiol blocking reagents, including N-ethyl maleimide [26]. In this set of experiments, we asked if the reaction of PRX3 with TS requires the Cys108 to be in the reduced form (Cys-SH) or as the Cys-sulfenic acid intermediate (Cys-SOH). To generate a stable Cys-sulfenic acid species, the PRX3 engineered dimer with the resolving Cys229 residue mutated to Ser was pre-reduced and reacted with 1.5 equivalents of H_2O_2. TS was then incubated with either reduced protein or the stabilized sulfenic acid intermediate at pH 8.0 at 37 °C for 45 min and unreacted TS was removed using a Bio-Gel P-6 column. The mass of the proteins was determined by MALDI-TOF mass spectrometry (Figure 4). Because MALDI-TOF is a relatively low-resolution instrument and the sulfenic acid intermediate is not stable during ionization, the presence of sulfenic acid was confirmed by the addition of dimedone, a small molecule that reacts with sulfenic acid but not thiol/thiolate [27]. Only the peroxide-oxidized samples showed an increase in mass consistent with the addition of one dimedone (143 Da vs. theoretical of 140 Da), indicating the presence of a stable sulfenic acid. An increase in the mass consistent with the addition of one TS molecule (1660 Da versus theoretical of 1664 Da) only occurred when PRX3 was in the reduced state, consistent with the reduced thiol but not the sulfenic acid acting as the nucleophile to attack TS.

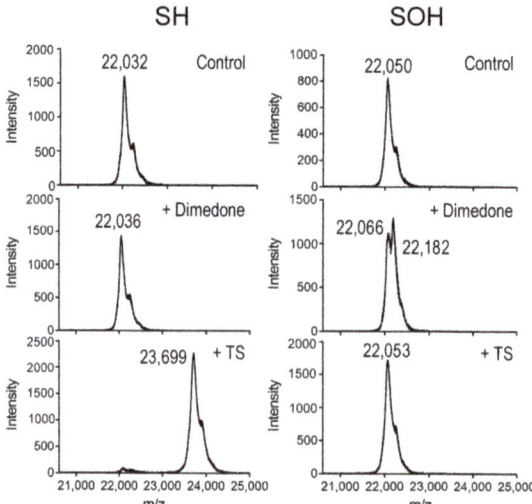

Figure 4. TS reacts with reduced Cys thiolate in PRX3, but not the sulfenic acid intermediate. MALDI-TOF MS analysis of the reaction of TS with untagged engineered dimer of PRX3 C229S in different oxidation states. Pre-reduced, untagged PRX3 engineered dimer lacking the Cys-S_R residue was oxidized with 1.5 equivalents of H_2O_2 to form a stable sulfenic acid intermediate. PRX3 with a thiol (SH) or sulfenic acid (SOH) were split and incubated with 1% DMSO (control), 20 mM dimedone, or 0.2 mM thiostrepton. Dimedone was added to confirm that sulfenic acid was present only in the samples treated with H_2O_2.

3.7. PRX3 Is More Likely to Be Found as Dimers than PRX1 or PRX2

The preference of TS for reduced and dimeric PRX is particularly interesting, as fully reduced PRXs 1–4 are predominantly found as decamers/dodecamers [4]. Based on our data we propose that PRX3 is more frequently found as a reduced dimer than PRX1 or PRX2 due to either differences in the oligomeric structure and/or differences in subcellular pH. In order to test this hypothesis, we used size-exclusion chromatography with multi-angle light scattering (SEC-MALS) with different pH buffers. For example, using this technique, one can separate the PRX3 dodecamer (~17 min) from the dimer (~21 min) and measure the mass of each species (Figure 5A). The oligomeric states of reduced and oxidized PRX1 and PRX2 were determined at pH 7.0, 7.5 and 8.0 (Figure 5B and Figure S3). PRX3 was tested only at pH 7.5 and 8.0 since it was not stable at lower pH values in our hands. Reduced PRXs 1–3 were fully decameric/dodecameric at all pH values tested. In contrast, the oligomeric state of the oxidized PRX proteins differed greatly as a function of pH. Oxidized PRX1 was predominantly decameric at all pH values. Oxidized PRX2 was predominantly decameric at pH 7.0, and the amount of dimer observed increased with pH, with dimer predominating at pH 8.0. In contrast, oxidized PRX3 was fully dimeric at both pH 7.5 and 8.0. We next tested the reactivity of the PRXs 1–3 engineered dimers across the pH range using the same SEC-MALS assay (Figure S3). All engineered dimers were dimeric at all pH values tested.

Taken together, these data support that for the oxidized wild-type proteins at the physiological relevant pH, the equilibrium for PRX3 is shifted more towards dimer than PRX1 and PRX2. The preceding experiments utilized either fully reduced or fully oxidized proteins, a state most likely not observed in cells when PRXs are constantly undergoing active turnover. It is also important to note, however, that some number of reduced active sites are necessary to react with TS (Figure 1). Therefore, TS would be most reactive when partial oxidation of PRX3 leads to dodecamer destabilization, while allowing a portion of the active sites to remain reduced. To test the hypothesis that the dodecameric structure of PRX3 is much less stable than the decameric structure of PRX2, the oligomeric status of PRX2 and PRX3 were measured by SEC-MALS analysis following partial oxidation at their respective cellular compartment pH. The pre-reduced proteins were treated with increasing substoichiometric amounts of H_2O_2, assuming that the H_2O_2 concentration will result in disulfide formation in an equal number of PRX active sites (Figure 5C and Figure S5). PRX1 was not measured since this isoform showed very little dimer formation even when fully oxidized (Figure 5B). At pH 8.0, PRX3 was dodecameric when fully reduced and a significant amount of dimer starts to appear upon the addition of 1/6 equivalents of H_2O_2 (enough to oxidize 2 of 12 active sites). PRX3 was fully dimeric after oxidation of 6 of the 12 active sites. In contrast, PRX2 still maintained a significant amount of decamer even when fully oxidized. This data and the higher pH of the mitochondria compared to the cytosol suggest that a much higher fraction of PRX3 will be dimeric than PRX2, which will be more frequently dimeric than PRX1. Therefore, PRX3 will have significantly more dimers with reduced active sites available to react with TS than other typical 2-Cys PRXs.

3.8. Gentian Violet Potentiates TS Adduction of PRX3 but Not PRX1 and PRX2

Treatment of MM tumor cells with GV leads to loss of TRX2 protein within 30 min [2]. When GV is used in combination with TS, the majority of PRX3 is irreversibly crosslinked by TS in MM cells [2,3]. To determine if GV can potentiate the formation of disulfide-bonded dimers in other PRX isoforms, we incubated MM cells with 1 µM GV and collected cell lysates after 24 h for immunoblotting analysis by non-reducing SDS-PAGE. Under these conditions PRXs migrate as 23–26 kDa reduced monomers and 46–50 kDa disulfide-bonded dimers (Figure 6A). Treatment with GV significantly increased the abundance of mitochondrial PRX3 disulfide-bonded dimers but had no observable effect of the formation of PRXs 1, 2, or 4 disulfide-bonded dimers (Figure 6A,B). To further evaluate the effects of GV, MM cells were incubated with increasing concentrations of GV in combination with a fixed concentration of TS for 24 h. These samples were then analyzed for TS induced PRX crosslinking by reducing SDS-PAGE and immunoblotting (Figure 6C,D). TS alone induced significant PRX3 crosslinking and minimal crosslinking of PRXs 1, 2 and 4, as described above. When TS was used in combination with GV, a dose dependent increase in PRX3 crosslinking was observed; at higher GV concentrations, all of the observed PRX3 formed covalent PRX3-TS-PRX3 adducts. No increase in PRXs 1, 2, or 4 crosslinking was observed with GV treatment. These data provide convincing evidence that TS and GV exert their cellular effects specifically on the mitochondrial TRX2/PRX3 antioxidant network.

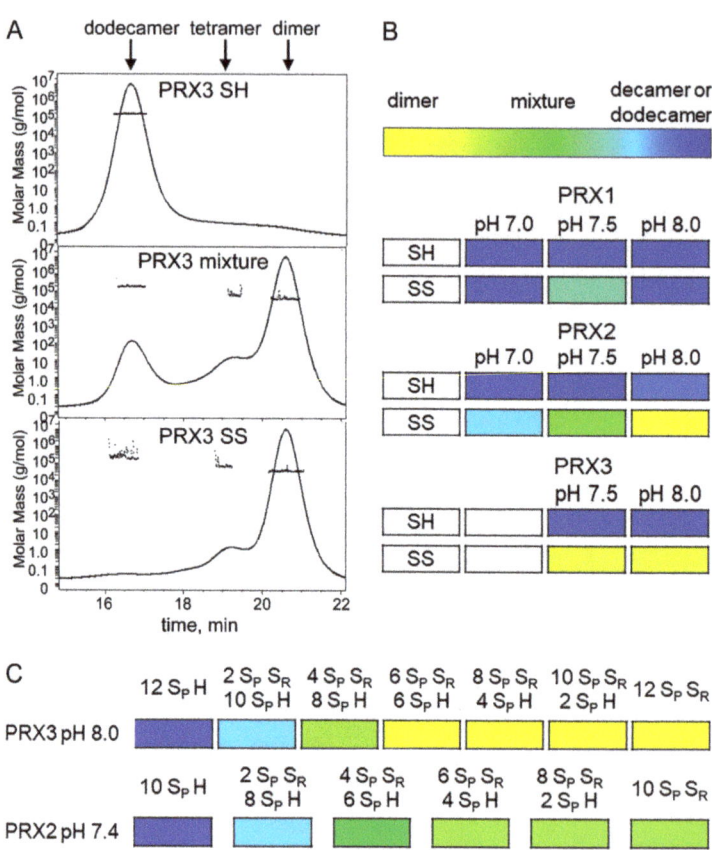

Figure 5. PRX3 is more likely to be dimer than PRX1 or PRX2. (A) SEC-MALS analysis of the influence of oxidation state on the distribution of oligomeric states for untagged wild-type PRX3 at pH 8.0. Shown is the elution profile OD_{280} trace for reduced (top), partially oxidized (middle panel) and oxidized (bottom panel). The dodecameric species elutes at ~17 min, while the dimer elutes at ~21 min. The mass for each species is indicated by the dots (left, y-axis). (B) Comparison of oligomeric states for PRX1, PRX2 and PRX3 as a function of pH and oxidation state (SH versus SS). The oligomeric state at each concentration ranged from fully dimeric (yellow) to fully (do)decameric (dark blue), with many samples exhibiting a mixture of the two species. The color gradient represents the approximate relative values of dimer and decamer within the mixtures. (Elution profiles for all samples are shown in Figure S3). All proteins were untagged. (C) Titration of PRX3 and PRX2 with peroxide at their typical cellular compartment values. Pre-reduced PRX2 and PRX3 were treated with increasing equivalents of peroxide. Relative amounts of dimer and (do)decamer in each sample are represented by the same color gradient as (B). The elution profiles for each sample are shown in Figure S5. PRX3 was not analyzed at pH 7.0 because of instability and precipitation at this pH.

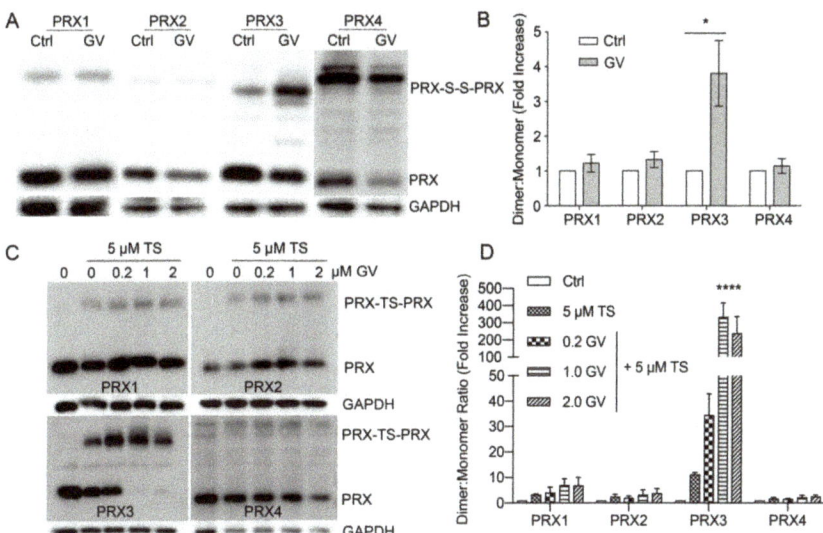

Figure 6. Specificity for Gentian violet (GV) to potentiate TS crosslinking of mitochondrial PRX3. (**A**) Western blots of PRXs 1–4 from MM tumor cells incubated with 1 µM GV for 24 h. Lysates were run on non-reducing SDS-PAGE gels. PRX-S-S-PRX represents the native intermolecular disulfide; the band above this indicated region in PRX4 is a non-specific band. (**B**) Quantification of PRXs 1–4 disulfide formation induced by GV under non-reducing conditions (n = 3). (**C**) Western blots of PRXs 1–4 from MM tumor cells incubated with 5 µM TS or 5 µM TS + indicated concentration of GV for 24 h. Lysates were run on reducing SDS-PAGE gels. (**D**) Quantification of PRXs 1–4 covalent crosslink by TS or TS + GV under reducing conditions. (* $p < 0.05$; **** $p < 0.0001$).

3.9. Disruption of the Mitochondrial Membrane Potential Does Not Affect TS-Mediated Crosslinking of PRX3

As mitochondrial membrane potential has been shown to play a significant role in the uptake and localization of compounds to the mitochondria [28], the effects of depolarizing the mitochondrial membrane potential on TS activity were evaluated. FCCP, a well-documented proton ionophore that rapidly dissipates mitochondrial membrane potential, depolarizes mitochondrial membranes rapidly in normal mesothelial and MM cells, as assessed by Seahorse Extracellular Flux Analysis (Figure S1C,D). Crosslinking of PRX3 by TS was unaffected at both early (4 h) and late (24 h) time points in normal and MM cell lines in the presence of FCCP (Figure 7A). The cytotoxic activity of TS in the presence of multiple concentrations of FCCP was also unaffected (Figure 7B). These data indicate that TS exerts cytotoxic activity through PRX3 inhibition independent of mitochondrial membrane potential.

To investigate the contribution of mitochondrial membrane potential on the ability of GV to act on mitochondrial targets, MM cells were incubated with GV and FCCP and cell lysates were collected over time. FCCP had minor effects on GV induced PRX1 and PRX2 disulfide-bonded dimer formation (Figure S6A,B). In contrast, GV induced PRX3 disulfide bonded dimers rapidly (15 min); the level of which was sustained throughout the time course (4 h) (Figure S6C). Loss of TRX2 expression was rapid, showing reduction in TRX2 protein levels by 30 min. Co-incubation of GV with 1 µM FCCP blunted TRX2 degradation and PRX3 disulfide-bonded dimer formation throughout the entirety of the experiment. These data indicate that unlike TS, GV activity against mitochondrial targets is sensitive to mitochondrial membrane potential. This is not unexpected due to the triphenyl-structure and the positive charge of GV [29,30].

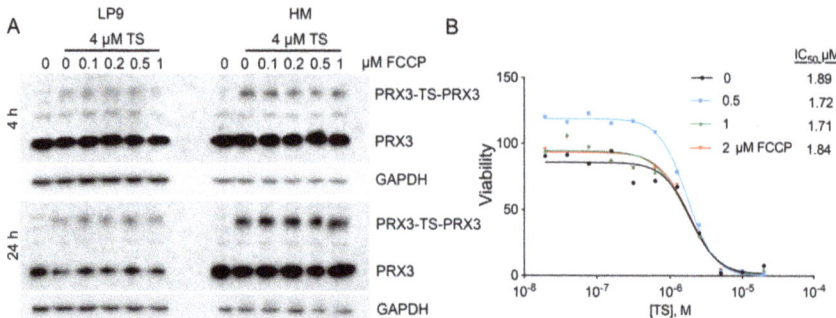

Figure 7. Intact mitochondrial membrane potential is not required for TS activity. (**A**) Western blots of normal LP9 and MM (HM cell line) cells incubated with 4 µM TS alone or in combination with indicated concentrations of FCCP. Lysates were collected at 4- and 24-h post incubation and separated by reducing SDS-PAGE. (**B**) Dose response curves of HM cells incubated with TS alone or in combination with indicated concentrations of FCCP. IC_{50} values (µM) are shown for indicated treatment groups.

4. Discussion

The goal of this study was to determine the molecular basis for the specificity of TS for human PRX3, one key component for this candidate redox-based cancer therapy. The origins of TS specificity could come from a combination of many variables, including normal versus cancer cell ROS levels, PRX3 levels, differences in the cellular localization of TS and/or PRX enzymes and differences in the reactivity and structural features of the PRX proteins. Since the PRXs have similar reaction mechanisms (Figure 1), detailed cellular and mechanistic studies evaluating multiple PRX isoforms within cells and with recombinant proteins were necessary.

PRX3 is over-expressed in MM cells and tumors [31], and PRX3 expression levels and mROS levels correlate with TS sensitivity (Figure 2). In MM cell culture, TS preferentially adducts mitochondrial PRX3 compared to the cytosolic enzymes PRX1 and PRX2 and ER-localized PRX4 (Figure 3). Additionally, GV exerts its effects on mitochondrial TRX2, specifically increasing the abundance of partially oxidized PRX3 disulfide-bonded dimers, the preferred target of TS, without any effect on PRXs 1, 2 or 4 (Figure 8). The data provided within argue that it is possible to target mitochondrial PRX3 specifically. Moreover, tumor types with genetic and phenotypic features of increased mitochondrial oxidative stress will be more susceptible to PRX3 and/or TRX2 inhibition [16].

We previously showed that TS targets PRX3 and provided preliminary evidence that PRX3 dimers, versus high molecular weight dodecamers, were the preferred target of TS [2,3]. Herein, we greatly expanded the analysis to determine the specificity of TS for PRX3 versus PRX1, PRX2 and PRX4 in cells and determined the structural and biochemical features of PRX3 that modulate this specificity. TS was able to crosslink all 2-Cys isoforms (PRXs 1–4) when the reactions were conducted at the pH of the mitochondrial compartment (~pH 8.0) (Figure 3). The engineered, dimeric forms of PRXs 1–3 were all more reactive than their native counterparts, particularly at pH 8.0. When the reaction was conducted at cytosolic pH (~7.4), crosslinking of all PRX isoforms by TS was significantly attenuated. These data provide novel evidence that TS activity against PRX3 is partially driven by the elevated pH found in the mitochondrial matrix. Of interest, elevated pH levels found in tumor cells may also contribute to the therapeutic window of TS in normal versus tumor cells [32].

These observations led us to determine which wild-type PRX isoform can form dimers containing some reduced active sites under physiological conditions. For these studies, we used a constant concentration of 100 µM PRX, which is physiologically relevant even if somewhat low for the estimates of PRX3 mitochondrial concentrations (48–125 µM) and slightly higher than the estimated concentration of PRX1 and PRX2 in the cytosol

(20–65 µM) [33–35]. A recent study using real-time monitoring of the PRX2 oligomerization state confirmed for the first time that PRX2 decamer-dimer oscillations occur and that oxidation favors dimers in cellulo. Of particular interest, this study confirmed that there was a measurable portion of reduced PRX2 dimers in cells, indicating that partial oxidation of PRX2 is sufficient to promote dimerization [36]. However, it should be noted that the oxidation state is only one factor and that the dimer/(do)decamer equilibrium can also be influenced by protein concentration, salt, pH and the presence of reporter and affinity tags.

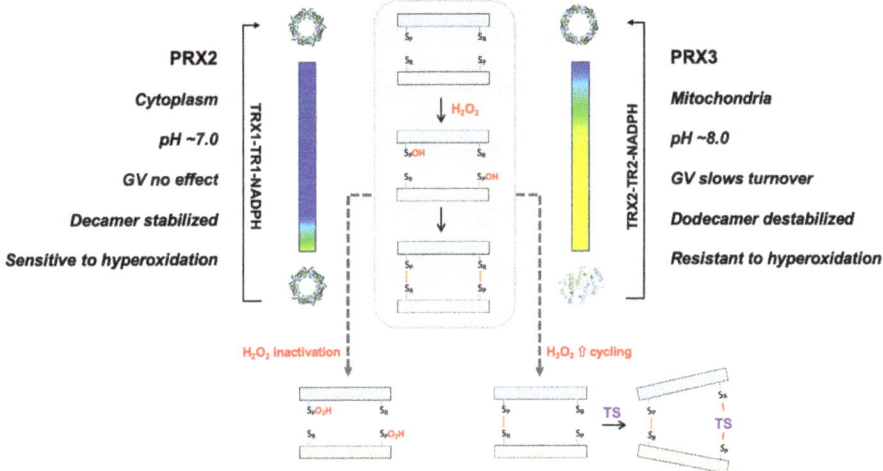

Figure 8. Summary of the biochemical, structural and environmental conditions that determine the specificity of TS for PRX3. The PRX3 dodecamer (blue) readily collapses to dimer (yellow; same coloring scheme used as in Figure 5), while the PRX2 decamer is more stable. In contrast to PRX2 where an increase in H_2O_2 cycling leads to hyperoxidation and inactivation, PRX3 can form an asymmetric dimer with one disulfide present. The other active site can then react with TS to form a covalent crosslink. Treatment with GV slows the reduction of the disulfide, further enhancing the formation of TS adducts. Double TS adducts have been observed with recombinant PRX3.

Our results showing that TS reacts with the reduced thiol/thiolate in PRXs and more efficiently with the PRX dimer, led us to hypothesize that the specificity of TS is driven by structural differences in PRX3 that facilitate collapse of the dodecamer toward dimer. Previous studies have shown that the equilibrium of other oxidized typical 2-Cys PRXs is shifted toward decamer at pH 7.0 and toward dimer at pH 8.0, with this transition driven by the protonation state of a conserved His residue within the dimer-dimer interface [37]. Here we show that the pH-dependence of the dimer/(do)decamer equilibrium differs between human PRXs 1–3. While oxidized (disulfide bonded) PRX2 shows a shift from decamer at pH 7 toward dimer at pH 8, the equilibrium for oxidized PRX1 is shifted toward decamer at all pH ranges, and the equilibrium for PRX3 is shifted toward dimer (Figure 5). Importantly, only a small proportion (2/12 possible disulfides) of the PRX3 active sites are needed to react with H_2O_2 to facilitate collapse of the dodecamer to the constituent dimeric units. This amount of peroxide required is even lower than reported earlier by colleagues [7]. The results from the panel of human PRXs tested herein supports the proposed concept from the former study that each PRX has its own "oxidation threshold" for dissociation to the dimeric subunits [36], with PRX3 exhibiting the strongest propensity to dissociation based on our data.

Taken together, these observations (Figure 8) are also consistent with the relative insensitivity of PRX3 to hyperoxidation and inactivation when compared to PRX1, PRX2 and bacterial 2-Cys PRX homologs [6–8,38]. Thus, under conditions of oxidative stress, PRX1 and PRX2 are more likely to become hyperoxidized and inactivated. Moreover, hyperoxidation of PRX1 and PRX2 stabilizes the decamer, further protecting the cytosolic proteins from TS inhibition (i.e., for the subunits within the decamer that were not hyperoxidized). In contrast, our data expands upon the observation that partial oxidation of PRX3 shifts it to dimer [7], which both protects it from hyperoxidation [22] and provides a pool of reduced Cys residues available to react with TS. Decreased TRX2 expression or activity would decrease the rate of disulfide reduction further, allowing for the accumulation of partially oxidized and dimeric PRX3, as seen in our experiments using the TRX2 inhibitor GV.

Given the requirement for mitochondrial pH, we also wondered if the mitochondrial membrane potential played a role in TS and GV activity. While disruption of the membrane potential did not affect TS cytotoxicity, it did blunt the ability of GV to reduce TRX2 protein levels and potentiate the adduction of PRX3 with TS (Figure S6). While it makes sense that the loss of membrane potential blocks the uptake of the positively charged GV molecule, the mechanism by which TS enters the mitochondria is currently unknown.

In conclusion, the primary drivers for the specific reaction of PRX3 with TS in cells include its mitochondrial localization with its higher pH and the unique biochemical and structural features that protect the protein from hyperoxidation and promote the facile collapse of the dodecamer to dimer (Figure 8). Thus, these observations add novel details to the mechanism of action of TS. The reaction of PRX3 with TS can be potentiated with GV by producing more dimeric species with only one disulfide bond, suggesting that other compounds or therapies that induce oxidative stress and lower the activity of the mitochondrial TRX2-TR2 system could also synergize. Indeed, several compounds with pro-oxidant features have been shown to synergize with TS [39–41]. The specific features of the TS-PRX3 interaction elucidated here provide mechanistic insight into this novel drug-target interaction, provide evidence inhibitors can specifically target the PRX3 isoform and support further development of this redox-based, prooxidant therapeutic strategy for cancer [4,42].

Supplementary Materials: The following are available online at https://www.mdpi.com/2076-3921/10/2/150/s1. Table S1: Sources and experimental conditions for the antibodies used in this study; Figure S1: TS sensitivity, PRX3 expression and Oxygen Consumption Rates (OCR) in MM cell lines and effect of membrane potential on TS activity; Figure S2: PRX5 does not react with TS; Figure S3: Comparison of oxidation- and pH-dependence of the oligomeric state for WT and engineered dimers of PRX1, PRX2 and PRX3; Figure S4: Comparison of the pH-dependence of TS adduct formation for WT and engineered dimers of PRXs 1–3; Figure S5: PRX3 dodecamer collapses to the dimeric form upon partial oxidation, while PRX2 decamer persists despite full oxidation; Figure S6: Effect of mitochondrial membrane potential on GV activity in MM cells (HM cell line).

Author Contributions: Conceptualization, K.J.N.; N.H.; W.T.L. and B.C.; methodology, K.J.N.; T.M.; U.G.; W.T.L. and B.C.; formal analysis, K.J.N.; T.M.; S.M, A.S.; S.B.; U.G.; T.L.S.J.; W.T.L. and B.C.; investigation, K.J.N.; T.M.; S.M.; A.S.; S.B.; U.G. and B.C.; resources, N.H, W.T.L. and B.C.; data curation, K.J.N.; T.M.; W.T.L. and B.C.; writing—original draft preparation, K.J.N.; T.M.; T.L.S.J.; W.T.L. and B.C.; writing—review and editing, K.J.N.; T.L.S.J.; W.T.L. and B.C.; visualization, K.J.N.; T.M.; S.M.; U.G.; W.T.L. and B.C.; supervision, K.J.N.; W.T.L. and B.C.; project administration, W.T.L. and B.C.; funding acquisition, N.H.; W.T.L. and B.C. All authors have read and agreed to the published version of the manuscript.

Funding: This work was supported by RS Oncology through Sponsored Research Agreements with B.C. and W.T.L.; development funds from the Department of Pathology and Laboratory Medicine (B.C.), the National Institutes of Health (GM072866 to W.T.L.), and Wake Forest Baptist Comprehensive Cancer Center Support Grant (P30CA012197).

Institutional Review Board Statement: Not applicable.

Informed Consent Statement: Not applicable.

Data Availability Statement: The data presented in this study are available on request from the corresponding authors.

Acknowledgments: We thank David Seward (UVM) for use of instrumentation in his laboratory and Arti Shukla (UVM) for providing mesothelial and malignant mesothelioma cell lines. Recombinant PRX5 was kindly provided by Derek Parsonage and Leslie Poole.

Conflicts of Interest: Cunniff and Heintz serve or have served as consultants for RS Oncology and have equity in the company. Heintz serves on the Board of Directors for RS Oncology The funders had no role in the design of the study; in the collection, analyses, or interpretation of data; in the writing of the manuscript, or in the decision to publish the results.

References

1. Corsello, S.M.; Nagari, R.T.; Spangler, R.D.; Rossen, J.; Kocak, M.; Bryan, J.G.; Humeidi, R.; Peck, D.; Wu, X.; Tang, A.A.; et al. Discovering the anticancer potential of non-oncology drugs by systematic viability profiling. *Nat. Cancer* **2020**, *1*, 235–248. [CrossRef] [PubMed]
2. Cunniff, B.; Newick, K.; Nelson, K.J.; Wozniak, A.N.; Beuschel, S.; Leavitt, B.; Bhave, A.; Butnor, K.; Koenig, A.; Chouchani, E.T.; et al. Disabling mitochondrial peroxide metabolism via combinatorial targeting of peroxiredoxin 3 as an effective therapeutic approach for malignant mesothelioma. *PLoS ONE* **2015**, *10*, e0127310. [CrossRef] [PubMed]
3. Newick, K.; Cunniff, B.; Preston, K.; Held, P.; Arbiser, J.; Pass, H.; Mossman, B.; Shukla, A.; Heintz, N. Peroxiredoxin 3 is a redox-dependent target of thiostrepton in malignant mesothelioma cells. *PLoS ONE* **2012**, *7*, e39404. [CrossRef] [PubMed]
4. Forshaw, T.E.; Holmila, R.; Nelson, K.J.; Lewis, J.E.; Kemp, M.L.; Tsang, A.W.; Poole, L.B.; Lowther, W.T.; Furdui, C.M. Peroxiredoxins in cancer and response to radiation therapies. *Antioxidants* **2019**, *8*, 11. [CrossRef]
5. Scalcon, V.; Bindoli, A.; Rigobello, M.P. Significance of the mitochondrial thioredoxin reductase in cancer cells: An update on role, targets and inhibitors. *Free Radic. Biol. Med.* **2018**, *127*, 62–79. [CrossRef]
6. Peskin, A.V.; Dickerhof, N.; Poynton, R.A.; Paton, L.N.; Pace, P.E.; Hampton, M.B.; Winterbourn, C.C. Hyperoxidation of peroxiredoxins 2 and 3: Rate constants for the reactions of the sulfenic acid of the peroxidatic cysteine. *J. Biol. Chem.* **2013**, *288*, 14170–14177. [CrossRef]
7. Poynton, R.A.; Peskin, A.V.; Haynes, A.C.; Lowther, W.T.; Hampton, M.B.; Winterbourn, C.C. Kinetic analysis of structural influences on the susceptibility of peroxiredoxins 2 and 3 to hyperoxidation. *Biochem. J.* **2016**, *473*, 411–421. [CrossRef]
8. Bolduc, J.A.; Nelson, K.J.; Haynes, A.C.; Lee, J.; Reisz, J.A.; Graff, A.H.; Clodfelter, J.E.; Parsonage, D.; Poole, L.B.; Furdui, C.M.; et al. Novel hyperoxidation resistance motifs in 2-Cys peroxiredoxins. *J. Biol. Chem.* **2018**, *293*, 11901–11912. [CrossRef]
9. Haynes, A.C.; Qian, J.; Reisz, J.A.; Furdui, C.M.; Lowther, W.T. Molecular basis for the resistance of human mitochondrial 2-Cys peroxiredoxin 3 to hyperoxidation. *J. Biol. Chem.* **2013**, *288*, 29714–29723. [CrossRef]
10. Ismail, T.; Kim, Y.; Lee, H.; Lee, D.S.; Lee, H.S. Interplay between mitochondrial peroxiredoxins and ROS in cancer development and progression. *Int. J. Mol. Sci.* **2019**, *20*, 4407. [CrossRef]
11. Reeves, S.A.; Parsonage, D.; Nelson, K.J.; Poole, L.B. Kinetic and thermodynamic features reveal that *Escherichia coli* BCP is an unusually versatile peroxiredoxin. *Biochemistry* **2011**, *50*, 8970–8981. [CrossRef] [PubMed]
12. Lin, Z.; Johnson, L.C.; Weissbach, H.; Brot, N.; Lively, M.O.; Lowther, W.T. Free methionine-(R)-sulfoxide reductase from *Escherichia coli* reveals a new GAF domain function. *Proc. Natl. Acad. Sci. USA* **2007**, *104*, 9597–9602. [CrossRef] [PubMed]
13. Hall, A.; Parsonage, D.; Poole, L.B.; Karplus, P.A. Structural evidence that peroxiredoxin catalytic power is based on transition-state stabilization. *J. Mol. Biol.* **2010**, *402*, 194–209. [CrossRef] [PubMed]
14. Nelson, K.J.; Parsonage, D.; Hall, A.; Karplus, P.A.; Poole, L.B. Cysteine pK(a) values for the bacterial peroxiredoxin AhpC. *Biochemistry* **2008**, *47*, 12860–12868. [CrossRef]
15. Weinberg, F.; Chandel, N.S. Reactive oxygen species-dependent signaling regulates cancer. *Cell Mol. Life Sci.* **2009**, *66*, 3663–3673. [CrossRef]
16. Gorrini, C.; Harris, I.S.; Mak, T.W. Modulation of oxidative stress as an anticancer strategy. *Nat. Rev. Drug Discov.* **2013**, *12*, 931–947. [CrossRef]
17. Yewdall, N.A.; Peskin, A.V.; Hampton, M.B.; Goldstone, D.C.; Pearce, F.G.; Gerrard, J.A. Quaternary structure influences the peroxidase activity of peroxiredoxin 3. *Biochem. Biophys. Res. Commun.* **2018**, *497*, 558–563. [CrossRef]
18. Cao, Z.; Roszak, A.W.; Gourlay, L.J.; Lindsay, J.G.; Isaacs, N.W. Bovine mitochondrial peroxiredoxin III forms a two-ring catenane. *Structure* **2005**, *13*, 1661–1664. [CrossRef]
19. Jonsson, T.J.; Johnson, L.C.; Lowther, W.T. Structure of the sulphiredoxin-peroxiredoxin complex reveals an essential repair embrace. *Nature* **2008**, *451*, 98–101. [CrossRef]
20. Jonsson, T.J.; Johnson, L.C.; Lowther, W.T. Protein engineering of the quaternary sulfiredoxin.peroxiredoxin enzyme.substrate complex reveals the molecular basis for cysteine sulfinic acid phosphorylation. *J. Biol. Chem.* **2009**, *284*, 33305–33310. [CrossRef]
21. Loberg, M.A.; Hurtig, J.E.; Graff, A.H.; Allan, K.M.; Buchan, J.A.; Spencer, M.K.; Kelly, J.E.; Clodfelter, J.E.; Morano, K.A.; Lowther, W.T.; et al. Aromatic residues at the dimer-dimer interface in the peroxiredoxin Tsa1 facilitate decamer formation and biological function. *Chem. Res. Toxicol.* **2019**, *32*, 474–483. [CrossRef] [PubMed]
22. Parsonage, D.; Youngblood, D.S.; Sarma, G.N.; Wood, Z.A.; Karplus, P.A.; Poole, L.B. Analysis of the link between enzymatic activity and oligomeric state in AhpC, a bacterial peroxiredoxin. *Biochemistry* **2005**, *44*, 10583–10592. [CrossRef] [PubMed]
23. Cho, H.; Cho, Y.Y.; Shim, M.S.; Lee, J.Y.; Lee, H.S.; Kang, H.C. Mitochondria-targeted drug delivery in cancers. *Biochim. Biophys. Acta Mol. Basis Dis.* **2020**, *1866*, 165808. [CrossRef] [PubMed]

24. Han, J.C.; Han, G.Y. A procedure for quantitative determination of tris(2-carboxyethyl)phosphine, an odorless reducing agent more stable and effective than dithiothreitol. *Anal. Biochem.* **1994**, *220*, 5–10. [CrossRef] [PubMed]
25. Setterdahl, A.T.; Chivers, P.T.; Hirasawa, M.; Lemaire, S.D.; Keryer, E.; Miginiac-Maslow, M.; Kim, S.K.; Mason, J.; Jacquot, J.P.; Longbine, C.C.; et al. Effect of pH on the oxidation-reduction properties of thioredoxins. *Biochemistry* **2003**, *42*, 14877–14884. [CrossRef] [PubMed]
26. Reisz, J.A.; Bechtold, E.; King, S.B.; Poole, L.B.; Furdui, C.M. Thiol-blocking electrophiles interfere with labeling and detection of protein sulfenic acids. *FEBS J.* **2013**, *280*, 6150–6161. [CrossRef]
27. Poole, L.B.; Furdui, C.M.; King, S.B. Introduction to approaches and tools for the evaluation of protein cysteine oxidation. *Essays Biochem.* **2020**, *64*, 1–17. [CrossRef]
28. Murphy, M.P.; Smith, R.A. Drug delivery to mitochondria: The key to mitochondrial medicine. *Adv. Drug Deliv. Rev.* **2000**, *41*, 235–250. [CrossRef]
29. Gadelha, F.R.; Moreno, S.N.; De Souza, W.; Cruz, F.S.; Docampo, R. The mitochondrion of *Trypanosoma cruzi* is a target of crystal violet toxicity. *Mol. Biochem. Parasitol.* **1989**, *34*, 117–126. [CrossRef]
30. Murphy, M.P. Targeting lipophilic cations to mitochondria. *Biochim. Biophys. Acta* **2008**, *1777*, 1028–1031. [CrossRef]
31. Kinnula, V.L.; Lehtonen, S.; Sormunen, R.; Kaarteenaho-Wiik, R.; Kang, S.W.; Rhee, S.G.; Soini, Y. Overexpression of peroxiredoxins I, II, III, V, and VI in malignant mesothelioma. *J. Pathol.* **2002**, *196*, 316–323. [CrossRef] [PubMed]
32. White, K.A.; Grillo-Hill, B.K.; Barber, D.L. Cancer cell behaviors mediated by dysregulated pH dynamics at a glance. *J. Cell. Sci.* **2017**, *130*, 663–669. [CrossRef] [PubMed]
33. Winterbourn, C.C. Reconciling the chemistry and biology of reactive oxygen species. *Nat. Chem. Biol.* **2008**, *4*, 278–286. [CrossRef] [PubMed]
34. Cox, A.G.; Pearson, A.G.; Pullar, J.M.; Jonsson, T.J.; Lowther, W.T.; Winterbourn, C.C.; Hampton, M.B. Mitochondrial peroxiredoxin 3 is more resilient to hyperoxidation than cytoplasmic peroxiredoxins. *Biochem. J.* **2009**, *421*, 51–58. [CrossRef] [PubMed]
35. Stein, K.T.; Moon, S.J.; Nguyen, A.N.; Sikes, H.D. Kinetic modeling of H_2O_2 dynamics in the mitochondria of HeLa cells. *PLoS Comput. Biol.* **2020**, *16*, e1008202. [CrossRef]
36. Pastor-Flores, D.; Talwar, D.; Pedre, B.; Dick, T.P. Real-time monitoring of peroxiredoxin oligomerization dynamics in living cells. *Proc. Natl. Acad. Sci. USA* **2020**, *117*, 16313–16323. [CrossRef]
37. Morais, M.A.; Giuseppe, P.O.; Souza, T.A.; Alegria, T.G.; Oliveira, M.A.; Netto, L.E.; Murakami, M.T. How pH modulates the dimer-decamer interconversion of 2-Cys peroxiredoxins from the Prx1 subfamily. *J. Biol. Chem.* **2015**, *290*, 8582–8590. [CrossRef]
38. Wood, Z.A.; Poole, L.B.; Karplus, P.A. Peroxiredoxin evolution and the regulation of hydrogen peroxide signaling. *Science* **2003**, *300*, 650–653. [CrossRef]
39. Cunniff, B.; Benson, K.; Stumpff, J.; Newick, K.; Held, P.; Taatjes, D.; Joseph, J.; Kalyanaraman, B.; Heintz, N.H. Mitochondrial-targeted nitroxides disrupt mitochondrial architecture and inhibit expression of peroxiredoxin 3 and FOXM1 in malignant mesothelioma cells. *J. Cell Physiol.* **2013**, *228*, 835–845. [CrossRef]
40. Qiao, S.; Lamore, S.D.; Cabello, C.M.; Lesson, J.L.; Munoz-Rodriguez, J.L.; Wondrak, G.T. Thiostrepton is an inducer of oxidative and proteotoxic stress that impairs viability of human melanoma cells but not primary melanocytes. *Biochem. Pharmacol.* **2012**, *83*, 1229–1240. [CrossRef]
41. Bowling, B.D.; Doudican, N.; Manga, P.; Orlow, S.J. Inhibition of mitochondrial protein translation sensitizes melanoma cells to arsenic trioxide cytotoxicity via a reactive oxygen species dependent mechanism. *Cancer Chemother. Pharmacol.* **2008**, *63*, 37–43. [CrossRef] [PubMed]
42. Chaiswing, L.; St Clair, W.H.; St Clair, D.K. Redox paradox: A novel approach to therapeutics-resistant cancer. *Antioxid. Redox Signal.* **2018**, *29*, 1237–1272. [CrossRef] [PubMed]

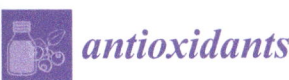

Article

Curcumin and Carnosic Acid Cooperate to Inhibit Proliferation and Alter Mitochondrial Function of Metastatic Prostate Cancer Cells

Saniya Ossikbayeva [1,2,†], Marina Khanin [3], Yoav Sharoni [3], Aviram Trachtenberg [3], Sultan Tuleukhanov [2], Richard Sensenig [4], Slava Rom [5], Michael Danilenko [3,*,‡] and Zulfiya Orynbayeva [1,‡,§]

1. Department of Surgery, Drexel University College of Medicine, Philadelphia, PA 19102, USA; ossikbayeva.s@kaznmu.kz (S.O.); zulfiya.orynbayeva@crl.com (Z.O.)
2. Department of Biophysics and Biomedicine, Al-Farabi Kazakh National University, Almaty 050040, Kazakhstan; sultan.tuleuhanov@kaznu.kz
3. Department of Clinical Biochemistry and Pharmacology, Faculty of Health Sciences, Ben-Gurion University of the Negev, Be'er Sheva 8410501, Israel; hanin@bgu.ac.il (M.K.); yoav@bgu.ac.il (Y.S.); aviramtr@post.bgu.ac.il (A.T.)
4. Department of Surgery, Cooper University Hospital, Camden, NJ 08103, USA; sensenigrb@verizon.net
5. Department of Pathology and Laboratory Medicine, Lewis Katz School of Medicine, Temple University, Philadelphia, PA 19140, USA; srom@temple.edu
* Correspondence: misha@bgu.ac.il; Tel.: +972-8-647-9969
† Current address: Kazakh Research Institute of Oncology and Radiology, Almaty 050022, Kazakhstan.
‡ Equal contribution.
§ Current address: Charles River Laboratories, Malvern, PA 19355, USA.

Citation: Ossikbayeva, S.; Khanin, M.; Sharoni, Y.; Trachtenberg, A.; Tuleukhanov, S.; Sensenig, R.; Rom, S.; Danilenko, M.; Orynbayeva, Z. Curcumin and Carnosic Acid Cooperate to Inhibit Proliferation and Alter Mitochondrial Function of Metastatic Prostate Cancer Cells. *Antioxidants* **2021**, *10*, 1591. https://doi.org/10.3390/antiox10101591

Academic Editor: Ana Sofia Fernandes

Received: 27 June 2021
Accepted: 7 October 2021
Published: 11 October 2021

Publisher's Note: MDPI stays neutral with regard to jurisdictional claims in published maps and institutional affiliations.

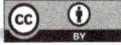

Copyright: © 2021 by the authors. Licensee MDPI, Basel, Switzerland. This article is an open access article distributed under the terms and conditions of the Creative Commons Attribution (CC BY) license (https://creativecommons.org/licenses/by/4.0/).

Abstract: Anticancer activities of plant polyphenols have been demonstrated in various models of neoplasia. However, evidence obtained in numerous in vitro studies indicates that proliferation arrest and/or killing of cancer cells require quite high micromolar concentrations of polyphenols that are difficult to reach in vivo and can also be (geno)toxic to at least some types of normal cells. The ability of certain polyphenols to synergize with one another at low concentrations can be used as a promising strategy to effectively treat human malignancies. We have recently reported that curcumin and carnosic acid applied at non-cytotoxic concentrations synergistically cooperate to induce massive apoptosis in acute myeloid leukemia cells, but not in normal hematopoietic and non-hematopoietic cells, via sustained cytosolic calcium overload. Here, we show that the two polyphenols can also synergistically suppress the growth of DU145 and PC-3 metastatic prostate cancer cell cultures. However, instead of cell killing, the combined treatment induced a marked inhibition of cell proliferation associated with G_0/G_1 cell cycle arrest. This was preceded by transient elevation of cytosolic calcium levels and prolonged dissipation of the mitochondrial membrane potential, without generating oxidative stress, and was associated with defective oxidative phosphorylation encompassing mitochondrial dysfunction. The above effects were concomitant with a significant downregulation of mRNA and protein expression of the oncogenic kinase SGK1, the mitochondria-hosted mTOR component. In addition, a moderate decrease in SGK1 phosphorylation at Ser422 was observed in polyphenol-treated cells. The mTOR inhibitor rapamycin produced a similar reduction in SGK1 mRNA and protein levels as well as phosphorylation. Collectively, our findings suggest that the combination of curcumin and carnosic acid at potentially bioavailable concentrations may effectively target different types of cancer cells by distinct modes of action. This and similar combinations merit further exploration as an anticancer modality.

Keywords: prostate cancer; curcumin; carnosic acid; cell cycle; OxPhos; SGK1

1. Introduction

Historically, phytochemicals have been one of the major foundations of drug development [1]. Curcumin (CUR), the principal curcuminoid of the Indian spice turmeric

(Supplementary Figure S1) has been the subject of numerous studies into its value as a cancer therapy that led to a number of clinical trials (e.g., [2–4]). The rationale for potential therapeutic applications of this compound is based on its pleiotropic effects on multiple cellular activities and regulatory pathways (see [4,5] for recent reviews), including the ability to induce oxidative stress [6–10] and/or endoplasmic reticulum stress [11–14] in various cancer cell types that lead to cell cycle arrest and cell death. However, the above effects are usually observed at high supraphysiological concentrations of CUR ($\geq$10 µM) that are difficult to reach in vivo due to a low bioavailability and extensive metabolism of this polyphenol [15,16]. Furthermore, at such concentrations CUR has been found to induce geno/cytotoxicity to at least some types of normal cells [17–21].

Combinations of CUR with different phytochemicals or drugs have demonstrated enhanced anticancer effects in various models of human malignancies, as compared to single agents (see [22–24] for recent reviews). For instance, pairing CUR with the polyphenols quercetin [25], resveratrol [26,27], epigallocatechin gallate [28] or ursolic acid [29] resulted in synergistic inhibitory effects on the growth and survival of colorectal, breast and prostate cancer cells. Our previous study has demonstrated that the combination of CUR and the carotenoid lycopene synergistically inhibited androgen receptor signaling in prostate cancer cells [30]. Such a combinatory approach has the potential to overcome therapeutic limitations of plant polyphenols by minimizing their effective concentrations in synergistically acting combinations while maintaining or increasing anticancer efficiency.

We have recently shown that co-treatment of acute myeloid leukemia (AML) cells with CUR and carnosic acid (CA), a phenolic diterpene from rosemary (Supplementary Figure S1) [31], at non-cytotoxic concentrations of each compound (2.5–5.0 µM CUR + 5–10 µM CA) results in a rapid and massive cell death through the synergistic activation of both extrinsic and intrinsic apoptotic pathways [32,33]. Interestingly, in contrast to CA, other plant phenolic compounds, such as silibinin, rosmarinic acid, resveratrol, quercetin or parthenolide, did not cooperate with CUR in AML cells [32,34]. In the present study, we examined whether the two polyphenols (CUR and CA) applied at similar low concentrations ($\leq$10 µM) would also synergize in inducing apoptotic cell death of DU145 and PC-3 cells, the most widely studied human metastatic prostate cancer cell lines [35]. Surprisingly, CUR + CA treatment caused only a slight or no induction of apoptosis in these cells; however, the combination dramatically inhibited clonal cell growth and G_1-to-S cell cycle transition in a synergistic manner.

Development of primary tumors and their further dissemination to metastatic loci are shown to be accompanied by metabolic reprogramming towards advancement of oxidative processes and loss of apoptotic potential [36–38]. Recent discoveries in this field indicate an active involvement of mitochondria in cancer progression and the development of chemoresistance [39–43]. Various plant polyphenols have been shown to target mitochondria in cancer cells (reviewed in [44]). Therefore, here, we focused on characterizing the effects of CUR and CA, alone and in combination, on mitochondrial function in DU145 and PC-3 cells. The data demonstrated that the marked inhibition of cell proliferation by CUR + CA was preceded by dissipation of the mitochondrial membrane potential ($\Delta\psi_m$) and suppression of all respiratory enzyme complexes. Notably, these effects were not accompanied by intracellular accumulation of reactive oxygen species (ROS).

2. Materials and Methods
2.1. Materials

Curcumin ($\geq$90%) and carnosic acid ($\geq$95%) were purchased from Cayman Chemical (Ann Arbor, MI, USA) and Enzo Life Sciences, Inc. (Farmingdale, NY, USA), respectively. Stock solutions of both polyphenols were prepared in DMSO and were refreshed every two weeks. DMSO was used as a vehicle throughout all experiments at a final concentration of 0.2%.

2.2. Cell Lines

Metastatic human prostate cancer cells (DU145 and PC-3) were purchased from ATCC (Manassas, VA, USA) at the available passage 60 and used up to passage 70. Cells were maintained in RPMI 1640 medium supplemented with 10% FBS. The cells were grown at 37 °C in a humidified 5% CO_2 atmosphere.

2.3. Alamar Blue Cell Viability Assay

Cells were seeded in a 96-well plate at a density of 9000 cells per well and treated with vehicle or polyphenols for 48 h. The cells were incubated with 100 µL of 3% Alamar Blue solution in a complete growth medium at 37 °C for 2 h [45]. The fluorescence signal of the Alamar Blue product resorufin (585 nm) was read on a BioTek Synergy 4 microplate reader (Winooski, VT, USA). In these and all the other experiments involving fluorescence, curcumin autofluorescence was subtracted from the signals obtained from cells treated with curcumin, alone and in combination with carnosic acid.

2.4. Assessment of Apoptosis

Apoptosis was evaluated using Annexin V-Propidium Iodide-based apoptosis kit (ThermoFisher Scientific, Waltham, MA, USA) and analyzed by flow cytometry on the BD Accuri C6 instrument. For each sample, 10,000 events were recorded. Annexin V-positive/PI-negative cells were considered to be in the early apoptotic phase; cells positive for both Annexin V and PI to be late apoptotic; and Annexin V-negative/PI-positive cells to be necrotic [46].

2.5. Colony Formation Assay

Clonogenic cell growth assay was performed with 20,000 PC-3 or DU145 cells seeded in a 6-well plate in the growth medium and incubated overnight. Cells were then treated with vehicle or polyphenols for 7 days. Colonies were fixed with 3.7% paraformaldehyde at room temperature for 5 min, rinsed with PBS, and stained with 0.05% crystal violet for 30 min. Cells were then washed with tap water and drained. The stained colonies were imaged on a Zeiss Axiovert 40 CFL inverted microscope with SPOT RT-SE™ digital camera (Diagnostic Instruments Inc., Sterling Heights, MI, USA) and analyzed using ImageJ program. Quantification of cell colonies per microscopic field of view was made using a density threshold.

2.6. Examination of Cell Cycle Distribution

Cells (1×10^6) were synchronized in serum-free growth medium for 24 h (DU145) or 48 h (PC-3) and incubated with polyphenols for 24 h. After treatment, cells were washed with ice-cold PBS and fixed in 70% ethanol at -20 °C for 24 h. Cells were then rinsed twice with PBS and incubated in 1 mL of PBS containing 0.1% Triton X-100 and 50 µg of RNAse at room temperature for 30 min. Propidium iodide (10 µg/mL) was added to the cells for 20 min followed by fluorescence analysis in BD Accuri C6 flow cytometer (BD Biosciences, San Jose, CA, USA). For each sample, 10,000 events were recorded.

2.7. Preparation of Whole Cell Lysates and Western Blotting

Cells rinsed with PBS were lysed in ice-cold buffer containing 50 mM, HEPES, pH 7.5, 150 mM NaCl, 10% glycerol, 1% Triton X-100, 1.5 mM EGTA, 2 mM sodium orthovanadate, 20 mM sodium pyrophosphate, 50 mM NaF, 1 mM DTT and 1:50 cOmplete™ protease inhibitor cocktail (Sigma-Aldrich-Merck, Rehovot, Israel). The lysates were incubated for 10 min on ice and centrifuged at $20,000 \times g$, 10 min, 4 °C. Supernatants (30 µg protein) were subjected to SDS-PAGE and blotted into nitrocellulose membrane (Whatman, Dassel, Germany). The membranes were blocked with 5% milk for 2 h and incubated with primary antibodies overnight at 4 °C, followed by incubation with HRP-conjugated secondary antibodies (Promega, Madison, WI, USA) for 1 h. The protein bands were visualized using Western Lightning™ Chemiluminescence Reagent Plus (PerkinElmer Life Sciences,

Inc., Boston, MA, USA). The Integrated Density Value (IDV) of each protein band was quantitated using the Image Quant LAS 4000 system (GE Healthcare, Little Chalfont, UK). The following primary antibodies were used. Cyclin D1 (sc-6281), cyclin E (sc-481), CDK2 (sc-163), CDK4 (sc-260), p21^{Cip1} (sc-6246) and p27^{Kip1} (sc-1641) were purchased from Santa Cruz Biotechnology (Dallas, TX, USA). Phospho-SGK1 (Ser78; #5599) and SGK1 (#12103) were obtained from Cell Signaling Technology (Danvers, MA, USA), and phospho-SGK (Ser422; #SAB4503834) from Merck-Sigma-Aldrich (Rehovot, Israel). Calreticulin (sc-11398) or GAPDH (sc-47724) from Santa Cruz Biotechnology (Dallas, TX, USA) was used as the loading control.

2.8. Evaluation of Cytosolic Calcium Levels

Cells (0.2×10^6) were trypsinized, washed with modified Krebs buffer (137 mM NaCl, 5 mM KCl, 1 mM KH_2PO_4, HEPES 20 mM, pH 7.4, 2 mM $MgCl_2$, 2 mM $CaCl_2$) and loaded with 2 µM Fluo-4AM at room temperature. After incubation for 15 min, cells were rinsed and kept in the buffer prior to measurements. For the Ca^{2+}-free experiments, the buffer was prepared without $CaCl_2$ and contained 1 mM EGTA. The changes in cytosolic calcium levels were analyzed for 30 min using BD Accuri C6 flow cytometer. For each sample, 1000 events were recorded per each one-minute time point. To assess the maximal calcium level, 10 µM ionophore ionomycin was added in the end of each measurement.

2.9. Evaluation of the Mitochondrial Membrane Potential

Harvested cells (0.2×10^6) were rinsed with modified Krebs buffer and loaded with 75 nM MitoRed (PromoCell GmbH, Heidelberg, Germany), the mitochondria membrane potential-sensitive indicator. After 30 min of incubation at room temperature, cells were rinsed and kept in the same buffer prior to examination. The signal was examined on a BD Accuri C6 flow cytometer. For the positive control, cells were treated with 2 µM FCCP (carbonyl cyanide-4-(trifluoromethoxy)phenylhydrazone), the dose which resulted in a collapse of the membrane potential. For each sample, 10,000 events were recorded.

2.10. Measurement of Oxidative Phosphorylation

Cellular respiration was analyzed at 37 °C using OROBOROS Oxygraph-2K (Innsbruck, Austria) [47,48]. Harvested cells were rinsed and resuspended in a modified Krebs buffer to assess the intact cells. Once the basal level of respiration was achieved, the ATPase inhibitor oligomycin (1 µg/mL) was added to evaluate the proton leak across the mitochondria inner membrane [49]. After inhibition, the 20 nM step FCCP titration was performed to "substitute" for the inhibited proton pump and stimulate respiration to its maximal rate. To examine OxPhos activity of individual respiratory enzymes, the permeabilized cell protocol was used. The addition of 10 µM digitonin compromises the plasma membrane enabling membrane impermeable modulators to enter cells and reach the mitochondria [50]. For this experiment, the cells were resuspended in the buffer, mimicking an intracellular environment (120 mM KCl, 10 mM NaCl, 1 mM KH_2PO_4, 20 mM MOPS, pH 7.2, 2 mM $MgCl_2$, 1 mM EGTA, 0.7 mM $CaCl_2$). The respiratory complexes were stimulated with 10 mM glutamate/2 mM malate (for complex I), 10 mM succinate (for complex II), 1 mM ascorbate/0.3 mM TMPD (for complex IV).

2.11. Measurement of the Levels of Reactive Oxygen Species

Harvested cells (0.2×10^6) were rinsed with modified Krebs buffer and loaded with 2 µM CM-H_2DCFDA, the indicator for cytosolic peroxides, or 5 µM MitoSox, the probe for mitochondrial superoxide (ThermoFisher Scientific, Waltham, MA, USA). After incubation for 30 min at room temperature, cells were rinsed with modified Krebs buffer and kept in the same buffer prior to examination. Fluorescence changes were analyzed on a BD Accuri C6 flow cytometer. H_2O_2 (100 µM) was used as a positive control in CM-H_2DCFDA-loaded samples, and 2.5 µM antimycin A in MitoSox-loaded samples.

2.12. Reverse Transcription and Quantitative PCR

Total cell RNA was extracted using RNeasy Mini kit (QIAGEN) followed by treatment with Ambion® Turbo DNase (ThermoFisher Scientific, Waltham, MA, USA). RNA quality and concentration were determined using a Nanodrop spectrophotometer (Nanodrop Technologies, Wilmington, DE, USA), and was adjusted to 50 ng/µL. RNA was converted to cDNA using the High-Capacity cDNA Reverse Transcriptase kit (Applied Biosystem, ThermoFisher Scientific, Waltham, MA, USA) and 1 µg RNA template, using Eppendorf Mastercycler Epigradient S (Hamburg, Germany). Initial gene profiling was performed on cDNA from DU145 cells using Human mTOR Signaling RT2 Profiler PCR Array (SA Biosciences, Qiagen, Germantown, MD, USA). GAPDH served as an internal control for gene expression normalization. To quantify gene expression in all cell lines, primers and TaqMan probes for SKG1 and GAPDH were acquired from Applied Biosystem (ThermoFisher Scientific, Waltham, MA, USA). qPCR was performed on ABI QuantStudio S3 real-time PCR system (ThermoFisher Scientific, Waltham, MA, USA). Data were analyzed with ABI DataAssist software (ThermoFisher Scientific, Waltham, MA, USA) using the $2^{-\Delta\Delta Ct}$ algorithm (relative quantification). Results are expressed in relative gene expression levels (fold regulation) compared with the untreated control. The qPCR was run in triplicate and repeated at least twice.

2.13. Statistical Analysis

Statistical analyses were performed using Prism GraphPad 7.0 software (San Diego, CA, USA). The cooperation between curcumin and carnosic acid was assessed by the Combination Index (CI) analysis using CompuSyn 1.0 software (ComboSyn Inc., Paramus, NJ, USA). The CI values were calculated on the basis of the levels of cell growth inhibition (fraction affected) by each agent individually and combination at non-constant ratios. CI values of <1, 1, and >1 show synergism, additivity and antagonism, respectively. Statistically significant differences between the means of several groups were assessed by one-way ANOVA with the Tukey multiple comparison post hoc analysis. The significance of the differences between two groups was estimated by unpaired, two-tailed Student's t-test. Differences were considered significant at $p < 0.05$.

3. Results

3.1. Concentration-Dependent Effects of Curcumin, Carnosic Acid and Their Combinations on Cell Growth and Viability

To evaluate the effects of curcumin (CUR) and carnosic acid (CA) on DU145 and PC-3 cells, we first employed the Alamar Blue assay to assess relative changes in the proportion of viable cells. Exposure to a range of (sub)micromolar concentrations of CUR (0.25–10 µM) for 48 h resulted in a dose-dependent decrease in cell growth/viability, with PC-3 cells being less responsive than DU145 cells (Figure 1a,c). When applied at the above concentrations, CA produced only minimal effects on both cell lines (Figure 1a,c). The data obtained in these experiments enabled us to select two relatively low concentrations of CUR (5 µM and 7 µM) for combined treatment with gradually increasing concentrations of CA. In DU145 cells, the combinations of 7 µM CUR and 1–5 µM CA produced a significantly enhanced reduction in the proportion of viable cells, as compared to the sum of the effects of single compounds (Figure 1a) or to the effect of CUR alone (Figure 1d). The combined effects of 5 µM CUR and CA were less pronounced, without an evidence for significant enhancement of the CUR effect by CA. Interestingly, when applied at lower concentrations (0.25–1.0 µM), CA even abolished the inhibitory effect of 5 µM CUR (Figure 1a,d). Detailed assessment of the cooperativity between the two polyphenols using the Combination Index (CI) analysis revealed a clear synergistic interaction between CUR and CA (CI < 1) at 7 µM CUR combined with 1–5 µM CA (Figure 1b), while the effects of 5 µM CUR combined with CA were additive at most (not shown). Therefore, the combination of 7 µM CUR and 5 µM CA, which produced the strongest synergistic reduction in cell viability (~50% compared to DMSO), was chosen for further studies. Surprisingly, these experiments showed no evidence of cooperation between the two polyphenols for PC-3 cells, i.e., the effects of CUR + CA combinations were similar to, or even weaker than, those of CUR alone. Again, the addition of CA at lower concentrations significantly abrogated the effects of CUR (Figure 1c,d).

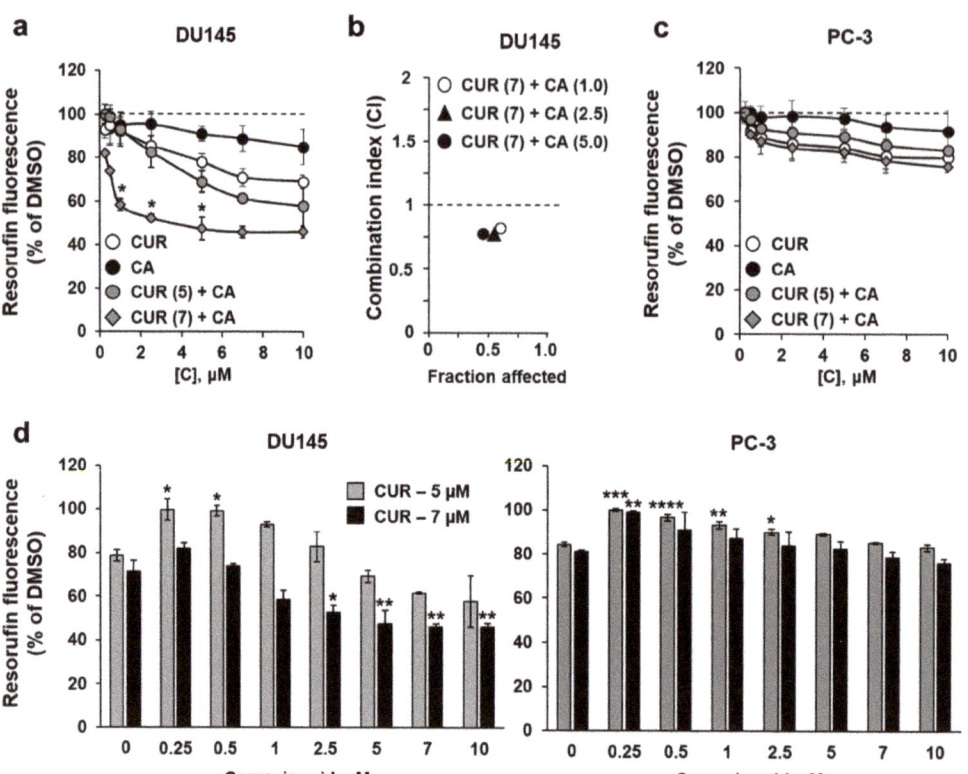

Figure 1. Effects of curcumin, carnosic acid and their combinations on the growth/viability of DU145 and PC-3 prostate cancer cells. (a,c) The Alamar Blue assay data obtained after 48 h of cell treatment with vehicle (DMSO) or the indicated concentrations of curcumin (CUR), carnosic acid (CA) and their combinations (CUR + CA). Values given in parentheses are concentrations (μM). Data are presented as mean ± SEM (n = 3). Statistically significant differences are indicated for CUR + CA vs. the sum of the effects of CUR and CA applied separately. * $p < 0.05$. (b) The Combination Index (CI) analysis of DU145 cell viability for the indicated CUR + CA (μM) combinations. The CI values are plotted against the levels of the fraction affected. (d) The Alamar Blue assay data demonstrating the effects of increasing concentrations of CA on DU145 and PC-3 cells treated with CUR at 5 μM or 7 μM. The values are derived from the data (mean ± SEM; n = 3) shown in panels (a,c). * $p < 0.05$; ** $p < 0.01$; *** $p < 0.001$ and **** $p < 0.0001$ vs. CUR alone (0 μM CA).

To examine whether the CUR ± CA-induced decreases in the relative quantity of viable cells were due to increased cell death, we evaluated the effects of the polyphenols using the annexin-V/PI assay in both DU145 and PC-3 cells. The results demonstrated that following 48 h of incubation, 7 μM CUR and 5 μM CA, alone or together, had a minimal or no apoptotic or necrotic effect on either cell line (Figure 2). For instance, treatment of PC-3 cells with CUR or CUR + CA resulted in a ≤10% increase in apoptotic cell death (Figure 2b), as compared to DMSO-treated cells ($p = 0.208$ or $p = 0.069$, respectively). This is unlike the previously observed rapid induction of massive apoptotic cell death in CUR + CA-treated AML cells [32,33].

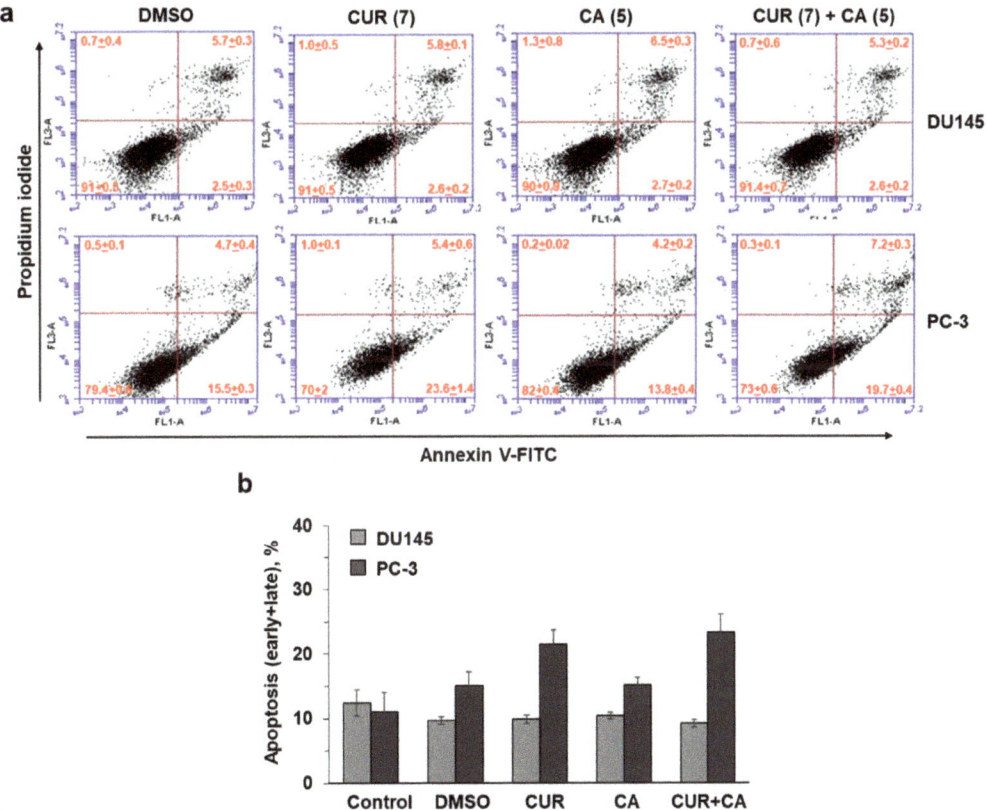

Figure 2. Effects of curcumin and carnosic acid on the induction of apoptosis. (**a**) Examples of primary flow cytometric data of annexin-V and propidium iodide binding to DU145 and PC-3 cells under the indicated treatment conditions (48 h). (**b**) Summarized data of apoptosis (early + late) induction, as exemplified in panel (**a**). Values given in parentheses are concentrations (μM). Data are presented as mean ± SEM (*n* = 3).

On the other hand, using the colony formation assay, we obtained strong support for the antiproliferative activity of the polyphenol combination in both cell lines tested. As shown in Figure 3, incubation of DU145 cells with CUR + CA for 7 days lead to an almost complete abrogation of clonal cell growth, whereas treatment with CUR or CA alone produced only a minor or no effect, respectively, as compared to untreated or vehicle-treated cells. Remarkably, while exhibiting no cooperativity in PC-3 cells when applied for 48 h (Figure 1c), the two polyphenols produced a marked synergistic suppression of clonal growth following 7 days of incubation (Figure 3), though the effect was somewhat less pronounced than that observed in DU145 cells.

3.2. Curcumin and Carnosic Acid Cooperate in Inducing Cell Cycle Arrest

To further characterize the cooperative antiproliferative activity of CUR and CA, we evaluated the effects of the polyphenols, alone or together, on cell cycle distribution following cell synchronization at G_1/S boundary by serum starvation. As exemplified in Figure 4a, incubation of synchronized DU145 cells with vehicle in 10% FBS-containing medium for 24 h resulted in a marked stimulation of G_1-to-S cell cycle progression. Treatment with 7 μM CUR or 5 μM CA resulted in a moderate decrease in the proportion of S phase without a noticeable accumulation of cells in the G_0/G_1 phase. However, the combined treatment produced a dramatic G_0/G_1 cell cycle arrest. The averaged data presented in Figure 4b demonstrate a significantly greater increase in the G_1/S ratio (indicative of G_0/G_1 arrest) by the combination compared to CUR or CA alone. Similar, but less pronounced effects were obtained in PC-3 cells (Figure 4b).

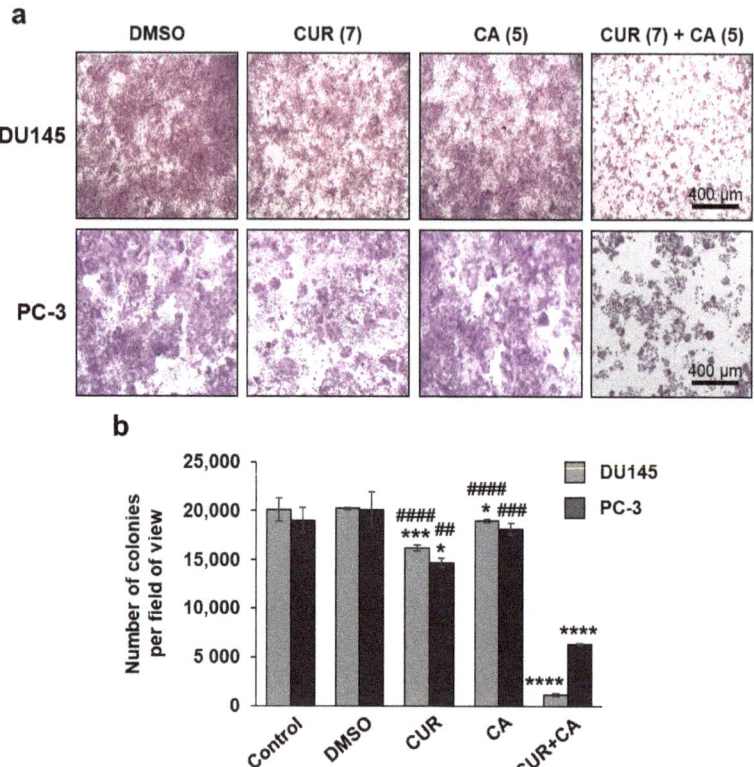

Figure 3. Colony formation analysis of the effects of curcumin and carnosic acid on cell growth. (**a**) Representative images of Crystal Violet-stained cell colonies obtained after 7 days of cell exposure to the indicated concentrations (in µM) of curcumin (CUR), carnosic acid (CA) and their combination (CUR + CA). Magnification: 40×; scale bar: 400 µm. (**b**) Quantitative evaluation of the colony formation data. The data are presented as averaged numbers of colonies per microscopic field of view (mean ± SEM; $n = 3$). Statistically significant differences for CUR, CA or CUR + CA vs. DMSO (* $p < 0.05$; *** $p < 0.001$ and **** $p < 0.0001$) and for CUR or CA applied separately vs. CUR + CA (## $p < 0.01$; ### $p < 0.001$ and #### $p < 0.0001$).

The G_0/G_1 cell cycle arrest induced by CUR + CA was accompanied by changes in the levels of several regulators of the G1-to-S transition, as determined in DU145 cells (Figure 4c and Supplementary Figure S2). Exposure to CUR and, especially, to its combination with CA for 15 h or 24 h resulted in an appreciable decrease in the level of D1 and E cyclins. The levels of CDK4 and CDK2 were not affected; however, those of the CDK inhibitors p21^{Cip1} and p27^{Kip1} were markedly elevated following combined treatments (Figure 4c,d).

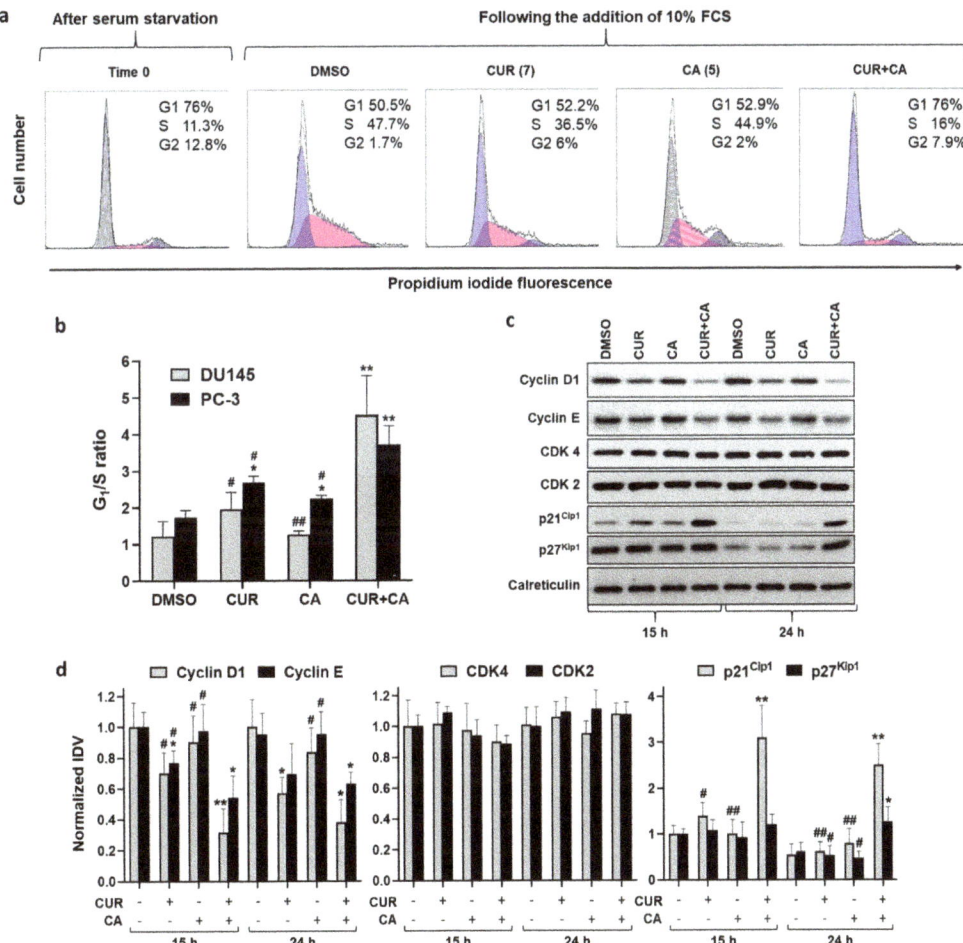

Figure 4. Modulation of cell cycle by curcumin, carnosic acid and their combination. (**a**) Representative flow cytometric data demonstrating inhibition of cell cycle progression in DU145 cells under the indicated treatment conditions (24 h). Values given in parentheses are concentrations (µM). (**b**) Quantitative data showing inhibition of G_1/S cell cycle transition. (**c**) Expression profile of cell cycle regulatory proteins. (**d**) Quantitative analysis of the protein expression data. Integrated Density Values (IDVs) of the indicated protein bands normalized to IDVs of respective calreticulin bands are shown. All IDV ratios are relative to that of the control (DMSO) sample at 15 h assumed as 1.0. Data are presented as mean ± SD (n = 3). Statistically significant differences for CUR, CA or CUR + CA vs. DMSO (* p < 0.05 and ** p < 0.01) and for CUR or CA vs. CUR + CA (# p < 0.05 and ## p < 0.01) determined separately at 15 h and 24 h.

3.3. Curcumin, Carnosic Acid and Their Combination Induce a Transient Rise of Cytosolic Calcium Levels

We have recently reported that in AML cells, CUR + CA-induced apoptosis is associated with a sustained elevation of cytosolic calcium levels ($[Ca^{2+}]_{cyt}$) [33]. Here, we also found that in prostate cancer cells this combination also evoked a $[Ca^{2+}]_{cyt}$ rise to higher levels than those observed after single treatments (Figure 5). However, in contrast to leukemia cells, the $[Ca^{2+}]_{cyt}$ elevation was transient and moderate, reaching only 30–40% of the maximal signal provoked by 10 µM calcium ionophore ionomycin (Supplementary Figure S3). Further, while in CUR+CA-treated AML cells, calcium was primarily mobilized from the endoplasmic reticulum [33], in prostate cancer cells it mainly influxed from the extracellular space since the use of Ca^{2+} free buffer resulted in an 80–90% decrease in the magnitude of the calcium signal (Figure 5).

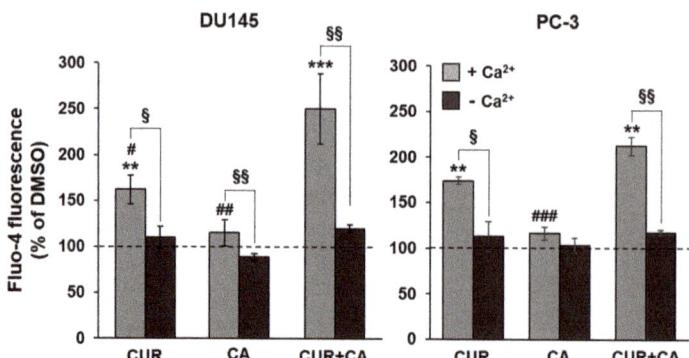

Figure 5. The combination of polyphenols induces elevation of cytosolic calcium levels in prostate cancer cells. Fluo-4 emission was recorded kinetically at 1 min intervals, starting immediately upon the addition of 7 µM CUR, 5 µM CA or their combination (CUR + CA). The bars show peak [Ca^{2+}]$_{cyt}$ signals recorded at 6–8 min (as in Supplementary Figure S3) relative to DMSO-treated cells. Data are presented as mean ± SEM (n = 3). Statistically significant differences for CUR, CA or CUR + CA vs. DMSO (** $p < 0.01$ and *** $p < 0.001$) and for CUR and CA vs. CUR + CA (# $p < 0.05$; ## $p < 0.01$ and ### $p < 0.001$). § $p < 0.05$ and §§ $p < 0.01$, significant difference between the two indicated groups (Student's t-test).

3.4. Effects of Polyphenols on Mitochondrial Functions

A modest elevation of calcium in the cytosol is sufficient to initiate calcium transport to the mitochondria [51]. The mitochondrial calcium uniport is an electrogenic process that occurs at the cost of the mitochondrial membrane potential ($\Delta\psi_m$). As shown in Figure 6, the addition of CUR or CA alone resulted in a slight reduction in $\Delta\psi_m$ in DU145 cells and was practically ineffective in PC-3 cells. However, the combination of these polyphenols markedly lowered the membrane potential to about 40% of the control level in DU145 cells, and to ~70% in PC-3 cells (Figure 6). This was a transient effect, echoing the transient cytosolic calcium elevation, as exemplified for DU145 cells in Supplementary Figure S3. The $\Delta\psi_m$ dropped within seconds after addition of the combination (0 h point in Figure 6) and partially recovered in 4–24 h.

The alterations in $\Delta\psi_m$, which are determinant of the electron transport, prompted us to evaluate the effects of polyphenols on oxidative phosphorylation (OxPhos). We applied the protocol of sequential addition of oligomycin, an inhibitor of ATPase, followed by titration of the protonophore FCCP to explore possible mitochondrial damage in intact (non-permeabilized) cells [48]. The original respirograms are available in the Supplementary Materials (Figure S4). The addition of the CUR + CA combination stimulated mitochondrial respiration in DU145 cells (Figure 7a) but decreased it in PC-3 cells (Figure 7b). Oligomycin did not strongly inhibit the respiration in DU145 cells. Subsequent addition of FCCP was not able to further stimulate respiration as it would under normal conditions, meaning that in the presence of the combination of polyphenols, the mitochondria function at their maximal respiratory capacity. These data correlate with a decrease in the membrane potential (Figure 6), indicating uncoupling of OxPhos in DU145 cells. On the other hand, the combination of polyphenols decreased the respiration in PC-3 cells (Figure 7b), so almost no further inhibition was produced by oligomycin, and no stimulation was induced by FCCP. Overall, the above data demonstrate that the presence of CUR + CA prevents the modulatory action of oligomycin and FCCP on OxPhos regardless of the mode of the mitochondrial respiratory response to the polyphenols, i.e., enhancement in DU145 cells or suppression in PC-3 cells (Figure 7a,b). These results suggest that the possible mechanisms of CUR + CA effects on the mitochondrial respiration include a protonophoric activity of the combination.

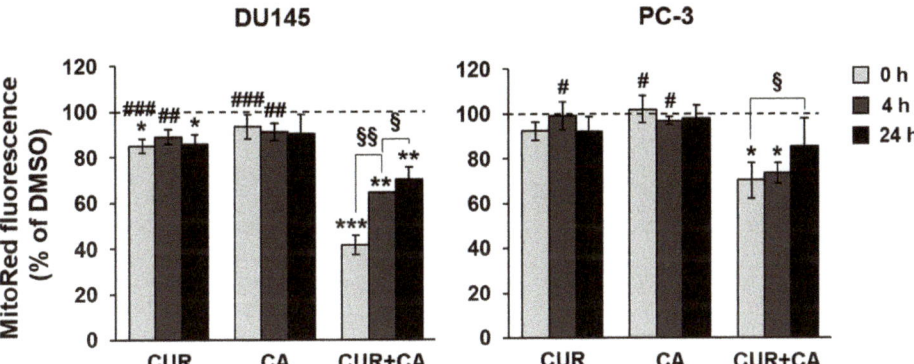

Figure 6. Combinatory effects of curcumin and carnosic acid on the mitochondrial membrane potential. Cells were treated with 7 µM CUR and 5 µM CA, alone and in combination (CUR + CA). The data were recorded at 5 min (0 h), 4 h and 24 h after the addition of DMSO or polyphenols. Data are presented as mean ± SEM (n = 3) relative to DMSO-treated cells. Statistically significant differences for CUR, CA or CUR + CA vs. DMSO (* $p < 0.05$; ** $p < 0.01$ and *** $p < 0.001$) and for CUR and CA vs. CUR + CA (# $p < 0.05$; ## $p < 0.01$ and ### $p < 0.001$). § $p < 0.05$ and §§ $p < 0.01$, significant difference between the indicated groups (Student's t-test).

The activities of individual respiratory complexes were evaluated using the cells permeabilized with the non-ionic detergent digitonin (Figure 7c,d) [50]. The integrated state 3 activities of the complexes I (Com I), I and II (Com I–II), and all complexes (Com I–IV) were assessed. Under permeabilized conditions, the contribution of calcium flow observed above is discounted, since in permeabilized cells the cytosolic content is diluted and, thus, the homeostatic integrity is compromised. This setting enables us to evaluate the potential direct effects of polyphenols on mitochondrial enzymes beyond plasma membrane-mediated calcium signaling.

In DU145 cells, the Com I activity was decreased by ~25% immediately (0 h) upon addition of the polyphenols, whereas the combined activities of Com I+II did not change significantly compared to DMSO-treated cells (Figure 7c). This is probably because of a higher rate of Com II respiration, as it is an electroneutral transporter and, therefore, it is less affected by membranotropic agents such as CUR. The combinatory activity of all complexes (Com I-IV) was elevated by ~20% over the control in agreement with a decrease in $\Delta\psi_m$ (Figure 6) and stimulated respiration observed in intact cells (Figure 7a). Following combined treatment of DU145 cells for 24 h, the OxPhos activities of all complexes were similarly reduced to the level of 60–70% of the control consistent with a decrease in $\Delta\psi_m$.

In PC-3 cells, the combination of polyphenols instantly (0 h) inhibited the activity of Com I to ~50%, of Com I+II to ~70% and of Com I-IV to ~80% of the control level (Figure 7d). These data are in consistence with the inhibited respiration observed in intact cells (Figure 7b). Following 24 h of incubation, the functionality of all PC-3 mitochondrial complexes constituted only about 60% of the control, also echoing a decreased $\Delta\psi_m$ at 24 h. Thus, regardless of differences in the initial responses of the mitochondria to the CUR + CA combination, in 24 h the resulting outcome in both DU145 and PC-3 cells was a decreased capacity of OxPhos (Figure 7c,d). The inhibitory effect of CUR + CA on Com I activity was common for the two cell lines (Figure 7c,d). One explanation for this finding is that the polyphenols may potentially interact with this complex in prostate cancer cells.

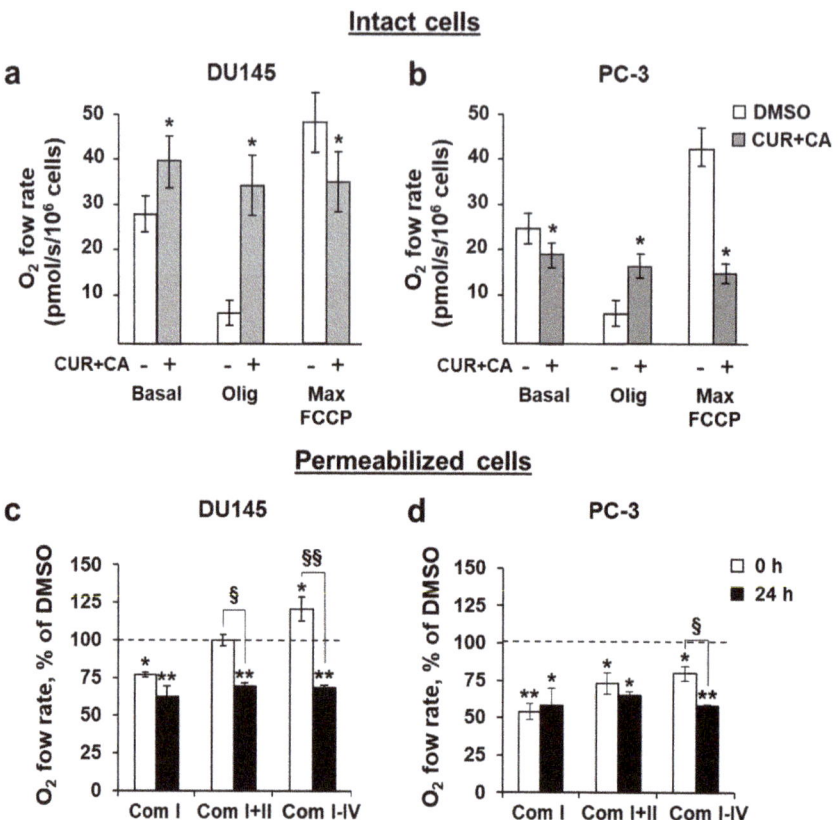

Figure 7. Combinatory effects of curcumin and carnosic acid on OxPhos. (**a,b**) Oxygen consumption in the presence or absence of 7 µM CUR and 5 µM CA (CUR + CA). Abbreviations: Basal, basal respiration; Olig, oligomycin-inhibited respiration; Max FCCP, the maximal respiratory capacity of mitochondria. (**c,d**) Respiration of permeabilized cells. The state 3 rates of OxPhos of complexes I, I+II, and I-IV measured upon addition (0 h) and after incubation (24 h) with the combination of CUR and CA, as compared to DMSO-treated cells. Data are presented as mean ± SEM ($n = 3$). Statistically significant differences in intact cell groups (**a,b**) treated with CUR + CA vs. DMSO: * $p < 0.05$. In permeabilized cell groups (**c,d**), statistically significant differences for the indicated groups vs. DMSO: * $p < 0.05$ and ** $p < 0.01$). § $p < 0.05$ and §§ $p < 0.01$, significant difference between the two indicated groups (Student's t-test).

3.5. Curcumin and Carnosic Acid Do Not Provoke Oxidative Stress in Prostate Cancer Cells

Retarded electron transport increases the chances of electron leakage and generation of superoxide [52]. We thus examined the levels of mitochondrial superoxide and cytosolic reactive oxygen species (ROS) in polyphenol-treated cells [53]. Within 5 min of the addition of CUR, alone or in combination with CA, a spike of superoxide signal was observed in both cancer cell lines (Figure 8a), which correlates with the drop in $\Delta\psi_m$ (Figure 6). This effect was transient and declined rapidly to the basal level, remaining so after 4 h and 24 h. CA alone had almost no effect on superoxide production but potentiated CUR-induced superoxide generation. In contrast to the mitochondrial superoxide, the cytosolic ROS levels did not significantly rise and even tended to slightly decrease with time (Figure 8b), suggesting that mitochondrial superoxide was effectively eliminated by endogenous scavengers preventing massive production of ROS.

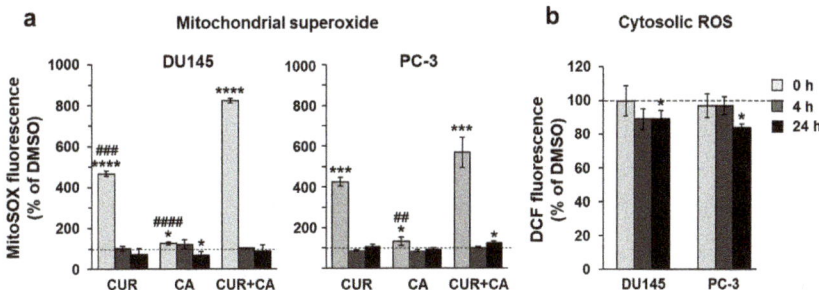

Figure 8. Effects of polyphenols on cellular production of reactive oxygen species. (**a**) Transient mitochondrial superoxide generation, as detected using the MitoSox probe following treatment with 7 µM CUR and 5 µM CA, alone and in combination (CUR + CA); (**b**) Cytosolic ROS assessed with the CM-H$_2$DCFDA probe in CUR + CA-treated cells. Changes in fluorescence were recorded at 5 min (0 h), 4 h and 24 h after the addition of DMSO or polyphenols. Data are presented as mean ± SEM (n = 3) relative to DMSO-treated cells. Statistically significant differences (**a**) for CUR, CA or CUR + CA vs. DMSO (* $p < 0.05$; *** $p < 0.001$ and **** $p < 0.0001$) and for CUR and CA vs. CUR + CA (## $p < 0.01$, ### $p < 0.001$ and #### $p < 0.0001$). In panel (**b**), significant differences for the indicated groups vs. DMSO: * $p < 0.05$.

3.6. Polyphenols Affect Mitochondria-Hosted mTOR Targets

The mammalian target of rapamycin (mTOR) has been shown to regulate mitochondrial function, e.g., by interacting with or stimulating translation of mitochondrial proteins [54,55]. As both CUR [56,57] and CA [58,59] individually were found to affect mTOR and its downstream effectors in various cancer cell types, we hypothesized that the polyphenol-induced changes in the mitochondrial activities observed in our study (Figures 6 and 7) may, at least in part, be related to the changes in mTOR signaling. To test this, we examined whether the effects of the CUR + CA combination on respiration of prostate cancer cells are influenced by rapamycin. Intact cells were incubated with 5 µM rapamycin [60] or vehicle for 1 h prior to addition of the combination of polyphenols. Due to lower rates of basal respiration in intact cells (Figure 7a,b), in order to demonstrate the cell responses to treatments the respiratory fluxes for each type of cells were normalized for their basal untreated respiration rates [61]. As shown in Figure 9a, rapamycin alone did not alter OxPhos in prostate cancer cells. However, the inhibitor caused a small but significant reduction in the stimulating effect of CUR + CA on DU145 respiration and prevented the drop in respiration in response to the combination in PC-3 cells (Figure 9a). The original respirograms are available in the Supplementary Materials (Figure S5).

The profile of the expression of mTOR genes that were affected by individual polyphenols, their combination, or rapamycin in DU145 cells after 24 h of treatment is shown in Figure 9b. The candidate genes that could physically be associated with mitochondria were searched among the transcripts of the mTOR downstream factors. Among the significantly altered genes, serum/glucocorticoid-regulated kinase 1 (SGK1) was the only one known to encode a protein localized in the mitochondrial outer membrane [62].

In DU145 cells, SGK1 gene expression was moderately down-regulated by rapamycin and CUR, and was not affected by CA, but when applied together the polyphenols caused a more pronounced downregulation of this tumor-promoting kinase (Figure 9b,c). In PC-3 cells, CA caused an elevation in SGK1 gene expression; however, CUR alone, the combination and rapamycin significantly reduced SGK1 expression (Figure 9c).

Consistent with the mRNA expression data (Figure 9b,c), treatment with the polyphenols, alone and in combination, or rapamycin resulted in a time-dependent reduction in SGK1 protein levels in both cell lines, as compared to DMSO-treated cells (Figure 10 and Supplementary Figure S6). Remarkably, in DU145 cells treated with CUR + CA or rapamycin for 24 h, SGK1 protein expression dropped to practically undetectable levels. In PC-3, the above treatments induced a moderate reduction in SGK1 levels (Figure 10).

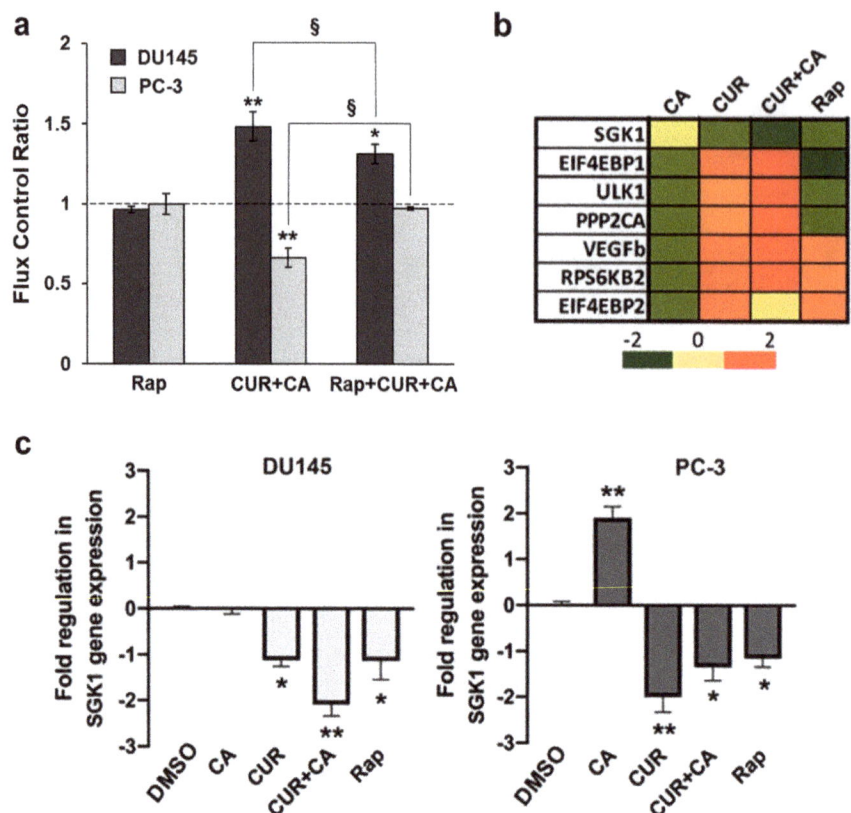

Figure 9. Effects of polyphenols and rapamycin on mitochondrial respiration and expression of mTOR downstream genes. (**a**) Rapamycin inhibits the effects of the polyphenol combination on mitochondrial respiration. Cells were pretreated with vehicle (DMSO) or 5 μM rapamycin (Rap) for 1 h followed by the addition of vehicle or 7 μM CUR and 5 μM CA (CUR + CA). Data are presented as mean ± SEM ($n = 3$) relative to DMSO. Statistically significant differences for the indicated groups vs. DMSO (* $p < 0.05$ and ** $p < 0.01$). § $p < 0.05$, significant differences between the indicated groups (Student's t-test). (**b**) Changes in mTOR downstream transcriptional profile upon treatment of DU145 cells with 5 μM rapamycin or 7 μM CUR, 5 μM CA or CUR + CA) for 24 h, relative to DMSO. (**c**) Quantitative analysis of SGK1 gene expression. Data are presented as fold regulation vs. DMSO (mean ± SEM; $n = 3$), where DMSO is set as 0. Statistically significant differences for treatments vs. control (DMSO): * $p < 0.05$ and ** $p < 0.01$.

The mTOR complex mTORC2 [63] and the 3-phosphoinositide-dependent protein kinase PDK2 [64] can activate SGK1 via phosphorylation at Ser422, and the mitogen-activated protein kinases (MAPKs) ERK5 [65] and p38 [66] via phosphorylation at Ser78. Here, we observed that treatment with CUR, CA or their combination resulted in a moderate reduction in SGK1 phosphorylation at Ser422 as compared to vehicle-treated cells. In DU145 cells, this effect was evidenced at both 6 h and 24 h, whereas in PC-3 cells a certain decrease in Ser422 phosphorylation was seen at 6 h, but not at 24 h (Figure 10 and Supplementary Figure S6). Interestingly, similar to the polyphenols, treatment with rapamycin also caused a decrease in Ser422 phosphorylation in both DU145 cells (at 6 h and 24 h) and PC-3 cells (at 6 h), implying that mTORC2, an indirect target of rapamycin [60,67,68], might be involved in the inhibitory effects of the polyphenols. The above treatments did not consistently affect SGK1 phosphorylation at Ser78, which mostly tended to increase slightly in the treated cells (Figure 10).

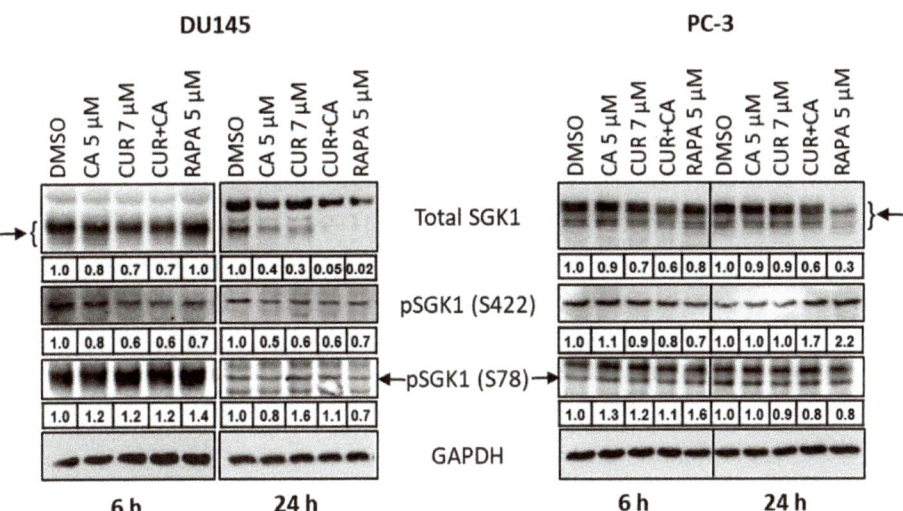

Figure 10. Effects of polyphenols and rapamycin on the protein expression and phosphorylation of serum- and glucocorticoid-regulated kinase 1 (SGK1) in prostate cancer cells. DU-145 and PC-3 cells were cultured with vehicle (DMSO), the indicated concentrations of curcumin (CUR) and carnosic acid (CA), alone and in combination, or the mTOR inhibitor rapamycin, for 6 or 24 h. Cells samples were then subjected to Western blot analysis. Integrated Density Values (IDVs) of the indicated protein bands normalized to IDVs of respective GAPDH bands are shown below corresponding blot images. Representative blots of 3 similar experiments are presented.

4. Discussion

The major finding of this study is that the plant polyphenols CUR and CA applied at low (<10 µM) concentrations, can synergistically cooperate to strongly suppress the growth of DU145 and PC-3 metastatic prostate cancer cell cultures in a time- and cell line-dependent manner. Notably, this effect was found to be essentially cytostatic (Figure 3), concomitant with G_0/G_1 cell cycle arrest (Figure 4), with only a negligible level of cell death (Figure 2). Inhibitory effects of various polyphenols, including CUR and CA, on cell cycle progression in cancer cells have been associated with the upregulation of both p21^{Cip1} and p27^{Kip1} (e.g., [69,70]). Importantly, some polyphenols, such as silibinin [71] or epigallocatechin gallate [72], were found to attenuate cellular degradation of these proteins, which was associated with cell cycle arrest, suggesting that a similar mechanism may, at least in part, account for the marked upregulation of p21^{Cip1} and p27^{Kip1} in CUR+CA-treated prostate cancer cells (Figure 4c,d).

The lack of cytotoxicity in CUR+CA-treated prostate cancer cells is strikingly different from the earlier-reported pronounced apoptotic cell death in AML cells [32–34]. Such distinct modes of CUR+CA action on prostate and blood cancer cells, coupled with the previously observed insusceptibility of untransformed hematopoietic and non-hematopoietic cells to this combination [32,33], indicate a remarkable cell-type dependence of the mechanisms underlying its anticancer effects. In AML cells, CUR+CA treatment results in a rapid (within 4–8 h) induction of apoptosis without inducing oxidative stress or changes in $\Delta\psi_m$ and is mediated solely by Ca^{2+} release from the endoplasmic reticulum leading to sustained $[Ca^{2+}]_{cyt}$ accumulation [33,34]. Although, similar to AML cells, CUR + CA treatment tended to lower cytosolic ROS in prostate cancer cells (Figure 8), prostate cancer cells exhibited a marked decrease in $\Delta\psi_m$ (Figure 6) and just a transient (within minutes) extracellular calcium-dependent $[Ca^{2+}]_{cyt}$ rise (Figure 5 and Figure S3). These cell type-dependent differences in regulatory responses might contribute to the observed distinct modes of CUR + CA action. Recently, Einbond et al. [73] have demonstrated that CUR (3.3–10.9) and CA (6.0–12.0 µM) can also cooperate in reducing the growth of triple-negative MDA-

MB-468 human breast cancer cells in culture. However, this cooperation was evaluated only on the basis of the 3-(4,5-dimethyl-2-thiazol)-2,5-diphenyl-2H tetrazolilum bromide (MTT) assay, which is unable to distinguish changes in cell proliferation from changes in the extent of cell death. Therefore, the mode and the mechanism of action of CUR + CA on these cells are unclear.

In general, the mechanisms of synergistic cell growth-inhibitory effects of CUR + CA at low concentrations appear to differ from those underlying the effects of CUR (e.g., [8,9,11,14]) or CA [74–77] alone at higher concentrations (> 10 µM) in that the latter effects are usually found to be mediated by the induction of generalized cellular stress responses. Interestingly, Rodriguez-Garcia [9] reported that while the apoptotic effect of CUR on LNCaP and PC-3 prostate cancer cells was ROS-dependent and was associated with thioredoxin oxidation, the polyphenol silibinin, which reduced ROS levels and prevented thioredoxin oxidation in these cells, produced only a cytostatic effect. The latter finding supports, though indirectly, our data, showing that the cytostatic effect of CUR + CA on DU145 and PC-3 cells occurs in the absence of oxidative stress and is even associated with a slight reduction in the cytosolic ROS levels (Figure 7b).

Synergistic anticancer effects of various polyphenol combinations have been demonstrated in several tumor cell types (see [23,78] for recent reviews); however, the nature of the synergy between these compounds has not been fully elucidated. Several mechanisms of cooperation between antioxidant phytochemicals, including polyphenols, have been proposed (reviewed in [79]). For instance, individual components of a combination may target distinct signaling/transcriptional pathways or different proteins in the same cellular regulatory pathway. Furthermore, one of the components may help regenerate or chemically stabilize the other outside and/or inside the cell. The latter effects as well as the ability of certain phytochemicals, e.g., CA and CUR, to suppress drug efflux/multidrug resistance systems [80–82] may facilitate intracellular accumulation of one or both compounds. Indeed, Nimiya et al. [83] have shown that different antioxidants, including the plant phenolic compounds gallic, caffeic and rosmarinic acids, increased CUR stability in phosphate buffer and serum-free cell culture medium at physiological pH, as measured by colorimetric and HPLC assays. Consistent with these data, we have recently found that the addition of CA increases intracellular CUR levels in AML cells [34]. This was demonstrated by flow cytometry on the basis of CUR fluorescent properties [84]. In a recent study, Levine et al. [85] also showed that combined treatment of canine cancer cell lines with CA-rich rosemary extract and CUR-rich turmeric extract markedly increased intracellular CUR accumulation.

The data obtained in the present study indicate that unlike CUR, CA alone had primarily a minor or no significant influence on various cellular responses, such as changes in cell growth (Figures 1 and 2), cell cycle distribution and regulatory protein levels (Figure 4), $[Ca^{2+}]_{cyt}$ levels (Figure 5 and Figure S3), mitochondrial superoxide production (Figure 8) and SGK1 gene expression (Figure 9). These results suggest that in metastatic prostate cancer cells, CA may act by potentiating CUR actions, likely by increasing its stability and/or cellular accumulation.

The metastatic ability of cancer cells is supported by the reprogramming of metabolic processes that include increases in the mitochondria membrane potential, rates of OxPhos, levels of ROS and calcium retention capacity [37,43]. Therefore, chemical agents that alter oxidative processes would perturb cancer metabolism and/or make neoplastic cells more susceptible to pharmacological factors. In this work, we specifically addressed the effects of CUR and CA on mitochondrial function. The immediate drop in $\Delta\psi_m$ observed in both prostate cancer cell lines treated with CUR + CA (Figure 6) could be associated with $[Ca^{2+}]_{cyt}$ elevation (Figure 5), which is pumped in the mitochondria at the cost of $\Delta\psi_m$. The mitochondria depolarization was likely the reason for prolonged suppression of all respiratory enzyme complexes, although initial respiratory responses of the two tested cancer cells to the combination of polyphenols differed—stimulation of the electron flow in DU145 cells and its inhibition in PC-3 (Figure 7). PC-3 cells were also less sensitive than

DU145 cells to alterations of the calcium signal and $\Delta\psi_m$ caused by CUR + CA treatment (Figures 5 and 6). The different responses of the mitochondria in the two prostate cancer cell lines to the polyphenols may be associated with their distinct metabolic features which include higher rates of glutamate/malate, citrate/malate and succinate oxidation and higher enzymatic activity of complex I in PC-3 cells compared to DU145 cells, as demonstrated in our previous study [43]. In addition, their mitochondrial membrane characteristics, e.g., variation of lipid content or the degree of saturation of acyl chains [86], may also differ. Earlier, using model membranes mimicking the mitochondria lipid bilayer we demonstrated a high affinity of CUR to cardiolipin, the mitochondria-unique phospholipid [87]. This in part explains the known curcumin's protonophoric activity [88] and overall potential benefits in the treatment of broad range of metabolic diseases and conditions with key involvement of mitochondria. Still, several studies have demonstrated that in CUR-treated non-neoplastic and cancer cells, the polyphenol primarily localizes in the endoplasmic reticulum and lysosomes and only modestly accumulates in the mitochondria (e.g., [89,90]). These data suggest that the effects of CUR on the mitochondria are likely to be indirect. Of note, it has recently been suggested that physicochemical properties of polyphenols are responsible for their anticancer properties by virtue of their protonophoric and pro-oxidant properties rather than their specific effects on downstream molecular targets [44].

The dissimilar sensitivity of the two prostate cancer cell lines to the antiproliferative effects of CUR + CA could be related to the above differences in mitochondrial performances as well as to genetic features linked to their metastatic loci, such as brain (DU145) and bone (PC-3). Albeit sharing common malignant identities, the PC-3 cells were reported to have higher metastatic potential compared to DU145 cells [91]. Prolonged energetic stress caused by the combination of polyphenols in prostate cancer cells correlated with cell cycle arrest (Figure 4). However, dissipation of $\Delta\psi_m$ and altered oxidative phosphorylation did not lead to oxidative stress, since the massive increase in the mitochondrial superoxide signal right after addition of the combination of polyphenols, was quickly eliminated (Figure 8).

A key metabolic regulator, mTOR, plays a significant role in tumorigenesis and has been shown to be spatially associated with mitochondria and to control mitochondrial functionality [54,55,68]. As an instrumental tool, we employed rapamycin, a selective mTOR inhibitor which directly targets the mTORC1 complex and also indirectly blocks mTORC2 activity [60,67,68]. While rapamycin did not alter cellular respiration in our experimental setting, it moderately but significantly prevented the cell type-dependent effects of the CUR + CA combination, i.e., stimulation of respiration in DU145 cells and inhibition in PC-3 cells (Figure 9a), suggesting that these effects were partially mediated by mTOR.

Our search for a possible modulation of mitochondria-destined mTOR downstream targets by CUR and CA revealed SGK1, a multifunctional kinase which primarily localizes in the outer mitochondria membrane [62,92] and is implicated in regulating the growth, survival, cell cycle and apoptosis resistance of cancer cells [93]. Increased expression of SGK1 has been shown in myeloma [94], breast [95] and prostate [96] cancer cell cultures. Downregulation of SGK1 expression or inhibition of its kinase activity results in antiproliferative and cytotoxic effects on various types of malignant cells [93], including prostate cancer cells [96–98]. In prostate cancer, SGK1 inhibition also has anti-androgen effects [97].

To the best of our knowledge, only one publication related to the effect of CUR on SGK1 has been cited in MEDLINE/PubMed so far, which showed that treatment of renal carcinoma cells with 20 µM CUR did not affect either SGK1 protein levels or its phosphorylation [99]. No evidence of SGK1 modulation by CA has yet been reported. However, antiproliferative and cytotoxic effects of other plant phenolic compounds, such as resveratrol [100] and genistein [101], were found to correlate with SGK1 downregulation. Particularly, resveratrol inhibited SGK1 activity in hepatocellular carcinoma cells and also in a cell-free kinase assay. Moreover, silencing SGK1 enhanced resveratrol-induced inhibition of cell growth and apoptotic cell death, whereas SGK1 overexpression attenuated these effects [100]. By analogy, our finding that, similar to rapamycin, CUR ± CA suppressed mRNA and protein expression of SGK1 in DU145 and PC-3 cells (Figures 9b,c and 10) suggests that SGK1 downregulation might contribute to the antiproliferative effect of these treatments, e.g., through upregulating p21^{Cip1} [94] and p27^{Kip1} [102]. There is accumulating evidence that SGK1 is an essential mediator of the phosphatidylinositol 3-kinase (PI3K)/mTOR signaling pathway (e.g., [93]). Thus, our finding that the polyphenols attenuate SGK1 phosphorylation at Ser422 (Figure 10), may suggest a role of the PI3K/mTOR pathway in the mechanism of the cytostatic effect of CUR + CA on prostate cancer cells. Further research is required to test this suggestion.

5. Conclusions

Our findings demonstrate that the combination of CUR and CA is more efficient than the individual compounds in arresting metastatic prostate cancer cell growth. The cytostatic effect of the combination was more pronounced in DU145 cells compared to PC-3 cells and was not accompanied by the induction of oxidative stress and cell death. CUR + CA-induced inhibition of cell growth was associated with G_0/G_1 cell cycle arrest and inhibition of mitochondrial function preceded by a rapid $[Ca^{2+}]_{cyt}$ rise and drop in $\Delta\psi_m$. Upon treatment with CUR±CA, the two cell lines mostly differed in the response magnitude and/or time course. Thus, while PC-3 cell growth was almost unaffected by CUR + CA at 48 h, the two cell lines responded similarly after 7 days of treatment (Figure 1 vs. Figure 3). Likewise, when compared to DU145 cells, PC-3 cells exhibited generally similar, though less pronounced changes in the cell cycle (Figure 4a), Ca^{2+}_{cyt} (Figure 5), $\Delta\psi_m$ (Figure 6), superoxide and ROS levels (Figure 8) and SGK1 expression (Figures 9c and 10). The main difference between DU145 and PC-3 cells was the dissimilar modulation of the mitochondrial respiration in response to polyphenol treatment (Figures 7 and 9a), which may or may not relate to the different sensitivity of the two cell lines to the polyphenols.

Prostate cancer is the second most common cancer in men worldwide, mainly in countries with high Human Development Index [103,104]. Although most patients with localized disease have high survival rates, patients with metastatic prostate cancer have poor prognosis, with a 5-year survival rate of about 30%. Therefore, our findings presented here warrant further testing of this combination in translational studies that may lead to clinical development. Synergistically acting combinations of low concentrations of plant polyphenols or related agents with enhanced anti-cancer capacities may represent a safe and efficient way of dietary and/or pharmacological intervention in human malignancies, including prostate cancer. We believe that under prolonged energetic stress caused by the combination of CUR and CA, the cancer cells may become more vulnerable projecting a better response to chemotherapeutic and/or radiation treatments. Still, deeper research is required to elucidate the molecular mechanism of the synergistic effects of CUR and CA on cellular signaling and integrated metabolic pathways in order to establish polyphenol-based combinatory cancer therapeutics or adjuvants to conventional treatment modalities. Characterization of the mechanistic interactions between the mitochondrial energetic machinery and the mitochondria-resident SGK1 expression and activity would be of great interest per se in understanding how the confined transcriptional control is exerted locally over the mitochondrial functions.

Supplementary Materials: The following are available online at https://www.mdpi.com/2076-3921/10/10/1591/s1. Figure S1: Chemical structures of curcumin and carnosic acid, Figure S2: Original images of the Western blots images shown in Figure 4c, Figure S3: Curcumin and carnosic acid cooperate in inducing moderate and transient cytosolic calcium elevation in DU145 prostate cancer cells, Figure S4: Combinatory effects of curcumin and carnosic acid on mitochondria respiration, Figure S5: Oxygraphic records of the effects of the combination of curcumin and carnosic acid on respiration of prostate cancer cells, Figure S6: Original images of the Western blots shown in Figure 10.

Author Contributions: Conceptualization, M.D., Y.S. and Z.O.; methodology, M.D., S.R. and Z.O.; validation, S.O., M.K., Y.S., S.T., R.S., M.D. and Z.O.; investigation, S.O., M.K., S.R., A.T. and Z.O.; resources, M.D. and S.T.; funding acquisition, Z.O., M.D. and Y.S.; writing—original draft preparation, R.S., M.D. and Z.O.; writing—review and editing, S.O., M.K., Y.S., S.T., R.S., M.D. and Z.O.; visualization, S.O., M.K., S.R., A.T. and Z.O.; supervision, M.D., Y.S. and Z.O. All authors have read and agreed to the published version of the manuscript.

Funding: This work was supported by Cornelius Beukenkamp endowment (to Z.O.) and by the Israel Science Foundation grant 226/16 (to M.D. and Y.S.).

Institutional Review Board Statement: Not applicable.

Informed Consent Statement: Not applicable.

Data Availability Statement: Data is contained within the article or supplementary material.

Conflicts of Interest: The authors declare no conflict of interest. The funders had no role in the study design, data acquisition and analysis, as well as in the manuscript preparation and making decision to publish the data.

Abbreviations

Abbreviations	
CA	Carnosic acid
CDK	Cyclin-dependent kinase
CM-H2DCFDA	5-(and-6)-chloromethyl-2′,7′-dichlorodihydrofluorescein diacetate, acetyl ester
CUR	Curcumin
DTT	Dithiothreitol
EGFR	Epidermal growth factor receptor
FBS	Fetal bovine serum
FCCP	Carbonyl cyanide-4-(trifluoromethoxy)phenylhydrazone
GAPDH	Glyceraldehyde phosphate dehydrogenase
HRP	Horseradish peroxidase
mTOR	Mammalian target of rapamycin
NFκB	Nuclear factor kappa B
OxPhos	Oxidative phosphorylation
ROS	Reactive oxygen species
SGK1	Serum/glucocorticoid regulated kinase 1
TMPD	N,N,N′,N′-Tetramethyl-p-phenylenediamine dihydrochloride

References

1. Newman, D.J.; Cragg, G.M. Natural products as sources of new drugs over the nearly four decades from 01/1981 to 09/2019. *J. Nat. Prod.* **2020**, *83*, 770–803. [CrossRef]
2. Dhillon, N.; Aggarwal, B.B.; Newman, R.A.; Wolff, R.A.; Kunnumakkara, A.B.; Abbruzzese, J.L.; Ng, C.S.; Badmaev, V.; Kurzrock, R. Phase II Trial of Curcumin in Patients with Advanced Pancreatic Cancer. *Clin. Cancer Res.* **2008**, *14*, 4491–4499. [CrossRef]
3. Choi, Y.H.; Han, D.H.; Kim, S.-W.; Kim, M.-J.; Sung, H.H.; Jeon, H.G.; Jeong, B.C.; Seo, S.I.; Jeon, S.S.; Lee, H.M.; et al. A randomized, double-blind, placebo-controlled trial to evaluate the role of curcumin in prostate cancer patients with intermittent androgen deprivation. *Prostate* **2019**, *79*, 614–621. [CrossRef]
4. Giordano, A.; Tommonaro, G. Curcumin and Cancer. *Nutrients* **2019**, *11*, 2376. [CrossRef]
5. Mortezaee, K.; Salehi, E.; Mahyari, H.M.; Motevaseli, E.; Najafi, M.; Farhood, B.; Rosengren, R.J.; Sahebkar, A. Mechanisms of apoptosis modulation by curcumin: Implications for cancer therapy. *J. Cell. Physiol.* **2019**, *234*, 12537–12550. [CrossRef]
6. Khan, M.A.; Gahlot, S.; Majumdar, S. Oxidative Stress Induced by Curcumin Promotes the Death of Cutaneous T-cell Lymphoma (HuT-78) by Disrupting the Function of Several Molecular Targets. *Mol. Cancer Ther.* **2012**, *11*, 1873–1883. [CrossRef]
7. Woo, J.-H.; Kim, Y.-H.; Choi, Y.-J.; Kim, D.-G.; Lee, K.-S.; Bae, J.H.; Min, D.S.; Chang, J.-S.; Jeong, Y.-J.; Lee, Y.H.; et al. Molecular mechanisms of curcumin-induced cytotoxicity: Induction of apoptosis through generation of reactive oxygen species, down-regulation of Bcl-XL and IAP, the release of cytochrome c and inhibition of Akt. *Carcinogenesis* **2003**, *24*, 1199–1208. [CrossRef] [PubMed]
8. Larasati, Y.; Yoneda-Kato, N.; Nakamae, I.; Yokoyama, T.; Meiyanto, E.; Kato, J.-Y. Curcumin targets multiple enzymes involved in the ROS metabolic pathway to suppress tumor cell growth. *Sci. Rep.* **2018**, *8*, 2039. [CrossRef] [PubMed]
9. Garcia, A.R.; Hevia, D.; Mayo, J.C.; Gonzalez-Menendez, P.; Coppo, L.; Lu, J.; Holmgren, A.; Sainz, R.M. Thioredoxin 1 modulates apoptosis induced by bioactive compounds in prostate cancer cells. *Redox Biol.* **2017**, *12*, 634–647. [CrossRef]

10. Wang, L.; Chen, X.; Du, Z.; Li, G.; Chen, M.; Chen, X.; Liang, G.; Chen, T. Curcumin suppresses gastric tumor cell growth via ROS-mediated DNA polymerase γ depletion disrupting cellular bioenergetics. *J. Exp. Clin. Cancer Res.* **2017**, *36*, 47. [CrossRef] [PubMed]
11. Lee, W.-J.; Chien, M.-H.; Chow, J.-M.; Chang, J.-L.; Wen, Y.-C.; Lin, Y.-W.; Cheng, C.-W.; Lai, G.-M.; Hsiao, M.; Lee, L.-M. Nonautophagic cytoplasmic vacuolation death induction in human PC-3M prostate cancer by curcumin through reactive oxygen species -mediated endoplasmic reticulum stress. *Sci. Rep.* **2015**, *5*, 10420. [CrossRef] [PubMed]
12. Wang, L.; Wang, L.; Song, R.; Shen, Y.; Sun, Y.; Gu, Y.; Shu, Y.; Xu, Q. Targeting Sarcoplasmic/Endoplasmic Reticulum Ca2+-ATPase 2 by Curcumin Induces ER Stress-Associated Apoptosis for Treating Human Liposarcoma. *Mol. Cancer Ther.* **2011**, *10*, 461–471. [CrossRef] [PubMed]
13. Kim, B.; Kim, H.S.; Jung, E.-J.; Lee, J.Y.; Tsang, B.K.; Lim, J.M.; Song, Y.S. Curcumin induces ER stress-mediated apoptosis through selective generation of reactive oxygen species in cervical cancer cells. *Mol. Carcinog.* **2016**, *55*, 918–928. [CrossRef] [PubMed]
14. Rivera, M.; Ramos, Y.; Rodríguez-Valentín, M.; López-Acevedo, S.; Cubano, L.A.; Zou, J.; Zhang, Q.; Wang, G.; Boukli, N.M. Targeting multiple pro-apoptotic signaling pathways with curcumin in prostate cancer cells. *PLoS ONE* **2017**, *12*, e0179587. [CrossRef]
15. Dei Cas, M.; Ghidoni, R. Dietary Curcumin: Correlation between Bioavailability and Health Potential. *Nutrients* **2019**, *11*, 2147. [CrossRef]
16. Sanchez, M.A.N.; González-Sarrías, A.; Vaquero, M.R.; Villalba, R.G.; Selma, M.V.; Tomas-Barberan, F.; García-Conesa, M.-T.; Espín, J.C. Dietary phenolics against colorectal cancer-From promising preclinical results to poor translation into clinical trials: Pitfalls and future needs. *Mol. Nutr. Food Res.* **2015**, *59*, 1274–1291. [CrossRef] [PubMed]
17. Gautam, S.C.; Xu, Y.X.; Pindolia, K.; Janakiraman, N.; Chapman, R.A. Nonselective Inhibition of Proliferation of Transformed and Nontransformed Cells by the Anticancer Agent Curcumin (Diferuloylmethane). *Biochem. Pharmacol.* **1998**, *55*, 1333–1337. [CrossRef]
18. Azqueta, A.; Collins, A. Polyphenols and DNA Damage: A Mixed Blessing. *Nutrients* **2016**, *8*, 785. [CrossRef]
19. Zikaki, K.; Aggeli, I.-K.; Gaitanaki, C.; Beis, I. Curcumin induces the apoptotic intrinsic pathway via upregulation of reactive oxygen species and JNKs in H9c2 cardiac myoblasts. *Apoptosis* **2014**, *19*, 958–974. [CrossRef]
20. Hollborn, M.; Chen, R.; Wiedemann, P.; Reichenbach, A.; Bringmann, A.; Kohen, L. Cytotoxic Effects of Curcumin in Human Retinal Pigment Epithelial Cells. *PLoS ONE* **2013**, *8*, e59603. [CrossRef]
21. Fox, J.T.; Sakamuru, S.; Huang, R.; Teneva, N.; Simmons, S.; Xia, M.; Tice, R.R.; Austin, C.P.; Myung, K. High-throughput genotoxicity assay identifies antioxidants as inducers of DNA damage response and cell death. *Proc. Natl. Acad. Sci. USA* **2012**, *109*, 5423–5428. [CrossRef] [PubMed]
22. Vue, B.; Zhang, S.; Chen, Q.-H. Synergistic Effects of Dietary Natural Products as Anti-Prostate Cancer Agents. *Nat. Prod. Commun.* **2015**, *10*, 2179–2188. [CrossRef] [PubMed]
23. Hosseini-Zare, M.S.; Sarhadi, M.; Zarei, M.; Thilagavathi, R.; Selvam, C. Synergistic effects of curcumin and its analogs with other bioactive compounds: A comprehensive review. *Eur. J. Med. Chem.* **2021**, *210*, 113072. [CrossRef] [PubMed]
24. Lin, S.R.; Chang, C.H.; Hsu, C.F.; Tsai, M.J.; Cheng, H.; Leong, M.K.; Sung, P.J.; Chen, J.C.; Weng, C.F. Natural compounds as potential adjuvants to cancer therapy: Preclinical evidence. *Br. J. Pharmacol.* **2020**, *177*, 1409–1423. [CrossRef] [PubMed]
25. Kundur, S.; Prayag, A.; Selvakumar, P.; Nguyen, H.; McKee, L.; Cruz, C.; Srinivasan, A.; Shoyele, S.; Lakshmikuttyamma, A. Synergistic anticancer action of quercetin and curcumin against triple-negative breast cancer cell lines. *J. Cell. Physiol.* **2019**, *234*, 11103–11118. [CrossRef] [PubMed]
26. Majumdar, A.P.N.; Banerjee, S.; Nautiyal, J.; Patel, B.B.; Patel, V.; Du, J.; Yu, Y.; Elliott, A.A.; Levi, E.; Sarkar, F.H. Curcumin Synergizes With Resveratrol to Inhibit Colon Cancer. *Nutr. Cancer* **2009**, *61*, 544–553. [CrossRef] [PubMed]
27. Gavrilas, L.I.; Cruceriu, D.; Ionescu, C.; Miere, D.; Balacescu, O. Pro-apoptotic genes as new targets for single and combinatorial treatments with resveratrol and curcumin in colorectal cancer. *Food Funct.* **2019**, *10*, 3717–3726. [CrossRef]
28. Eom, D.-W.; Lee, J.H.; Kim, Y.-J.; Hwang, G.S.; Kim, S.-N.; Kwak, J.H.; Cheon, G.J.; Kim, K.H.; Jang, H.-J.; Ham, J.; et al. Synergistic effect of curcumin on epigallocatechin gallate-induced anticancer action in PC3 prostate cancer cells. *BMB Rep.* **2015**, *48*, 461–466. [CrossRef]
29. Lodi, A.; Saha, A.; Lu, X.; Wang, B.; Sentandreu, E.; Collins, M.; Kolonin, M.G.; DiGiovanni, J.; Tiziani, S. Combinatorial treatment with natural compounds in prostate cancer inhibits prostate tumor growth and leads to key modulations of cancer cell metabolism. *NPJ Precis. Oncol.* **2017**, *1*, 1–12. [CrossRef]
30. Linnewiel-Hermoni, K.; Khanin, M.; Danilenko, M.; Zango, G.; Amosi, Y.; Levy, J.; Sharoni, Y. The anti-cancer effects of carotenoids and other phytonutrients resides in their combined activity. *Arch. Biochem. Biophys.* **2015**, *572*, 28–35. [CrossRef]
31. Bahri, S.; Jameleddine, S.; Shlyonsky, V. Relevance of carnosic acid to the treatment of several health disorders: Molecular targets and mechanisms. *Biomed. Pharmacother.* **2016**, *84*, 569–582. [CrossRef]
32. Pesakhov, S.; Khanin, M.; Studzinski, G.P.; Danilenko, M. Distinct Combinatorial Effects of the Plant Polyphenols Curcumin, Carnosic Acid, and Silibinin on Proliferation and Apoptosis in Acute Myeloid Leukemia Cells. *Nutr. Cancer* **2010**, *62*, 811–824. [CrossRef]
33. Pesakhov, S.; Nachliely, M.; Barvish, Z.; Aqaqe, N.; Schwartzman, B.; Voronov, E.; Sharoni, Y.; Studzinski, G.P.; Fishman, D.; Danilenko, M. Cancer-selective cytotoxic Ca2+ overload in acute myeloid leukemia cells and attenuation of disease progression in mice by synergistically acting polyphenols curcumin and carnosic acid. *Oncotarget* **2016**, *7*, 31847–31861. [CrossRef]

34. Trachtenberg, A.; Muduli, S.; Sidoryk, K.; Cybulski, M.; Danilenko, M. Synergistic Cytotoxicity of Methyl 4-Hydroxycinnamate and Carnosic Acid to Acute Myeloid Leukemia Cells via Calcium-Dependent Apoptosis Induction. *Front. Pharmacol.* **2019**, *10*, 507. [CrossRef]
35. Namekawa, T.; Ikeda, K.; Horie-Inoue, K.; Inoue, S. Application of Prostate Cancer Models for Preclinical Study: Advantages and Limitations of Cell Lines, Patient-Derived Xenografts, and Three-Dimensional Culture of Patient-Derived Cells. *Cells* **2019**, *8*, 74. [CrossRef] [PubMed]
36. Palmberg, C.; Rantala, I.; Tammela, T.L.; Helin, H.; Koivisto, P.A. Low apoptotic activity in primary prostate carcinomas without response to hormonal therapy. *Oncol. Rep.* **2000**, *7*, 1141–1144. [CrossRef] [PubMed]
37. Freitas, M.; Baldeiras, I.; Proença, T.; Alves, V.; Mota-Pinto, A.; Sarmento-Ribeiro, A. Oxidative stress adaptation in aggressive prostate cancer may be counteracted by the reduction of glutathione reductase. *FEBS Open Bio* **2012**, *2*, 119–128. [CrossRef] [PubMed]
38. Koivisto, P.; Visakorpi, T.; Rantala, I.; Isola, J. Increased cell proliferation activity and decreased cell death are associated with the emergence of hormone-refractory recurrent prostate cancer. *J. Pathol.* **1997**, *183*, 51–56. [CrossRef]
39. Kaambre, T.; Chekulayev, V.; Shevchuk, I.; Karu-Varikmaa, M.; Timohhina, N.; Tepp, K.; Bogovskaja, J.; Kütner, R.; Valvere, V.; Saks, V. Metabolic control analysis of cellular respiration in situ in intraoperational samples of human breast cancer. *J. Bioenerg. Biomembr.* **2012**, *44*, 539–558. [CrossRef] [PubMed]
40. Koit, A.; Shevchuk, I.; Ounpuu, L.; Klepinin, A.; Chekulayev, V.; Timohhina, N.; Tepp, K.; Puurand, M.; Truu, L.; Heck, K.; et al. Mitochondrial Respiration in Human Colorectal and Breast Cancer Clinical Material Is Regulated Differently. *Oxidative Med. Cell. Longev.* **2017**, *2017*, 1372640. [CrossRef]
41. Martinez-Outschoorn, U.E.; Pestell, R.G.; Howell, A.; Tykocinski, M.L.; Nagajyothi, F.; Machado, F.S.; Tanowitz, H.B.; Sotgia, F.; Lisanti, M.P. Energy transfer in "parasitic" cancer metabolism. *Cell Cycle* **2011**, *10*, 4208–4216. [CrossRef]
42. Wallace, D.C. Mitochondria and cancer. *Nat. Rev. Cancer* **2012**, *12*, 685–698. [CrossRef]
43. Panov, A.; Orynbayeva, Z. Bioenergetic and Antiapoptotic Properties of Mitochondria from Cultured Human Prostate Cancer Cell Lines PC-3, DU145 and LNCaP. *PLoS ONE* **2013**, *8*, e72078. [CrossRef]
44. Stevens, J.F.; Revel, J.S.; Maier, C.S. Mitochondria-Centric Review of Polyphenol Bioactivity in Cancer Models. *Antioxid. Redox Signal.* **2018**, *29*, 1589–1611. [CrossRef] [PubMed]
45. Rampersad, S.N. Multiple Applications of Alamar Blue as an Indicator of Metabolic Function and Cellular Health in Cell Viability Bioassays. *Sensors* **2012**, *12*, 12347–12360. [CrossRef] [PubMed]
46. Galluzzi, L.; Vitale, I.; Abrams, J.M.; Alnemri, E.S.; Baehrecke, E.H.; Blagosklonny, M.V.; Dawson, T.M.; Dawson, V.L.; El-Deiry, W.S.; Fulda, S.; et al. Molecular definitions of cell death subroutines: Recommendations of the Nomenclature Committee on Cell Death 2012. *Cell Death Differ.* **2012**, *19*, 107–120. [CrossRef]
47. Gnaiger, E.; Steinlechner-Maran, R.; Méndez, G.; Eberl, T.; Margreiter, R. Control of mitochondrial and cellular respiration by oxygen. *J. Bioenerg. Biomembr.* **1995**, *27*, 583–596. [CrossRef]
48. Pesta, D.; Gnaiger, E. High-resolution respirometry: OXPHOS protocols for human cells and permeabilized fibers from small biopsies of human muscle. *Methods Mol. Biol.* **2012**, *810*, 25–58. [CrossRef]
49. Brand, M.D.; Nicholls, D.G. Assessing mitochondrial dysfunction in cells. *Biochem. J.* **2011**, *435*, 297–312. [CrossRef]
50. Kuznetsov, A.V.; Veksler, V.; Gellerich, F.N.; Saks, V.; Margreiter, R.; Kunz, W.S. Analysis of mitochondrial function in situ in permeabilized muscle fibers, tissues and cells. *Nat. Protoc.* **2008**, *3*, 965–976. [CrossRef]
51. Duchen, M.R. Mitochondria and calcium: From cell signalling to cell death. *J. Physiol.* **2000**, *529 Pt 1*, 57–68. [CrossRef]
52. Murphy, M.P. How mitochondria produce reactive oxygen species. *Biochem. J.* **2009**, *417*, 1–13. [CrossRef]
53. Kalyanaraman, B.; Darley-Usmar, V.; Davies, K.J.; Dennery, P.A.; Forman, H.J.; Grisham, M.B.; Mann, G.E.; Moore, K.; Roberts, L.J., 2nd; Ischiropoulos, H. Measuring reactive oxygen and nitrogen species with fluorescent probes: Challenges and limitations. *Free Radic. Biol. Med.* **2012**, *52*, 1–6. [CrossRef]
54. Ramanathan, A.; Schreiber, S.L. Direct control of mitochondrial function by mTOR. *Proc. Natl. Acad. Sci. USA* **2009**, *106*, 22229–22232. [CrossRef]
55. Morita, M.; Gravel, S.-P.; Hulea, L.; Larsson, O.; Pollak, M.; St-Pierre, J.; Topisirovic, I. mTOR coordinates protein synthesis, mitochondrial activity and proliferation. *Cell Cycle* **2015**, *14*, 473–480. [CrossRef]
56. Beevers, C.S.; Li, F.; Liu, L.; Huang, S. Curcumin inhibits the mammalian target of rapamycin-mediated signaling pathways in cancer cells. *Int. J. Cancer* **2006**, *119*, 757–764. [CrossRef]
57. Yu, S.; Shen, G.; Khor, T.O.; Kim, J.H.; Kong, A.-N.T. Curcumin inhibits Akt/mammalian target of rapamycin signaling through protein phosphatase-dependent mechanism. *Mol. Cancer Ther.* **2008**, *7*, 2609–2620. [CrossRef] [PubMed]
58. El-Huneidi, W.; Bajbouj, K.; Muhammad, J.; Vinod, A.; Shafarin, J.; Khoder, G.; Saleh, M.; Taneera, J.; Abu-Gharbieh, E. Carnosic Acid Induces Apoptosis and Inhibits Akt/mTOR Signaling in Human Gastric Cancer Cell Lines. *Pharmaceuticals* **2021**, *14*, 230. [CrossRef] [PubMed]
59. Gao, Q.; Liu, H.; Yao, Y.; Geng, L.; Zhang, X.; Jiang, L.; Shi, B.; Yang, F. Carnosic acid induces autophagic cell death through inhibition of the Akt/mTOR pathway in human hepatoma cells. *J. Appl. Toxicol.* **2015**, *35*, 485–492. [CrossRef] [PubMed]
60. Schieke, S.M.; Phillips, D.; McCoy, J.P.; Aponte, A.M.; Shen, R.-F.; Balaban, R.S.; Finkel, T. The Mammalian Target of Rapamycin (mTOR) Pathway Regulates Mitochondrial Oxygen Consumption and Oxidative Capacity. *J. Biol. Chem.* **2006**, *281*, 27643–27652. [CrossRef]

61. Gnaiger, E. Polarographic oxygen sensors, the oxygraph, and high-resolution respirometry to assess mitochondrial functions. In *Drug-Induced Mitochondrial Dysfunction*; Dykens, J., Will, Y., Eds.; John Wiley & Sons, Inc.: Hoboken, NJ, USA, 2008; pp. 327–352.
62. Engelsberg, A.; Kobelt, F.; Kuhl, D. The N-terminus of the serum- and glucocorticoid-inducible kinase Sgk1 specifies mitochondrial localization and rapid turnover. *Biochem. J.* **2006**, *399*, 69–76. [CrossRef]
63. García-Martínez, J.M.; Alessi, D. mTOR complex 2 (mTORC2) controls hydrophobic motif phosphorylation and activation of serum- and glucocorticoid-induced protein kinase 1 (SGK1). *Biochem. J.* **2008**, *416*, 375–385. [CrossRef]
64. Kobayashi, T.; Cohen, P. Activation of serum- and glucocorticoid-regulated protein kinase by agonists that activate phosphatidylinositide 3-kinase is mediated by 3-phosphoinositide-dependent protein kinase-1 (PDK1) and PDK2. *Biochem. J.* **1999**, *339 Pt 2*, 319–328. [CrossRef]
65. Hayashi, M.; Tapping, R.I.; Chao, T.-H.; Lo, J.-F.; King, C.; Yang, Y.; Lee, J.-D. BMK1 Mediates Growth Factor-induced Cell Proliferation through Direct Cellular Activation of Serum and Glucocorticoid-inducible Kinase. *J. Biol. Chem.* **2001**, *276*, 8631–8634. [CrossRef] [PubMed]
66. Meng, F.; Yamagiwa, Y.; Taffetani, S.; Han, J.; Patel, T. IL-6 activates serum and glucocorticoid kinase via p38α mitogen-activated protein kinase pathway. *Am. J. Physiol. Cell Physiol.* **2005**, *289*, C971–C981. [CrossRef] [PubMed]
67. Sarbassov, D.D.; Ali, S.M.; Sengupta, S.; Sheen, J.-H.; Hsu, P.P.; Bagley, A.F.; Markhard, A.L.; Sabatini, D.M. Prolonged Rapamycin Treatment Inhibits mTORC2 Assembly and Akt/PKB. *Mol. Cell* **2006**, *22*, 159–168. [CrossRef] [PubMed]
68. Szwed, A.; Kim, E.; Jacinto, E. Regulation and metabolic functions of mTORC1 and mTORC2. *Physiol. Rev.* **2021**, *101*, 1371–1426. [CrossRef]
69. Steiner, M.; Priel, I.; Giat, J.; Levy, J.; Sharoni, Y.; Danilenko, M. Carnosic Acid Inhibits Proliferation and Augments Differentiation of Human Leukemic Cells Induced by 1,25-Dihydroxyvitamin D3 and Retinoic Acid. *Nutr. Cancer* **2001**, *41*, 135–144. [CrossRef] [PubMed]
70. Srivastava, R.K.; Chen, Q.; Siddiqui, I.; Sarva, K.; Shankar, S. Linkage of Curcumin-Induced Cell Cycle Arrest and Apoptosis by Cyclin-Dependent Kinase Inhibitor p21/WAF1/CIP1. *Cell Cycle* **2007**, *6*, 2953–2961. [CrossRef]
71. Roy, S.; Kaur, M.; Agarwal, C.; Tecklenburg, M.; Sclafani, R.A.; Agarwal, R. p21 and p27 induction by silibinin is essential for its cell cycle arrest effect in prostate carcinoma cells. *Mol. Cancer Ther.* **2007**, *6*, 2696–2707. [CrossRef]
72. Huang, H.-C.; Way, T.-D.; Lin, C.-L.; Lin, J.-K. EGCG Stabilizes p27kip1 in E2-Stimulated MCF-7 Cells through Down-Regulation of the Skp2 Protein. *Endocrinology* **2008**, *149*, 5972–5983. [CrossRef] [PubMed]
73. Einbond, L.S.; Wu, H.-A.; Kashiwazaki, R.; He, K.; Roller, M.; Su, T.; Wang, X.; Goldsberry, S. Carnosic acid inhibits the growth of ER-negative human breast cancer cells and synergizes with curcumin. *Fitoterapia* **2012**, *83*, 1160–1168. [CrossRef] [PubMed]
74. Mahmoud, N.; Saeed, M.E.; Sugimoto, Y.; Klinger, A.; Fleischer, E.; Efferth, T. Putative molecular determinants mediating sensitivity or resistance towards carnosic acid tumor cell responses. *Phytomedicine* **2020**, *77*, 153271. [CrossRef] [PubMed]
75. Zhang, X.; Chen, Y.; Cai, G.; Li, X.; Wang, D. Carnosic acid induces apoptosis of hepatocellular carcinoma cells via ROS-mediated mitochondrial pathway. *Chem. Biol. Interact.* **2017**, *277*, 91–100. [CrossRef] [PubMed]
76. Su, K.; Wang, C.-F.; Zhang, Y.; Cai, Y.-J.; Zhang, Y.-Y.; Zhao, Q. The inhibitory effects of carnosic acid on cervical cancer cells growth by promoting apoptosis via ROS-regulated signaling pathway. *Biomed. Pharmacother.* **2016**, *82*, 180–191. [CrossRef] [PubMed]
77. Kim, D.-H.; Park, K.-W.; Chae, I.G.; Kundu, J.; Kim, E.-H.; Kundu, J.K.; Chun, K.-S. Carnosic acid inhibits STAT3 signaling and induces apoptosis through generation of ROS in human colon cancer HCT116 cells. *Mol. Carcinog.* **2016**, *55*, 1096–1110. [CrossRef]
78. Fantini, M.; Benvenuto, M.; Masuelli, L.; Frajese, G.V.; Tresoldi, I.; Modesti, A.; Bei, R. In Vitro and in Vivo Antitumoral Effects of Combinations of Polyphenols, or Polyphenols and Anticancer Drugs: Perspectives on Cancer Treatment. *Int. J. Mol. Sci.* **2015**, *16*, 9236–9282. [CrossRef]
79. Chen, X.; Li, H.; Zhang, B.; Deng, Z. The synergistic and antagonistic antioxidant interactions of dietary phytochemical combinations. *Crit. Rev. Food Sci. Nutr.* **2021**, *61*, 1–20. [CrossRef]
80. Nabekura, T.; Yamaki, T.; Hiroi, T.; Ueno, K.; Kitagawa, S. Inhibition of anticancer drug efflux transporter P-glycoprotein by rosemary phytochemicals. *Pharmacol. Res.* **2010**, *61*, 259–263. [CrossRef]
81. Li, H.; Krstin, S.; Wink, M. Modulation of multidrug resistant in cancer cells by EGCG, tannic acid and curcumin. *Phytomedicine* **2018**, *50*, 213–222. [CrossRef]
82. Costea, T.; Vlad, O.C.; Miclea, L.-C.; Ganea, C.; Szöllősi, J.; Mocanu, M.-M. Alleviation of Multidrug Resistance by Flavonoid and Non-Flavonoid Compounds in Breast, Lung, Colorectal and Prostate Cancer. *Int. J. Mol. Sci.* **2020**, *21*, 401. [CrossRef]
83. Nimiya, Y.; Wang, W.; Du, Z.; Sukamtoh, E.; Zhu, J.; Decker, E.; Zhang, G. Redox modulation of curcumin stability: Redox active antioxidants increase chemical stability of curcumin. *Mol. Nutr. Food Res.* **2016**, *60*, 487–494. [CrossRef]
84. Hope-Roberts, M.; Horobin, R.W. A review of curcumin as a biological stain and as a self-visualizing pharmaceutical agent. *Biotech. Histochem.* **2017**, *92*, 315–323. [CrossRef]
85. Levine, C.B.; Bayle, J.; Biourge, V.; Wakshlag, J.J. Cellular effects of a turmeric root and rosemary leaf extract on canine neoplastic cell lines. *BMC Veter. Res.* **2017**, *13*, 388. [CrossRef]
86. Sapandowski, A.; Stope, M.B.; Evert, K.; Evert, M.; Zimmermann, U.; Peter, D.; Päge, I.; Burchardt, M.; Schild, L. Cardiolipin composition correlates with prostate cancer cell proliferation. *Mol. Cell. Biochem.* **2015**, *410*, 175–185. [CrossRef]

87. Ben-Zichri, S.; Kolusheva, S.; Danilenko, M.; Ossikbayeva, S.; Stabbert, W.J.; Poggio, J.L.; Stein, D.E.; Orynbayeva, Z.; Jelinek, R. Cardiolipin mediates curcumin interactions with mitochondrial membranes. *Biochim. Biophys. Acta BBA Biomembr.* **2019**, *1861*, 75–82. [CrossRef] [PubMed]
88. Lim, H.W.; Lim, H.Y.; Wong, K.P. Uncoupling of oxidative phosphorylation by curcumin: Implication of its cellular mechanism of action. *Biochem. Biophys. Res. Commun.* **2009**, *389*, 187–192. [CrossRef] [PubMed]
89. Nazıroğlu, M.; Çiğ, B.; Yazğan, Y.; Schwaerzer, G.K.; Theilig, F.; Pecze, L. Albumin evokes Ca^{2+}-induced cell oxidative stress and apoptosis through TRPM2 channel in renal collecting duct cells reduced by curcumin. *Sci. Rep.* **2019**, *9*, 12403. [CrossRef]
90. Moustapha, A.; Peretout, P.A.; Rainey, N.E.; Sureau, F.; Geze, M.; Petit, J.M.; Dewailly, E.; Slomianny, C.; Petit, P.X. Curcumin induces crosstalk between autophagy and apoptosis mediated by calcium release from the endoplasmic reticulum, lysosomal destabilization and mitochondrial events. *Cell Death Discov.* **2015**, *1*, 15017. [CrossRef]
91. Keer, H.N.; Gaylis, F.D.; Kozlowski, J.M.; Kwaan, H.C.; Bauer, K.D.; Sinha, A.A.; Wilson, M.J. Heterogeneity in plasminogen activator (PA) levels in human prostate cancer cell lines: Increased PA activity correlates with biologically aggressive behavior. *Prostate* **1991**, *18*, 201–214. [CrossRef] [PubMed]
92. O'Keeffe, B.A.; Cilia, S.; Maiyar, A.C.; Vaysberg, M.; Firestone, G.L. The serum- and glucocorticoid-induced protein kinase-1 (Sgk-1) mitochondria connection: Identification of the IF-1 inhibitor of the F1F0-ATPase as a mitochondria-specific binding target and the stress-induced mitochondrial localization of endogenous Sgk-1. *Biochimie* **2013**, *95*, 1258–1265. [CrossRef]
93. Zhu, R.; Yang, G.; Cao, Z.; Shen, K.; Zheng, L.; Xiao, J.; You, L.; Zhang, T. The prospect of serum and glucocorticoid-inducible kinase 1 (SGK1) in cancer therapy: A rising star. *Ther. Adv. Med. Oncol.* **2020**, *12*, 1758835920940946. [CrossRef]
94. Fagerli, U.-M.; Ullrich, K.; Stühmer, T.; Holien, T.; Köchert, K.; Holt, R.U.; Bruland, Ø.S.; Chatterjee, M.; Nogai, H.; Lenz, G.; et al. Serum/glucocorticoid-regulated kinase 1 (SGK1) is a prominent target gene of the transcriptional response to cytokines in multiple myeloma and supports the growth of myeloma cells. *Oncogene* **2011**, *30*, 3198–3206. [CrossRef]
95. Sahoo, S.; Brickley, D.R.; Kocherginsky, M.; Conzen, S.D. Coordinate expression of the PI3-kinase downstream effectors serum and glucocorticoid-induced kinase (SGK-1) and Akt-1 in human breast cancer. *Eur. J. Cancer* **2005**, *41*, 2754–2759. [CrossRef]
96. Liu, W.; Wang, X.; Wang, Y.; Dai, Y.; Xie, Y.; Ping, Y.; Yin, B.; Yu, P.; Liu, Z.; Duan, X.; et al. SGK1 inhibition-induced autophagy impairs prostate cancer metastasis by reversing EMT. *J. Exp. Clin. Cancer Res.* **2018**, *37*, 73. [CrossRef] [PubMed]
97. Sherk, A.B.; Frigo, D.; Schnackenberg, C.G.; Bray, J.D.; Laping, N.J.; Trizna, W.; Hammond, M.; Patterson, J.R.; Thompson, S.K.; Kazmin, D.; et al. Development of a Small-Molecule Serum- and Glucocorticoid-Regulated Kinase-1 Antagonist and Its Evaluation as a Prostate Cancer Therapeutic. *Cancer Res.* **2008**, *68*, 7475–7483. [CrossRef] [PubMed]
98. Liu, W.; Wang, X.; Liu, Z.; Wang, Y.; Yin, B.; Yu, P.; Duan, X.; Liao, Z.; Chen, Y.; Liu, C.; et al. SGK1 inhibition induces autophagy-dependent apoptosis via the mTOR-Foxo3a pathway. *Br. J. Cancer* **2017**, *117*, 1139–1153. [CrossRef] [PubMed]
99. Seo, S.U.; Woo, S.M.; Lee, H.-S.; Kim, S.H.; Min, K.-J.; Kwon, T.K. mTORC1/2 inhibitor and curcumin induce apoptosis through lysosomal membrane permeabilization-mediated autophagy. *Oncogene* **2018**, *37*, 5205–5220. [CrossRef] [PubMed]
100. Catalogna, G.; Moraca, F.; D'Antona, L.; Dattilo, V.; Perrotti, G.; Lupia, A.; Costa, G.; Ortuso, F.; Iuliano, R.; Trapasso, F.; et al. Review about the multi-target profile of resveratrol and its implication in the SGK1 inhibition. *Eur. J. Med. Chem.* **2019**, *183*, 111675. [CrossRef] [PubMed]
101. Qin, J.; Chen, J.X.; Zhu, Z.; Teng, J.A. Genistein Inhibits Human Colorectal Cancer Growth and Suppresses MiR-95, Akt and SGK1. *Cell. Physiol. Biochem.* **2015**, *35*, 2069–2077. [CrossRef]
102. Liang, X.; Lan, C.; Jiao, G.; Fu, W.; Long, X.; An, Y.; Wang, K.; Zhou, J.; Chen, T.; Li, Y.; et al. Therapeutic inhibition of SGK1 suppresses colorectal cancer. *Exp. Mol. Med.* **2017**, *49*, e399. [CrossRef] [PubMed]
103. Bray, F.; Ferlay, J.; Soerjomataram, I.; Siegel, R.L.; Torre, L.A.; Jemal, A. Global cancer statistics 2018: GLOBOCAN estimates of incidence and mortality worldwide for 36 cancers in 185 countries. *CA Cancer J. Clin.* **2018**, *68*, 394–424. [CrossRef] [PubMed]
104. Rebello, R.J.; Oing, C.; Knudsen, K.E.; Loeb, S.; Johnson, D.C.; Reiter, R.E.; Gillessen, S.; Van der Kwast, T.; Bristow, R.G. Prostate cancer. *Nat. Rev. Dis. Primers* **2021**, *7*, 9. [CrossRef] [PubMed]

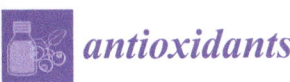

Review

Fighting Oxidative Stress with Sulfur: Hydrogen Sulfide in the Renal and Cardiovascular Systems

Joshua J. Scammahorn [1], Isabel T. N. Nguyen [1], Eelke M. Bos [2], Harry Van Goor [3,*] and Jaap A. Joles [1]

1. Department of Nephrology & Hypertension, University Medical Center Utrecht, 3508 GA Utrecht, The Netherlands; j.j.scammahorn@umcutrecht.nl (J.J.S.); T.N.Nguyen-4@umcutrecht.nl (I.T.N.N.); J.A.Joles@umcutrecht.nl (J.A.J.)
2. Department of Neurosurgery, Erasmus Medical Center Rotterdam, 3015 CN Rotterdam, The Netherlands; e.bos@erasmusmc.nl
3. Department of Pathology and Medical Biology, University Medical Center Groningen and University of Groningen, 9713 GZ Groningen, The Netherlands
* Correspondence: h.van.goor@umcg.nl

Abstract: Hydrogen sulfide (H_2S) is an essential gaseous signaling molecule. Research on its role in physiological and pathophysiological processes has greatly expanded. Endogenous enzymatic production through the transsulfuration and cysteine catabolism pathways can occur in the kidneys and blood vessels. Furthermore, non-enzymatic pathways are present throughout the body. In the renal and cardiovascular system, H_2S plays an important role in maintaining the redox status at safe levels by promoting scavenging of reactive oxygen species (ROS). H_2S also modifies cysteine residues on key signaling molecules such as keap1/Nrf2, NFκB, and HIF-1α, thereby promoting anti-oxidant mechanisms. Depletion of H_2S is implicated in many age-related and cardiorenal diseases, all having oxidative stress as a major contributor. Current research suggests potential for H_2S-based therapies, however, therapeutic interventions have been limited to studies in animal models. Beyond H_2S use as direct treatment, it could improve procedures such as transplantation, stem cell therapy, and the safety and efficacy of drugs including NSAIDs and ACE inhibitors. All in all, H_2S is a prime subject for further research with potential for clinical use.

Keywords: hydrogen sulfide; reactive oxygen species; H_2S donors; cardiorenal syndrome; thiosulfate

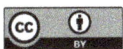

1. Introduction

Hydrogen sulfide (H_2S) was first described as a pungent toxic gas in "De Morbis Artificum Diatriba", Bernardino Ramazzini's treatise on worker's diseases [1]. Today, we have come to better understand the toxic effect of H_2S and have determined that this is most likely the result of cytochrome C oxidase (mitochondrial Complex IV), monoamine oxidase, -and/or Na^+-K^+-ATPase inhibition [1–3]. A brief overview of H_2S toxicity is given in Table 1. In short, high concentrations disrupt the oxidative metabolism process of cells leading to impairment of organs most reliant on these processes [1]. During research on its toxicity, several groups reported the presence of H_2S in tissues of healthy humans and laboratory animals [4–6]. Although the transsulfuration pathway was described in mammals more than fifty years ago, it was not until 1996 that the role of H_2S as an endogenous gaseous signaling molecule was proposed [7,8]. Since then, research has expanded on the topic, revealing its role in many physiological processes including those of the renal and cardiovascular system [9,10].

In the body, the kidneys are believed to be the third largest producer of H_2S, after the liver and gut [9]. All of the known pathways leading to the production of H_2S have been described in the kidneys. Furthermore, renal homeostasis appears to be under control of H_2S to some degree, with H_2S levels contributing to the glomerular filtration rate (GFR), Na^+ excretion, and K^+ excretion [11]. Various effects mediated by H_2S have been observed with consequences in both the renal and cardiovascular systems including epigenetic regulation of apoptosis, immunoregulatory effects, cellular protein homeostasis, and its role as an oxygen sensor and/or inducing hypometabolism in cells [12]. These have been extensively reviewed elsewhere [9,12]. H_2S has also been shown to have powerful antioxidant properties. Indeed, it is part of the reactive species interactome, as defined by Cortese-Krott et al. as the chemical interactions between reactive oxygen, nitrate and sulfur species (resp. ROS, RNS and RSS) and their downstream targets [13–15]. In general, H_2S has shown potential as a biomarker for disease; the reduction of H_2S levels correlates with renal/cardiovascular disease progression and general mortality [16,17].

Table 1. A brief overview of the toxic effects of hydrogen sulfide gas exposure.

Concentration	20–50 ppm	100–200 ppm	250–500 ppm	500+ ppm	1000+ ppm
Effects	Kerato-conjunctivitis, Airway agitation	Olfactory paralysis (smell disappears), Eye and airway agitation becomes severe	Lung edema that worsens with longer exposure time	Serious eye damage within 30 min Unconscious or dead within 8 h Amnesia	Immediate collapse due to respiratory failure

The complex interplay between the cardiovascular and renal system leads to pathologies affecting one having consequences for the other [18,19]}. This can lead to new diseases developing or worsening existing ones [20]. This has led to the classification system based on the syndrome created by these interactions, known as the cardiorenal syndrome (CRS) [19,21]. A major component of this syndrome is related to blood pressure control, in which renal renin–angiotensin–aldosterone system (RAAS) activation, sympathetic nervous system, and the pump function of the heart can fall into a vicious circle [22]. However, this does not fully explain the CRS with chronic inflammation, persistent RAAS activation, and ROS signaling being further implicated [20]. Notably, H_2S has been shown to affect various aspects of cardiorenal interactions [9,10]. Furthermore, H_2S can be beneficial in the individual pathologies that fall under CRS: heart failure, cardiac hypertrophy, ischemia, chronic kidney disease (CKD), angiotensin related hypertension, and diabetes related renal pathology to name a few [23–25]. The antioxidant effects of H_2S specifically in renal-cardiovascular systems might hold the key to a better understanding or treatment of CRS [11,26–28]. Considering the potential role of oxidative stress in this syndrome, it is important to further explore this in a dedicated review.

2. Endogenous Production of Hydrogen Sulfide

There are four known pathways resulting in the production of H_2S in mammals, with the kidneys showing notable activity in all three enzymatic ones [9,29]. Blood vessels also show the activity of these enzymes [30]. Two enzymatic pathways, that of cystathionine-β-synthase (CBS) and cystathionine gamma-lyase (CSE), are grouped together under the broader transsulfuration pathway, discussed in Section 2.1. A third enzymatic pathway exists primarily in the mitochondria, the cysteine catabolic pathway mediated by 3-mercaptopyruvate sulfurtransferase (3-MST), and is expanded upon in Section 2.2. Another non-enzymatic pathway leading to the production of H_2S has been explored recently and is covered in Section 2.3. The presence of H_2S throughout the body is thought to be regulated by the hypothalamic–pituitary axis (at least in mice) and diet [31,32].

2.1. Transsulfuration Pathway

The transsulfuration pathway was described in mammals during the mid-twentieth century, later rising to prominence due to the unravelling of H_2S's potential as a signaling molecule [1]. The result of this pathway is the biosynthesis of L-cysteine from homocysteine, as shown in Figure 1, a process central in the metabolism of sulfur and regulation of cellular redox [33,34]. The enzymes CBS and CSE are essential to this pathway, being able to produce H_2S independently as well as in concert with each other. CBS, present in the kidney, but less so in the heart, uses a combination of cysteine and homocysteine to generate H_2S [29]. It can also produce cystathionine from serine and homocysteine. CSE, notably active in the kidney and vasculature, but not the heart (in mice), takes cystationine created from CBS to produce cysteine, which it can also use to generate H_2S [35,36]. It is important to note that CSE expression is induced by endoplasmic reticulum stress and oxidative stress among other stimuli, whereas CBS is inhibited by the other gaseous signaling molecules, NO, and carbon monoxide (CO). For more details on transsulfuration pathway and its regulation, see Sbodio et al. [33].

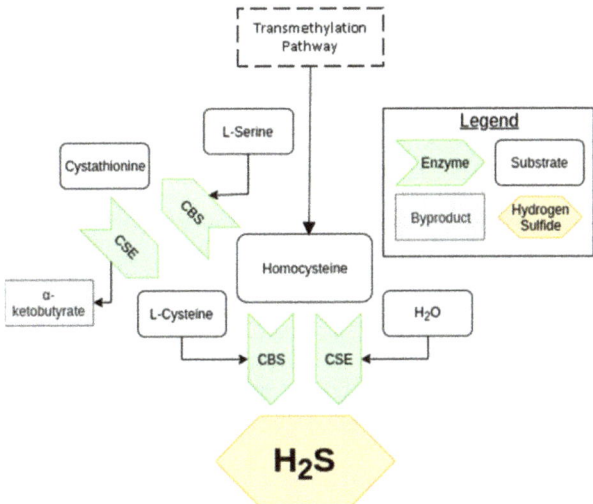

Figure 1. An overview of the transsulfuration pathway. The arrow, representing an enzyme, points toward the product of the reaction it catalyzes.

2.2. Cysteine Catabolism Pathway

Cysteine can be used to generate H_2S via the cysteine catabolic pathway. D-cysteine is processed by D-amino acid oxidase (DOA) in the peroxisomes to produce 3-mercaptopyruvate (3MP), while L-cysteine and α-ketobutyrate produced from the transsulfuration pathway are turned into 3MP by cysteine aminotransferase (CAT) in the mitochondria, as shown in Figure 2 [37].

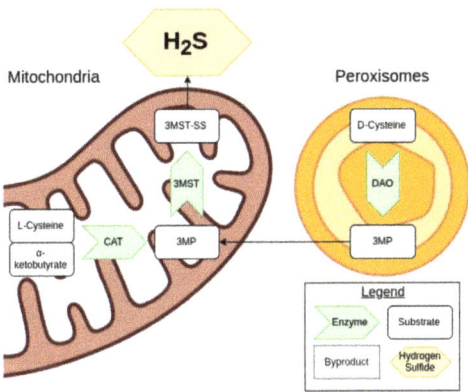

Figure 2. An overview of the cysteine catabolism pathway.

The enzyme 3-MST then comes into play, producing sulfides and polysulfides including H_2S. In turn, H_2S can reduce these various products. 3-MST is also capable of converting H_2S into a hydrogen polysulfide. When 3MP is not present in sufficient concentrations for the 3-MST activity, antioxidant cysteine and glutathione concentrations drop, suggesting that these are consumed [37].

2.3. Nonenzymatic Pathways

Recently, non-enzymatic production of H_2S has also been described in blood and in vitro [35]. This process appears to require the presence of iron (Fe^{3+} form) and vitamin B6 in blood. Interestingly, the enzymatic pathway is most prominent in the liver and the kidney, while non-enzymatic production plays a greater role in other tissues [35]. The optimal substrate for this form of production appears to be cysteine, regardless of the D/L-isomer [35]. How this process relates to the redox aspect of H_2S remains to be explored. Besides this novel pathway, various molecules found naturally in the body can donate H_2S including thiocysteine, thiosulfate, and polysulfides [38]. Such molecules therefore provide natural leads for therapeutic drugs.

3. Antioxidant Mechanisms of Hydrogen Sulfide

Cardiovascular and renal research on H_2S in rodents indicate that it has the potential to modulate oxidative stress at the tissue and organ level [34]. At the cellular level, H_2S has been shown to influence cellular redox via four mechanisms [39]. The first is the scavenging of ROS by induction of major antioxidants [27]. Second, cysteine residues in proteins can be modulated by H_2S, resulting in persulfidation, which, in combination with thioredoxin, potentially protects proteins from oxidative stress [40,41]. Third, H_2S plays a role in the mitochondria and oxidative respiration production of adenosine triphosphate (ATP) [42–44]. Finally, H_2S can react with metals including iron in the heme of cytochrome c oxidase [3]. Xie et al. have published an extensive review on the topic of H_2S and cellular redox [27]. Beyond these interactions, it has become clear that there is an interplay with NO, another gaseous signaling molecule [45].

3.1. Reactive Oxygen Species Scavenging

Downstream of the transsulfuration pathway, cysteine also acts as an important antioxidant and can be used to produce the major antioxidant glutathione [33]. Glutathione is a thiol produced by combining L-glutamate and L-cysteine by glutamate cysteine ligase and then combining the product (γ-glutamyl-L-cysteine) with L-glycine by glutathione synthase. H_2S, cysteine, and glutathione can all scavenge ROS by forming disulfide bonds from their –SH residue [33]. However, H_2S's role in direct scavenging is thought to be limited, as the concentrations present in vivo are too low for that to be its primary mode of antioxidant activity. Thus, antioxidant effects related to CBS and CSE are not necessarily directly related to H_2S production, but to other products resulting from the transsulfuration pathway. It is more likely that effects seen at the cellular level are a result of H_2S's signaling capabilities. Indeed, the production of glutathione is regulated by known targets of H_2S signaling including the Keap1/Nrf2 pathway.

3.2. Protein Modification

H_2S has the ability to modify many proteins including Keap1, NFκb, and HIF-1α. One of the major antioxidant pathways is the Keap1/Nrf2 pathway, a simplified version of which can be found in Figure 3. H_2S has been shown to modulate Nrf2 through sulfuration of Keap1, leading to activation of Nrf2 [27]. In this way, H_2S contributes to protecting the cell from oxidative stress related injury [46]. Nrf2 in turn regulates the production of major ROS scavengers such as glutathione and thioredoxin, as discussed previously [27,47]. Keap1 also leads to transcription of various antioxidant enzymes such as superoxide dismutase, catalase, and glutathione peroxidase [27]. These aspects of Nrf2 signaling are important for preventing oxidative stress induced senescence [12]. H_2S also activates NFκb, a cornerstone of the inflammatory pathways activated by ROS signaling, as summarized in Figure 3 [10,30]. NFκb leads to transcription of some of the same antioxidant enzymes that are stimulated by Keap1 [27]. HIF-1α is a third important signaling molecule that is potentially activated or downregulated by H_2S [48,49]. The signaling pathway of HIF-1α is briefly presented in Figure 3. The regulation is H_2S-dose dependent, as lower doses appear to upregulate and stabilize HIF-1α while a higher dose downregulates and destabilizes it [48,50].

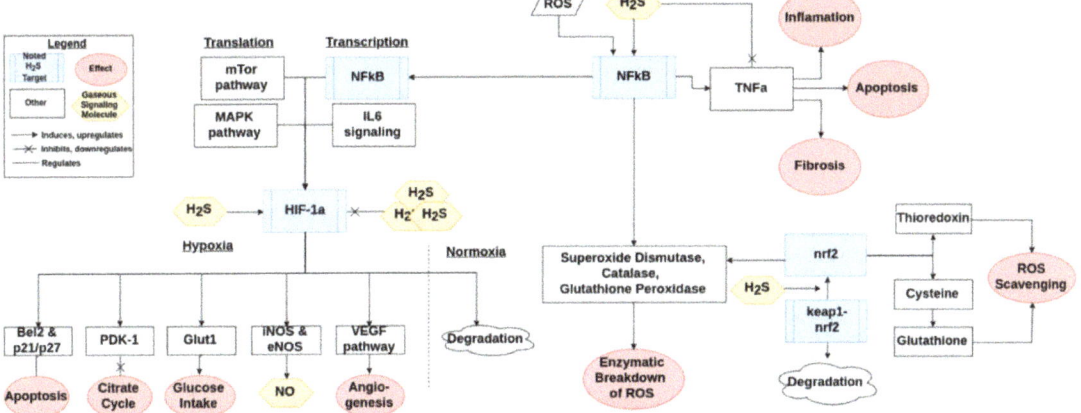

Figure 3. An overview of how H_2S interacts with the Keap1/Nrf2, NFκb, and HIF-1α pathways. The conglomerate of three H_2S indicates supraphysiological levels of H_2S.

3.3. Mitochondria and Respiratory Oxidation

The major cellular production of ROS is due to oxidative respiration and therefore located in the mitochondria. H_2S is an essential molecule for mitochondria and regulates the amounts of ROS produced [43]. ROS are in turn important for regulating adaptation in order to promote tissue survival, however, this comes at the cost of proper function when ROS induces oxidative stress [51]. There is a particularly interesting effect in tissues that express the enzyme CSE and/or CBS. This is due to translocation of these enzymes to the mitochondria in response to hypoxia and forced calcium release to the cytoplasm, at least in vitro [43,52]. Translocation of CSE under the influence of calcium increases ATP production under normoxic and hypoxic conditions at the cost of cysteine. However, addition of extra H_2S through donors leads to decreased ATP production in normoxic conditions [43]. Recently, normoxic perfusion of H_2S donors in whole ex vivo porcine kidneys resulted in renal oxygen consumption being reduced by over 60% with corresponding decreases in mitochondrial activity [53]. This would suggest that ROS production is reduced by H_2S through hypometabolism.

Despite the hypometabolism induced by H_2S, ATP levels, renal function, and histological structure were unaffected, providing evidence that H_2S can partially substitute oxygen in ATP production, thus reducing the amount of ROS generated by the mitochondria [53]. In the mitochondria, H_2S interacts with the heme group of cytochrome c and the metal cofactors of cytochrome c oxidase. Located in the intermembrane compartment, cytochrome c transfers electrons between cytochrome c reductase (complex III) and cytochrome c oxidase (IV). H_2S is able to donate electrons in the mitochondrial ATP production machinery through its interaction with cytochrome c as well as reducing complex IV directly without interacting with complex III [54]. Beyond the implications for ROS production, cytochrome c plays an important role in inducing apoptosis in which H_2S intervenes.

4. Hydrogen Sulfide in Cardiovascular and Renal Physiology

Considering the interactions found between H_2S and ROS, it is important to note the role of the two in maintaining cellular homeostasis. ROS is a necessary signaling molecule that is maintained at an optimal concentration under physiological circumstances, with too little or too much being potentially problematic [55]. For an overview of the consequences of reduced ROS, see the reviews by Sies et al. [51,55]. Increased ROS at oxidative stress levels forms an essential part of our understanding of the biological role of H_2S. Under physiological circumstances in the cardiovascular system, H_2S interacts with the balance between NO and ROS [56]. Renal H_2S, on the other hand, seems to be under the influence of higher enzyme concentrations [9,29]. In both cases, cell proliferation and functions are influenced by the degree of sulfuration versus oxidation of various proteins [9,29,56]. In this section, we focus on how these cellular and signaling mechanisms take place in the cardiovascular and renal systems and what effects result at the tissue and organ level under physiological circumstances.

4.1. Cardiovascular

The production of ROS, in particular hydrogen peroxide (H_2O_2), in the heart is important for its ability to adapt to environmental stress [56]. In cardiomyocytes, stimulation of the alpha-adrenergic receptors by noradrenaline leads to the production of ROS through NAPDH oxidase (NOX) [56]. ROS can then in turn oxidize cysteine residues in important signaling pathways such as NFκb and Nrf2. The cysteine residues are sulfurated by H_2S, providing fine control over these activations considering that the effects of oxidation are dependent on which residues are oxidized [57]. NFκb, a pro-inflammatory pathway, is also activated by angiotensin II (ANG II) and/or mechanical stretch via NOX and in turn ROS can regulate NOX activation through oxidation [30]. This, combined with the ability of H_2S to activate these pathways without the inflammatory effect, would suggest that the role of H_2S is in part to limit ROS signaling to physiological levels.

At the tissue level, H_2S protects against dysfunction through cellular senescence and apoptosis while allowing for adaptation in the form of controlled inflammation, angiogenesis, and proliferation enacted by physiological levels of ROS [49,58]. This is supported by aging studies in rats where the levels of H_2S were followed. Aged hearts in general are more prone to disease than younger hearts and tend to have lower levels of H_2S [59]. Furthermore, when looking solely at aged hearts, those with lower levels of H_2S are more prone to age related pathologies than those that have retained more H_2S [60]. One of the major driving mechanisms of these types of pathologies appears to be oxidative stress, the state in which ROS supersedes the safe adaptive range [12]. Going a step further, intervening with H_2S treatment in hearts undergoing oxidative stress can restore redox balance [61].

When it comes to the vasculature, ROS are well established signaling molecules under physiological circumstances in the blood vessels, with different ROS having different properties in how they distribute in and out of the cell [55]. In the long-term, H_2S prevents and reverses vascular remodeling through preventing smooth muscle proliferation and apoptosis [55]. H_2S also interacts with NO for more rapid changes such as control of the vessel diameter, particularly when NO is depleted [62,63]. H_2O_2 and NO can cause vasodilation, whereas ROS other than H_2O_2 such as superoxide (O_2^-) causes vasoconstriction [56]. Overall, H_2S appears to be a vasodilator [30,63]. However, the interactions are much more complex than their individual effects. Indeed, stimulation of the angiotensin receptor I or endothelin (ET) receptor A leads to NADPH production of ROS and vasoconstriction while ET receptor B causes vasodilation [62]. It may be possible that H_2S regulation has the strongest effect on the dominant ROS being produced (be that O_2^- or H_2O_2), resulting in an opposite effect on the vessels.

4.2. Renal

The kidneys are a major producer of H$_2$S, as indicated by their expression of CBS, CSE, and 3-MST [9,11]. H$_2$S causes similar effects to those of the cardiovascular system due to the interactions with the same pathways to protect against inflammation and apoptosis by regulating ROS signaling [9,64]. Likewise, the defenses that H$_2$S provides against oxidative stress are important for maintaining cellular function in the kidneys. Furthermore, renal H$_2$S is also reduced due to the effects of aging in the kidneys [65]. One of the mechanisms behind this effect is the modification of p21 regulated senescence [65]. On the matter of NO–ROS interactions, there is indication that H$_2$S works in tandem with NO in the kidneys by upregulating endothelial NO synthase and thus stimulating NO production [9]. However, there are also effects that are unique to the kidneys.

H$_2$S is involved in renal homeostasis by increasing GFR and the excretion of Na+ and K+ through inhibition of the Na$^+$–K$^+$–2Cl$^-$-cotransporter and Na$^+$–K$^+$–ATPase [11]. This explains part of H$_2$S's ability to regulate blood pressure, in combination with its role in the RAAS system through cyclic adenosine monophosphate (cAMP) regulated renin release and its aforementioned regulation of blood vessels [66–68]. However, research has shown that H$_2$S is metabolized in the presence of oxygen (O$_2$) in renal tissue [69]. In this sense, it acts as a sensor for O$_2$, becoming more active under hypoxic conditions and enhancing renal blood flow to alleviate hypoxia in the kidneys [9,11]. Hypoxia also leads to systemic signaling from the kidney to increase the number of red blood cells through erythropoietin (EPO) [70]. In other words, under physiological circumstances, there is a balance between the gases H$_2$S, O$_2$, and NO that help maintain hemopoiesis and renal homeostasis [64,71].

5. Role in Cardiorenal Syndrome Pathologies

H$_2$S production levels have been implicated as potential disease markers in various pathologies [38]. Furthermore, reduced sulfate excretion has been shown to be a potential biomarker for renal and cardiovascular diseases as well as overall mortality in the general population [16]. When examining renal and cardiovascular pathologies in regard to H$_2$S research, there is a clear overlap with aging-associated pathologies, but also pathologies related to cardiorenal syndrome (CRS) [12,20]. These include heart failure, kidney failure, ischemic events, cardiomyopathy, hypertension, and diabetes, an overview of which is given in Figure 4. While the definition of CRS has not been fully developed, the current definitions provide a useful framework for an examination of H$_2$S [20]. Following Ronco et al.'s classification of CRS, pathologies were grouped in the criteria of acute/chronic and the initial location of the syndrome: heart, kidney, or systemic [18]. By examining the changes found in these diseases in the context of the previously discussed physiological balance of H$_2$S and other redox molecules, this section addresses the potential role of the antioxidant aspect of H$_2$S.

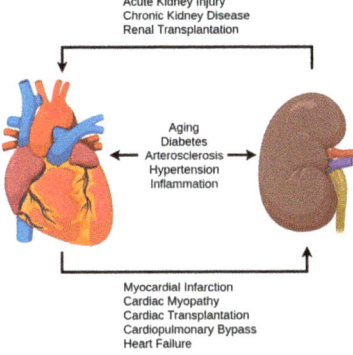

Figure 4. A simplified overview of pathologies and events contributing to the cardiorenal syndrome.

5.1. Cardiac Cardiorenal Syndrome (CRS) Pathologies

A well-known effect of aging in humans is the switch from steady increase to a decrease in diastolic pressure after passing middle age (as opposed to the continuous increase of systolic pressure). This is attributed to increased arterial stiffness and hypertrophy of the heart with preserved end diastolic volume [72]. One of the major mechanisms behind this and other afflictions of the heart is uncoupling of NOS, leading to production of O_2^-, where H_2S has been shown to be restored in the experimental setting using rat models [59]. During aging, the level of H_2S in heart tissue was reduced in rats [60]. Hearts with lower H_2S levels have been shown to be more prone to disease as well as having reduced functionality and experience uncoupling [59,73]. In other words, it is possible that H_2S's antioxidant capabilities are a key aspect of the cardiac pathologies of aging. Notably, such pathologies tend to fall under the CRS.

Acute pathologies initiating in the heart related to CRS include myocardial infarction, heart transplantation, surgery, and acute heart failure from cardiomyopathy [20]. In general, these fall under ischemic events or maladaptation to the environment. In both cases, ROS signaling and H_2S have been shown to play a role. The role of ROS in pathology is one of overproduction, in which the adaptive processes turn into damaging ones in the form of oxidative stress [55]. H_2S mitigates the negative effects to a degree in acute disease, however, it can easily become depleted. The amount of H_2S reserves is indicative of the severity of the disease and damage, as shown by studies on aged rat hearts. This effect is also observed within aging; when comparing aged hearts, the levels of H_2S also predicted the severity of the disease at the same (calendar) age [74].

Direct ROS scavenging is not the only potential path for H_2S to mitigate the damage in acute cardiac problems. Inflammation plays a crucial role in the extent of damage that takes place and is responsible for increased ROS levels. In turn, ROS modifies important signaling pathways such as NFκB and Keap1/Nrf2/, which are also targets for H_2S modification, as previously discussed. H_2S reduces inflammation, fibrosis, and hypertrophy induced by these pathways, however, it can become rapidly depleted during prolonged or intense oxidative stress [75,76]. Notably, H_2S has been shown to play an essential role in autophagy, a major underlying mechanism of cardiac injury [77]. In cardiac autophagy, oxidative stress leads to the degradation of mitochondria, the primary source of that stress, as a form of self-survival [78]. H_2S has the ability to prevent autophagy in experimental settings, thus reducing the long-term effects of acute damage [78].

The chronic CRS pathology initiating in the heart is primarily chronic heart failure [20]. Oxidative stress has been indicated as a major player in heart failure, with much research focused on the activation of matrix metallopeptidases (MMPs), which downregulates the production of H_2S [54]. The importance of H_2S in heart failure is demonstrated by the study of Koning et al. on 'the fate of sulfate' [25]. In this study, patients with chronic heart failure were followed and their sulfate levels in blood and urine were measured. Patients showed higher plasma levels of sulfate and lower urinary excretion of sulfate compared to healthy controls [22]. While this research shows that sulfate may be useful as a biomarker, it does beg the question of what the extra sulfate is indicative of, especially considering that higher H_2S in the tissues of rodent models suggests protection. It may be possible that the reduced sulfate excretion in the urine is indicative of renal malfunction in these patients, as low excretion is also correlated with certain forms of renal disease progression [17]. Reduced sulfate excretion will clearly increase plasma levels. It is also possible that the sulfate found in the plasma might be in the form of polysulfides that are produced from the interactions with free radicals [79].

5.2. Renal CRS Pathologies

Acute renal initiators of CRS fall under the broad clinical observation of acute kidney injury (AKI), characterized by the loss of kidney function within one week [80]. AKI can be further classified into groups based on the location of the underlying cause, namely prerenal, renal (intrinsic), and postrenal. Interestingly, H_2S has been found to play a role in pathologies belonging to each of these categories. AKI has the potential to develop into CKD, with oxidative stress, hypoxia, and fibrosis being implicated in the transition [64]. Furthermore, the kidney signals its distress to the rest of the body and attempts to rectify the situation by reducing vascular resistance through various mechanisms [81]. This activation can have long-term consequences for the kidney, as it can lead to renal inflammation and fibrosis [81]. RAAS activation also leads to more workload on the heart due to increased blood volume and vascular resistance, thus contributing to the development or exacerbation of CRS and related cardiac pathologies [81].

Prerenal AKI is characterized by a sharp decrease in blood flow to the kidneys and is therefore not an initiating event in CRS, but is rather secondary to problems of the heart and vasculature. The most common cause of AKI is prerenal caused by surgery, with cardiac surgery, namely cardiopulmonary bypass, having the highest associations [82,83]. This type of ischemic event is similar to direct renal injury by transplantation, which results in an ischemic/reperfusion event [11,34]. Direct injury by transplantation is a potential initiator of CRS [20]. In both cases, the role of H_2S as an oxygen sensor and regulator of metabolism is essential [9,84]. At the cellular level, reduced O_2 leads to reduction in the metabolism of H_2S, thereby increasing its levels. H_2S then regulates the mitochondria and oxidative signaling to bring the cell into a lower energetic state [85]. In the case of the renal stem cells, located in the papilla and possibly in the tubules, this brings them into a quiescent state. This protects the tissues from cell depletion in the hypoxic environment, assuming the hypoxia is transient. However, the capacity of endogenous levels of H_2S to perform this crucial ability is limited and crossing that limit leads to pathology.

Renal AKI also includes various conditions in which the kidney is directly affected [20] such as acute interstitial nephritis [86]. Acute interstitial nephritis is the result of an acute autoimmune reaction or response to an infection (pyelonephritis), or, most commonly, a variety of medications [86,87]. Regardless of the instigator, the cause of disease is inflammation, which in turn can lead to fibrosis in the long-term [87]. Despite having various potent targets for H_2S, little research has been done on the topic. Chen et al. showed that sepsis induced AKI, a different major inflammatory type of injury, corresponds with H_2S levels and that renal damage can be ameliorated by introducing more H_2S [88]. While there are to the best of our knowledge no publications on H_2S related medication-instigated interstitial nephritis, H_2S has been shown to improve the safety of nonsteroidal anti-inflammatory drugs (NSAIDs) in other organs [89,90]. NSAIDs are a known potential instigator of interstitial nephritis, while also increasing the chance of developing AKI, particularly in individuals with CKD [91]. On a tangent, acute nephrotoxicity caused by acetaminophen overdose depletes glutathione (and therefore H_2S) in the kidneys, whilst supplementation with H_2S donors reduces inflammation and damage [92,93].

Acute tubular necrosis, another cause of intrinsic AKI, can be induced by cisplatin. H_2S, in turn, has been shown to be protective in cisplatin-induced renal disease [94]. Recent research suggests that the protective effect is a result of SIRT3 modification, leading to attenuation of mitochondrial damage [95]. It is important to note that not all donors create this effect, indeed, the slow releasing H_2S donor GYY4137 worsens the renal damage by promoting increased oxidative stress [96]. Furthermore, cisplatin is thought to downregulate CSE, leading to reduced levels of H_2S in renal cells, potentially the mechanism for its nephrotoxicity [94]. Other forms of tubular necrosis also result from ischemia and/or inflammatory processes, again suggesting a potential role for H_2S signaling.

Postrenal AKI is caused by the blockage of the urinary tract, causing backflow and/or build-up of urine in the kidneys [97]. This blockage can be caused by a variety of problems, from kidney stones to bacterial infection [97]. The causes may not be directly related to the redox control by H_2S, however, H_2S plays an important role in mitigating the damage resulting from this type of injury. Rats undergoing unilateral ureteral obstruction suffer fibrosis and loss of function that can be ameliorated by H_2S treatment [98]. In particular, GYY4137 seems to mitigate fibrosis via the TGF-B1 mediated pathway, which is involved in crosstalk with NFκB and inflammation [98]. Furthermore, H_2S speeds up recovery time in the rats that recover from the damage [98]. Should the acute obstruction become a chronic one, then TGF-B1 and ANG II are upregulated, causing an epithelial–mesenchymal transition in the kidney [99]. H_2S mitigates this effect and has been shown to be protective in ANG II related pathologies [23,99].

CKD is characterized by increased levels of oxidative stress and chronic hypoxia [64]. Nrf2 plays an important role in regulating the oxidative stress under physiological circumstances, however, in CKD, the activation seems to be insufficient [64]. This could be due to the complex interactions that can cause or propagate CKD such as hyperglycemia and hypoxia [64]. In any case, the result is hypoxia, fibrosis, inflammation, oxidative stress, and/or anemia [50]. It is clear, however, that in CKD, H_2S production capacity is reduced in the kidneys as well as the liver [100]. This is mirrored by homocysteine levels being elevated while H_2S levels are reduced in patients with CKD, suggesting that the transsulfuration pathway is disrupted [101]. H_2S interactions with the HIF-1α pathway could be important, as HIF-1α protects against hypoxic injury initially and is downregulated in CKD [50]. Prolonged exposure to HIF-1α activation, however, leads to fibrosis of the kidneys [50]. H_2S's dose dependent activation or downregulation could prove important to potential treatment. This, together with H_2S's ability to alleviate inflammation, fibrosis oxidative stress, and anemia (through increased EPO synthesis) makes it a solid candidate for future research on CKD. For an in-depth review of H_2S and CKD, we refer to the extensive paper by Dugbartey [50].

5.3. Systemic CRS Pathologies

While not a primary disease of the heart or kidney, the various forms of diabetes mellitus (DM) play an important role in the development and severity of various CRS pathologies. ROS is induced and antioxidant pathways downregulated by advanced glycation end products resulting from hyperglycemia [102]. An example of one such pathway is cAMP, which leads to increased ROS in DM type II and is also regulated by H_2S [67,103]. At the glomerulus, blood is filtered and excretion products including water and small molecules are transferred to Bowman's capsule for further processing in the tubuli. Specialized cells called podocytes serve a crucial role in this filtration process and are damaged by hyperglycemia, resulting in reduced GFR. This damage and other forms of diabetic nephropathy (DN) can be prevented by H_2S [104]. Furthermore, the damage caused by hyperglycemic conditions in diabetic kidney disease (DKD) in general can be relieved by H_2S [96]. H_2S production is reduced in hyperglycemic conditions due to excessive MMP-9 activity, thus paving the way for oxidative stress to develop [11]. However, H_2S serves another role and increases insulin sensitivity and cellular glucose uptake, thus potentially tackling the hyperglycemia at its source [105,106]. Altogether, H_2S should be considered an important topic of research when it comes to the pathology and treatment of diabetic CRS.

Hypertension is an important pathology due in part to its role as a risk factor for various other pathologies, some with significant morbidity and/or mortality rates [107]. It can be categorized as the more common primary hypertension with no directly attributable cause [108] or the rarer secondary hypertension, in which an underlying disorder such as renal dysfunction is the culprit [23,107]. An important clinical distinction is resistant hypertension, defined as hypertension that does not respond to combination therapy of the four major antihypertensive drugs [107]. An estimated 9–18% of hypertensive cases are resistant and can be either essential or secondary, indicating a societal need for better understanding and treatment options for these patients [107,109]. As discussed in the previous section, blood pressure is in part controlled by redox signaling [63,110]. Higher levels of ROS signaling predispose to hypertension and CSE knockout mice develop hypertension [9]. The few studies in humans on H_2S in diabetes and transplantation that also included blood pressure measurements show H_2S levels to be inversely associated with blood pressure [24]. The animal models in which H_2S can effectively reduce blood pressure are numerous including ANG II-induced hypertension [23,111], spontaneously hypertensive rats [112], and L-NNA induced hypertension (inhibition of NO synthesis) [26]. When existing antihypertensive drugs such as angiotensin-converting enzyme inhibitors (ACE-inhibitors) are modified by sulfhydrylation, they act as a donor for H_2S [112]. In the case of sulfhydrylated ACE-inhibitors, their safety is improved as well as having greater potential in treating hypertension than their standard counterparts through direct effects in the vascular tissue [112]. Due to its various mechanisms of antioxidant activity and numerous effects related to blood pressure control, H_2S could potentially serve as a new treatment for both kidney-induced secondary hypertension as well as essential hypertension.

Atherosclerosis is a common pathology of aging and comes with potentially debilitating consequences, monitored clinically primarily through concentrations of low density lipoprotein (LDL) and total cholesterol in the blood. Much like hypertension, treatment and prevention of this mostly asymptomatic process is essential for promoting cardiovascular health in the long-term. The endogenous production of H_2S is perhaps a double-edged sword in atherosclerosis, however, as shown in Figure 5 [30]. Endogenously produced H_2S is connected to atherosclerosis as a CSE knockout shows accelerated atherosclerosis development, rescuable by H_2S treatment [113]. Preexisting plaques, on the other hand, can develop micro-vessels through CSE/H_2S mediated angiogenesis, which increases the risk of plaque ruptures [114]. Exogenous treatment has shown more promise on the whole through suggested mechanisms such as dilating the vessels to restore flow, interactions with the Keap1/Nrf2 redox balance, protecting endothelial functionality from cell senescence, bypassing affected vessels through angiogenesis, protecting against (mitochondrial) DNA damage, and possibly foam cell formation via SIRT1 [115]. H_2S is also important in the liver's metabolism of lipids, an essential part of atherosclerosis, and oxidized LDL levels are inversely related to H_2S [30,115]. While more research is needed in this area before its application in humans, tentative optimism can be had for the potential of H_2S in preventing atherosclerosis as well as treating early stages, but should be considered with more caution for advanced disease.

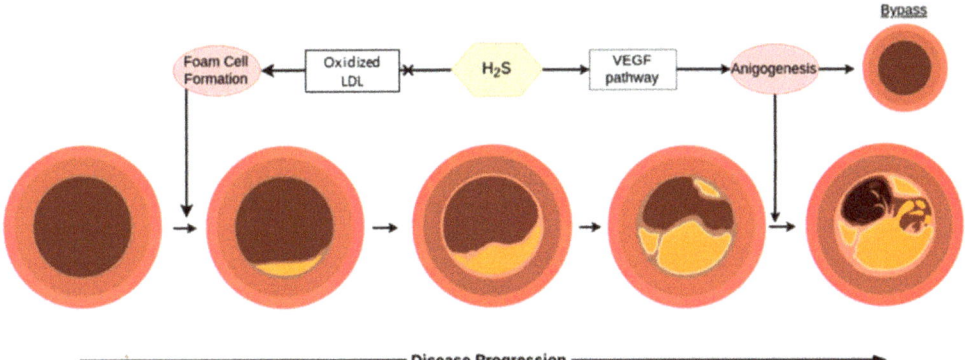

Figure 5. H_2S is helpful in early stages for the prevention of disease, however, it can be detrimental in later stages of atherosclerosis. In the figure, LDL is low density lipoprotein, and VEGF is vascular endothelial growth factor.

6. Therapeutic Potential in Cardiovascular and Renal Disease

Considering the wide variety of diseases in which H_2S has been implicated during recent years, it is not surprising that research has also started on exploiting its potential as a therapeutic drug [116]. A major line of study are the therapeutic applications during ischemic/reperfusion events of both the heart and kidneys [34,84,85,117]. Notably, H_2S treatment leads to amelioration of aging, sclerosis, and fibrosis in these organ systems. Furthermore, existing medications that interact with the renal-cardiovascular system interplay such as NSAIDs and ACE inhibitors are being modified with sulfur to induce H_2S production. One such modification, ATB-346, has been shown to improve the safety of

NSAIDs and is currently at stage II trials [118]. Beyond direct administration, the combination of H_2S and precursors present in food and produced by the gut biome open the way for diet potential [32,119,120]. Indeed, H_2S has been recognized as the primary effector of antioxidant behavior in foods such as garlic and onion [32,119,120]. Another lifestyle change, regular aerobic exercise, has been shown to induce H_2S in vivo [76]. In short, there is not only a wide variety of targets for H_2S treatment, but also a wide variety of treatment possibilities (Table 2). However, how much of the therapeutic potential for renal and cardiovascular disease is explained by the antioxidant effect of H_2S?

Table 2. An overview of some of the potential treatments using hydrogen sulfide.

Administration Type	Examples	Considerations
Donors	NaHS, Na_2S	Easy to use in vitro and in animal models. Phase 1 clinical trials.
	Sodium Thiosulfate ($Na_2S_2O_3$)	Already used in the clinic, increasingly tested in animal models.
Modified Drugs	ACE-inhibitors (Zofenopril, Captopril)	Improved safety and efficacy.
	NSAIDS (Diclonefac, Ibuprofen, Naproxen)	Improved safety.
Gas	H_2S	Non-oral administration, potentially dangerous.
Modified Treatments	Transplantation	Improvements over cold preservation with greater success rates.
	Stem Cell Treatments	Protection from oxidative stress during processing. Better treatment results.

6.1. Treatments Using H_2S Donors

H_2S donors are widely used in various recent studies. While NaHS or Na_2S is convenient for preclinical experiments, sodium thiosulfate ($Na_2S_2O_3$) is already registered for use in humans as a treatment for cyanide poisoning as well as being used off-label for calciphylaxis [121,122]. NaHS has been promising in the treatment of atherosclerosis in rat models [113] and hypertension in spontaneously hypertensive rats, Dahl salt sensitive rats, ANG II infusion, and NO synthesis inhibition [24]. It has been shown to improve renal function, reduce extent of injury, improve recovery rate after injury, treat diabetic renal disease, and increase tubular regeneration [9,105,123]. NaHS has also been used to ameliorate aging of various tissues including the kidneys and heart [12,65]. Sodium thiosulfate is beneficial in treating ANG II induced hypertension, renal damage, and heart disease [23,26,111,124]. It has also shown promise in rat models of cardiac ischemia [125,126] and preeclampsia [127] as well as mouse models of cardiomyopathy [128]. Sodium thiosulfate has been shown to be safe in intravenous doses up to at least 15 grams in patients with acute coronary syndrome undergoing coronary angiography [129]. In all of these cases, evidence is mounting that the interactions of H_2S and redox signaling is the main mechanism leading to these benefits [74,76,88,111,130].

6.2. Improving Transplantation Success

Along the same lines as its use in the treatment of ischemia/reperfusion events, H_2S has been shown to improve solid organ transplantation success in rats [131]. This is an important finding considering the limited supply of organs and the role of transplantation to treat end stage kidney or heart disease. As described in Section 4, H_2S protects tissue from ischemic/reperfusion events by reducing the resulting oxidative stress [84,85]. From a therapeutic standpoint, this would mean that administering H_2S or upregulating its production could reduce the damage of infarctions, ischemic events, and transplantation [116]. An important point to consider is that H_2S can be used in the perfusion of donor organs, and when doing so, it induces a hypometabolic state. This state can be used to replace the normal cooling method for transporting the organ, reducing the damage caused by the cooling on top of its benefits regarding oxidative stress. Beyond the success rate of the transplantation, it would be valuable if future research could investigate if H_2S reduces the prerenal kidney injuries that come with transplantation of other organs, in particular heart transplants, as these can lead to the development of CRS (see Section 5.2).

6.3. Diet and Exercise

Recently, H_2S has been shown to be involved in the benefits exercise and diet can have on cardiovascular health. In the case of exercise, it has been shown that long-term regular aerobic exercise is beneficial in attenuating age-related fibrosis of the heart. Recently, the mechanism of this attenuation was related to H_2S levels [76]. In the case of diet, the benefits of the allium genus (onions), in particular allium sativum (garlic), has been connected to H_2S released from diallyl disulfide [50,58]. Diallyl sulfide has been shown to have CSE-dependent benefits related to HIF-1a expression in cellular hypoxia responses [50,58]. Many of the benefits of these foods have been attributed to their antioxidant properties [32,119,120]. As H_2S's protective effects depend upon activation of endogenous antioxidant capacity, it may surpass the disappointing results that direct antioxidant treatment have shown thus far [132].

6.4. Regenerative Medicine

Stem cell treatment has shown promise in treating serious heart disease including heart failure [133]. There are several proposed mechanisms of this benefit including differentiation, immunomodulatory factor, and H_2S secretion [134]. However, its effectiveness can vary greatly between individuals. Indeed, many clinical trials on stem cell treatment focus on using stem cells obtained from the patient, which can be of low quality considering the condition of these patients [133]. The quality of stem cells and their ability to differentiate requires a minimum level of ROS, however, high levels lead to oxidative stress that results in senescence or death of the stem cells [135]. This can be particularly challenging due to simple matters that might take place in a treatment protocol such as exposure to air, resulting in an increase of ROS in readily available stem cell sources such as mesenchymal stem cells (MSCs) [134]. Considering the previously discussed ways that H_2S antagonizes ROS, it stands to reason that H_2S co-therapy might create a synergistic effect by better enabling stem cells to reach greater therapeutic potential while at the same time providing protection on its own. Indeed initial research in bone indicates that H_2S does indeed preserve MSC function [135]. Recently, Abdelmonem et al. found that preconditioning in vitro or co-delivery in vivo using NaHS both resulted in improved outcomes in treating rats with heart failure over MSC treatment alone [136]. Any combination of NaHS and/or MSCs resulted in no notable fibrosis. All combinations improved ejection fraction, fractional shortening, and the left ventricle diameter in heart failure with the preconditioned MSC treatment coming closest to healthy controls. Furthermore, preconditioned MSCs were able to restore QRS duration and QT intervals to healthy control levels, whereas NaHS alone or in combination with MSCs did not [136]. While still in an early phase, combination therapy of stem cells and H_2S has the potential to become a novel therapy.

7. Discussion

All in all, H_2S research has thus far opened new avenues of research into important diseases of the cardiovascular and renal systems, many of which need more or better treatment options. A great deal of H_2S's potential lies in its antioxidant properties. H_2S's ability to activate endogenous antioxidant production, modify key signaling proteins that are also targeted by ROS, and regulate the metabolism of mitochondria make it a complex and interesting puzzle. This complexity may also underlie the benefits seen in the treatment of rodent models of disease and the observations of H_2S associations with different aspects of various diseases in humans.

Although most of the research has been done in cell lines and in rodent models, we are reaching the point in which translation to the clinic is underway. The existing research in humans has initially mostly been observational, exploring changes in sulfate under various circumstances. Currently a handful of drugs modified to be H_2S donors are in varying phases of clinical trials. While the focus of these trials is on improving the safety profile of the original drug, the safety data in humans may ease the way for trials aimed specifically on the use of H_2S donors as a treatment. Sodium thiosulfate is also in various clinical trials, for example, it has proven safe in phase II trials for treatment of acute coronary syndrome (ClinicalTrials.gov identifier NCT03017963) and is undergoing phase III trials. Hopefully, the results in animal models to directly treat pathologies such as those belonging to CRS as well as indirectly by improving other treatment options such as transplantation and stem cell therapies can be replicated in humans.

It is also important to realize that while H_2S is reduced in cardiovascular and renal pathologies, H_2S and the transsulfuration enzymes are increased in other pathologies such as cancer and certain genetic neurological disorders [38]. When considering its use in humans, one should be careful to take this into consideration, as it could very well have implications for use in some subpopulations. From the other perspective of treating those pathologies with overproduction, care must also be taken to avoid making the heart and kidneys more vulnerable to oxidative stress related pathologies, exacerbating the already growing CRS problem. A diagram depicting dose-response relationships of H_2S can be found in Figure 6. However, even if such problems exist, they are not insurmountable, and we remain optimistic about H_2S's therapeutic potential.

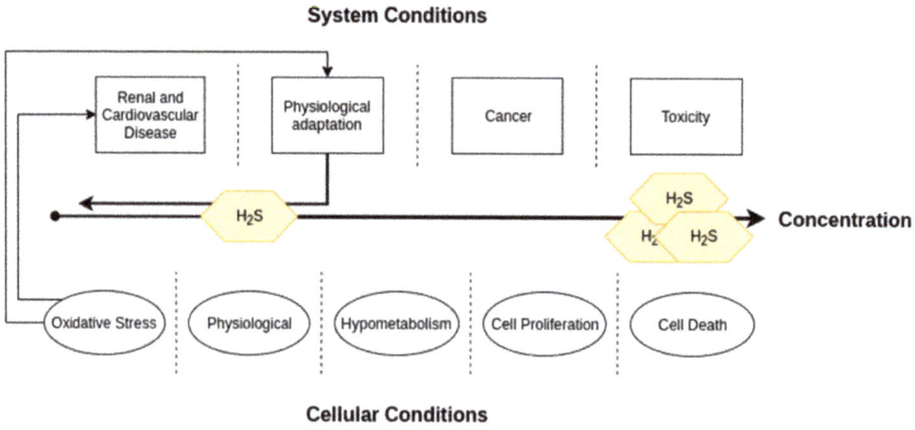

Figure 6. A diagram depicting dose-response relationships of H_2S concentrations. This review focused on the renal and cardiovascular systems, in which levels of H_2S lower than physiological amounts can lead to disease. However, it is important to note that high levels are characteristic of cancer and can also lead to toxicity.

8. Conclusions

H_2S is a gaseous signaling molecule that plays an important role in redox signaling. Research has exploded on its role in a broad spectrum of biological processes, both physiological and pathological. In the case of the renal and cardiovascular systems, H_2S plays an important role in maintaining ROS signaling at safe levels by promoting scavenging of ROS as well as competitively modifying cysteine residues on key signaling molecules. As such, depletion of H_2S is implicated in a variety of age-related pathologies as well as pathologies that fall under CRS. A number of these pathologies are difficult to treat and require novel therapies. Current research suggests potential for H_2S-based therapies, however, this has been limited primarily to studies in rodents. Fortunately, one donor of H_2S, sodium thiosulfate, is already registered for use in humans, thus easing the way for translational studies. Furthermore, H_2S shows potential for improving other forms of treatment such as the safety of NSAIDs, transplantation success, and stem cell therapies. Considering all these points, H_2S is a prime target for further research with potentially a large clinical impact.

Author Contributions: Conceptualization, J.J.S., I.T.N.N., H.V.G. and J.A.J.; resources, J.J.S.; writing—original draft preparation, J.J.S.; writing—review and editing, J.J.S., I.T.N.N., E.M.B.; H.V.G. and J.A.J.; visualization, J.J.S.; supervision, H.V.G. and J.A.J.; project administration, H.V.G.; funding acquisition, H.V.G. and J.A.J. All authors have read and agreed to the published version of the manuscript.

Funding: This research was funded by a grant from the Netherlands CardioVascular Research Initiative: An initiative with support of the Dutch Heart Foundation (CVON2014-11 [RECONNECT]). This research was also supported by a grant from the Dutch Kidney Foundation (#17O16).

Acknowledgments: Figures 2, 5 and 6 were created using BioRender.com.

Conflicts of Interest: The authors declare no conflict of interest.

References

1. Szabo, C. A timeline of hydrogen sulfide (H(2)S) research: From environmental toxin to biological mediator. *Biochem. Pharm.* **2018**, *149*, 5–19. [CrossRef] [PubMed]
2. Guidotti, T.L. Hydrogen sulphide. *Occup. Med.* **1996**, *46*, 367–371. [CrossRef]
3. Dorman, D.C.; Moulin, F.J.; McManus, B.E.; Mahle, K.C.; James, R.A.; Struve, M.F. Cytochrome oxidase inhibition induced by acute hydrogen sulfide inhalation: Correlation with tissue sulfide concentrations in the rat brain, liver, lung, and nasal epithelium. *Toxicol. Sci.* **2002**, *65*, 18–25. [CrossRef] [PubMed]
4. Warenycia, M.W.; Goodwin, L.R.; Benishin, C.G.; Reiffenstein, R.J.; Francom, D.M.; Taylor, J.D.; Dieken, F.P. Acute hydrogen sulfide poisoning. Demonstration of selective uptake of sulfide by the brainstem by measurement of brain sulfide levels. *Biochem. Pharm.* **1989**, *38*, 973–981. [CrossRef]
5. Goodwin, L.R.; Francom, D.; Dieken, F.P.; Taylor, J.D.; Warenycia, M.W.; Reiffenstein, R.J.; Dowling, G. Determination of sulfide in brain tissue by gas dialysis/ion chromatography: Postmortem studies and two case reports. *J. Anal. Toxicol.* **1989**, *13*, 105–109. [CrossRef] [PubMed]
6. Savage, J.C.; Gould, D.H. Determination of sulfide in brain tissue and rumen fluid by ion-interaction reversed-phase high-performance liquid chromatography. *J. Chromatogr.* **1990**, *526*, 540–545. [CrossRef]
7. Binkley, F.; Du Vigneaud, V. The Formation of Cysteine from Homocysteine and Serine by Liver Tissue of Rats. *J. Biol. Chem.* **1942**, *144*, 507–511. [CrossRef]
8. Abe, K.; Kimura, H. The possible role of hydrogen sulfide as an endogenous neuromodulator. *J. Neurosci.* **1996**, *16*, 1066–1071. [CrossRef]
9. Cao, X.; Bian, J.S. The Role of Hydrogen Sulfide in Renal System. *Front. Pharm.* **2016**, *7*, 385. [CrossRef]
10. Wu, D.; Hu, Q.; Zhu, D. An Update on Hydrogen Sulfide and Nitric Oxide Interactions in the Cardiovascular System. *Oxidative Med. Cell. Longev.* **2018**, *2018*, 4579140. [CrossRef]
11. Koning, A.M.; Frenay, A.R.; Leuvenink, H.G.; Van Goor, H. Hydrogen sulfide in renal physiology, disease and transplantation–the smell of renal protection. *Nitric Oxide* **2015**, *46*, 37–49. [CrossRef] [PubMed]
12. Perridon, B.W.; Leuvenink, H.G.; Hillebrands, J.L.; Van Goor, H.; Bos, E.M. The role of hydrogen sulfide in aging and age-related pathologies. *Aging (Albany Ny.)* **2016**, *8*, 2264–2289. [CrossRef] [PubMed]
13. Cortese-Krott, M.M.; Fernandez, B.O.; Kelm, M.; Butler, A.R.; Feelisch, M. On the chemical biology of the nitrite/sulfide interaction. *Nitric Oxide* **2015**, *46*, 14–24. [CrossRef] [PubMed]
14. Fukuto, J.M.; Ignarro, L.J.; Nagy, P.; Wink, D.A.; Kevil, C.G.; Feelisch, M.; Cortese-Krott, M.M.; Bianco, C.L.; Kumagai, Y.; Hobbs, A.J.; et al. Biological hydropersulfides and related polysulfides—A new concept and perspective in redox biology. *FEBS Lett.* **2018**, *592*, 2140–2152. [CrossRef]
15. Cortese-Krott, M.M.; Koning, A.; Kuhnle, G.G.C.; Nagy, P.; Bianco, C.L.; Pasch, A.; Wink, D.A.; Fukuto, J.M.; Jackson, A.A.; Van Goor, H.; et al. The Reactive Species Interactome: Evolutionary Emergence, Biological Significance, and Opportunities for Redox Metabolomics and Personalized Medicine. *Antioxid Redox Signal.* **2017**, *27*, 684–712. [CrossRef] [PubMed]
16. Van den Born, J.C.; Frenay, A.S.; Koning, A.M.; Bachtler, M.; Riphagen, I.J.; Minović, I.; Feelisch, M.; Dekker, M.M.; Bulthuis, M.L.C.; Gansevoort, R.T.; et al. Urinary Excretion of Sulfur Metabolites and Risk of Cardiovascular Events and All-Cause Mortality in the General Population. *Antioxid Redox Signal.* **2019**, *30*, 1999–2010. [CrossRef] [PubMed]
17. Van den Born, J.C.; Frenay, A.R.; Bakker, S.J.; Pasch, A.; Hillebrands, J.L.; Lambers Heerspink, H.J.; van Goor, H. High urinary sulfate concentration is associated with reduced risk of renal disease progression in type 2 diabetes. *Nitric Oxide* **2016**, *55–56*, 18–24. [CrossRef]
18. Ronco, C.; Haapio, M.; House, A.A.; Anavekar, N.; Bellomo, R. Cardiorenal syndrome. *J. Am. Coll. Cardiol.* **2008**, *52*, 1527–1539. [CrossRef]

19. House, A.A.; Anand, I.; Bellomo, R.; Cruz, D.; Bobek, I.; Anker, S.D.; Aspromonte, N.; Bagshaw, S.; Berl, T.; Daliento, L.; et al. Definition and classification of Cardio-Renal Syndromes: Workgroup statements from the 7th ADQI Consensus Conference. *Nephrol. Dial. Transpl.* **2010**, *25*, 1416–1420. [CrossRef] [PubMed]
20. Braam, B.; Joles, J.A.; Danishwar, A.H.; Gaillard, C.A. Cardiorenal syndrome–current understanding and future perspectives. *Nat. Rev. Nephrol.* **2014**, *10*, 48–55. [CrossRef]
21. Uduman, J. Epidemiology of Cardiorenal Syndrome. *Adv. Chronic Kidney Dis.* **2018**, *25*, 391–399. [CrossRef] [PubMed]
22. Ronco, C.; Bellasi, A.; Di Lullo, L. Cardiorenal Syndrome: An Overview. *Adv. Chronic Kidney Dis.* **2018**, *25*, 382–390. [CrossRef] [PubMed]
23. Snijder, P.M.; Frenay, A.R.; Koning, A.M.; Bachtler, M.; Pasch, A.; Kwakernaak, A.J.; Van den Berg, E.; Bos, E.M.; Hillebrands, J.L.; Navis, G.; et al. Sodium thiosulfate attenuates angiotensin II-induced hypertension, proteinuria and renal damage. *Nitric Oxide* **2014**, *42*, 87–98. [CrossRef] [PubMed]
24. Van Goor, H.; Van den Born, J.C.; Hillebrands, J.L.; Joles, J.A. Hydrogen sulfide in hypertension. *Curr. Opin. Nephrol. Hypertens.* **2016**, *25*, 107–113. [CrossRef] [PubMed]
25. Koning, A.M.; Meijers, W.C.; Minović, I.; Post, A.; Feelisch, M.; Pasch, A.; Leuvenink, H.G.; De Boer, R.A.; Bakker, S.J.; Van Goor, H. The fate of sulfate in chronic heart failure. *Am. J. Physiol. Heart Circ. Physiol.* **2017**, *312*, H415–H421. [CrossRef]
26. Nguyen, I.T.N.; Klooster, A.; Minnion, M.; Feelisch, M.; Verhaar, M.C.; Van Goor, H.; Joles, J.A. Sodium thiosulfate improves renal function and oxygenation in L-NNA-induced hypertension in rats. *Kidney Int.* **2020**, *98*, 366–377. [CrossRef] [PubMed]
27. Xie, Z.Z.; Liu, Y.; Bian, J.S. Hydrogen Sulfide and Cellular Redox Homeostasis. *Oxidative Med. Cell. Longev.* **2016**, *2016*, 6043038. [CrossRef] [PubMed]
28. Kalyanaraman, B. Teaching the basics of redox biology to medical and graduate students: Oxidants, antioxidants and disease mechanisms. *Redox Biol.* **2013**, *1*, 244–257. [CrossRef]
29. Bao, L.; Vlcek, C.; Paces, V.; Kraus, J.P. Identification and tissue distribution of human cystathionine beta-synthase mRNA isoforms. *Arch. Biochem. Biophys.* **1998**, *350*, 95–103. [CrossRef]
30. Kanagy, N.L.; Szabo, C.; Papapetropoulos, A. Vascular biology of hydrogen sulfide. *Am. J. Physiol. Cell Physiol.* **2017**, *312*, C537–C549. [CrossRef]
31. Hine, C.; Kim, H.J.; Zhu, Y.; Harputlugil, E.; Longchamp, A.; Matos, M.S.; Ramadoss, P.; Bauerle, K.; Brace, L.; Asara, J.M.; et al. Hypothalamic-Pituitary Axis Regulates Hydrogen Sulfide Production. *Cell Metab.* **2017**, *25*, 1320–1333.e1325. [CrossRef]
32. Hine, C.; Zhu, Y.; Hollenberg, A.N.; Mitchell, J.R. Dietary and Endocrine Regulation of Endogenous Hydrogen Sulfide Production: Implications for Longevity. *Antioxid Redox Signal.* **2018**, *28*, 1483–1502. [CrossRef]
33. Sbodio, J.I.; Snyder, S.H.; Paul, B.D. Regulators of the transsulfuration pathway. *Br. J. Pharm.* **2019**, *176*, 583–593. [CrossRef]
34. Bos, E.M.; Wang, R.; Snijder, P.M.; Boersema, M.; Damman, J.; Fu, M.; Moser, J.; Hillebrands, J.L.; Ploeg, R.J.; Yang, G.; et al. Cystathionine γ-lyase protects against renal ischemia/reperfusion by modulating oxidative stress. *J. Am. Soc. Nephrol.* **2013**, *24*, 759–770. [CrossRef]
35. Yang, J.; Minkler, P.; Grove, D.; Wang, R.; Willard, B.; Dweik, R.; Hine, C. Non-enzymatic hydrogen sulfide production from cysteine in blood is catalyzed by iron and vitamin B(6). *Commun. Biol.* **2019**, *2*, 194. [CrossRef]
36. Xu, S.; Liu, Z.; Liu, P. Targeting hydrogen sulfide as a promising therapeutic strategy for atherosclerosis. *Int. J. Cardiol.* **2014**, *172*, 313–317. [CrossRef] [PubMed]
37. Kimura, Y.; Koike, S.; Shibuya, N.; Lefer, D.; Ogasawara, Y.; Kimura, H. 3-Mercaptopyruvate sulfurtransferase produces potential redox regulators cysteine- and glutathione-persulfide (Cys-SSH and GSSH) together with signaling molecules H(2)S(2), H(2)S(3) and H(2)S. *Sci. Rep.* **2017**, *7*, 10459. [CrossRef] [PubMed]
38. Cao, X.; Ding, L.; Xie, Z.Z.; Yang, Y.; Whiteman, M.; Moore, P.K.; Bian, J.S. A Review of Hydrogen Sulfide Synthesis, Metabolism, and Measurement: Is Modulation of Hydrogen Sulfide a Novel Therapeutic for Cancer? *Antioxid Redox Signal.* **2019**, *31*, 1–38. [CrossRef] [PubMed]
39. Pal, V.K.; Bandyopadhyay, P.; Singh, A. Hydrogen sulfide in physiology and pathogenesis of bacteria and viruses. *Iubmb Life* **2018**, *70*, 393–410. [CrossRef]
40. Wedmann, R.; Onderka, C.; Wei, S.; Szijártó, I.A.; Miljkovic, J.L.; Mitrovic, A.; Lange, M.; Savitsky, S.; Yadav, P.K.; Torregrossa, R.; et al. Improved tag-switch method reveals that thioredoxin acts as depersulfidase and controls the intracellular levels of protein persulfidation. *Chem. Sci.* **2016**, *7*, 3414–3426. [CrossRef]
41. Palde, P.B.; Carroll, K.S. A universal entropy-driven mechanism for thioredoxin-target recognition. *Proc. Natl. Acad. Sci. USA* **2015**, *112*, 7960–7965. [CrossRef]
42. Ahmad, A.; Olah, G.; Szczesny, B.; Wood, M.E.; Whiteman, M.; Szabo, C. AP39, A Mitochondrially Targeted Hydrogen Sulfide Donor, Exerts Protective Effects in Renal Epithelial Cells Subjected to Oxidative Stress in Vitro and in Acute Renal Injury in Vivo. *Shock* **2016**, *45*, 88–97. [CrossRef]
43. Fu, M.; Zhang, W.; Wu, L.; Yang, G.; Li, H.; Wang, R. Hydrogen sulfide (H2S) metabolism in mitochondria and its regulatory role in energy production. *Proc. Natl. Acad. Sci. USA* **2012**, *109*, 2943–2948. [CrossRef]
44. Strutyns'ka, N.A.; Semenykhina, O.M.; Chorna, S.V.; Vavilova, H.L.; Sahach, V.F. Hydrogen sulfide inhibits Ca(2+)-induced mitochondrial permeability transition pore opening in adult and old rat heart. *Fiziol. Zh.* **2011**, *57*, 3–14. [CrossRef]
45. Bruce King, S. Potential biological chemistry of hydrogen sulfide (H2S) with the nitrogen oxides. *Free Radic. Biol. Med.* **2013**, *55*, 1–7. [CrossRef]

46. Zhang, J.; Shi, C.; Wang, H.; Gao, C.; Chang, P.; Chen, X.; Shan, H.; Zhang, M.; Tao, L. Hydrogen sulfide protects against cell damage through modulation of PI3K/Akt/Nrf2 signaling. *Int. J. Biochem. Cell Biol.* **2019**, *117*, 105636. [CrossRef] [PubMed]
47. Amaral, J.H.; Rizzi, E.S.; Alves-Lopes, R.; Pinheiro, L.C.; Tostes, R.C.; Tanus-Santos, J.E. Antioxidant and antihypertensive responses to oral nitrite involves activation of the Nrf2 pathway. *Free Radic. Biol. Med.* **2019**, *141*, 261–268. [CrossRef]
48. Kai, S.; Tanaka, T.; Daijo, H.; Harada, H.; Kishimoto, S.; Suzuki, K.; Takabuchi, S.; Takenaga, K.; Fukuda, K.; Hirota, K. Hydrogen sulfide inhibits hypoxia- but not anoxia-induced hypoxia-inducible factor 1 activation in a von hippel-lindau- and mitochondria-dependent manner. *Antioxid Redox Signal.* **2012**, *16*, 203–216. [CrossRef]
49. Wang, M.; Yan, J.; Cao, X.; Hua, P.; Li, Z. Hydrogen sulfide modulates epithelial-mesenchymal transition and angiogenesis in non-small cell lung cancer via HIF-1α activation. *Biochem. Pharm.* **2020**, *172*, 113775. [CrossRef] [PubMed]
50. Dugbartey, G.J. The smell of renal protection against chronic kidney disease: Hydrogen sulfide offers a potential stinky remedy. *Pharm. Rep.* **2018**, *70*, 196–205. [CrossRef] [PubMed]
51. Sies, H.; Berndt, C.; Jones, D.P. Oxidative Stress. *Annu. Rev. Biochem.* **2017**, *86*, 715–748. [CrossRef]
52. Zhu, H.; Blake, S.; Chan, K.T.; Pearson, R.B.; Kang, J. Cystathionine β-Synthase in Physiology and Cancer. *BioMed Res. Int.* **2018**, *2018*, 3205125. [CrossRef] [PubMed]
53. Maassen, H.; Hendriks, K.D.W.; Venema, L.H.; Henning, R.H.; Hofker, S.H.; Van Goor, H.; Leuvenink, H.G.D.; Coester, A.M. Hydrogen sulphide-induced hypometabolism in human-sized porcine kidneys. *PLoS ONE* **2019**, *14*, e0225152. [CrossRef] [PubMed]
54. Vitvitsky, V.; Miljkovic, J.L.; Bostelaar, T.; Adhikari, B.; Yadav, P.K.; Steiger, A.K.; Torregrossa, R.; Pluth, M.D.; Whiteman, M.; Banerjee, R.; et al. Cytochrome c Reduction by H(2)S Potentiates Sulfide Signaling. *ACS Chem. Biol.* **2018**, *13*, 2300–2307. [CrossRef] [PubMed]
55. Sies, H.; Jones, D.P. Reactive oxygen species (ROS) as pleiotropic physiological signalling agents. *Nat. Rev. Mol. Cell Biol.* **2020**, *21*, 363–383. [CrossRef]
56. Madamanchi, N.R.; Runge, M.S. Redox signaling in cardiovascular health and disease. *Free Radic. Biol. Med.* **2013**, *61*, 473–501. [CrossRef]
57. Foster, D.B.; Van Eyk, J.E.; Marbán, E.; O'Rourke, B. Redox signaling and protein phosphorylation in mitochondria: Progress and prospects. *J. Bioenerg. Biomembr.* **2009**, *41*, 159–168. [CrossRef]
58. Flannigan, K.L.; Agbor, T.A.; Motta, J.P.; Ferraz, J.G.; Wang, R.; Buret, A.G.; Wallace, J.L. Proresolution effects of hydrogen sulfide during colitis are mediated through hypoxia-inducible factor-1α. *Faseb. J.* **2015**, *29*, 1591–1602. [CrossRef]
59. Drachuk, K.O.; Dorofeyeva, N.A.; Sagach, V.F. The role of hydrogen sulfide in diastolic function restoration during aging. *Fiziol. Zh.* **2016**, *62*, 9–18. [CrossRef]
60. Jin, S.; Pu, S.X.; Hou, C.L.; Ma, F.F.; Li, N.; Li, X.H.; Tan, B.; Tao, B.B.; Wang, M.J.; Zhu, Y.C. Cardiac H2S Generation Is Reduced in Ageing Diabetic Mice. *Oxidative Med. Cell Longev.* **2015**, *2015*, 758358. [CrossRef]
61. Mys, L.A.; Budko, A.Y.; Strutynska, N.A.; Sagach, V.F. Pyridoxal-5-phosphate restores hydrogen sulfide synthes and redox state of heart and blood vessels tissue in old animals. *Fiziol. Zh.* **2017**, *63*, 3–9. [CrossRef] [PubMed]
62. Majzunova, M.; Dovinova, I.; Barancik, M.; Chan, J.Y. Redox signaling in pathophysiology of hypertension. *J. BioMed. Sci.* **2013**, *20*, 69. [CrossRef] [PubMed]
63. Berenyiova, A.; Drobna, M.; Cebova, M.; Kristek, F.; Cacanyiova, S. Changes in the vasoactive effects of nitric oxide, hydrogen sulfide and the structure of the rat thoracic aorta: The role of age and essential hypertension. *J. Physiol. Pharm.* **2018**, *69*. [CrossRef]
64. Honda, T.; Hirakawa, Y.; Nangaku, M. The role of oxidative stress and hypoxia in renal disease. *Kidney Res. Clin. Pr.* **2019**, *38*, 414–426. [CrossRef] [PubMed]
65. Lee, H.J.; Feliers, D.; Barnes, J.L.; Oh, S.; Choudhury, G.G.; Diaz, V.; Galvan, V.; Strong, R.; Nelson, J.; Salmon, A.; et al. Hydrogen sulfide ameliorates aging-associated changes in the kidney. *Geroscience* **2018**, *40*, 163–176. [CrossRef]
66. Kurtz, A. Control of renin synthesis and secretion. *Am. J. Hypertens.* **2012**, *25*, 839–847. [CrossRef] [PubMed]
67. Cao, X.; Wu, Z.; Xiong, S.; Cao, L.; Sethi, G.; Bian, J.S. The role of hydrogen sulfide in cyclic nucleotide signaling. *Biochem. Pharm.* **2018**, *149*, 20–28. [CrossRef]
68. Luo, R.; Hu, S.; Liu, Q.; Han, M.; Wang, F.; Qiu, M.; Li, S.; Li, X.; Yang, T.; Fu, X.; et al. Hydrogen sulfide upregulates renal AQP-2 protein expression and promotes urine concentration. *Faseb. J.* **2019**, *33*, 469–483. [CrossRef]
69. Olson, K.R. Hydrogen sulfide as an oxygen sensor. *Clin. Chem. Lab. Med.* **2013**, *51*, 623–632. [CrossRef]
70. Leigh, J.; Juriasingani, S.; Akbari, M.; Shao, P.; Saha, M.N.; Lobb, I.; Bachtler, M.; Fernandez, B.; Qian, Z.; Van Goor, H.; et al. Endogenous H(2)S production deficiencies lead to impaired renal erythropoietin production. *Can. Urol. Assoc. J.* **2018**, *13*, E210–E219. [CrossRef]
71. Ratliff, B.B.; Abdulmahdi, W.; Pawar, R.; Wolin, M.S. Oxidant Mechanisms in Renal Injury and Disease. *Antioxid Redox Signal.* **2016**, *25*, 119–146. [CrossRef]
72. Maksuti, E.; Westerhof, N.; Westerhof, B.E.; Broomé, M.; Stergiopulos, N. Contribution of the Arterial System and the Heart to Blood Pressure during Normal Aging—A Simulation Study. *PLoS ONE* **2016**, *11*, e0157793. [CrossRef]
73. Strutynska, N.A.; Kotsiuruba, A.V.; Budko, A.Y.; Mys, L.A.; Sagach, V.F. Mitochondrial dysfunction in the aging heart is accompanied by constitutive no-synthases uncoupling on the background of oxidative and nitrosative stress. *Fiziol. Zh.* **2016**, *62*, 3–11. [CrossRef]

74. Wei, C.; Zhao, Y.; Wang, L.; Peng, X.; Li, H.; Zhao, Y.; He, Y.; Shao, H.; Zhong, X.; Li, H.; et al. H2 S restores the cardioprotection from ischemic post-conditioning in isolated aged rat hearts. *Cell Biol. Int.* **2015**, *39*, 1173–1176. [CrossRef]
75. Liang, M.; Jin, S.; Wu, D.D.; Wang, M.J.; Zhu, Y.C. Hydrogen sulfide improves glucose metabolism and prevents hypertrophy in cardiomyocytes. *Nitric Oxide* **2015**, *46*, 114–122. [CrossRef]
76. Ma, N.; Liu, H.M.; Xia, T.; Liu, J.D.; Wang, X.Z. Chronic aerobic exercise training alleviates myocardial fibrosis in aged rats through restoring bioavailability of hydrogen sulfide. *Can. J. Physiol. Pharm.* **2018**, *96*, 902–908. [CrossRef] [PubMed]
77. Zhang, Q.Y.; Jin, H.F.; Chen, S.; Chen, Q.H.; Tang, C.S.; Du, J.B.; Huang, Y.Q. Hydrogen Sulfide Regulating Myocardial Structure and Function by Targeting Cardiomyocyte Autophagy. *Chin. Med. J.* **2018**, *131*, 839–844. [CrossRef] [PubMed]
78. Wohlgemuth, S.E.; Calvani, R.; Marzetti, E. The interplay between autophagy and mitochondrial dysfunction in oxidative stress-induced cardiac aging and pathology. *J. Mol. Cell. Cardiol.* **2014**, *71*, 62–70. [CrossRef] [PubMed]
79. Iciek, M.; Bilska-Wilkosz, A.; Górny, M. Sulfane sulfur—New findings on an old topic. *Acta Biochim. Pol.* **2019**, *66*, 533–544. [CrossRef] [PubMed]
80. Ronco, C.; Bellomo, R.; Kellum, J.A. Acute kidney injury. *Lancet* **2019**, *394*, 1949–1964. [CrossRef]
81. Dudoignon, E.; Dépret, F.; Legrand, M. Is the Renin-Angiotensin-Aldosterone System Good for the Kidney in Acute Settings? *Nephron* **2019**, *143*, 179–183. [CrossRef] [PubMed]
82. Meersch, M.; Schmidt, C.; Zarbock, A. Perioperative Acute Kidney Injury: An Under-Recognized Problem. *Anesth Analg.* **2017**, *125*, 1223–1232. [CrossRef] [PubMed]
83. Thiele, R.H.; Isbell, J.M.; Rosner, M.H. AKI associated with cardiac surgery. *Clin. J. Am. Soc. Nephrol.* **2015**, *10*, 500–514. [CrossRef] [PubMed]
84. Azizi, F.; Seifi, B.; Kadkhodaee, M.; Ahghari, P. Administration of hydrogen sulfide protects ischemia reperfusion-induced acute kidney injury by reducing the oxidative stress. *Ir. J. Med. Sci.* **2016**, *185*, 649–654. [CrossRef] [PubMed]
85. Bos, E.M.; Leuvenink, H.G.; Snijder, P.M.; Kloosterhuis, N.J.; Hillebrands, J.L.; Leemans, J.C.; Florquin, S.; Van Goor, H. Hydrogen sulfide-induced hypometabolism prevents renal ischemia/reperfusion injury. *J. Am. Soc. Nephrol.* **2009**, *20*, 1901–1905. [CrossRef]
86. Caravaca-Fontán, F.; Fernández-Juárez, G.; Praga, M. Acute kidney injury in interstitial nephritis. *Curr. Opin. Crit. Care* **2019**, *25*, 558–564. [CrossRef]
87. Clark, M.R.; Trotter, K.; Chang, A. The Pathogenesis and Therapeutic Implications of Tubulointerstitial Inflammation in Human Lupus Nephritis. *Semin. Nephrol.* **2015**, *35*, 455–464. [CrossRef]
88. Chen, Y.; Jin, S.; Teng, X.; Hu, Z.; Zhang, Z.; Qiu, X.; Tian, D.; Wu, Y. Hydrogen Sulfide Attenuates LPS-Induced Acute Kidney Injury by Inhibiting Inflammation and Oxidative Stress. *Oxid Med. Cell Longev.* **2018**, *2018*, 6717212. [CrossRef]
89. Wallace, J.L.; Vaughan, D.; Dicay, M.; MacNaughton, W.K.; De Nucci, G. Hydrogen Sulfide-Releasing Therapeutics: Translation to the Clinic. *Antioxid Redox Signal.* **2018**, *28*, 1533–1540. [CrossRef]
90. Van Dingenen, J.; Pieters, L.; Vral, A.; Lefebvre, R.A. The H2S-Releasing Naproxen Derivative ATB-346 and the Slow-Release H2S Donor GYY4137 Reduce Intestinal Inflammation and Restore Transit in Postoperative Ileus. *Front. Pharmacol.* **2019**, *10*. [CrossRef]
91. Zhang, X.; Donnan, P.T.; Bell, S.; Guthrie, B. Non-steroidal anti-inflammatory drug induced acute kidney injury in the community dwelling general population and people with chronic kidney disease: Systematic review and meta-analysis. *Bmc Nephrol.* **2017**, *18*, 256. [CrossRef]
92. Ozkaya, O.; Genc, G.; Bek, K.; Sullu, Y. A case of acetaminophen (paracetamol) causing renal failure without liver damage in a child and review of literature. *Ren. Fail.* **2010**, *32*, 1125–1127. [CrossRef]
93. Ozatik, F.Y.; Teksen, Y.; Kadioglu, E.; Ozatik, O.; Bayat, Z. Effects of hydrogen sulfide on acetaminophen-induced acute renal toxicity in rats. *Int. Urol. Nephrol.* **2019**, *51*, 745–754. [CrossRef] [PubMed]
94. Cao, X.; Zhang, W.; Moore, P.K.; Bian, J. Protective Smell of Hydrogen Sulfide and Polysulfide in Cisplatin-Induced Nephrotoxicity. *Int. J. Mol. Sci.* **2019**, *20*, 313. [CrossRef]
95. Yuan, Y.; Zhu, L.; Li, L.; Liu, J.; Chen, Y.; Cheng, J.; Peng, T.; Lu, Y. S-Sulfhydration of SIRT3 by Hydrogen Sulfide Attenuates Mitochondrial Dysfunction in Cisplatin-Induced Acute Kidney Injury. *Antioxid Redox Signal.* **2019**, *31*, 1302–1319. [CrossRef]
96. Liu, M.; Jia, Z.; Sun, Y.; Zhang, A.; Yang, T. A H 2 S Donor GYY4137 Exacerbates Cisplatin-Induced Nephrotoxicity in Mice. *Mediat. Inflamm.* **2016**, *2016*, 8145785. [CrossRef] [PubMed]
97. Farrar, A. Acute Kidney Injury. *Nurs. Clin. North Am.* **2018**, *53*, 499–510. [CrossRef] [PubMed]
98. Lin, S.; Lian, D.; Liu, W.; Haig, A.; Lobb, I.; Hijazi, A.; Razvi, H.; Burton, J.; Whiteman, M.; Sener, A. Daily therapy with a slow-releasing H(2)S donor GYY4137 enables early functional recovery and ameliorates renal injury associated with urinary obstruction. *Nitric Oxide* **2018**, *76*, 16–28. [CrossRef] [PubMed]
99. Lin, S.; Visram, F.; Liu, W.; Haig, A.; Jiang, J.; Mok, A.; Lian, D.; Wood, M.E.; Torregrossa, R.; Whiteman, M.; et al. GYY4137, a Slow-Releasing Hydrogen Sulfide Donor, Ameliorates Renal Damage Associated with Chronic Obstructive Uropathy. *J. Urol.* **2016**, *196*, 1778–1787. [CrossRef] [PubMed]
100. Aminzadeh, M.A.; Vaziri, N.D. Downregulation of the renal and hepatic hydrogen sulfide (H2S)-producing enzymes and capacity in chronic kidney disease. *Nephrol. Dial. Transpl.* **2012**, *27*, 498–504. [CrossRef] [PubMed]
101. Karmin, O.; Siow, Y.L. Metabolic Imbalance of Homocysteine and Hydrogen Sulfide in Kidney Disease. *Curr. Med. Chem.* **2018**, *25*, 367–377. [CrossRef]
102. Nowotny, K.; Jung, T.; Höhn, A.; Weber, D.; Grune, T. Advanced glycation end products and oxidative stress in type 2 diabetes mellitus. *Biomolecules* **2015**, *5*, 194–222. [CrossRef]

103. Isoni, C.A.; Borges, E.A.; Veloso, C.A.; Mattos, R.T.; Chaves, M.M.; Nogueira-Machado, J.A. cAMP activates the generation of reactive oxygen species and inhibits the secretion of IL-6 in peripheral blood mononuclear cells from type 2 diabetic patients. *Oxidative Med. Cell Longev.* **2009**, *2*, 317–321. [CrossRef] [PubMed]
104. Liu, Y.; Zhao, H.; Qiang, Y.; Qian, G.; Lu, S.; Chen, J.; Wang, X.; Guan, Q.; Liu, Y.; Fu, Y. Effects of hydrogen sulfide on high glucose-induced glomerular podocyte injury in mice. *Int. J. Clin. Exp. Pathol.* **2015**, *8*, 6814–6820. [PubMed]
105. Xue, R.; Hao, D.D.; Sun, J.P.; Li, W.W.; Zhao, M.M.; Li, X.H.; Chen, Y.; Zhu, J.H.; Ding, Y.J.; Liu, J.; et al. Hydrogen sulfide treatment promotes glucose uptake by increasing insulin receptor sensitivity and ameliorates kidney lesions in type 2 diabetes. *Antioxid Redox Signal.* **2013**, *19*, 5–23. [CrossRef] [PubMed]
106. Cai, J.; Shi, X.; Wang, H.; Fan, J.; Feng, Y.; Lin, X.; Yang, J.; Cui, Q.; Tang, C.; Xu, G.; et al. Cystathionine γ lyase-hydrogen sulfide increases peroxisome proliferator-activated receptor γ activity by sulfhydration at C139 site thereby promoting glucose uptake and lipid storage in adipocytes. *Biochim. Biophys. Acta* **2016**, *1861*, 419–429. [CrossRef] [PubMed]
107. Yaxley, J.P.; Thambar, S.V. Resistant hypertension: An approach to management in primary care. *J. Fam. Med. Prim. Care* **2015**, *4*, 193–199. [CrossRef]
108. Van Der Sande, N.G.C.; Blankestijn, P.J.; Visseren, F.L.J.; Beeftink, M.M.; Voskuil, M.; Westerink, J.; Bots, M.L.; Spiering, W. Prevalence of potential modifiable factors of hypertension in patients with difficult-to-control hypertension. *J. Hypertens.* **2019**, *37*, 398–405. [CrossRef] [PubMed]
109. Doroszko, A.; Janus, A.; Szahidewicz-Krupska, E.; Mazur, G.; Derkacz, A. Resistant Hypertension. *Adv. Clin. Exp. Med.* **2016**, *25*, 173–183. [CrossRef] [PubMed]
110. Al-Magableh, M.R.; Kemp-Harper, B.K.; Hart, J.L. Hydrogen sulfide treatment reduces blood pressure and oxidative stress in angiotensin II-induced hypertensive mice. *Hypertens. Res.* **2015**, *38*, 13–20. [CrossRef] [PubMed]
111. Snijder, P.M.; Frenay, A.R.; De Boer, R.A.; Pasch, A.; Hillebrands, J.L.; Leuvenink, H.G.; Van Goor, H. Exogenous administration of thiosulfate, a donor of hydrogen sulfide, attenuates angiotensin II-induced hypertensive heart disease in rats. *Br. J. Pharm.* **2015**, *172*, 1494–1504. [CrossRef] [PubMed]
112. Bucci, M.; Vellecco, V.; Cantalupo, A.; Brancaleone, V.; Zhou, Z.; Evangelista, S.; Calderone, V.; Papapetropoulos, A.; Cirino, G. Hydrogen sulfide accounts for the peripheral vascular effects of zofenopril independently of ACE inhibition. *Cardiovasc. Res.* **2014**, *102*, 138–147. [CrossRef] [PubMed]
113. Mani, S.; Li, H.; Untereiner, A.; Wu, L.; Yang, G.; Austin, R.C.; Dickhout, J.G.; Lhoták, Š.; Meng, Q.H.; Wang, R. Decreased endogenous production of hydrogen sulfide accelerates atherosclerosis. *Circulation* **2013**, *127*, 2523–2534. [CrossRef] [PubMed]
114. Van den Born, J.C.; Mencke, R.; Conroy, S.; Zeebregts, C.J.; Van Goor, H.; Hillebrands, J.L. Cystathionine γ-lyase is expressed in human atherosclerotic plaque microvessels and is involved in micro-angiogenesis. *Sci. Rep.* **2016**, *6*, 34608. [CrossRef] [PubMed]
115. Wang, Z.J.; Wu, J.; Guo, W.; Zhu, Y.Z. Atherosclerosis and the Hydrogen Sulfide Signaling Pathway—Therapeutic Approaches to Disease Prevention. *Cell Physiol. Biochem.* **2017**, *42*, 859–875. [CrossRef] [PubMed]
116. Wen, Y.D.; Wang, H.; Zhu, Y.Z. The Drug Developments of Hydrogen Sulfide on Cardiovascular Disease. *Oxidative Med. Cell Longev.* **2018**, *2018*, 4010395. [CrossRef]
117. Snijder, P.M.; De Boer, R.A.; Bos, E.M.; Van den Born, J.C.; Ruifrok, W.P.; Vreeswijk-Baudoin, I.; van Dijk, M.C.; Hillebrands, J.L.; Leuvenink, H.G.; Van Goor, H. Gaseous hydrogen sulfide protects against myocardial ischemia-reperfusion injury in mice partially independent from hypometabolism. *PLoS ONE* **2013**, *8*, e63291. [CrossRef] [PubMed]
118. Wallace, J.L.; Nagy, P.; Feener, T.; Allain, T.; Ditrói, T.; Vaughan, D.; Muscara, M.; De Nucci, G.; Buret, A. A3 A proof-of-concept, phase 2 clinical trial of the gi safety of a hydrogen sulfide-releasing anti-inflammatory drug (ATB-346). *J. Can. AsSoc. Gastroenterol.* **2019**, *2*, 7–8. [CrossRef]
119. Capasso, A. Antioxidant action and therapeutic efficacy of *Allium sativum* L. *Molecules* **2013**, *18*, 690–700. [CrossRef]
120. Kim, S.; Kim, D.B.; Jin, W.; Park, J.; Yoon, W.; Lee, Y.; Kim, S.; Lee, S.; Kim, S.; Lee, O.H.; et al. Comparative studies of bioactive organosulphur compounds and antioxidant activities in garlic (*Allium sativum* L.), elephant garlic (*Allium ampeloprasum* L.) and onion (*Allium cepa* L.). *Nat. Prod. Res.* **2018**, *32*, 1193–1197. [CrossRef] [PubMed]
121. Parker-Cote, J.L.; Rizer, J.; Vakkalanka, J.P.; Rege, S.V.; Holstege, C.P. Challenges in the diagnosis of acute cyanide poisoning. *Clin. Toxicol.* **2018**, *56*, 609–617. [CrossRef]
122. Nigwekar, S.U.; Brunelli, S.M.; Meade, D.; Wang, W.; Hymes, J.; Lacson, E., Jr. Sodium thiosulfate therapy for calcific uremic arteriolopathy. *Clin. J. Am. Soc. Nephrol.* **2013**, *8*, 1162–1170. [CrossRef] [PubMed]
123. Sun, H.J.; Wu, Z.Y.; Cao, L.; Zhu, M.Y.; Liu, T.T.; Guo, L.; Lin, Y.; Nie, X.W.; Bian, J.S. Hydrogen Sulfide: Recent Progression and Perspectives for the Treatment of Diabetic Nephropathy. *Molecules* **2019**, *24*, 2857. [CrossRef] [PubMed]
124. Oosterhuis, N.R.; Frenay, A.R.; Wesseling, S.; Snijder, P.M.; Slaats, G.G.; Yazdani, S.; Fernandez, B.O.; Feelisch, M.; Giles, R.H.; Verhaar, M.C.; et al. DL-propargylglycine reduces blood pressure and renal injury but increases kidney weight in angiotensin-II infused rats. *Nitric Oxide* **2015**, *49*, 56–66. [CrossRef] [PubMed]
125. Kannan, S.; Boovarahan, S.R.; Rengaraju, J.; Prem, P.; Kurian, G.A. Attenuation of cardiac ischemia-reperfusion injury by sodium thiosulfate is partially dependent on the effect of cystathione beta synthase in the myocardium. *Cell Biochem. Biophys.* **2019**, *77*, 261–272. [CrossRef]
126. Ravindran, S.; Jahir Hussain, S.; Boovarahan, S.R.; Kurian, G.A. Sodium thiosulfate post-conditioning protects rat hearts against ischemia reperfusion injury via reduction of apoptosis and oxidative stress. *Chem. Biol. Interact.* **2017**, *274*, 24–34. [CrossRef]

127. Terstappen, F.; Clarke, S.M.; Joles, J.A.; Ross, C.A.; Garrett, M.R.; Minnion, M.; Feelisch, M.; Goor, H.V.; Sasser, J.M.; Lely, A.T. Sodium Thiosulfate in the Pregnant Dahl Salt-Sensitive Rat, a Model of Preeclampsia. *Biomolecules* **2020**, *10*, 302. [CrossRef]
128. Mizuta, Y.; Tokuda, K.; Guo, J.; Zhang, S.; Narahara, S.; Kawano, T.; Murata, M.; Yamaura, K.; Hoka, S.; Hashizume, M.; et al. Sodium thiosulfate prevents doxorubicin-induced DNA damage and apoptosis in cardiomyocytes in mice. *Life Sci.* **2020**, *257*, 118074. [CrossRef]
129. De Koning, M.L.Y.; Assa, S.; Maagdenberg, C.G.; Van Veldhuisen, D.J.; Pasch, A.; Van Goor, H.; Lipsic, E.; Van der Harst, P. Safety and Tolerability of Sodium Thiosulfate in Patients with an Acute Coronary Syndrome Undergoing Coronary Angiography: A Dose-Escalation Safety Pilot Study (SAFE-ACS). *J. Interv. Cardiol.* **2020**, *2020*, 6014915. [CrossRef]
130. Li, H.; Wang, Y.; Wei, C.; Bai, S.; Zhao, Y.; Li, H.; Wu, B.; Wang, R.; Wu, L.; Xu, C. Mediation of exogenous hydrogen sulfide in recovery of ischemic post-conditioning-induced cardioprotection via down-regulating oxidative stress and up-regulating PI3K/Akt/GSK-3β pathway in isolated aging rat hearts. *Cell Biosci.* **2015**, *5*, 11. [CrossRef]
131. Snijder, P.M.; Van den Berg, E.; Whiteman, M.; Bakker, S.J.; Leuvenink, H.G.; Van Goor, H. Emerging role of gasotransmitters in renal transplantation. *Am. J. Transpl.* **2013**, *13*, 3067–3075. [CrossRef] [PubMed]
132. Bjelakovic, G.; Nikolova, D.; Gluud, C. Antioxidant supplements and mortality. *Curr. Opin. Clin. Nutr Metab. Care* **2014**, *17*, 40–44. [CrossRef] [PubMed]
133. Tehzeeb, J.; Manzoor, A.; Ahmed, M.M. Is Stem Cell Therapy an Answer to Heart Failure: A Literature Search. *Cureus* **2019**, *11*, e5959. [CrossRef] [PubMed]
134. Tan, D.Q.; Suda, T. Reactive Oxygen Species and Mitochondrial Homeostasis as Regulators of Stem Cell Fate and Function. *Antioxid. Redox Signal.* **2018**, *29*, 149–168. [CrossRef]
135. Liu, Y.; Yang, R.; Liu, X.; Zhou, Y.; Qu, C.; Kikuiri, T.; Wang, S.; Zandi, E.; Du, J.; Ambudkar, I.S.; et al. Hydrogen sulfide maintains mesenchymal stem cell function and bone homeostasis via regulation of Ca(2+) channel sulfhydration. *Cell Stem Cell* **2014**, *15*, 66–78. [CrossRef]
136. Abdelmonem, M.; Shahin, N.N.; Rashed, L.A.; Amin, H.A.A.; Shamaa, A.A.; Shaheen, A.A. Hydrogen sulfide enhances the effectiveness of mesenchymal stem cell therapy in rats with heart failure: In vitro preconditioning versus in vivo co-delivery. *BioMed. Pharm.* **2019**, *112*, 108584. [CrossRef] [PubMed]

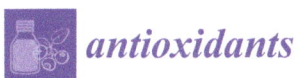

Article

The Phosphodiesterase Type 5 Inhibitor Sildenafil Improves DNA Stability and Redox Homeostasis in Systemic Sclerosis Fibroblasts Exposed to Reactive Oxygen Species

Luigi Di Luigi [1,†], Guglielmo Duranti [2,†], Ambra Antonioni [3], Paolo Sgrò [1], Roberta Ceci [2], Clara Crescioli [1], Stefania Sabatini [2], Andrea Lenzi [4], Daniela Caporossi [3], Francesco Del Galdo [5], Ivan Dimauro [3,‡] and Cristina Antinozzi [1,*,‡]

1. Unit of Endocrinology, Department of Movement, Human and Health Sciences, University of Rome "Foro Italico", Piazza Lauro de Bosis 15, 00135 Rome, Italy; luigi.diluigi@uniroma4.it (L.D.L.); paolo.sgro@uniroma4.it (P.S.); clara.crescioli@uniroma4.it (C.C.)
2. Unit of Biochemistry, Department of Movement, Human and Health Sciences, University of Rome "Foro Italico", Piazza Lauro de Bosis 15, 00135 Rome, Italy; guglielmo.duranti@uniroma4.it (G.D.); roberta.ceci@uniroma4.it (R.C.); stefania.sabatini@uniroma4.it (S.S.)
3. Unit of Biology and Genetics, Department of Movement, Human and Health Sciences, University of Rome "Foro Italico", Piazza Lauro de Bosis 15, 00135 Rome, Italy; ambra.anto@hotmail.it (A.A.); daniela.caporossi@uniroma4.it (D.C.); ivan.dimauro@uniroma4.it (I.D.)
4. Department of Experimental Medicine, Sapienza University of Rome, Viale Regina Elena 324, 00161 Rome, Italy; andrea.lenzi@uniroma1.it
5. Division of Rheumatic and Musculoskeletal Diseases, Leeds Institute of Molecular Medicine, University of Leeds, Woodhouse, Leeds LS2 9JT, UK; F.DelGaldo@leeds.ac.uk
* Correspondence: cristina.antinozzi@uniroma4.it
† These authors contributed equally to this work.
‡ These authors contributed equally to this work.

Received: 5 August 2020; Accepted: 22 August 2020; Published: 25 August 2020

Abstract: Systemic sclerosis (SSc) is a multi-system connective tissue disease characterized by the increased deposition of extracellular matrix proteins such as collagen and fibronectin. Although the pathogenesis is not completely understood, a number of studies suggest that free radicals could be the major contributors to the disease. Indeed, different studies demonstrated how oxidative stress could contribute to the fibrotic process activation at the level of the skin and visceral organs. Emerging evidences highlight the beneficial effects of sildenafil, a phosphodiesterase type 5 inhibitor (PDE5i), which protects different cell lines from the cell damage induced by reactive oxygen species (ROS). These data make sildenafil a good candidate for therapeutic treatment aimed to protect biological macromolecules against oxidative damage, thus preserving cell viability. The purpose of this study was to evaluate the sensitivity of SSc dermal fibroblasts to an oxidative insult and the ability for sildenafil to prevent/reduce the DNA damage due to ROS action. Additionally, we evaluated the capacity for sildenafil to influence redox homeostasis and cytotoxicity, as well as cell proliferation and cell cycle progression. We demonstrated that SSc fibroblasts have an increased sensitivity to a pro-oxidant environment in comparison to healthy controls. The sildenafil treatment reduced ROS-induced DNA damage, counteracted the negative effects of ROS on cell viability and proliferation, and promoted the activity of specific enzymes involved in redox homeostasis maintenance. To our knowledge, in this report, we demonstrate, for the first time, that sildenafil administration prevents ROS-induced instability in human dermal fibroblasts isolated by SSc patients. These results expand the use of PDE5i as therapeutic agents in SSc by indicating a protective role in tissue damage induced by oxidative insult.

Keywords: oxidative stress; sildenafil; DNA damage; systemic sclerosis

1. Introduction

Systemic sclerosis (SSc) is a multi-system connective tissue disorder characterized by the increased deposition of extracellular matrix proteins, where increased oxidative stress plays a role in the activation of the fibrotic process at the level of the skin and visceral organs [1–3].

In fact, it is known that excessive oxidative stress contributes to vascular damage, jeopardizes the function of the endothelial system, leading to immune system involvement, and it participates in the establishment and maintenance of fibroblast activation [4,5].

Several authors have shown that SSc patients have a reduced antioxidant capacity; however, the exact stage of the disease at which the increase in reactive oxygen species (ROS) occurs is still uncertain [6,7]. The plasma levels of ascorbic acid, α-tocopherol, β-carotene, and selenium were found lower in SSc patients than in healthy controls [6,7]. Moreover, patients with SSc have shown a high rate of chromosomal breakages, consistent with the known clastogenic activity of ROS, and increased levels of plasma markers of oxidative stress [8,9]. In particular, several authors have demonstrated that the systemic oxidative imbalance occurring in SSc patients induces changes in different subcellular components and macromolecules, oxidative denaturation, and derangement, as well as the loss of lipid asymmetry in membranes and DNA damage [10,11]. These are considered cellular changes that can induce premature cell senescence or cell death.

Controversial results exist about the possible beneficial effects of the treatment with different antioxidants in patients with SSc. The favorable outcome depends on the nature of the antioxidant substance, stage of the disease, and the duration of treatment [12–18].

Emerging evidences suggest specific protective effects of phosphodiesterase type 5 (PDE5) inhibition with sildenafil in protecting them from genotoxic damage induced by ROS in different cell lines [19–21]. Phosphodiesterases (PDE) are a group of ubiquitous enzymes that hydrolyze the nucleotides cyclic adenosine monophosphate (cAMP) or cyclic guanosine monophosphate (cGMP) to their inactive forms AMP and GMP [22]. In mammalians, PDE enzymes are classified into 11 families—namely, PDE1-PDE11. The use of PDE5 inhibitors (PDE5i) has been established in Raynaud's phenomenon and pulmonary arterial hypertension, and they are emerging as antifibrotic agents in interstitial lung disease [23–25].

The high potential antioxidant capability of sildenafil [26,27] makes this PDE5 inhibitor a good candidate for therapeutic treatment aimed to reduce oxidative damage to biological macromolecules, thus preserving cell viability.

The objective of this study was to evaluate the sensitivity of SSc dermal fibroblasts to oxidative stress and the ability for sildenafil to prevent/reduce the DNA damage induced by ROS. Additionally, we evaluated the capacity of sildenafil to influence redox homeostasis and cytotoxicity, as well as cell proliferation and cell cycle progression. To our knowledge, this is the first study on the redox characterization of SSc fibroblasts and their response to ROS-induced DNA damage, where it also highlights the possible capacity of sildenafil to determine an increased protection against oxidative stress-related alterations

2. Materials and Methods

2.1. Chemicals

Dulbecco's modified Eagle's medium (DMEM)/Ham's F-12 medium (1:1) (with and without phenol red), phosphate-buffered saline (PBS) Ca^{2+}/Mg^{2+}-free, bovine serum albumin (BSA) fraction V, glutamine, antibiotics, collagenase type IV, NaOH, Bradford reagent, 4′,6-Diamidino-2-phenylindole (DAPI), hydrogen peroxide, sildenafil citrate salts (98%), propidium iodide, ribonuclease enzyme, a redox-sensitive probe, and all reagents for Western blotting were from Sigma Aldrich (St. Louis, MO, USA). Fetal calf serum was from Gibco® (Grand Island, NY, USA). 2-mercaptoethanol was from Life Technologies, Inc. Laboratories (Grand Island, NY, USA). Cy3-labeled secondary antibodies (Abs) were from Jackson Laboratory (Bar Harbor, ME, USA); peroxidase secondary Abs and all reagents for Sodium Dodecyl Sulphate-PolyAcrylamide Gel Electrophoresis (SDS-PAGE) were from Millipore (Billerica, MA, USA). Plastic ware for cell cultures and disposable filtration units for growth media preparation were purchased from Corning (Milan, Italy).

2.2. Cell Culture

Human dermal fibroblasts (Hfbs) were isolated at the SSc clinic within the Leeds Institute of Rheumatic and Musculoskeletal Medicine (Leeds, UK) and processed as previously described [28]. Cells were derived from excisional skin biopsies of 3 patients with early diffuse cutaneous SSc (SSc) (mean age 61.9 ± 9.2 years) and 3 healthy controls (H) (mean age 55.6 ± 8.0 years) [28]. Informed consent was obtained and approved by the National Research Ethics Service (NRES) Committee (REC 10/H1306/88). The combined treatment with sildenafil and hydrogen peroxide was performed by adding this PDE5i to the culture medium 0.5 h before treatment with the pro-oxidant. The sildenafil concentration (1 µM) was chosen on the basis of the near-therapeutic doses utilized to treat erectile dysfunction, according to its pharmacokinetics (maximum drug concentration, Cmax and area under the time–concentration curves, AUC) [29].

2.3. Protein Expression Analysis

Healthy and SSc fibroblasts were treated for 24 h with H_2O_2 (50 and 100 µM) in the presence or absence of sildenafil. Cells were then lysed in Radioimmunoprecipitation assay (RIPA) buffer (150 mM NaCl, 50 mM tris-HCl pH 8, 1 mM Ethylenediaminetetraacetic acid (EDTA), 1% nonyl phenoxypolyethoxylethanol (NP40), 0.25% sodium deoxycholate, and 0.1% SDS, water to volume) supplemented with protease and phosphatase inhibitor cocktails (Sigma-Aldrich, Darmstadt, Germany).

For the immunoblot analysis, an equal amount of proteins (20–30 µg) was resolved in SDS-polyacrylamide (Bio-Rad Laboratories, Inc., Hercules, CA, USA) gels and transferred on polyvinylidene fluoride (PVDF) or nitrocellulose membranes, as previously described [30,31]. Thereafter, membranes were incubated with primary antibodies (Abs) appropriately diluted in Tween Tris-buffered saline (TTBS), followed by peroxidase-conjugated secondary immunoglobulin (Ig)G (1:10,000). Proteins were revealed by the enhanced chemiluminescence system (ECL plus, Millipore, Burlington, MA, USA). Image acquisition was performed with Image Quant Las 4000 software (GE Healthcare, Chicago, IL, USA). Densitometric analysis was performed with Quantity One® software version 4.6.8 (Bio-Rad Laboratories, Inc., Hercules, CA, USA). Western blot analysis was performed for three/four independent experiments. The list of primary antibodies utilized for the Western blot is reported in Table 1.

Table 1. List of primary antibodies utilized.

Antigen	Product Number	Dilution	Manufacturer
Superoxide dismutase (SOD) 1	sc-101523	1:1000	Santa Cruz (Santa Cruz, CA, USA)
Superoxide dismutase (SOD) 2	sod-110	1:1000	StressGen (San Diego, CA, USA)
Protein light chain (LC3) I-II	sc-271625	1:1000	Santa Cruz
Phospho-checkpoint kinase (p-CHK) 2	2197	1:1000	Cell Signaling (Leiden, The Netherlands)
Checkpoint kinase (CHK) 2	sc-5278	1:1000	Santa Cruz
Caspase (CASP) 3	sc-56053	1:1000	Santa Cruz
BCL2 associated X (BAX)	sc-526	1:1000	Santa Cruz
B-cell lymphoma-2 (BCL-2)	50E3	1:1000	Cell signaling
Phospho-extracellular signal-regulated kinases (p-ERK) 1/2	sc-7383	1:1000	Santa Cruz

Table 1. Cont.

Antigen	Product Number	Dilution	Manufacturer
Extracellular signal-regulated kinases (ERK) 2	sc-154	1:1000	Santa Cruz
Sequestosome 1 (P62)	sc-48402	1:1000	Santa Cruz
Catalase (CAT)	sc-271803	1:1000	Santa Cruz
β-actin	sc-47778	1:5000	Santa Cruz
γ-histone family member X (γH2AX)	ab26350	1:100	Abcam (Cambridge, UK)
DNA repair protein RAD51 (RAD51)	ab63801	1:1000	Abcam

2.4. Immunofluorescence Microscopy

A total of 1×10^4 cells were seeded onto glass coverslips in the growth medium. For γH2aX and RAD51 localization, healthy and SSc fibroblasts were treated with sildenafil and then stimulated for 0.5 h or 1 h with 50 µM or 100 µM H_2O_2. After stimulation, cells were washed out from the drugs and maintained in a drug-free medium for 4 h. Next, cells were washed and fixed with 95% ethanol and 5% acetic acid for 5 min and incubated with a blocking buffer containing 3% BSA/TBS for 30 min at room temperature. Primary Abs were incubated 1 h in blocking buffer, followed by the Cy3-conjugated secondary Ab (1.500). For method specificity, slides lacking the primary Abs were processed. Details on the primary antibodies are reported in Table 1. DAPI nucleic acid stain (1:10,000) was used to mark nuclei. Images were acquired at the magnification of 60×, and slides were examined with a Zeiss Z1 microscope (Zeiss International, Oberkochen, Germany) and Leica TCS SP2 (Leica, Milano, Italy). Experiments were performed three times.

2.5. 3-(4,5-Dimethylthiazol-2-yl)-2,5-Diphenyl-2H-Tetrazolium Bromide (MTT) Assay

Healthy and SSc fibroblasts (4×10^3 cells/well) were seeded in 96-well plates and incubated 1 h (T0) or 24 h (T24) with 50 µM or 100 µM H_2O_2 in the presence or absence of sildenafil. As previously described [32], the MTT assay was performed using Cell Proliferation Kit I (MTT) (Roche, Basilea, Switzerland), according to the manufacturer's instructions. Experiments were performed in triplicate with different cell preparations.

2.6. Cell Viability

For the cell viability assay, healthy and SSc fibroblasts were seeded in 6-well plates and incubated for 1 h with 50 µM or 100 µM H_2O_2 in the presence or absence of sildenafil. At the end of the incubation, drugs were washed out, and cells were either harvested (T0) or cultured for 7 (7 d) and 14 days (14 d) in drug-free media. Cell viability was assessed each day by trypan blue (0.05% v/v solution in PBS) exclusion mixed in a ratio of 1:1. Cell number counting was assayed by a hemocytometer, and only cells excluding trypan blue dye were analyzed. The number of viable cells at each time point was derived, averaging at least five different fields for each well. Each experimental point was repeated in duplicate or triplicate. Results are expressed as the number of cells. Experiments were performed four times with different cell preparations.

2.7. Cell Cycle Analysis

To evaluate the cell cycle progression, 25×10^4 healthy and SSc fibroblasts were seeded, with or without sildenafil, and then stimulated for 24 h with 50 µM or 100 µM H_2O_2. Propidium iodide (PI) assay was performed as previously described [33]. Briefly, cells were harvested, washed with PBS, suspended into 50% fetal bovine serum (FBS)-PBS solution, and fixed with 70% (v/v) alcohol at −20 °C overnight. After centrifugation, cells were suspended with 50 µM PI solution and ribonuclease A. DNA content was analyzed with FACScan CytoFLEX (Beckman Coulter, Brea, CA, USA). Experiments were performed in triplicate with different cell preparations.

2.8. Measurement of Intracellular ROS Levels

For intracellular ROS levels analysis, healthy and SSc fibroblasts were seeded at 5×10^3/mL in 6-well plates and incubated for 1 h with H_2O_2 50 µM or 100 µM in the presence or absence of sildenafil. At the end of treatment, cells were loaded with 200 µL of 5 µM dichloro-dihydro-fluorescein diacetate (DCFH-DA) dissolved in dimethylsulfoxide (DMSO) in PBS solution and maintained at 37 °C in the dark. The loading buffer was removed after 40 min, and the cells were incubated at 37 °C for an additional 30 min in a prewarmed growth medium. Then, the cell layer was washed with serum-free DMEM, and the level of ROS was determined by a Spark® fluorescence plate reader (Biocompare, South San Francisco, CA, USA) at 488/525 nm. Results obtained were expressed as absorbance arbitrary units/mg of proteins tested.

2.9. Thiobarbituric Acid Reactive Substances (TBARS)

TBARS levels were assayed by spectrophotometric analysis, as previously described [34]. The methodology calculates malondialdehyde (MDA) and other aldehydes generated by lipid peroxidation induced by hydroxyl free radicals. Briefly, healthy and SSc fibroblasts, treated with sildenafil and then stimulated for 1 h with 50 µM or 100 µM H_2O_2, were lysed in RIPA buffer. Cell lysate (150 µL) was added to 25 µL 0.2% butylated hydroxytoluene (BHT) and 600 µL of 15% aqueous trichloroacetic acid (TCA). Then, the mixture was centrifuged at 4000× g for 15 min at 4 °C. The deproteinized supernatant was transferred in a cryotube and added with 600 µL of thiobarbituric acid (TBA, 0.375% in 0.25 M HCl). Samples were then heated at 100 °C for 15 min in boiling water. The absorbance was determined at 535 nm by a spectrophotometric method and compared to standard MDA (1,1,3,3-tetramethoxypropane) solution. The levels of TBARS were expressed as nmol/mg of proteins.

2.10. Glutathione Homeostasis

Intracellular reduced (GSH) and oxidized (GSSG) glutathione amounts were evaluated by a 5,5'-dithio-bis(2-nitrobenzoic acid) (DTNB)-glutathione reductase recycling assay, as previously described [35]. Briefly, 1×10^7 healthy and SSc fibroblasts, treated with sildenafil and then stimulated for 1 h with 50 µM or 100 µM H_2O_2, were collected and suspended in 1:1 (v/v) 5% sulfosalicylic acid (SSA). Cells were lysed by freezing and thawing and, then, were centrifuged at 10,000× g for 5 min at 4 °C. The deproteinized supernatant was analyzed for the total glutathione content. Oxidized glutathione (GSSG) was measured in samples where reduced GSH was masked by pretreatment with 2-vinylpyridine (2%). Ten microliters of the sample were added to the reaction buffer (700 µL nicotinamide adenine dinucleotide phosphate (NADPH) (0.3 mM), 100 µL DTNB (6 mM), and 190 µL H_2O). The reaction was started by adding 2.66 U/mL glutathione reductase and followed at 412 nm by the TNB stoichiometric formation. Samples Δ optical density (ΔOD)/min412 were compared to those obtained by using glutathione standards. Results were normalized for protein contents.

2.11. Enzymatic Activities

Healthy and SSc fibroblasts were treated with sildenafil and then stimulated for 1 h with 50 µM or 100 µM H_2O_2. After treatment, cells were immediately collected. Intracellular superoxide dismutase (SOD) and catalase (CAT) activities were measured using commercial assay kits (Cayman Chemical Company, Ann Arbor, MI, USA), as previously described [35]. Experiments were performed at different times using different cell preparations. Results obtained as units/mg of proteins tested were expressed as fold over controls.

2.12. Cytokine Assay

Healthy and SSc fibroblasts were plated at 2×10^4 cells/mL in 96-well tissue culture plates and incubated 1 h with 50 µM or 100 µM H_2O_2 in the presence or absence of sildenafil. Cell culture supernatants were assayed for the macrophage migration inhibitor factor (MIF) by the magnetic bead-based multiplex assay according to the manufacturer's protocol. As previously described [36], data acquisition was performed by the Bio-Plex 200 System™ (Bio-Rad Laboratories, Inc., Hercules, CA, USA). Data analysis was performed by Bio-Plex Manager™ 6.0 software (Bio-Rad Laboratories, Inc., Hercules, CA, USA). Quality control pools of low, normal, and high concentrations for all parameters were included in each assay. Data were expressed as pg/mL. Cells supernatants were run in triplicate.

2.13. Statistical Analysis

The statistical analysis was conducted using GraphPad Prism software 8.0 (GraphPad Software, San Diego, CA, USA). To test the normality of the quantitative variables, the Kolmogorov-Smirnov or Shapiro-Wilk tests were applied. Normally distributed, continuous variables were analyzed using one- or two-way ANOVA and a Student's t-test. In all cases, p-value ≤ 0.05 was considered significant. All data were expressed as the mean ± SE.

3. Results

3.1. SSc Fibroblasts Appeared More Sensitive to Oxidative Stress-Induced DNA Double-Strand Breaks (DSBs) in Comparison to the Healthy Control Cells

The immunofluorescence analysis demonstrated that, already to the lowest doses tested (50 µM H_2O_2 for 0.5 h), SSc Hfbs showed higher sensitivity to oxidative stress compared to healthy ones, with a percentage of γH2aX-positive cells of 46.4 ± 17.9% after 30 min ($p < 0.05$ vs. control (ctr)), reaching 93.0 ± 5.7% after 1 h ($p < 0.01$ vs. ctr and $p < 0.01$ vs. healthy) (Figure 1A). At the highest dose of the pro-oxidant (100 µM H_2O_2), SSc Hfbs showed increased γH2aX by 62.9 ± 12.7% after 30 min ($p < 0.01$ vs. ctr and $p < 0.05$ vs. healthy) and 82.7 ± 9.1% after 1 h ($p < 0.01$ vs. ctr) (Figure 1A). Differently, healthy Hfbs showed a significant increase of γH2aX by 65.1 ± 6.1% only after 1 h with the H_2O_2 100 µM ($p < 0.01$ vs. ctr) (Figure 1A).

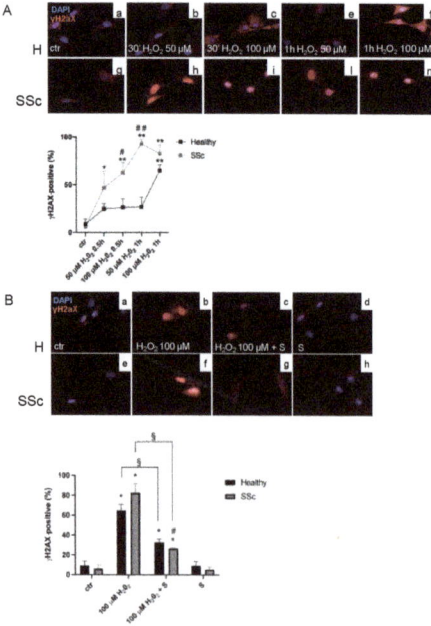

Figure 1. Analysis of H2aX phosphorylation in healthy controls (H) and systemic sclerosis (SSc) fibroblasts exposed to a pro-oxidant environment. (**A**) Immunofluorescence analysis of γH2aX in H

and SSc fibroblasts treated with 50 and 100 µM H_2O_2 for 0.5 and 1 h. (**B**) Exposure of H and SSc fibroblasts to the highest dose of H_2O_2 (100 µM for 1 h) in the presence or in absence of sildenafil (1 µM). Nuclei were stained with 4′,6-diamidino-2-phenylindole (DAPI) (blue). Pictures are representative of at least three separate experiments; magnification 60×. Diagrams represent the percentage of γH2aX-positive cells in the healthy controls (black lines/columns) and SSc (grey lines/columns) fibroblasts. * $p < 0.05$, ** $p < 0.01$ vs. ctr, # $p < 0.05$, ## $p < 0.01$ healthy vs. SSc, and § $p < 0.05$ H_2O_2 vs. H_2O_2 + S. Data represent mean ± SE. Results are derived from three separate experiments using different cell preparations. S, sildenafil.

3.2. Sildenafil Improved the DNA Repair Activation Process in H_2O_2-Damaged Healthy and SSc Fibroblasts

To assess the effects of sildenafil on γH2AX induced by the higher dose of hydrogen peroxide, we performed an immunofluorescence analysis in healthy and SSc Hfbs treated with H_2O_2 100 µM for 1 h in the presence or not of sildenafil. As shown in Figure 1B, a pro-oxidant environment induced a significant increase of γH2AX in both healthy (ctr vs. 100 µM H_2O_2: 8.8% ± 5.2% vs. 65.5 ± 12.2%, $p < 0.05$) and SSc fibroblasts (ctr vs. 100 µM H_2O_2: 6.2 ± 3.6% vs. 82.7 ± 9.1%, $p < 0.05$); however, the presence of sildenafil significantly decreased the percentage of γH2AX-positive cells by 32.8 ± 4.9% in healthy (100 µM H_2O_2 vs. 100 µM H_2O_2 + S, 65.5 ± 12.2% vs. 32.7 ± 3.5%, $p < 0.05$) and 56.1 ± 0.9% in SSc fibroblasts (100 µM H_2O_2 vs. 100 µM H_2O_2 + S, 82.7 ± 9.1% vs. 26.6 ± 0.7%, $p < 0.05$), respectively. When the same analysis was extended to RAD51, a protein involved in DNA repair mechanisms [37], we found that, at the basal condition, SSc already showed a higher number of RAD51 foci per cell than healthy Hfbs (healthy vs. SSc: 0.5 ± 0.2 vs. 17.2 ± 4.2, $p < 0.01$) (Figure 2A). Exposure to 50 µM of H_2O_2 induced a significant increase of RAD51 foci per cell either in healthy (ctr vs. 50 µM H_2O_2: 0.5 ± 0.2 vs. 41.3 ± 4.2, $p < 0.01$) or in SSc fibroblasts (ctr vs. 50 µM H_2O_2: 17.2 ± 4.2 vs. 66.3 ± 5.3, $p < 0.01$), although the number of RAD51 foci was significantly higher in the SSc ($p < 0.01$). Of interest, the highest dose of H_2O_2 (100 µM) induced major recruitment of RAD51 only in healthy Hfbs (ctr vs. 100 µM H_2O_2: 0.5 ± 0.2 vs. 22.1 ± 3.6 foci/cell, $p < 0.01$) (Figure 2A). The pretreatment with sildenafil reduced significantly the recruitment of RAD51 in the presence of low doses of H_2O_2 (50 µM) only in SSc Hfbs (50 µM H_2O_2 vs. 50 µM H_2O_2 + S: 66.3 ± 5.3 vs. 46.1 ± 4.3, $p < 0.01$), whereas no differences were observed in healthy Hfbs, where the level of RAD51 remained quite similar to that without sildenafil ($p > 0.05$) (Figure 2A). At high doses of H_2O_2 (100 µM), the presence of sildenafil increased RAD51 recruitment exclusively in SSc Hfbs (100 µM H_2O_2 vs. 100 µM H_2O_2 + S: 15.8 ± 3.6 vs. 32.0 ± 3.9, $p < 0.01$). No significant changes were observed in healthy Hfbs exposed to the pro-oxidant condition between the presence and absence of sildenafil ($p > 0.05$). Finally, the analysis of serine/threonine kinase (CHK2) modulation, a key component of the DNA damage response, highlighted that, in a pro-oxidant environment (50 µM and 100 µM H_2O_2 for 24 h), there was an increase of its phosphorylated form in SSc Hfbs (50 µM H_2O_2: 5.4 ± 2.1 and 100 µM H_2O_2: 5.5 ± 1.5, $p < 0.05$), independently of the presence of sildenafil ($p > 0.05$) (Figure 2B). No significant effects were demonstrated in healthy Hfbs (data not shown).

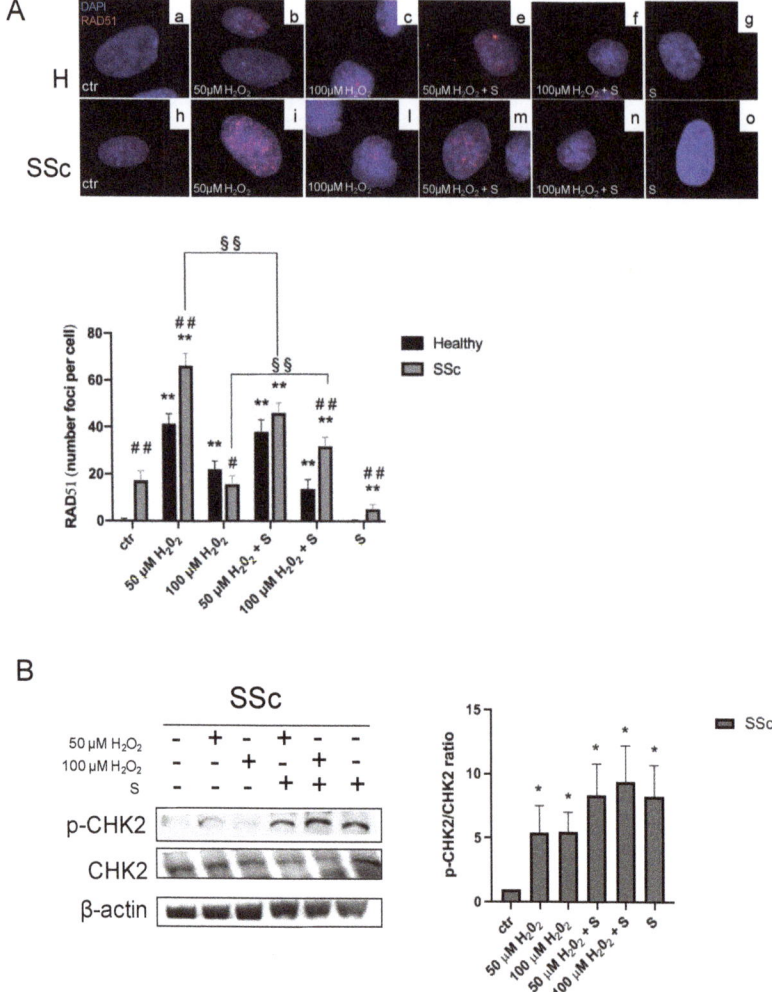

Figure 2. Analysis of DNA repair ability in healthy control (H) and SSc fibroblasts exposed to a pro-oxidant environment. (**A**) Representative immunofluorescence analysis of RAD51 in H and SSc fibroblasts treated with 50 and 100 μM H_2O_2 for 1h in the presence or in absence of sildenafil 1 μM. The diagram represents the number of RAD51 foci per cell in healthy (black columns) and SSc (grey columns) fibroblasts. (**B**) Western blot analysis for a serine/threonine kinase (CHK2) phosphorylation in SSc fibroblasts. Diagram depicted a densitometric analysis expressed as the ratio p-CHK2/total CHK2. * $p < 0.05$, ** $p < 0.01$ vs. ctr, # $p < 0.05$, ## $p < 0.01$ healthy vs. SSc, §§ $p < 0.01$ H_2O_2 vs. H_2O_2 + S. Data represent mean ± SE. Results are derived from three separate experiments using different cell preparations. S, sildenafil.

3.3. Sildenafil Sustained the Cell Viability and Ameliorated the Cell Proliferation in SSc Fibroblasts

To evaluate the effect of sildenafil on the cell cycle progression following H_2O_2 administration (50 μM and 100 μM H_2O_2 for 24 h), a flow cytometric analysis was performed. As shown in Figure 3A and Figure S1, at each experimental point, no significant differences in the various phases of the cell cycle were observed in both types of Hfbs ($p > 0.05$). However, in SSc, the highest dose of pro-oxidant induced an increase of cells blocked in the G1 sub-phase (6.5% after H_2O_2 50 μM, $p > 0.05$ and 14.4%

after H_2O_2 100 µM, $p < 0.05$). Furthermore, the pretreatment with sildenafil reduced the proportion of cells in the G1 subphase by 77% after H_2O_2 50 µM (from 6.5% to 1.9%, $p < 0.05$) and by 83% after H_2O_2 100 µM (from 14.4% to 2.4%, $p < 0.05$) (Figure 3B).

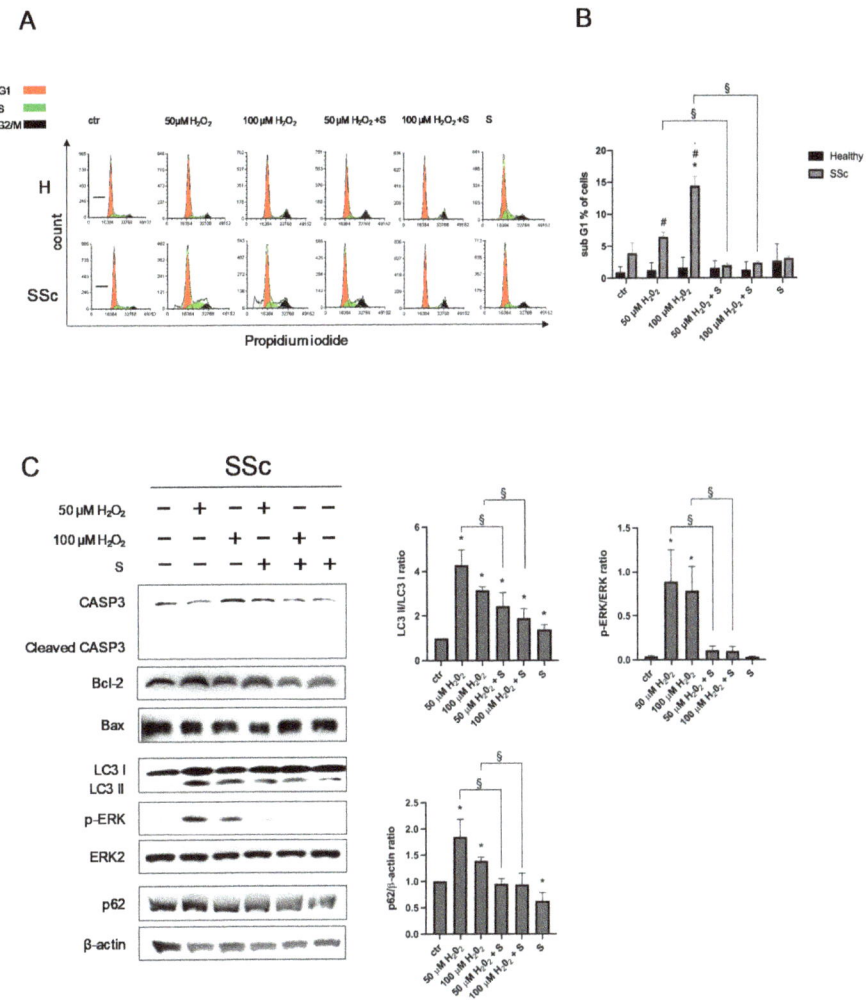

Figure 3. Analysis of the cell viability in healthy control (H) and SSc fibroblasts exposed to a pro-oxidant environment. (**A**) The cell cycle progression of H and SSc fibroblasts stimulated with 50 and 100 µM H_2O_2 for 24 h in the presence or in absence of sildenafil 1 µM. (**B**) Histogram represented the percentage of cells in the G1 subphase in healthy (black columns) and in SSc (grey columns) fibroblasts. (**C**) At the same experimental conditions, CASP3, cleaved CASP3, Bcl-2, Bax, and LC3 I and II, as well as ERK2, p-ERK, and P62, were analyzed in SSc fibroblasts though immunoblotting. Histograms depicted the densitometric analysis (mean ± SE) expressed as ratios of LC3 II/LC3 I, p-ERK/total ERK2, and P62/β-actin. * $p < 0.05$ vs. ctr, # $p < 0.05$ healthy vs. SSc, and § $p < 0.05$ H_2O_2 vs. H_2O_2 + S. S, sildenafil, and CASP3, CASPASE3.

To better characterize this phenomenon, specific protein markers of the apoptotic and autophagic processes were analyzed. As shown in Figure 3C, at the same experimental conditions, there was an increase of the cleaved form of LC3B (LC3 II), p62 expression, and ERK phosphorylation levels ($p < 0.05$). No significant effects were observed for CASPASE 3 cleavage, Bcl-2, or Bax ($p > 0.05$). The presence of sildenafil reduced the activation of LC3 II, the level of p62, and ERK phosphorylation ($p < 0.05$).

A further analysis of cell proliferation at T0 and T24, on both types of fibroblasts, highlighted a generalized reduction of cell proliferation following H_2O_2 exposure ($p < 0.05$ and $p < 0.01$) independently from the presence of sildenafil, although at 24 h, the presence of sildenafil showed a trend towards improving the cell proliferation ($p = 0.0523$) (Figure 4A,B). Long-term analysis of the cell viability after 7 d and 14 d demonstrated a different effect between the experimental groups (Figure 4C). In healthy Hfbs, the most significant effect of sildenafil was observed with the higher (100 µM) H_2O_2 exposure at 7 d (H_2O_2 vs. H_2O_2 + S: $(2.9 \pm 0.5) \times 10^4$ vs. $(4.1 \pm 0.7) \times 10^4$, $p < 0.05$) and 14 d (H_2O_2 vs. H_2O_2 + S: $(3.2 \pm 0.7) \times 10^4$ vs. $(5.9 \pm 0.1) \times 10^4$, $p < 0.05$), whereas, in SSc Hfbs, it was observed with both H_2O_2 doses at 7 d (50 µM H_2O_2 vs. 50 µM H_2O_2 + S: $(1.7 \pm 0.5) \times 10^4$ vs. $(3.0 \pm 0.4) \times 10^4$, $p < 0.05$ and 100 µM H_2O_2 vs. 100 µM H_2O_2 + S: $(1.0 \pm 0.2) \times 10^4$ vs. $(2.2 \pm 0.3) \times 10^4$, $p < 0.01$) and 14 d (50 µM H_2O_2 vs. 50 µM H_2O_2 + S: $(2.3 \pm 0.6) \times 10^4$ vs. $(4.0 \pm 0.6) \times 10^4$, $p < 0.05$ and 100 µM H_2O_2 vs. 100 µM H_2O_2 + S: $(1.3 \pm 0.3) \times 10^4$ vs. $(2.8 \pm 0.8) \times 10^4$, $p < 0.05$) (Figure 4C).

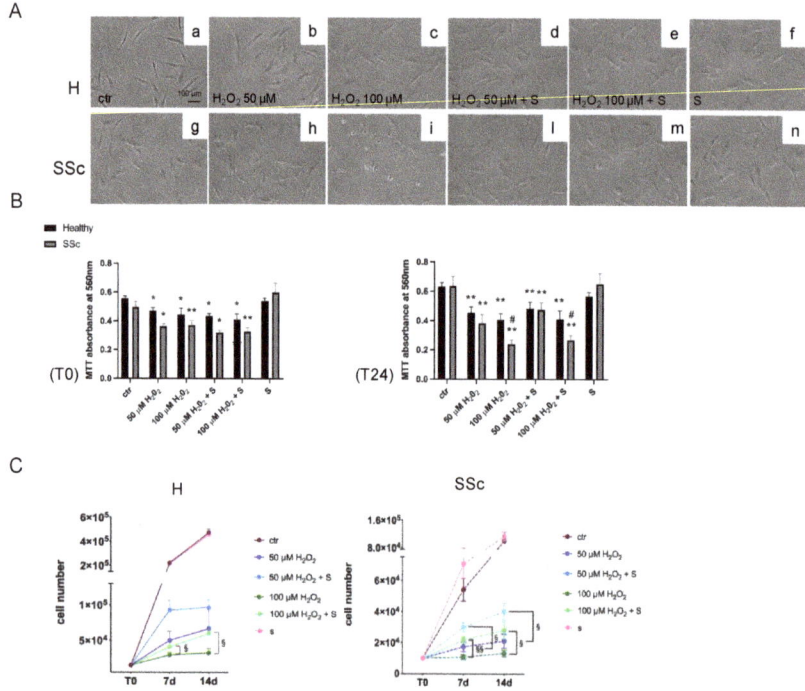

Figure 4. Analysis of the cell proliferation in healthy control (H) and SSc fibroblasts exposed to a pro-oxidant environment. (A) Morphological changes in H and SSc fibroblasts at the basal level (panels a,g) treated with 50 (panels b,h) and 100 µM H_2O_2 (panels c,i) for 24 h in the presence or in absence of sildenafil 1 µM (panels d–f,l–n). Scale Bar = 100 µm. (B) Cell viability was measured in healthy (black columns) and SSc fibroblasts (grey columns) stimulated with 50 and 100 µM H_2O_2 for 1 h (T0, left panel) and 24 h (T24, right panel) in the presence or in absence of sildenafil 1 µM. (C) Cell proliferation analysis in H (left panel) and SSc fibroblasts (right panel) treated with 50 and 100 µM H_2O_2 for 1 h in the presence or in absence of sildenafil 1 µM at the basal level (T0) after 7 days (7 d) and 14 days (14 d) of washing from the treatment. * $p < 0.05$, ** $p < 0.01$ vs. ctr, # $p < 0.05$ healthy vs. SSc, § $p < 0.05$, and §§ $p < 0.01$ H_2O_2 vs. H_2O_2 + S. Data are expressed as mean ± SE. S, sildenafil.

3.4. Sildenafil Reduces the ROS Levels in Healthy and SSc Fibroblasts

Previous experiments have been performed to demonstrate that sildenafil per se did not retain scavenger activity on oxygen-derived free radicals when added to the culture medium (data not shown).

As shown in Figure 5A, already at the basal level, SSc showed higher intracellular ROS levels when compared to healthy fibroblasts (healthy vs. SSc: 1.2 ± 0.0 vs. 1.6 ± 0.0, $p < 0.05$). Hydrogen peroxide administration induced a significant dose-dependent increase in ROS levels, particularly in SSc fibroblasts (healthy, 50 µM H_2O_2: 1.7 ± 0.0, $p < 0.05$ vs. ctr and 100 µM H_2O_2: 2.8 ± 0.1, $p < 0.01$ vs. ctr and SSc, 50 µM H_2O_2: 2.3 ± 0.1, $p < 0.05$ vs. ctr and 100 µM H_2O_2: 3.7 ± 0.2, $p < 0.01$ vs. ctr). Interestingly, the combined treatment with sildenafil reduced H_2O_2-induced ROS levels in healthy fibroblasts at both doses tested (50 µM H_2O_2 vs. 50 µM H_2O_2 + S: 1.7 ± 0.0 vs. 1.2 ± 0.1, $p > 0.05$ and 100 µM H_2O_2 vs. 100 µM H_2O_2 + S: 2.8 ± 0.1 vs. 1.3 ± 0.1, $p < 0.01$), whereas, in SSc cells, there was a significant reduction of ROS only at the highest dose (100 µM H_2O_2 vs. 100 µM H_2O_2 + S: 3.7 ± 0.2 vs. 1.9 ± 0.1, $p < 0.01$), respectively. No significant differences were found with sildenafil administration alone ($p > 0.05$) (Figure 5A).

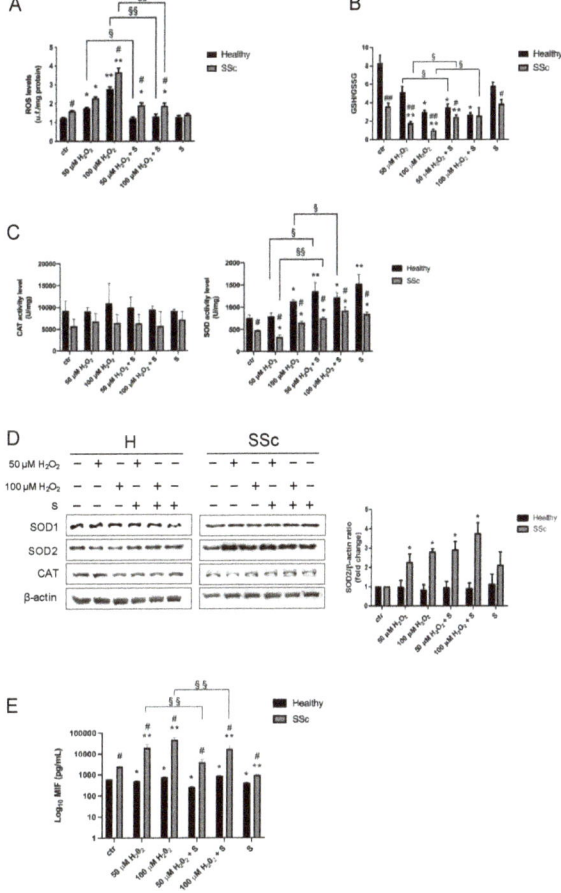

Figure 5. Analysis of the redox status in healthy control (H) and SSc fibroblasts after hydrogen peroxide administration. Healthy (black columns) and SSc (grey columns) fibroblasts were treated for 1 h with 50 and 100 µM H_2O_2 in the presence or in absence of sildenafil 1 µM and then analyzed for (**A**) ROS

amount; (**B**) GSH/GSSG; (**C**) catalase (CAT) and superoxide dismutase (SOD) activity; (**D**) CAT, SOD1, and SOD2 protein contents; and (**E**) MIF level. * $p < 0.05$, ** $p < 0.01$ vs. ctr, ## $p < 0.01$, # $p < 0.05$ healthy vs. SSc, § $p < 0.05$, and §§ $p < 0.05$ H_2O_2 vs. H_2O_2 + S. Data are expressed as mean ± SE. S, sildenafil; ROS, reactive oxygen species; GSSG, glutathione oxidized states; GSH, glutathione reduced states; SOD1 and 2, manganese superoxide dismutase isoforms 1 and 2; and MIF, macrophage migration inhibitory factor.

3.5. Sildenafil Ameliorates an Antioxidant Response in SSc Fibroblasts

The evaluation of the glutathione homeostasis revealed significant differences in the GSH/GSSG ratio between the experimental groups. In particular, in SSc, the total glutathione levels were already found lower compared with the counterpart healthy ones at the basal level (healthy vs. SSc: 164.9 ± 8.6 vs. 109.3 ± 5.8, $p < 0.01$) (Figure S2A), also showing a greater reduction of the GSH/GSSG ratio when exposed to both concentrations of H_2O_2 (ctr vs. 50 µM H_2O_2: 3.6 ± 0.3 vs. 1.7 ± 0.2, $p < 0.01$ and ctr vs. 100 µM H_2O_2: 3.6 ± 0.3 vs. 0.9 ± 0.1, $p < 0.01$). Differently, healthy Hfbs showed a significant reduction of the GSH/GSSG ratio only after exposure to the highest dose of H_2O_2 (ctr vs. 50 µM H_2O_2: 8.3 ± 0.8 vs. 5.1 ± 0.6, $p > 0.05$ and ctr vs. 100 µM H_2O_2: 8.3 ± 0.8 vs. 2.9 ± 0.3, $p < 0.05$) (Figure 5B). Pretreatment with sildenafil has proved particularly effective in SSc fibroblasts where it counteracts the reduction of the GSH/GSSH ratio induced by free radicals (50 µM H_2O_2 vs. 50 µM H_2O_2 + S: 1.7 ± 0.2 vs. 2.4 ± 0.2, $p < 0.05$ and 100 µM H_2O_2 vs. 100 µM H_2O_2 + S: 0.9 ± 0.1 vs. 2.6 ± 0.8, $p < 0.05$) (Figure 5B). Both types of fibroblasts showed no difference after the administration of sildenafil alone ($p > 0.05$). At the level of the antioxidant enzyme activities, we found substantial differences between two types of fibroblasts depending on the enzyme examined (Figure 5C). In particular, while catalase (CAT) activity showed only a tendency to be lower in SSc cells compared to the healthy counterparts ($p = 0.0938$), and its level was not influenced by the presence of H_2O_2 and/or sildenafil ($p > 0.05$), the analysis of superoxide dismutase (SOD) activity highlighted distinct and significant differences between the two groups. Indeed, SOD activity was ≈ 37.7% lower in SSc compared with the counterpart healthy (ctr: healthy vs. SSc, 754.9 ± 41.3 vs. 473.8 ± 6.2, $p < 0.05$). In the presence of ROS, both cell lines were responsive, with a significant increase of SOD activity only at the higher dose (healthy, 100 µM H_2O_2: 1127.8 ± 21.3 and SSc, 100 µM H_2O_2 647.2 ± 19.9, $p < 0.05$). Moreover, while in healthy ones, the combined treatment with sildenafil induced a major increase in SOD activity in both H_2O_2 doses tested (50 µM H_2O_2 vs. 50 µM H_2O_2 + S: 791.0 ± 46.7 vs. 1356.4 ± 112.9, $p < 0.05$ and 100 µM H_2O_2 vs. 100 µM H_2O_2 + S: 1127.8 ± 21.3 vs. 1213.8 ± 61.5, $p < 0.05$), in SSc, this increase was present only at the low dose (50 µM H_2O_2 vs. 50 µM H_2O_2 + S: 330.0 ± 22.5 vs. 745.7 ± 12.3, $p < 0.05$) (Figure 5C). The presence of sildenafil alone induced a significant increase in SOD activity in both cell types compared with unstimulated cells (healthy, ctr vs. S: 754.9 ± 41.3 vs. 1521.2 ± 11.7, $p < 0.01$ and SSc, ctr vs. S: 473.8 ± 6.2 vs. 839.8 ± 24.9, $p < 0.05$).

At the protein level, no effects were detected for CAT and SOD1 ($p > 0.05$), whereas SOD2 was significantly upregulated only in SSc cells exposed to H_2O_2 ($p < 0.05$), independently from the presence of sildenafil ($p > 0.05$) (Figure 5D).

3.6. Macrophage Migration Inhibitory Factor Level

As already demonstrated by Kim et al. (2008) [38], the analysis of the macrophage migration inhibitory factor (MIF) revealed already at the basal level profound differences, with SSc cells showing higher levels compared with the healthy control (healthy vs. SSc: 586.3 ± 5.1 vs. 2448.0 ± 30.1, $p < 0.05$) (Figure 5E). The presence of hydrogen peroxide evoked in our cellular models a different response of this inflammatory cytokine. In particular, we found a slight decrease of MIF in healthy ones (50 µM H_2O_2: 508.8 ± 3.8, $p < 0.05$ and 100 µM H_2O_2: 749.5 ± 24.8, $p < 0.05$) and a massive increase in SSc ones (50 µM H_2O_2: 19,685.0 ± 9135.0, $p < 0.01$ and 100 µM H_2O_2: 47,417.0 ± 15,026.0, $p < 0.01$) (Figure 5E). Interestingly, the concomitant treatment with sildenafil produced significant effects only in SSc cells reducing the MIF secretion induced by hydrogen peroxide (50 µM H_2O_2 vs. 50 µM H_2O_2 + S: 19,685.0

± 9135.0 vs. 4127.0 ± 1367.0, $p < 0.01$ and 100 µM H_2O_2 vs. 100 µM H_2O_2 + S: 47,417.0 ± 15,026.0 vs. 17,285.0 ± 6374.0, $p < 0.01$) (Figure 5E).

3.7. Sildenafil Mitigates the Effect of Oxidative Insult on TBAR Levels

As shown in Figure S2C, no differences in the TBAR levels were observed at the basal level between healthy and SSc cells ($p > 0.05$). Under pro-oxidant conditions, TBAR levels increased in both cell types tested, showing the greatest sensitivity of SSc. Indeed, already at a low dose of H_2O_2, there was a significant increase in TBAR in SSc cells (ctr vs. 50 µM H_2O_2: 0.6 ± 0.0 vs. 0.8 ± 0.0, $p < 0.01$). Only at the highest concentration of hydrogen peroxide, there was a significant increase in TBAR in both cell types (healthy, ctr vs. 100 µM H_2O_2: 0.5 ± 0.0 vs. 0.9 ± 0.1, $p < 0.01$ and SSc, ctr vs. 100 µM H_2O_2: 0.6 ± 0.0 vs. 1.0 ± 0.1, $p < 0.01$). The concomitant presence of sildenafil induced no significant variation in TBAR levels after the low dose of H_2O_2 ($p > 0.05$), whereas, at the highest dose, sildenafil reported TBARS levels similar to the control in both experimental groups ($p < 0.01$). No significant differences were found with sildenafil administration alone ($p > 0.05$).

4. Discussion

The present study demonstrates for the first time that the PDE5 inhibitor sildenafil reduces the sensitivity to DNA damage of human SSc fibroblasts exposed to a pro-oxidant environment, improving their genomic stability. In addition, sildenafil counteracts the negative effects of ROS on cell viability and proliferation, inhibiting the activation of the autophagic pathway and modulating the activity of specific enzymes involved in redox homeostasis. Taken together, these results suggest that sildenafil may be a possible candidate for therapeutic treatment aimed at counteracting oxidative stress adverse effects.

There is considerable evidence implicating sildenafil as a key molecule capable of preventing ROS-induced DNA damage in several different types of cells, a condition present during the progression of many diseases—as, for example, in atherosclerosis, cardiovascular diseases, and systemic sclerosis [7,20,21,39].

In the present study, we utilized a cell culture of human dermal fibroblasts from healthy and SSc patients already validated as a useful model to investigate the mechanisms involved in SSc fibrosis [23,40,41]. We found that SSc fibroblasts were more sensitive to exogenous exposure to ROS compared with the healthy counterparts. In fact, a brief exposure to low concentrations of hydrogen peroxide (50 µM) already induced an increased nuclear accumulation of γH2aX, a marker of single and double DNA stranded breaks (SSBs and DSBs) [42]. Moreover, we observed that the accumulation of γH2aX induced by the high dose of hydrogen peroxide (100 µM) both in healthy and in SSc ones was less evident in the presence of sildenafil. Therefore, as already suggested by others in different pathological conditions [19–21], here, we showed that sildenafil reduced ROS-induced DNA damage in SSc and healthy fibroblasts. Additionally, our data demonstrated that the presence of sildenafil modifies the nuclear distribution of RAD51, a central player in homologous recombination (HR) and DSBs repair [43,44]. The RAD51 redistribution to chromatin and nuclear foci formations, mainly induced by DSBs, is crucial to HR repair. In particular, the formation of RAD51 nuclear foci was dramatically enhanced by H_2O_2, indicating the proceeding of HR repair; however, and more markedly in SSc cells, sildenafil modified ROS-induced effects. In particular, in the presence of low levels of DNA damage, the PDE5i determined a reduced redistribution of RAD51. Presumably, the extent of DNA damage did not exceed the intrinsic capacity of the cells to repair themselves. Differently, in the presence of massive DNA damage, sildenafil improved the cellular response by increasing the efficiency of cell repair systems.

CHK2 is a checkpoint kinase and a key component of the DNA damage response regulating the binding of RAD51 to DNA [45,46]. Genotoxic stress triggering CHK2 phosphorylation regulates a variety of downstream effectors, inducing a proper cellular response as cell cycle checkpoint activation [47], cell death, and DNA repair [48,49]. The analysis of the cell cycle progression, along with the analysis of specific markers of cell death, further highlighted the greater sensitivity of SSc fibroblasts to ROS insult. In particular, our results suggested that these cells were unstable, less proliferative, and with a significant number of cells that undergo autophagic cell death compared to the healthy cells. Among the beneficial pleiotropic effects of sildenafil, its ability to preserve the cell cycle kinetics under oxidative stress conditions has already been demonstrated in vivo and in vitro on different cell lines [20,21,50–52]; however, this is the first study showing that sildenafil treatment rescued SSc cells from the sub-G1 phase, restoring their normal cell cycle distribution and protecting them from autophagy. The lack of effect of sildenafil on CHK2 modulation was not surprising, since it could already be maximally activated by other cellular pathways responsive to ROS [53]. All these data were further confirmed by the data on cell proliferation, showing a partial recovery when sildenafil was concomitant to oxidative stress (Figure 4).

There are evidences of antioxidative effects of sildenafil on different cell lines and animal models [19–21,26,27,54–56], and very recently, our group has shown that sildenafil was involved in ROS-mediated signaling through the modulation of Signal transducer and activator of transcription (STAT) 3, ERK, nuclear factor kappa-light-chain-enhancer of activated B cells (NF-Kb), and protein kinase B (PKB/AKT), as well as in reducing the expression/secretion of proinflammatory and profibrotic cytokines in SSc fibroblasts exposed to H_2O_2 [23]. Here, for the first time, we successfully demonstrated that the presence of sildenafil ameliorates the management of redox imbalance in SSc fibroblasts exposed to a pro-oxidant environment, reducing ROS levels and improving the efficiency of the glutathione system, as well as increasing the level of SOD and its activity. These results were further supported by the reduced production of both the macrophage inhibitory factor (MIF), a pleiotropic inflammatory cytokine with broad target cell specificity that is secreted following several stimuli, including oxidative stress [57], and thiobarbituric acid reactive substances (TBARS), formed as a bioproduct of lipid peroxidation [58].

The molecular mechanism behind the pharmacologic actions of this PDE5i relates to its potential to increase intracellular cyclic guanosine monophosphate (cGMP) [59]. The regulations of cell function by extrinsic factors occurs through a series of second-messenger signals starting by a ligand-receptor interaction and, then, modulating both the intensity and the nature of immediate and delayed cellular responses. Thus, second messengers exert control over principal cellular events. There is evidence that biological responses triggered by oxidative products are able to provoke various pathogenic intracellular signals involving calcium, G-proteins, cAMP, cGMP, phospholipase C and D, protein kinase C, ceramide, and the mitogen-activated protein kinase (MAP) kinase cascade, leading to cellular dysfunction [60]. Thus, as suggested by Abdollahi et al. (2003) [56], increasing cyclic nucleotides by the use of phosphodiesterase inhibitors could overcome oxidative stress-induced cellular dysfunctions. To confirm this hypothesis, recently, it has been demonstrated that the augmentation of the cGMP/Protein Kinase G (cGMP/PKG) pathway ameliorated the antioxidant response of retinal cells cultured in hypoxic conditions, increasing the superoxide dismutase and catalase enzyme activities [61]. However, considering the complexity of cellular oxidative stress associated with this pathology, it stands to reason that a complete mechanism of action for sildenafil could require additional cellular pathways involved in the regulation of inflammation, proliferation, cell death, and antioxidant defenses [62–64].

5. Conclusions

Although our in vitro system represents a simplified model reproducing the alteration of the redox homeostasis determined by the pathological state [65–67], we believe that our research extends the scope of sildenafil as a therapeutic agent in oxidative stress-related pathologies for SSc.

Particularly, our findings offer compelling evidences indicating that the administration of sildenafil in SSc fibroblasts exposed to a pro-oxidant: (i) protects against ROS-induced DNA damage, (ii) preserves the cell cycle kinetics, and (iii) improves redox homeostasis (Figure 6).

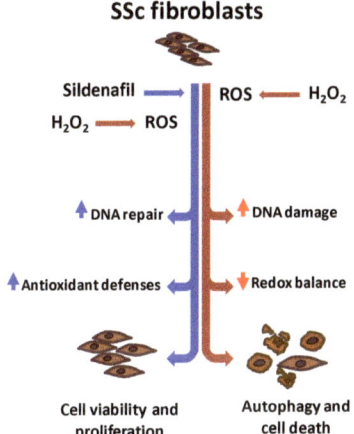

Figure 6. Reactive oxygen species (ROS) resulting from pro-oxidant exposure (H_2O_2, red arrows) increase the DNA damage and affect the redox homeostasis in systemic sclerosis fibroblasts (SSc). As a consequence, cells undergo cell death by autophagy. In the same pro-oxidant environment, the presence of the phosphodiesterase type 5 inhibitor sildenafil (blue arrows) counteracts the negative effects of ROS on cell viability and proliferation, inhibiting the activation of the autophagic pathway and modulating the activity of specific enzymes involved in redox homeostasis.

Therefore, the aforementioned effects suggest a possible positive impact of sildenafil not only on the treatment of the first signs of the disease, such as endovascular damage and decreased blood flow in the digital vein (Raynaud's phenomenon), but, also, on the last stages when skin fibrosis occurs.

However, further studies are needed to deepen the molecular mechanisms by which sildenafil acts as an antigenotoxic drug and antioxidant, as well as to establish the feasibility and efficacy of this PDE5i in the clinical setting of patients at risk of developing SSc and in those where the pathology is already in progress.

Supplementary Materials: The following are available online at http://www.mdpi.com/2076-3921/9/9/786/s1: Figure S1: Analysis of the cell cycle progression of healthy control (H) and SSc fibroblasts exposed to a pro-oxidant agent. Figure S2: Analysis of the redox status in healthy control and SSc fibroblasts treated with hydrogen peroxide.

Author Contributions: Conceptualization, C.A. and I.D.; methodology, C.A., I.D., and G.D.; formal analysis, L.D.L.; investigation, C.A., I.D., and G.D; resources, C.A.; writing—original draft preparation, C.A., I.D., and G.D.; writing—review and editing, L.D.L., R.C., D.C., S.S., C.C., A.L., F.D.G., A.A., and P.S.; and funding acquisition, C.A. All authors have read and agreed to the published version of the manuscript.

Funding: This work was supported by the Italian Ministry of Education, University and Research (MIUR) in the Scientific Independence of Young Researchers (SIR) program (grant n° RBSI14D5NX).

Acknowledgments: The authors would like to thank Manuela Cervelli (Department of Sciences, Università degli Studi di Roma TRE) for technical assistance in ROS determinations. GD supports AILS (Associazione Italiana Lotta alla Sclerodermia Onlus).

Conflicts of Interest: The authors declare no conflict of interest.

References

1. Denton, C.P.; Black, C.M.; Abraham, D.J. Mechanisms and consequences of fibrosis in systemic sclerosis. *Nat. Clin. Pract. Rheumatol.* **2006**, *2*, 134–144. [CrossRef] [PubMed]
2. Black, C.M.; Stephen, C. Systemic sclerosis (scleroderma) and related disorders. In *Oxford Textbook of Rheumatology*; Maddison, P.J., Isenberg, D.A., Woo, P., Glass, D.N., Eds.; Oxford University Press: Oxford, UK, 1993; pp. 771–789.

3. Colletti, M.; Galardi, A.; De Santis, M.; Guidelli, G.M.; Di Giannatale, A.; Di Luigi, L.; Antinozzi, C. Exosomes in Systemic Sclerosis: Messengers Between Immune, Vascular and Fibrotic Components? *Int. J. Mol. Sci.* **2019**, *20*, 4337. [CrossRef] [PubMed]
4. Sena, C.M.; Leandro, A.; Azul, L.; Seiça, R.; Perry, G. Vascular Oxidative Stress: Impact and Therapeutic Approaches. *Front. Physiol.* **2018**, *9*, 1668. [CrossRef]
5. Cano Sanchez, M.; Lancel, S.; Boulanger, E.; Neviere, R. Targeting Oxidative Stress and Mitochondrial Dysfunction in the Treatment of Impaired Wound Healing: A Systematic Review. *Antioxidants* **2018**, *7*, 98. [CrossRef]
6. Bruckdorfer, K.R.; Hillary, J.B.; Bunce, T.; Vancheeswaran, R.; Black, C.M. Increased susceptibility to oxidation of low-density lipoproteins isolated from patients with systemic sclerosis. *Arthritis Rheumatol.* **1995**, *38*, 1060–1067. [CrossRef]
7. Herrick, A.L.; Cerinic, M.M. The emerging problem of oxidative stress and the role of antioxidants in systemic sclerosis. *Clin. Exp. Rheumatol.* **2001**, *19*, 4–8.
8. Parlanti, E.; Pietraforte, D.; Iorio, E.; Visentin, S.; de Nuccio, C.; Zijno, A.; D'Errico, M.; Simonelli, V.; Sanchez, M.; Fattibene, P.; et al. An altered redox balance and increased genetic instability characterize primary fibroblasts derived from xeroderma pigmentosum group A patients. *Mutat. Res.* **2015**, *782*, 34–43. [CrossRef]
9. Emerit, I.; Filipe, P.; Meunier, P.; Auclair, C.; Freitas, J.; Deroussent, A.; Gouyette, A.; Fernandes, A. Clastogenic activity in the plasma of scleroderma patients: A biomarker of oxidative stress. *Dermatology* **1997**, *194*, 140–146. [CrossRef]
10. Giovannetti, A.; Gambardella, L.; Pietraforte, D.; Rosato, E.; Giammarioli, A.M.; Salsano, F.; Malorni, W.; Straface, E. Red blood cell alterations in systemic sclerosis: A pilot study. *Cell Physiol. Biochem.* **2012**, *30*, 418–427. [CrossRef] [PubMed]
11. Svegliati, S.; Cancello, R.; Sambo, P.; Luchetti, M.; Paroncini, P.; Orlandini, G.; Discepoli, G.; Paterno, R.; Santillo, M.; Cuozzo, C.; et al. Platelet derived growth factor and reactive oxygen species (ROS) regulate Ras protein levels in primary human fibroblasts via ERK1/2. Amplification of ROS and Ras in systemic sclerosis fibroblasts. *J. Biol. Chem.* **2005**, *280*, 36474–36482. [CrossRef]
12. Dooley, A.; Shi-Wen, X.; Aden, N.; Tranah, T.; Desai, N.; Denton, C.P.; Abraham, D.J.; Bruckdorfer, R. Modulation of collagen type I, fibronectin and dermal fibroblast function and activity, in systemic sclerosis by the antioxidant epigallocatechin-3-gallate. *Rheumatology* **2010**, *49*, 2024–2036. [CrossRef] [PubMed]
13. Denton, C.P.; Bunce, T.D.; Darado, M.B.; Roberts, Z.; Wilson, H.; Howell, K.; Bruckdorfer, R.; Black, C.M. Probucol improves symptoms and reduces lipoprotein oxidation susceptibility in patients with Raynaud's phenomenon. *Rheumatology* **1999**, *38*, 309–315. [CrossRef] [PubMed]
14. Cracowski, J.L.; Girolet, S.; Imbert, B.; Seinturier, C.; Stanke-Labesque, F.; Bessard, J.; Boignard, A.; Bessard, G.; Carpentier, P.H. Effects of short-term treatment with vitamin E in systemic sclerosis: A double blind, randomized, controlled clinical trial of efficacy based on urinary isoprostane measurement. *Free Radic. Biol. Med.* **2005**, *38*, 98–103. [CrossRef] [PubMed]
15. Mavrikakis, M.E.; Lekakis, J.P.; Papamichael, C.M.; Stamatelopoulos, K.S.; Kostopoulos, C.; Stamatelopoulos, S.F. Ascorbic acid does not improve endothelium-dependent flow-mediated dilatation of the brachial artery in patients with Raynaud's phenomenon secondary to systemic sclerosis. *Int. J. Vitam. Nutr. Res.* **2003**, *73*, 3–7. [CrossRef] [PubMed]
16. Dooley, A.; Bruckdorfer, K.R.; Abraham, D.J. Modulation of fibrosis in systemic sclerosis by nitric oxide and antioxidants. *Cardiol. Res. Pract.* **2012**, *2012*, 521958. [CrossRef]
17. Rosato, E.; Borghese, F.; Pisarri, S.; Salsano, F. The treatment with Nacetylcysteine of Raynaud's phenomenon and ischemic ulcers therapy in sclerodermic patients: A prospective observational study of 50 patients. *Clin. Rheumatol.* **2009**, *28*, 1379–1384. [CrossRef]
18. Herrick, A.L.; Hollis, S.; Schofield, D.; Rieley, F.; Blann, A.; Griffin, K.; Moore, T.; Braganza, J.M.; Jayson, M.I. A double-blind placebo-controlled trial of antioxidant therapy in limited cutaneous systemic sclerosis. *Clin. Exp. Rheumatol.* **2000**, *18*, 349–356.
19. Bernardes, F.P.; Batista, A.T.; Porto, M.L.; Vasquez, E.C.; Campagnaro, B.P.; Meyrelles, S.S. Protective effect of sildenafil on the genotoxicity and cytotoxicity in apolipoprotein E-deficient mice bone marrow cells. *Lipids Health Dis.* **2016**, *15*, 100. [CrossRef]

20. Dias, A.T.; Rodrigues, B.P.; Porto, M.L.; Gava, A.L.; Balarini, C.M.; Freitas, P.S.F.; Palomino, A.; Casarini, E.D.; Campagnaro, P.B.; Pereira, M.C.T.; et al. Sildenafil ameliorates oxidative stress and DNA damage in the stenotic kidneys in mice with renovascular hypertension. *J. Transl. Med.* **2014**, *12*, 35. [CrossRef]
21. Rodrigues, B.P.; Campagnaro, B.P.; Balarini, C.M.; Pereira, T.M.; Meyrelles, S.S.; Vasquez, E.C. Sildenafil ameliorates biomarkers of genotoxicity in an experimental model of spontaneous atherosclerosis. *Lipids Health Dis.* **2013**, *12*, 128. [CrossRef]
22. Jeon, Y.H.; Heo, Y.S.; Kim, C.M.; Hyun, Y.L.; Lee, T.G.; Ro, S.; Cho, J.M. Phosphodiesterase: Overview of protein structures, potential therapeutic applications and recent progress in drug development. *Cell. Mol. Life Sci.* **2005**, *62*, 1198–1220. [CrossRef] [PubMed]
23. Di Luigi, L.; Sgrò, P.; Duranti, G.; Sabatini, S.; Caporossi, D.; Del Galdo, F.; Dimauro, I.; Antinozzi, C. Sildenafil Reduces Expression and Release of IL-6 and IL-8 Induced by Reactive Oxygen Species in Systemic Sclerosis Fibroblasts. *Int. J. Mol. Sci.* **2020**, *21*, 3161. [CrossRef] [PubMed]
24. Herrick, A.L.; van den Hoogen, F.; Gabrielli, A.; Tamimi, N.; Reid, C.; O'Connell, D.; Vázquez-Abad, M.D.; Denton, P.D. Modified-release sildenafil reduces Raynaud's phenomenon attack frequency in limited cutaneous systemic sclerosis. *Arthritis Rheum.* **2011**, *63*, 775–782. [CrossRef] [PubMed]
25. Fries, R.; Shariat, K.; von Wilmowsky, H.; Böhm, M. Sildenafil in the treatment of Raynaud's phenomenon resistant to vasodilatory therapy. *Circulation* **2005**, *112*, 2980–2985. [CrossRef]
26. Menezes, T.N.; Naumann, G.B.; Mendonça, A.B.; Leal, A.M.; Porto, L.M.; Teixeira-Ferreira, A.; Perales, J.; Meyrelles, S.S.; Figueiredo, G.S.; Vasquez, C.E. Antioxidant effect of sildenafil: Potential hepatoprotection via differential expression of mitochondrial proteins in apolipoprotein E knockout mice. *Pharmacol. Rep.* **2019**, *71*, 422–429. [CrossRef]
27. Ebrahimi, F.; Shafaroodi, H.; Asadi, S.; Nezami, B.G.; Ghasemi, M.; Rahimpour, S.; Hashemi, M.; Doostar, Y.; Dehpour, A.R. Sildenafil decreased cardiac cell apoptosis in diabetic mice: Reduction of oxidative stress as a possible mechanism. *Can. J. Physiol. Pharmacol.* **2009**, *87*, 556–564. [CrossRef]
28. Del Galdo, F.; Sotgia, F.; de Almeida, C.J.; Jasmin, J.F.; Musick, M.; Lisanti, M.P.; Jiménez, S.A. Decreased expression of caveolin 1 in patients with systemic sclerosis: Crucial role in the pathogenesis of tissue fibrosis. *Arthritis Rheumatol.* **2008**, *58*, 2854–2865. [CrossRef]
29. Giannattasio, S.; Corinaldesi, C.; Colletti, M.; Di Luigi, L.; Antinozzi, C.; Filardi, T.; Scolletta, S.; Basili, S.; Lenzi, A.; Morano, S.; et al. The phosphodiesterase 5 inhibitor sildenafil decreases the proinflammatory chemokine IL-8 in diabetic cardiomyopathy: In vivo and in vitro evidence. *J. Endocrinol. Invest.* **2019**, *42*, 715–725. [CrossRef]
30. Mercatelli, N.; Fittipaldi, S.; De Paola, E.; Dimauro, I.; Paronetto, M.P.; Jackson, M.J.; Caporossi, D. MiR-23-TrxR1 as a novel molecular axis in skeletal muscle differentiation. *Sci. Rep.* **2017**, *7*, 7219. [CrossRef]
31. Marampon, F.; Antinozzi, C.; Corinaldesi, C.; Vannelli, G.B.; Sarchielli, E.; Migliaccio, S.; Di Luigi, L.; Lenzi, A.; Crescioli, C. The phosphodiesterase 5 inhibitor tadalafil regulates lipidic homeostasis in human skeletal muscle cell metabolism. *Endocrine* **2018**, *59*, 602–613. [CrossRef]
32. Fittipaldi, S.; Mercatelli, N.; Dimauro, I.; Jackson, M.J.; Paronetto, M.P.; Caporossi, D. Alpha B-crystallin induction in skeletal muscle cells under redox imbalance is mediated by a JNK-dependent regulatory mechanism. *Free Radic. Biol. Med.* **2015**, *86*, 331–342. [CrossRef] [PubMed]
33. Shen, Y.; Vignali, P.; Wang, R. Rapid Profiling Cell Cycle by Flow Cytometry Using Concurrent Staining of DNA and Mitotic Markers. *Bio. Protoc.* **2017**, *7*, e2517. [CrossRef] [PubMed]
34. Duranti, G.; Ceci, R.; Sgrò, P.; Sabatini, S.; Di Luigi, L. Influence of the PDE5 inhibitor tadalafil on redox status and antioxidant defense system in C2C12 skeletal muscle cells. *Cell Stress Chaperones* **2017**, *22*, 389–396. [CrossRef] [PubMed]
35. Duranti, G.; Ceci, R.; Patrizio, F.; Sgrò, P.; Di Luigi, L.; Sabatini, S.; Felici, F.; Bazzucchi, I. Chronic consumption of quercetin reduces erythrocytes oxidative damage: Evaluation at resting and after eccentric exercise in humans. *Nutr. Res.* **2018**, *50*, 73–81. [CrossRef]
36. Crescioli, C.; Corinaldesi, C.; Riccieri, V.; Raparelli, V.; Vasile, M.; Del Galdo, F.; Valesini, G.; Lenzi, A.; Basili, S.; Antinozzi, C. Association of circulating CXCL10 and CXCL11 with systemic sclerosis. *Ann. Rheum. Dis.* **2018**, *77*, 1845–1846. [CrossRef]
37. Illert, A.L.; Kawaguchi, H.; Antinozzi, C.; Bassermann, F.; Quintanilla-Martinez, L.; von Klitzing, C.; Hiwatari, M.; Peschel, C.; de Rooij, D.G.; Morris, S.W.; et al. Targeted inactivation of nuclear interaction partner of ALK disrupts meiotic prophase. *Development* **2012**, *139*, 2523–2534. [CrossRef]

38. Kim, J.Y.; Kwok, S.K.; Hur, K.H.; Kim, H.J.; Kim, N.S.; Yoo, S.A.; Kim, W.U.; Cho, C.S. Up-regulated macrophage migration inhibitory factor protects apoptosis of dermal fibroblasts in patients with systemic sclerosis. *Clin. Exp. Immunol.* **2008**, *152*, 328–335. [CrossRef]
39. Tonini, C.L.; Campagnaro, B.P.; Louro, L.P.; Pereira, T.M.; Vasquez, E.C.; Meyrelles, S.S. Effects of aging and hypercholesterolemia on oxidative stress and DNA damage in bone Marrow mononuclear cells in apolipoprotein E-deficient mice. *Int. J. Mol. Sci.* **2013**, *14*, 3325–3342. [CrossRef]
40. Gillespie, J.; Ross, R.L.; Corinaldesi, C.; Esteves, F.; Derrett-Smith, E.; McDermott, M.F.; Doody, G.M.; Denton, C.P.; Emery, P.; Del Galdo, F. Transforming Growth Factor β Activation Primes Canonical Wnt Signaling Through Down-Regulation of Axin-2. *Arthritis Rheumatol.* **2018**, *70*, 932–942. [CrossRef]
41. Kapanadze, B.; Morris, E.; Smith, E.; Trojanowska, M. Establishment and characterization of scleroderma fibroblast clonal cell lines by introduction of the hTERT gene. *J. Cell. Mol. Med.* **2010**, *14*, 1156–1165. [CrossRef]
42. Kuo, L.J.; Yang, L.X. Gamma-H2AX—A novel biomarker for DNA double-strand breaks. *Vivo* **2008**, *22*, 305–309.
43. Symington, L.S. Mechanism and regulation of DNA end resection in eukaryotes. *Crit. Rev. Biochem. Mol. Biol.* **2016**, *51*, 195–212. [CrossRef] [PubMed]
44. Testa, E.; Nardozi, D.; Antinozzi, C.; Faieta, M.; Di Cecca, S.; Caggiano, C.; Fukuda, T.; Bonanno, E.; Zhenkun, L.; Maldonado, A.; et al. H2AFX and MDC1 promote maintenance of genomic integrity in male germ cells. *J. Cell Sci.* **2018**, *131*, jcs214411. [CrossRef] [PubMed]
45. Zannini, L.; Delia, D.; Buscemi, G. CHK2 kinase in the DNA damage response and beyond. *J. Mol. Cell Biol.* **2014**, *6*, 442–457. [CrossRef]
46. Bahassi, E.M.; Ovesen, J.L.; Riesenberg, A.L.; Bernstein, W.Z.; Hasty, P.E.; Stambrook, P.J. The Checkpoint Kinases Chk1 and Chk2 Regulate the Functional Associations Between hBRCA2 and Rad51 in Response to DNA Damage. *Oncogene* **2008**, *27*, 3977–3985. [CrossRef]
47. Yu, Q.; Rose, J.H.; Zhang, H.; Pommier, Y. Antisense inhibition of Chk2/hCds1 expression attenuates DNA damage-induced S and G2 checkpoints and enhances apoptotic activity in HEK-293 cells. *FEBS Lett.* **2001**, *505*, 7–12. [CrossRef]
48. Ghosh, J.C.; Dohi, T.; Raskett, C.M.; Kowalik, T.F.; Altieri, D.C. Activated checkpoint kinase 2 provides a survival signal for tumor cells. *Cancer Res.* **2006**, *66*, 11576–11579. [CrossRef]
49. Wang, H.C.; Chou, W.C.; Shieh, S.Y.; Shen, C.Y. Ataxia telangiectasia mutated and checkpoint kinase 2 regulate BRCA1 to promote the fidelity of DNA end-joining. *Cancer Res.* **2006**, *66*, 1391–1400. [CrossRef]
50. Leal, M.A.; Balarini, C.M.; Dias, A.T.; Porto, M.L.; Gava, A.L.; Pereira, T.M.; Meyrelles, S.S.; Vasquez, E.C. Mechanisms of enhanced vasoconstriction in the mouse model of atherosclerosis: The beneficial effects of sildenafil. *Curr. Pharm. Biotechnol.* **2015**, *16*, 517–530. [CrossRef]
51. Fahning, B.M.; Dias, A.T.; Oliveira, J.P.; Gava, A.L.; Porto, M.L.; Gomes, I.B.; Nogueira, B.V.; Campagnaro, B.P.; Pereira, T.M.; Vasquez, E.C.; et al. Sildenafil improves vascular endothelial structure and function in renovascular hypertension. *Curr. Pharm. Biotechnol.* **2015**, *16*, 823–831. [CrossRef]
52. Dias, A.T.; Cintra, A.S.; Frossard, J.C.; Palomino, Z.; Casarini, D.E.; Gomes, I.B.; Balarini, C.M.; Gava, A.L.; Campagnaro, B.P.; Pereira, T.M.; et al. Inhibition of phosphodiesterase 5 restores endothelial function in renovascular hypertension. *J. Transl. Med.* **2014**, *12*, 250. [CrossRef] [PubMed]
53. Chang, J.F.; Hsu, J.L.; Sheng, Y.H.; Leu, W.J.; Yu, C.C.; Chan, S.H.; Chan, M.L.; Hsu, L.C.; Liu, S.P.; Guh, J.H. Phosphodiesterase Type 5 (PDE5) Inhibitors Sensitize Topoisomerase II Inhibitors in Killing Prostate Cancer Through PDE5-Independent Impairment of HR and NHEJ DNA Repair Systems. *Front. Oncol.* **2019**, *8*, 681. [CrossRef] [PubMed]
54. Semen, K.; Yelisyeyeva, O.; Jarocka-Karpowicz, I.; Kaminskyy, D.; Solovey, L.; Skrzydlewska, E.; Yavorskyi, O. Sildenafil reduces signs of oxidative stress in pulmonary arterial hypertension: Evaluation by fatty acid composition, level of hydroxynonenal and heart rate variability. *Redox Biol.* **2016**, *7*, 48–57. [CrossRef] [PubMed]
55. Balarini, C.M.; Leal, M.A.; Gomes, I.B.S.; Pereira, T.M.; Gava, A.L.; Meyrelles, S.S.; Vasquez, E.C. Sildenafil restores endothelial function in the apolipoprotein E knockout mouse. *J. Transl. Med.* **2013**, *11*, 3. [CrossRef]
56. Abdollahi, M.; Fooladian, F.; Emami, B.; Zafari, K.; Bahreini-Moghadam, A. Protection by sildenafil and theophylline of lead acetateinduced oxidative stress in rat submandibular gland and saliva. *Hum. Exp. Toxicol.* **2003**, *22*, 587–592. [CrossRef]

57. Yukitake, H.; Takizawa, M.; Kimura, H. Macrophage Migration Inhibitory Factor as an Emerging Drug Target to Regulate Antioxidant Response Element System. *Oxid. Med. Cell. Longev.* **2017**, *2017*, 8584930. [CrossRef]
58. Knight, J.A.; Pieper, R.K.; McClellan, L. Specificity of the thiobarbituric acid reaction: Its use in studies of lipid peroxidation. *Clin. Chem.* **1988**, *34*, 2433–2438. [CrossRef]
59. Glossmann, H.; Petrischor, G.; Bartsch, G. Molecular Mechanisms of the Effects of Sildenafil (VIAGRA). *Exp. Gerontol.* **1999**, *34*, 305–318. [CrossRef]
60. Leonarduzzi, G.; Arkan, M.C.; Basaga, H.; Chiarpotto, E.; Sevanian, A.; Poli, G. Lipid oxidation products in cell signaling. *Free Radic. Biol. Med.* **2000**, *28*, 1370–1378. [CrossRef]
61. Olivares-González, L.; Martínez-Fernández de la Cámara, C.; Hervás, D.; Marín, M.P.; Lahoz, A.; Millán, J.M.; Rodrigo, R. cGMP-Phosphodiesterase Inhibition Prevents Hypoxia-Induced Cell Death Activation in Porcine Retinal Explants. *PLoS ONE* **2016**, *11*, e0166717. [CrossRef]
62. Hemnes, A.R.; Zaiman, A.; Champion, H.C. PDE5A inhibition attenuates bleomycin-induced pulmonary fibrosis and pulmonary hypertension through inhibition of ROS generation and RhoA/Rho kinase activation. *Am. J. Physiol. Lung Cell. Mol. Physiol.* **2008**, *294*, L24–L33. [CrossRef] [PubMed]
63. Liu, X.M.; Peyton, K.J.; Wang, X.; Durante, W. Sildenafil stimulates the expression of gaseous monoxide-generating enzymes in vascular smooth muscle cells via distinct signaling pathways. *Biochem. Pharmacol.* **2012**, *84*, 1045–1054. [CrossRef] [PubMed]
64. Park, H.S.; Park, J.W.; Kim, H.J.; Choi, C.W.; Lee, H.J.; Kim, B.I.; Chun, Y.S. Sildenafil alleviates bronchopulmonary dysplasia in neonatal rats by activating the hypoxia-inducible factor signaling pathway. *Am. J. Respir. Cell Mol. Biol.* **2013**, *48*, 105–113. [CrossRef]
65. Gabrielli, A.; Svegliati, S.; Moroncini, G.; Amico, D. New insights into the role of oxidative stress in scleroderma fibrosis. *Open Rheumatol. J.* **2012**, *6*, 87–95. [CrossRef]
66. Grygiel-Gorniak, B.; Puszczewicz, M. Oxidative damage and antioxidative therapy in systemic sclerosis. *Mediat. Inflamm.* **2014**, *2014*, 389582. [CrossRef]
67. Gabrielli, A.; Svegliati, S.; Moroncini, G.; Pomponio, G.; Santillo, M.; Avvedimento, V.E. Oxidative stress and the pathogenesis of scleroderma: The Murrell's hypothesis revisited. *Semin. Immunopathol.* **2008**, *30*, 329–337. [CrossRef] [PubMed]

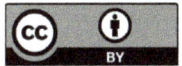

© 2020 by the authors. Licensee MDPI, Basel, Switzerland. This article is an open access article distributed under the terms and conditions of the Creative Commons Attribution (CC BY) license (http://creativecommons.org/licenses/by/4.0/).

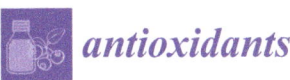

Article

Comparison of Anti-Oxidative Effect of Human Adipose- and Amniotic Membrane-Derived Mesenchymal Stem Cell Conditioned Medium on Mouse Preimplantation Embryo Development

Kihae Ra [1], Hyun Ju Oh [1,2], Eun Young Kim [3], Sung Keun Kang [3], Jeong Chan Ra [3], Eui Hyun Kim [1], Se Chang Park [4,*] and Byeong Chun Lee [1,*]

1. Department of Theriogenology and Biotechnology, College of Veterinary Medicine, Seoul National University, Seoul 08826, Korea; ragh1102@snu.ac.kr (K.R.); ohj@mkbiotech.co.kr (H.J.O.); hyun9214@snu.ac.kr (E.H.K.)
2. Research and Development Center, MKbiotech Co., Ltd., 99 Daehak-ro, Daejeon 34134, Korea
3. Biostar Stem Cell Research Institute, R Bio Co., Ltd., Seoul 08506, Korea; naraokke@stemcellbio.com (E.Y.K.); kangsk@stemcellbio.com (S.K.K.); jcra@stemcellbio.com (J.C.R.)
4. Laboratory of Aquatic Biomedicine, College of Veterinary Medicine, Seoul National University, Seoul 08826, Korea
* Correspondence: parksec@snu.ac.kr (S.C.P.); bclee@snu.ac.kr (B.C.L.)

Abstract: Oxidative stress is a major cause of damage to the quantity and quality of embryos produced in vitro. Antioxidants are usually supplemented to protect embryos from the suboptimal in vitro culture (IVC) environment. Amniotic membrane-derived mesenchymal stem cells (AMSC) have emerged as a promising regenerative therapy, and their paracrine factors with anti-oxidative effects are present in AMSC conditioned medium (CM). We examined the anti-oxidative potential of human AMSC-CM treatment during IVC on mouse preimplantation embryo development and antioxidant gene expression in the forkhead box O (FoxO) pathway. AMSC-CM (10%) was optimal for overall preimplantation embryo developmental processes and upregulated the expression of FoxOs and their downstream antioxidants in blastocysts (BL). Subsequently, compared to adipose-derived mesenchymal stem cell (ASC)-CM, AMSC-CM enhanced antioxidant gene expression and intracellular GSH levels in the BL. Total antioxidant capacity and SOD activity were greater in AMSC-CM than in ASC-CM. Furthermore, SOD and catalase were more active in culture medium supplemented with AMSC-CM than in ASC-CM. Lastly, the anti-apoptotic effect of AMSC-CM was observed with the regulation of apoptosis-related genes and mitochondrial membrane potential in BL. In conclusion, the present study established AMSC-CM treatment at an optimal concentration as a novel antioxidant intervention for assisted reproduction.

Keywords: adipose-derived mesenchymal stem cell; amniotic membrane-derived mesenchymal stem cell; antioxidants; assisted reproductive technology; conditioned medium; embryo; in vitro culture; in vitro fertilization; oxidative stress

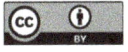

1. Introduction

The success rate of assisted reproductive technologies (ART) to surmount infertility has increased with the improvement of conditions for embryo in vitro production [1]. The balance of reactive oxygen species (ROS) and antioxidants is maintained at physiologically normal levels in female reproductive systems, but is disrupted in vitro, resulting in an increase in exposure to oxidative damage risk [2]. In the process of assisted reproduction, a number of external factors causing oxidative stress appear from technical procedures to environmental sources [3]. Subsequently, oxidative stress due to accumulated ROS in in vitro-produced embryos impairs the efficiency of embryonic development and induces reproductive failure due to an increase in embryo fragmentation and apoptosis, and a decrease in fertilization rate and blastocyst (BL) development [4–6]. Accordingly, the application of antioxidants to ART can be an effective intervention to counteract the oxidative damage in in vitro-produced embryos [7], especially to improve the in vitro culture (IVC) medium for favorable outcomes in preimplantation embryo development. Accumulating studies have indicated that the addition of antioxidants to IVC medium improves preimplantation embryo development by regulating the embryonic environment and protecting embryos from oxidative damage [8–11], which leads to the decrease in developmental competence of embryos produced in vitro compared to that of embryos developed in vivo [12].

Mesenchymal stem cells (MSCs) are known to ameliorate oxidative stress through the upregulation of enzymatic antioxidants [13]. MSCs isolated from multiple tissue sources have common but various features, which emphasize their importance as regenerative medicine [14]. Among multiple sources, adipose-derived MSCs (ASCs) are the most widely studied, forming the basis of research on MSC-based therapy [15] and is representatively known a strong antioxidant [6,13,16–18]. Contemporarily, amniotic membrane-derived MSCs (AMSC) have emerged as a novel candidate in the field of regenerative medicine because of their unique advantages, including noninvasive isolation, stable immunogenicity, abundant availability, multipotency for all three germ layers, and no associated ethical issues [19]. The amniotic membrane is a constituent of the placenta with its essential function of nutrient supplementation and physical protection for the fetus during pregnancy, but is generally discarded post-partum and infrequently utilized compared to other MSCs [20]. However, AMSCs retain the anti-microbial, anti-tumorigenic, immunomodulatory, and anti-inflammatory characteristics of amniotic membrane [21]. Recent studies on potential therapeutic features of human AMSCs have focused on their role in immunomodulation, suppressing inflammation, and inhibiting oxidative damage [22–25]. Although diverse studies support the anti-oxidative effect of AMSCs in diseases models, the therapeutic applications of AMSCs were restricted to cell transplantation [22,26,27]. The regenerative effect of stem cell therapy is mainly facilitated by its paracrine factors, such as cytokines and growth factors, rather than by direct regenerative mechanisms [28,29]. These stem cell-derived paracrine factors are secreted during cell culture and are present in the stem cell-conditioned medium (CM) [30]. The therapeutic efficacy of the CM is comparable to that of the conventional cell-based therapy. Furthermore, the use of CM offers several advantages over conventional stem cell-therapy, such as improved reproducibility, no requirement to match the donors and recipients, and no risk of immune rejection [31].

In the present study, we aimed to investigate the anti-oxidative potential of AMSC-CM and establish the optimal concentration for AMSC-CM treatment during embryo IVC. Consequently, the anti-oxidative and anti-apoptotic effects of AMSC-CM were evaluated as compared to ASC-CM in the development of mouse preimplantation embryos.

2. Materials and Methods

2.1. Chemicals and Reagents

All materials were purchased from Sigma-Aldrich (St. Louis, MO, USA), unless otherwise specified.

2.2. Culture and Characterization of ASCs and AMSCs

Both ASCs and AMSCs were obtained from R Bio Stem Cell Research Center under GMP conditions. All subjects gave their informed consent for inclusion before they participated in the study. The protocol was approved by the Ethics Committee of Biostar Stem Cell Technology (IRB NO. 2019-03). ASCs were cultured and characterized as previously described [6]. For the establishment of AMSCs, cryopreserved AMSCs (1×10^6) from the amnion tissue of three female donors were cultured in T-175 flasks containing RPME-P (R BIO, Seoul, Korea) supplemented with 1% antibiotic-antimycotic solution at 37 °C with 5% CO_2. The AMSCs were cultured in AMSC medium (R BIO) until 80–90% confluency and non-adherent cells were discarded through medium change. The immunophenotypic markers of cultured AMSCs was characterized by flow cytometry. AMSCs (1×10^6) were suspended in phosphate-buffered saline (PBS) and labeled with fluorescein isothiocyanate and phycoerythrin isotype controls. The labeled cells were incubated for 30–60 min with the following antibodies against human antigens: MSC positive markers (CD73, CD90, CD105, CD29, and CD44) and negative markers (CD31, CD34, and CD45) (BD Biosciences, San Jose, CA, USA). After the cells were washed with PBS, the analysis was conducted with FACSCalibur™ flow cytometer (BD Biosciences) and CellQuest Pro software (BD Biosciences).

2.3. Preparation of ASC-CM and AMSC-CM

ASC-CM were collected using the same method as previously described [6]. AMSCs per donor (passage 6) were cultured in RPME-P until 90% confluency, and then the medium was replaced to Dulbecco's modified Eagle's medium (DMEM) after washing twice with PBS. The culture medium was collected every 24 h and then DMEM was added to the original flask. Supernatants were collected for 5 days and then pooled. To obtain CM, the pooled supernatant was centrifuged (1700 rpm, 5 min) and then filtered in a 0.22-μm filter. Lastly, filtered CM of donors was equally mixed and concentrated 10× by centrifugation at $3000 \times g$ for 90 min using a filter tube (Vivaspin 20, GE healthcare, Chicago, IL, USA).

2.4. Experimental Animals

All experiments using experimental animals in this study were approved by the Institutional Animal Care and Use Committee of Seoul National University (SNU-170511-2-4). Seven-week-old female and 10-week-old male ICR mice were purchased from Orient Bio (Gapyeong, Korea). Mice were kept in an animal facility under conventional environment with the light/dark cycle, humidity and temperature regulated.

2.5. In Vitro Fertilization and Culture

After cervical dislocation of mature male mice, caudal epididymides were removed and the duct of the caudal epididymis was incised. The sperm stored inside were dispersed into a droplet of CARD medium (Cosmo Bio Co., Tokyo, Japan). Sperm were incubated for an hour at 36 °C to enable capacitation. The induction of superovulation of mature female mice was conducted by an intraperitoneal injection of 10 IU pregnant mare serum gonadotropin and human chorionic gonadotropin (hCG) after 47 h. The cumulus-oocyte complexes (COCs) were recovered from the oviductal ampulla of the mice 16 h after hCG injection and transferred to a droplet of CARD medium. The sperm suspension was treated with COCs for insemination and incubated for 3 h at 36 °C. In vitro fertilized embryos were washed and cultured in fresh human tubal fluid (Cosmo Bio Co., Tokyo, Japan) at 36 °C for 24 h. Embryos that cleaved to the 2- or 4-cell were randomly divided and then cultured in the groups as described in experimental design for 96 h. The embryo development was evaluated by assessing the number of 4-cell, 16-cell, BL, and hatched BL using a stereomicroscope. The temperature was set based on the literature and our preliminary study. The literature demonstrated that slightly lower temperature could be physiologically relevant to reproductive tissues [32–34] and comparable to traditional 37 °C for reproductive outcomes [35–37]. In our preliminary study, developmental rate to BL at 36 °C showed no difference to that at 37 °C, and both rates were observed within the normal range.

2.6. Experimental Design

First, fertilized embryos were cultured in continuous single culture-NX (CSCM-NX; FUJIFILM Irvine Scientific, Santa Ana, CA, USA) containing 10%, 20%, and 50% (v/v) AMSC-CM. After determining the optimal concentration of AMSC-CM for IVC supplementation, embryos were cultured followed by in vitro fertilization in CSCM-NX containing ASC-CM or AMSC-CM. The optimal concentration of ASC-CM was set 5% (v/v) as previously reported [6]. The control group was cultured in CSCM-NX medium without CM supplementation.

2.7. Quantitative Reverse Transcription-Polymerase Chain Reaction (qRT-PCR)

RNA was extracted from BLs using an RNAqueous™-Micro Total RNA Isolation Kit (Ambion, Austin, TX, USA), according to the manufacturer's instructions. The concentration of extracted total RNA was quantified by a NanoDrop 2000 Spectrophotometer (Thermo Fisher Scientific, Wilmington, DE, USA) and presented in Table S1. Using the RNA, complementary DNA (cDNA) was synthesized by a Maxime RT premix kit (iNtRON, Gyeonggi, Korea). qRT-PCR was carried out using a StepOnePlus Real-Time PCR System (Applied Biosystems, Foster City, CA, USA) and the protocol in detail was previously described [18]. The expression of target genes was measured and normalized relative to the control house-keeping gene, 18S rRNA [38–40]. The gene expression values were calculated as previously described [18]. The list of primers is presented in Table 1.

Table 1. List of primer and sequence used for quantitative reverse transcription-polymerase chain reaction.

Gene	Accession No.	Primer Sequence
18S rRNA	NR_003278.3	F: ACCGCGGTTCTATTTTGTTG R: CCCTCTTAATCATGGCCTCA
AMPK	NM_001013367.3	F: GCTGTGGCTCACCCAATTAT R: ATCAAAAGGGAGGGTTCCAC
JNK	NM_016700.4	F: CGGAACACCTTGTCCTGAAT R: GAGTCAGCTGGGAAAAGCAC
AKT	NM_001165894.1	F: ACTCATTCCAGACCCACGAC R: GTCCAGGGCAGACACAATCT
SIRT1	NM_001159589.2	F: AGTTCCAGCCGTCTCTGTGT R: GATCCTTTGGATTCCTGCAA
FoxO1	NM_019739.3	F: ACATTTCGTCCTCGAACCAG R: CAGGTCATCCTGCTCTGTCA
FoxO3	NM_019740.3	F: ATGGGAGCTTGGAATGTGAC R: TTAAAATCCAACCCGTCAGC
SOD2	NM_013671.3	F: CTGTCTTCAGCCACACCAGA R: CTGCTCTTCCAAAGGTCCTG
Catalase	NM_009804.2	F: TTGACAGAGAGCGGATTCCT R: TCTGGTGATATCGTGGGTGA
GPx1	NM_008160.6	F: CCGACCCCAAGTACATCATT R: CCCACCAGGAACTTCTCAAA
Bax	NM_007527.3	F: ACCAAGAAGCTGAGCGAGTG R: TGCAGCTCCATATTGCTGTC
Bcl2	NM_009741.5	F: ATGATAACCGGGAGATCGTG R: AGCCCCTCTGTGACAGCTTA
Caspase3	NM_001284409.1	F: TGTCATCTCGCTCTGGTACG R: ATTTCAGGCCCATGAATGTC

F, Forward primer; R, Reverse primer.

2.8. Intracellular ROS and Glutathione (GSH) Detection

The levels of intracellular ROS and GSH were measured in BLs from the control, ASC-CM, and AMSC-CM groups by staining respectively with H_2DCFDA (2,7′-dichlorodihydrofluorescein diacetate) and CellTracker Blue (4-chloromethyl-6,8-difluoro-7-hydroxycoumarin; CMF_2HC). BLs from each group were incubated in 1% polyvinyl alcohol (PVA)-PBS containing 10 μM H_2DCFDA or CellTracker Blue in the dark at 25 °C. After 30 min, BLs were washed and moved to a droplet of PVA-PBS covered with mineral oil. The quantitative intensity of fluorescence was evaluated under an epifluorescence microscope (TE2000-S; Nikon, Tokyo, Japan) using filters (ROS: 460 nm, GSH: 370 nm) and analyzed by Image J software version 1.52 (National Institutes of Health, Bethesda, MO, USA).

2.9. Antioxidant Capacity and Enzyme Activity Assays

The total antioxidant capacity (TAC), superoxide dismutase (SOD), and catalase activity were measured using OxiSelect™ assay kits (Cell Biolabs Inc., San Diego, CA, USA) according to the manufacturer's protocol. Non-conditioned medium as control, ASC-CM and AMSC-CM were assessed for TAC, SOD, and CAT activity levels. Culture medium of the control, ASC-CM, and AMSC-CM groups before and after IVC were assessed for SOD and CAT activity levels. The results of each colorimetric assay were assessed using measured absorbances at 490 nm for TAC and SOD activity, and 520 nm for CAT activity.

2.10. Mitochondrial Membrane Potential Assay

BLs from the control, ASC-CM, and AMSC-CM groups were washed in 1% PVA-PBS and fixed in 4% paraformaldehyde-PBS for 1 h. After washing in 1% PVA-PBS, BLs were incubated in 1% PVA-PBS containing 2 µL JC-1 solution (Abcam, Cambridge, UK) and then washed in fresh 1% PVA-PBS. After 30 min, BLs were placed on a droplet of glycerol on a microscope glass slide with a coverslip. The fluorescence intensity of JC-1 aggregate at 590 nm and JC-1 monomer at 530 nm was evaluated using epifluorescence microscope and analyzed using Image J software version 1.52.

2.11. Statistical Analysis

A Kolmogorov–Smirnov test was conducted as normality test. Unpaired t-test was used to compare two groups. One-way ANOVA followed by Newman–Keuls or Tukey's post-hoc test and two-way ANOVA test with Bonferroni post-test were used to compare more than two groups. GraphPad Prism version 5 (GraphPad Software, San Diego, CA, USA) was used for statistical analyses. Data are presented as mean ± standard error of the mean (SEM), and a p-value < 0.05 was considered statistically significant among the groups. All experiments were performed with at least three replicates.

3. Results

3.1. Characterization of AMSC and ASC

AMSCs were analyzed with flow cytometry to identify the expression of phenotypic markers (Figure 1) and confirmed that AMSCs from all donors were positive for mesenchymal markers (CD73, CD90, CD105, CD29, and CD44), and negative for the endothelial marker (CD31) and hematopoietic markers (CD34 and CD45). The result of ASC characterization was previously described [6].

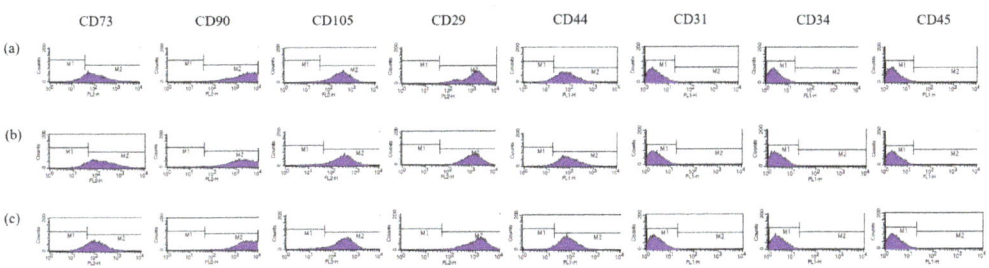

Figure 1. Characterization of human amniotic membrane-derived mesenchymal stem cell (AMSC). AMSCs isolated from three donors (**a**–**c**) were positive for CD73, CD90, CD105, CD29, CD44, and negative for CD31, CD34, and CD45.

3.2. Effects of Various Concentrations of AMSC-CM on Embryo Development

Embryo development to 4-, 16-cell stages, BL, and hatched BL was evaluated to determine the optimal concentration of AMSC-CM supplementation among the three different concentrations of AMSC-CM (10%, 20%, and 50%). As shown in Table 2, embryo development rate to the 4-cell stage was significantly lower in the 50% AMSC-CM group (79.6 ± 4.0) than in the control (91.8 ± 1.8, $p < 0.05$), 10% (92.5 ± 4.8, $p < 0.05$), and 20% AMSC-CM (93.4 ± 3.0, $p < 0.05$) groups. Moreover, the embryo development rate to the 16-cell stage was significantly higher in the 10% AMSC-CM group (74.3 ± 4.8) than in the 20% (61.2 ± 3.5, $p < 0.05$) and 50% AMSC-CM (59.5 ± 3.8, $p < 0.05$) groups. The rate of BL formation in the 10% AMSC-CM group (51.7 ± 4.1) was significantly higher than that in the control (38.6 ± 4.5, $p < 0.05$), 20% (30.7 ± 5.5, $p < 0.05$), and 50% AMSC-CM (28.3 ± 6.8, $p < 0.05$) groups. BL hatching rate in the 10% AMSC-CM group (32.6 ± 5.9) was also significantly higher than that in the control (19.4 ± 4.6, $p < 0.05$), 20% (19.1 ± 3.5, $p < 0.05$), and 50% AMSC-CM (18.8 ± 3.4, $p < 0.05$) groups.

Table 2. Effect of human amniotic membrane-derived mesenchymal stem cell conditioned medium (AMSC-CM) on in vitro fertilized mouse embryos development.

Group	No. of Cultured Embryos	No. of Embryos Developed to (%)			
		4-Cell	16-Cell	Blastocyst	Hatched Blastocyst
Control	72	66 (91.8 ± 1.8) [b]	51 (71.1 ± 2.6) [ab]	28 (38.6 ± 4.5) [a]	14 (19.4 ± 4.6) [a]
10% AMSC-CM	74	69 (92.5 ± 4.8) [b]	55 (74.3 ± 4.8) [b]	39 (51.7 ± 4.1) [b]	25 (32.6 ± 5.9) [b]
20% AMSC-CM	74	69 (93.4 ± 3.0) [b]	45 (61.2 ± 3.5) [a]	23 (30.7 ± 5.5) [a]	15 (19.1 ± 3.5) [a]
50% AMSC-CM	76	61 (79.6 ± 4.0) [a]	46 (59.5 ± 3.8) [a]	24 (28.3 ± 6.8) [a]	16 (18.8 ± 3.4) [a]

Experiments were repeated at least 3 times. [a,b] Mean ± SEM with different superscript letters indicate significant differences (at least $p < 0.05$).

3.3. Comparison of the Effects of ASC-CM and AMSC-CM on Embryo Development

Following the former experiment, which confirmed 10% as the optimal concentration of AMSC-CM treatment, the effects of ASC-CM and AMSC-CM during IVC on embryo development to the 4-, 16-cell stages, BL, and hatched BL were compared. As presented in Table 3, the developmental rate of embryos to the 4-cell stage was similar among groups, but the rate to the 16-cell stage was significantly increased in the AMSC-CM group (87.6 ± 5.1) compared to the control group (73.7 ± 3.3, $p < 0.05$). In addition, BL formation rate of AMSC-CM group (65.7 ± 3.3) was significantly higher than that of the control group (44.4 ± 5.2, $p < 0.05$). The developmental rates of 16-cell and BL in the ASC-CM groups (79.2 ± 4.0 and 56.4 ± 2.8, respectively) showed no difference from those of the other groups. The rate of hatched BL in the AMSC-CM group was greater than that in the other groups, although the difference was not statistically significant.

Table 3. Effect of human adipose-derived mesenchymal stem cell conditioned medium (ASC-CM) and amniotic membrane-derived mesenchymal stem cell conditioned medium (AMSC-CM) on in vitro fertilized mouse embryos development.

Group	No. of Cultured Embryos	Number of Embryos Developed to (%)			
		4-Cell	16-Cell	Blastocyst	Hatched Blastocyst
Control	135	127 (93.1 ± 2.0)	101 (73.7 ± 3.3) [a]	62 (44.4 ± 5.2) [a]	40 (27.4 ± 8.0)
ASC-CM	134	124 (91.9 ± 1.7)	108 (79.2 ± 4.0) [ab]	76 (56.4 ± 2.8) [ab]	44 (32.2 ± 4.0)
AMSC-CM	130	125 (95.7 ± 1.4)	117 (87.6 ± 5.1) [b]	85 (65.7 ± 3.3) [b]	53 (39.7 ± 2.8)

Experiments were repeated at least 3 times. [a,b] Mean ± SEM with different superscript letters indicate significant differences (at least $p < 0.05$).

3.4. Comparative Effects of ASC-CM and AMSC-CM on Antioxidant Gene Expression in BL

BLs developed in the control, ASC-CM, and AMSC-CM groups were analyzed for the expression of the antioxidant genes in the forkhead box O (FoxO) pathway and apoptosis-related genes, as presented in Figure 2. First, the expression of upstream regulators of FoxO was evaluated; the expression of AMP-activated protein kinase (AMPK), c-Jun N-terminal kinase (JNK), and protein kinase B (AKT) exhibited no significant differences among groups. Next, the level of sirtuin (SIRT) 1, a mediator of FoxO, was shown to be significantly higher in the AMSC-CM group (2.7 ± 0.4) than in the control (1.0 ± 0.0, $p < 0.05$) and ASC-CM group (1.4 ± 0.3, $p < 0.05$). FoxO1 and FoxO3 levels were significantly increased in the AMSC-CM group (3.0 ± 0.4 and 2.4 ± 0.4, respectively) compared to the control group (1.0 ± 0.0, $p < 0.05$). Furthermore, FoxO1 expression in the AMSC-CM group (3.0 ± 0.4) was significantly higher than that in the ASC-CM group (1.4 ± 0.2, $p < 0.05$) but FoxO3 levels were similar between two groups. The level of SOD2 was significantly greater in the ASC-CM and AMSC-CM groups (2.6 ± 0.1 and 2.7 ± 0.1, respectively) than in the control group (1.0 ± 0.0, $p < 0.05$). Catalase and glutathione peroxidase (GPx) 1 levels were significantly increased in the AMSC-CM group (3.4 ± 0.6 and 2.6 ± 0.2, respectively) compared to the control (1.0 ± 0.0, $p < 0.05$) and ASC-CM groups (1.1 ± 0.2 and 1.2 ± 0.2, respectively, $p < 0.05$).

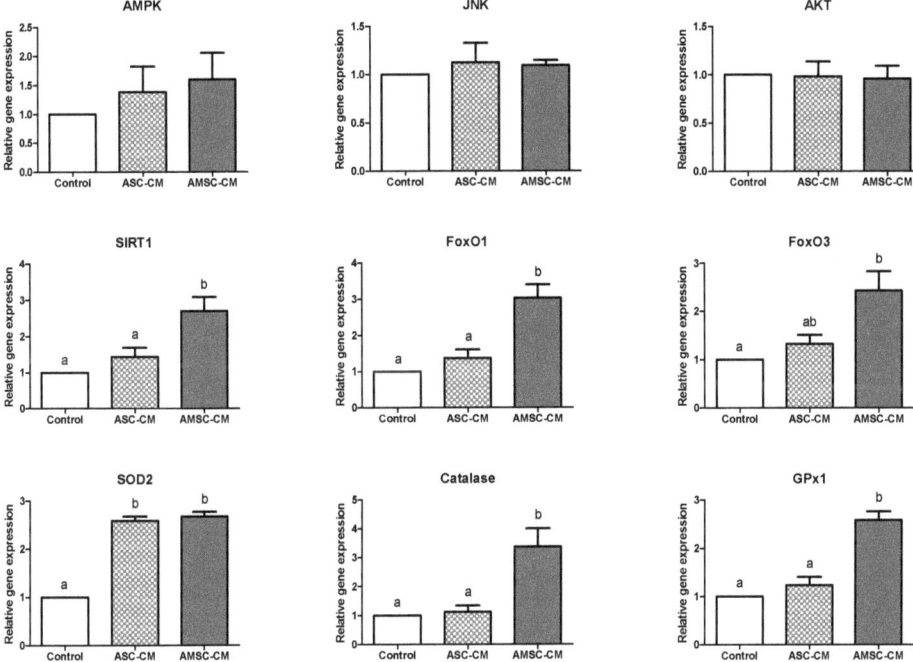

Figure 2. Relative antioxidant gene expression in blastocysts cultured in control, human adipose-derived mesenchymal stem cell conditioned medium (ASC-CM) and amniotic membrane-derived mesenchymal stem cell conditioned medium (AMSC-CM). Data are normalized to housekeeping gene 18S rRNA and presented as mean ± standard error of the mean (SEM). Superscript letters in each column indicate significant differences ($p < 0.05$).

3.5. Comparative Effects of ASC-CM and AMSC-CM on Intracellular Oxidative Stress in BL

Anti-oxidative effects of ASC-CM and AMSC-CM were evaluated through the measurement of ROS and GSH in BL. ROS levels in the BL of the AMSC-CM group (0.7 ± 0.1) were significantly lower than those in the control group (1.0 ± 0.0, $p < 0.05$), but the ASC-

CM group showed no significant difference with the other groups (Figure 3a). As shown in Figure 3b, GSH levels in the BL in both ASC-CM (1.2 ± 0.0) and AMSC-CM (1.3 ± 0.0) groups were significantly increased compared to the control group (1.0 ± 0.0, $p < 0.05$).

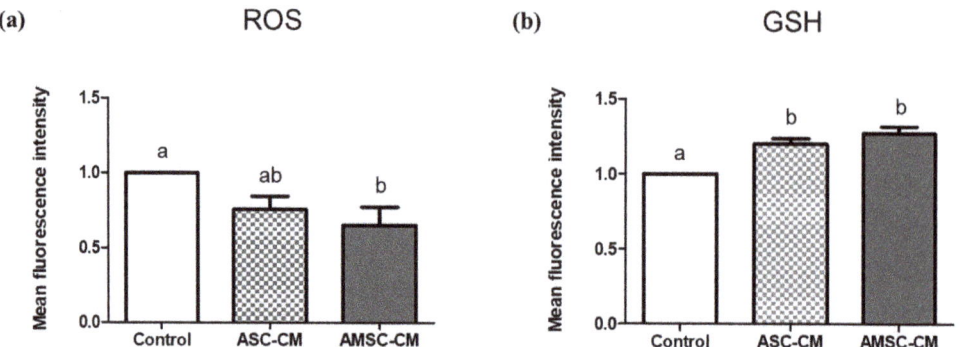

Figure 3. Evaluation of intracellular reactive oxygen species (ROS) and glutathione (GSH) in blastocysts (BL) cultured with human adipose-derived mesenchymal stem cell conditioned medium (ASC-CM) and amniotic membrane-derived mesenchymal stem cell conditioned medium (AMSC-CM). (a) ROS and (b) GSH level in BL. Data are presented as the mean ± SEM. Superscript letters in each column indicate significant differences ($p < 0.05$).

3.6. Comparison of Antioxidant Biomarkers in ASC-CM and AMSC-CM

TAC and SOD activity of both ASC-CM (2.8 ± 0.2 and 2.6 ± 0.1) and AMSC-CM (7.0 ± 0.2 and 3.5 ± 0.2) were significantly higher when compared to the control (1.0 ± 0.0 and 1.0 ± 0.2, respectively, $p < 0.05$, Figure 4a,b). Comparing ASC-CM and AMSC-CM, TAC and SOD activity of AMSC-CM was significantly greater than ASC-CM ($p < 0.05$, Figure 4a,b). Catalase activities in ASC-CM (1.1 ± 0.0) and AMSC-CM (1.1 ± 0.0) were similar but significantly higher than the control (1.0 ± 0.0, $p < 0.05$, Figure 4c).

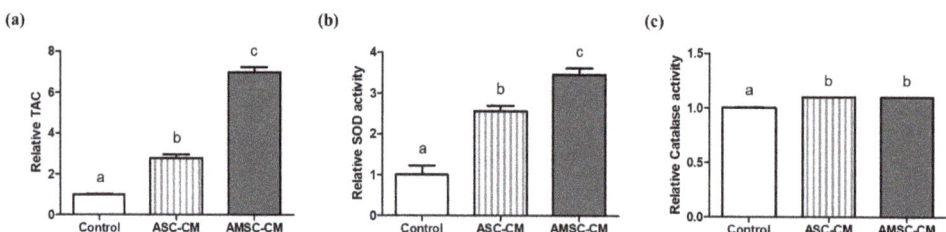

Figure 4. Comparison of antioxidant biomarkers level in human adipose-derived mesenchymal stem cell conditioned medium (ASC-CM) and amniotic membrane-derived mesenchymal stem cell conditioned medium (AMSC-CM). (a) Total antioxidant capacity (TAC), (b) superoxide dismutase (SOD) activity, and (c) catalase activity. Data are normalized to average value of control and presented as the mean ± SEM. Superscript letters in each column indicate significant differences ($p < 0.05$).

3.7. Comparison of Antioxidant Biomarkers in Culture Medium with ASC-CM and AMSC-CM

Catalase activity was significantly increased in pre-IVC medium supplemented with AMSC-CM (1.02 ± 0.0) compared to the control (1.0 ± 0.0, $p < 0.05$) and ASC-CM (1.0 ± 0.0, $p < 0.05$, Figure 5b). Likewise, SOD activity in post-IVC medium supplemented with AMSC-CM (1.7 ± 0.2) was significantly greater than that in the control and ASC-CM groups (1.0 ± 0.1 and 1.0 ± 0.1, respectively, $p < 0.05$, Figure 6a). Furthermore, catalase activity was significantly higher in post-IVC medium supplemented with AMSC-CM

(1.0 ± 0.0) than in ASC-CM (0.9 ± 0.0, $p < 0.05$, Figure 6b) but not when compared to the control.

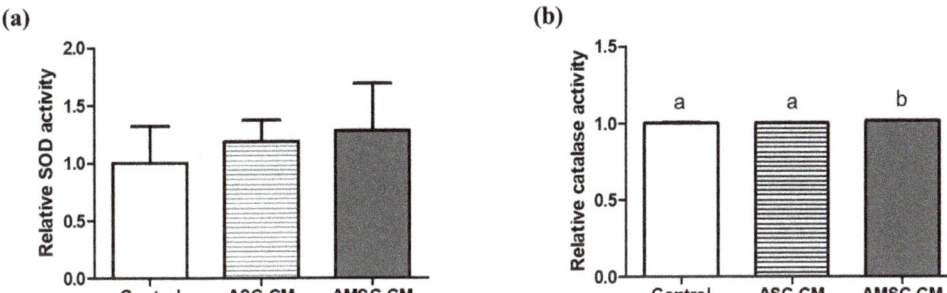

Figure 5. Comparison of antioxidant biomarkers level in fresh culture medium supplemented with human adipose-derived mesenchymal stem cell conditioned medium (ASC-CM) and amniotic membrane-derived mesenchymal stem cell conditioned medium (AMSC-CM). (a) Superoxide dismutase (SOD) and (b) catalase activity. Data are normalized to average value of control and presented as the mean ± SEM. Superscript letters in each column indicate significant differences ($p < 0.05$).

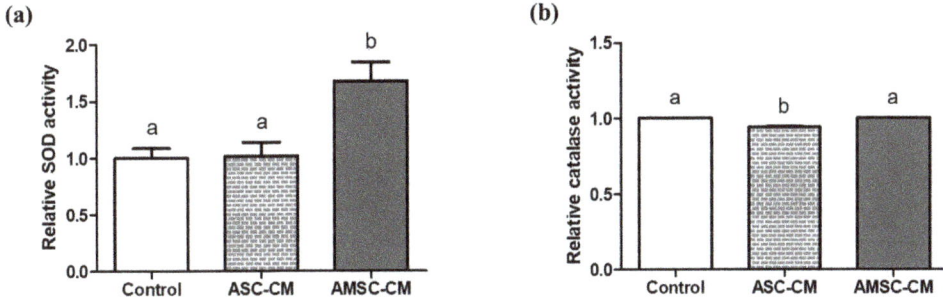

Figure 6. Comparison of antioxidant biomarker levels in culture medium supplemented with human adipose-derived mesenchymal stem cell conditioned medium (ASC-CM) and amniotic membrane-derived mesenchymal stem cell conditioned medium (AMSC-CM) which was collected after 5 days of embryo culture. (a) Superoxide dismutase (SOD) and (b) catalase activity. Data are normalized to average value of control and presented as the mean ± SEM. Superscript letters in each column indicate significant differences ($p < 0.05$).

3.8. Comparative Effects of ASC-CM and AMSC-CM on Apoptosis-Related Gene Expression in BL

To assess not only oxidative stress but also the consequent apoptosis of BL, the relative expression of the anti-apoptotic and pro-apoptotic genes was analyzed. The expression levels of B cell leukemia/lymphoma 2 (Bcl2) in both ASC-CM (1.8 ± 0.1) and AMSC-CM (1.7 ± 0.1) groups were significantly greater than those of the control (1.0 ± 0.0, $p < 0.05$, Figure 7). The ratio of Bcl2-associated X (Bax) to Bcl2 expression level in both ASC-CM (0.5 ± 0.1) and AMSC-CM (0.3 ± 0.1) groups was significantly lower than those of the control (1.0 ± 0.0, $p < 0.05$, Figure 7). Although no differences were found between the relative gene expression level of Bax among groups, Caspase 3 levels were significantly lower in the AMSC-CM group (0.6 ± 0.1) than in the ASC-CM group (1.1 ± 0.2, $p < 0.05$, Figure 7).

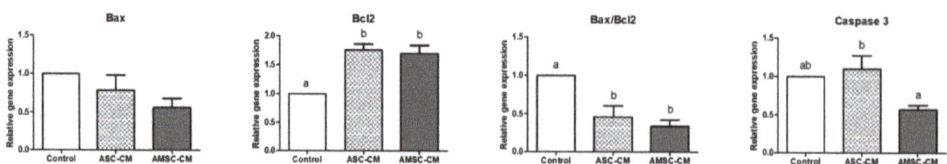

Figure 7. Relative apoptosis-related gene expression in blastocysts cultured in the control, human adipose-derived mesenchymal stem cell conditioned medium (ASC-CM) and amniotic membrane-derived mesenchymal stem cell conditioned medium (AMSC-CM) group. Data are normalized to housekeeping gene 18S rRNA and presented as mean ± standard error of the mean (SEM). Superscript letters in each column indicate significant differences ($p < 0.05$).

3.9. Comparative Effects of ASC-CM and AMSC-CM on Intracellular Apoptosis in BL

Mitochondrial membrane potential was visualized and measured as an indicator of intracellular apoptosis using JC-1 fluorescence staining of BLs from the control, ASC-CM, and AMSC-CM groups (Figure 8a). The ratio of JC-1 aggregate to JC-1 monomer in BLs of the AMSC-CM group (1.3 ± 0.1) was significantly higher than that of the control group (1.0 ± 0.0, $p < 0.05$). However, the ratio in BLs from the ASC-CM group was similar to that of the other groups (Figure 8b).

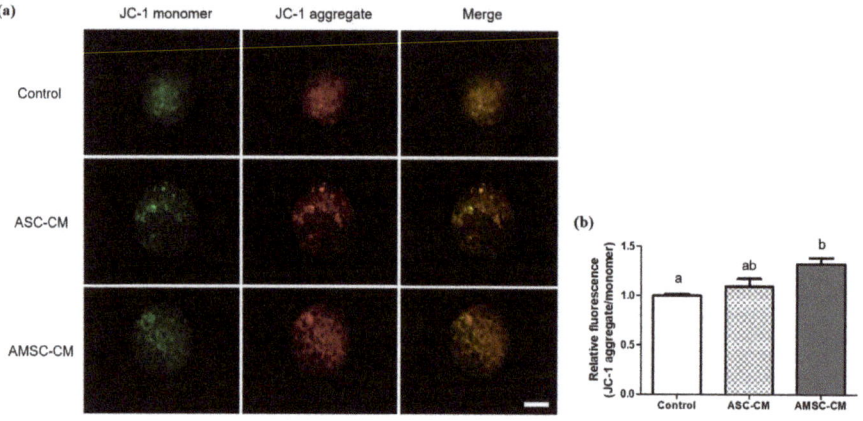

Figure 8. Assessment of mitochondrial membrane potential in blastocysts (BL) cultured with human adipose-derived mesenchymal stem cell conditioned medium (ASC-CM) and amniotic membrane-derived mesenchymal stem cell conditioned medium (AMSC-CM). (a) Representative fluorescent images of JC-1 monomer (green) and aggregate (red) stained BL. Original magnification 400×. Scale bar = 50 μm. (b) The ratio of JC-1 aggregate (red) to JC-1 monomer (green) presented by quantifying fluorescence intensity of JC-1 mitochondrial membrane potentials in BL. Data are expressed as the mean ± standard error of the mean (SEM). Superscript letters in each column indicate significant differences ($p < 0.05$).

4. Discussion

The present study was conducted with the purpose of (1) examining the anti-oxidative effect of human AMSC-CM treatment during IVC on mouse preimplantation embryo development, while simultaneously evaluating antioxidant gene expression, more specifically, the genes in the FoxO pathway, and (2) comparing human ASC-CM and AMSC-CM as supplementation for mouse embryo culture with regard to their anti-oxidative and anti-apoptotic effects.

At first, the effect of various concentrations of AMSC-CM treatment (10%, 20%, and 50%) during IVC was investigated to establish the optimal concentration for the development of in vitro fertilized mouse embryos. The rate of embryos that developed to the 4-cell and 16-cell stage were significantly lower in the 50% AMSC-CM group than in the 10%

AMSC-CM group. These results indicate that a high CM concentration does not ensure better efficiency of embryo development regardless of the large quantity of cytokines as previously explained [6]. Remarkably, we found that 10% AMSC-CM significantly improved BL formation rate (Table 2), which is an index for embryo developmental potential and consequently determines the success of implantation [41], compared to the control group as well as the other higher concentration of AMSC-CM treated groups. In addition, the 10% AMSC-CM group showed the most enhanced BL hatching ability, a crucial precondition for successful implantation and pregnancy rates [42]. Together, our results indicated that 10% AMSC-CM treatment during IVC is optimal for overall preimplantation embryo developmental processes from early cleavage to BL hatching.

A few studies have compared the characteristics and proliferation rate of ASC and AMSC [43–45], but to the best of our knowledge, the comparison between anti-oxidative effects of ASC-CM and AMSC-CM has never been reported, particularly on the embryo and its culture medium. Therefore, the effects of ASC-CM and AMSC-CM treatment at the respective confirmed optimal concentrations in embryo IVC medium were compared. As validated by the results presented in Table 2, AMSC-CM treatment improved embryo development compared to the control. The embryo developmental rate of the AMSC-CM group was greater than that of the ASC-CM group at all the assessed stages (Table 3), but the difference was not statistically significant. The expression of antioxidant genes in the FoxO signaling pathway was analyzed to evaluate the quality of BLs cultured with ASC-CM or AMSC-CM. FoxO transcription factors modulate various cellular functions, including differentiation, growth, metabolism, and apoptosis [46]. These factors predominantly regulate the oxidative stress response by controlling the expression of manganese-dependent SOD (SOD2), catalase, and GPx1 that constitute the primary defense mechanism against ROS [47]. FoxO is considered as a therapeutic target for infertility and is critical for the preimplantation embryo development in mice [46]. Specifically, among the mammalian FoxO family, FoxO1 and FoxO3 are key players in female reproductive processes [48]. We found that the relative expression of FoxO1 and FoxO3 was significantly increased in the BLs cultured with AMSC-CM as compared to those of the control group. Furthermore, the expression levels of SOD2, catalase, and GPx1, downstream targets of the FoxO subfamily, were significantly greater in the AMSC-CM group than in the control group (Figure 2). Remarkably, compared with ASC-CM, AMSC-CM promoted the expression of FoxO1, catalase, and GPx1 (Figure 2). We also analyzed genes that function as upstream regulators of FoxO such as AMPK [49] and JNK [50], as well as AKT [51], but none of the genes exhibited notable differences in expression, which seems to have an ambiguous influence on FoxO activity in that FoxO receives various signals from growth factors, metabolic and oxidative stress [52] and involves numerous mechanisms for its regulation [53]. However, we found an increase in SIRT1 expression in BL cultured with AMSC-CM, which is a crucial regulator of oxidative stress that protects cells by upregulating antioxidant activity through FoxO-dependent mechanisms and, in particular, the interaction of SIRT1 and FOXO3a mainly functions in protecting oocytes against loss of developmental competence from reproductive aging [54]. GSH is a representative non-enzymatic antioxidant that is essential for embryo development after fertilization up to the BL stage [55]. In this study, intracellular GSH levels were increased in BLs with ASC-CM and AMSC-CM treatment, but ROS levels were decreased only in the AMSC-CM group (Figure 3). ROS are attenuated by a collaborative defense system comprising enzymatic and non-enzymatic antioxidants [56]. Collectively, the results described above suggest that AMSC-CM exerts an anti-oxidative effect during embryo culture by improving the expression of both enzymatic and non-enzymatic antioxidants in BL.

We then investigated the antioxidant biomarker activity in CM, pre- and post-IVC medium containing different CM. In addition to TAC, a complex indicator showing the comprehensive activity of various antioxidants [57], the activities of SOD and catalase were all greater in both ASC-CM and AMSC-CM when compared to non-conditioned medium (Figure 4). Notably, we found evident difference that AMSC-CM showed greater level of antioxidant biomarkers than ASC-CM. The results are consistent with various studies that reported the factors secreted from MSC contain antioxidants as one of the predominant elements, which are included in CM and exert anti-oxidative effects in paracrine mechanisms [13,58–60]. In particular, numerous growth factors found in CM of human amnion tissue and AMSC [61] have been identified to function as antioxidants including insulin-like growth factor [62], platelet-derived growth factor [63], epidermal growth factor [64], hepatocyte growth factor [65] and fibroblast growth factor [66]. Moreover, pre- and post-IVC medium analysis revealed that the activities of SOD and catalase were higher in culture medium supplemented with AMSC-CM than the medium with ASC-CM (Figures 5 and 6). Therefore, the improvement in embryo developmental rate and antioxidant expression in BLs could be explained by the favorable culture conditions from the active antioxidants in AMSC-CM.

In addition, apoptosis, which is generally accompanied by oxidative damage, was evaluated in BLs. The anti-apoptotic effect of AMSC-CM was confirmed in that pro-apoptotic gene expression was decreased and anti-apoptotic gene expression was increased. More specifically, an upregulation of the anti-apoptotic gene Bcl2 was observed not only in the AMSC-CM group, but also in the ASC-CM group, indicating that both CMs have anti-apoptotic effects. However, Caspase 3 which is known as an apoptosis executioner [67] was downregulated in the AMSC-CM group compared to the ASC-CM group (Figure 7). The caspase signaling pathway is activated by apoptosis-inducing factors released from the mitochondrial intermembrane space to the cytoplasm following the decrease of mitochondrial membrane potential, which is induced by oxidative damage in cells [68]. The effect of ASC-CM on mitochondrial membrane potential was not significant; however, as predicted, the ratio of JC-1 aggregate to JC-1 monomer was found to be higher in BLs cultured with AMSC-CM than in the control (Figure 8), indicating both anti-oxidative and anti-apoptotic effects of AMSC-CM on in vitro produced BL with enhanced mitochondrial membrane potential.

The present study compared antioxidant competence of CM obtained from two different types of MSC, ASC-CM and AMSC-CM, and suggested that AMSC-CM may be more efficient for embryo culture rather than ASC-CM. Our findings are supported by previous studies demonstrating that the quantity and variety of secretome from MSC can alter depending on different tissue sources of origin [29,69,70]. A point to be considered is that, to date, it is uncertain that MSC-CM can outperform chemical antioxidant compounds. To cite an example, several studies indicated that resveratrol, one of the chemically defined antioxidants which has been extensively studied [71], achieved less effective outcomes than MSC in pathological condition and diseases related to oxidative damage [72–74]. However, a direct comparison of MSC-CM and other antioxidant compounds has never been conducted to the best of our knowledge, especially in terms of assisted reproduction, and further studies are expected for clarification.

5. Conclusions

In conclusion, this study established that AMSC-CM treatment, at the optimal concentration, acts as an antioxidant during IVC of mouse preimplantation embryos. Furthermore, AMSC-CM treatment had a beneficial effect on embryo developmental rate and upregulated the FoxO-mediated expression of antioxidant enzymes in BLs cultured with AMSC-CM. Compared with ASC-CM, as a conventional antioxidant, AMSC-CM demonstrated enhanced expression of both enzymatic and non-enzymatic antioxidants, promotion of anti-oxidative culture conditions, and anti-apoptotic effects on developed embryos. These findings indicate that AMSC-CM can be developed as a novel and competent antioxidant interventions for the improvement of assisted reproductive technologies.

Supplementary Materials: The following are available online at https://www.mdpi.com/2076-3921/10/2/268/s1, Table S1: Analysis of the quantity and quality of the extracted RNA.

Author Contributions: Conceptualization, K.R., H.J.O., E.Y.K., S.K.K. and J.C.R.; Data curation, K.R.; Formal analysis, K.R.; Funding acquisition, S.C.P. and B.C.L.; Investigation, K.R., E.Y.K., and E.H.K.; Methodology, K.R. and H.J.O.; Project administration, S.K.K., J.C.R., S.C.P. and B.C.L.; Resources, J.C.R., S.C.P. and B.C.L.; Supervision, S.C.P. and B.C.L.; Validation, S.C.P. and B.C.L.; Visualization, K.R.; Writing—original draft, K.R.; Writing—review and editing, K.R. All authors have read and agreed to the published version of the manuscript.

Funding: This research was supported by Nature Cell (#550-20170028, #550-20200076) and the BK21 plus program, and Research Institute for Veterinary Science.

Institutional Review Board Statement: The study was conducted according to the guidelines of the Declaration of Helsinki, and approved by the Ethics Committee of Biostar Stem Cell Technology (IRB NO. 2019-03). All experiments using experimental animals in this study were approved by the Institutional Animal Care and Use Committee of Seoul National University (SNU-170511-2-4).

Informed Consent Statement: Informed consent was obtained from all subjects involved in the study.

Conflicts of Interest: K.R., H.J.O., E.H.K., S.C.P. and B.C.L. declare that they have no conflict of interest. E.Y.K., S.K.K. and J.C.R. have been employees of Nature Cell and declare no intervention in data analysis, interpretation and presentation as stated in author contributions. All authors never inappropriately influence or bias the results of this study.

References

1. Chronopoulou, E.; Harper, J.C. IVF culture media: Past, present and future. *Hum. Reprod. Update* **2015**, *21*, 39–55. [CrossRef]
2. Agarwal, A.; Allamaneni, S.S. Role of free radicals in female reproductive diseases and assisted reproduction. *Reprod. Biomed. Online* **2004**, *9*, 338–347. [CrossRef]
3. Du Plessis, S.S.; Makker, K.; Desai, N.R.; Agarwal, A. Impact of oxidative stress on IVF. *Expert Rev. Obstet. Gynecol.* **2008**, *3*, 539–554. [CrossRef]
4. Yang, H.W.; Hwang, K.J.; Kwon, H.C.; Kim, H.S.; Choi, K.W.; Oh, K.S. Detection of reactive oxygen species (ROS) and apoptosis in human fragmented embryos. *Hum. Reprod.* **1998**, *13*, 998–1002. [CrossRef] [PubMed]
5. Oyawoye, O.; Abdel Gadir, A.; Garner, A.; Constantinovici, N.; Perrett, C.; Hardiman, P. Antioxidants and reactive oxygen species in follicular fluid of women undergoing IVF: Relationship to outcome. *Hum. Reprod.* **2003**, *18*, 2270–2274. [CrossRef]
6. Ra, K.; Oh, H.J.; Kim, E.Y.; Kang, S.K.; Ra, J.C.; Kim, E.H.; Lee, B.C. Anti-Oxidative Effects of Human Adipose Stem Cell Conditioned Medium with Different Basal Medium during Mouse Embryo In Vitro Culture. *Animals* **2020**, *10*, 1414. [CrossRef]
7. Agarwal, A.; Said, T.M.; Bedaiwy, M.A.; Banerjee, J.; Alvarez, J.G. Oxidative stress in an assisted reproductive techniques setting. *Fertil. Steril.* **2006**, *86*, 503–512. [CrossRef]
8. Cambra, J.M.; Martinez, C.A.; Rodriguez-Martinez, H.; Martinez, E.A.; Cuello, C.; Gil, M.A. N-(2-mercaptopropionyl)-glycine enhances in vitro pig embryo production and reduces oxidative stress. *Sci. Rep.* **2020**, *10*, 18632. [CrossRef] [PubMed]
9. Wang, X.; Falcone, T.; Attaran, M.; Goldberg, J.M.; Agarwal, A.; Sharma, R.K. Vitamin C and vitamin E supplementation reduce oxidative stress-induced embryo toxicity and improve the blastocyst development rate. *Fertil. Steril.* **2002**, *78*, 1272–1277. [CrossRef]
10. Abdelrazik, H.; Sharma, R.; Mahfouz, R.; Agarwal, A. L-carnitine decreases DNA damage and improves the in vitro blastocyst development rate in mouse embryos. *Fertil. Steril.* **2009**, *91*, 589–596. [CrossRef] [PubMed]
11. Wang, F.; Tian, X.; Zhang, L.; He, C.; Ji, P.; Li, Y.; Tan, D.; Liu, G. Beneficial effect of resveratrol on bovine oocyte maturation and subsequent embryonic development after in vitro fertilization. *Fertil. Steril.* **2014**, *101*, 577–586. [CrossRef] [PubMed]
12. Gruber, I.; Klein, M. Embryo culture media for human IVF: Which possibilities exist? *J. Turk. Ger. Gynecol. Assoc.* **2011**, *12*, 110–117. [CrossRef] [PubMed]
13. Stavely, R.; Nurgali, K. The emerging antioxidant paradigm of mesenchymal stem cell therapy. *Stem Cells Transl. Med.* **2020**, *9*, 985–1006. [CrossRef]
14. Ullah, I.; Subbarao, R.B.; Rho, G.J. Human mesenchymal stem cells—Current trends and future prospective. *Biosci. Rep.* **2015**, *35*. [CrossRef]
15. Pittenger, M.F.; Discher, D.E.; Peault, B.M.; Phinney, D.G.; Hare, J.M.; Caplan, A.I. Mesenchymal stem cell perspective: Cell biology to clinical progress. *NPJ Regen. Med.* **2019**, *4*, 22. [CrossRef]
16. Kim, W.S.; Park, B.S.; Sung, J.H. The wound-healing and antioxidant effects of adipose-derived stem cells. *Expert Opin. Biol. Ther.* **2009**, *9*, 879–887. [CrossRef]
17. Kim, W.S.; Park, B.S.; Kim, H.K.; Park, J.S.; Kim, K.J.; Choi, J.S.; Chung, S.J.; Kim, D.D.; Sung, J.H. Evidence supporting antioxidant action of adipose-derived stem cells: Protection of human dermal fibroblasts from oxidative stress. *J. Dermatol. Sci.* **2008**, *49*, 133–142. [CrossRef]

18. Ra, K.; Oh, H.J.; Kim, G.A.; Kang, S.K.; Ra, J.C.; Lee, B.C. High Frequency of Intravenous Injection of Human Adipose Stem Cell Conditioned Medium Improved Embryo Development of Mice in Advanced Maternal Age through Antioxidant Effects. *Animals* **2020**, *10*, 978. [CrossRef]
19. Toda, A.; Okabe, M.; Yoshida, T.; Nikaido, T. The potential of amniotic membrane/amnion-derived cells for regeneration of various tissues. *J. Pharmacol. Sci.* **2007**, *105*, 215–228. [CrossRef]
20. Kim, E.Y.; Lee, K.B.; Kim, M.K. The potential of mesenchymal stem cells derived from amniotic membrane and amniotic fluid for neuronal regenerative therapy. *BMB Rep.* **2014**, *47*, 135–140. [CrossRef] [PubMed]
21. Diaz-Prado, S.; Muinos-Lopez, E.; Hermida-Gomez, T.; Rendal-Vazquez, M.E.; Fuentes-Boquete, I.; de Toro, F.J.; Blanco, F.J. Multilineage differentiation potential of cells isolated from the human amniotic membrane. *J. Cell Biochem.* **2010**, *111*, 846–857. [CrossRef]
22. Abbasi-Kangevari, M.; Ghamari, S.H.; Safaeinejad, F.; Bahrami, S.; Niknejad, H. Potential Therapeutic Features of Human Amniotic Mesenchymal Stem Cells in Multiple Sclerosis: Immunomodulation, Inflammation Suppression, Angiogenesis Promotion, Oxidative Stress Inhibition, Neurogenesis Induction, MMPs Regulation, and Remyelination Stimulation. *Front. Immunol.* **2019**, *10*, 238. [CrossRef]
23. Bulati, M.; Miceli, V.; Gallo, A.; Amico, G.; Carcione, C.; Pampalone, M.; Conaldi, P.G. The Immunomodulatory Properties of the Human Amnion-Derived Mesenchymal Stromal/Stem Cells Are Induced by INF-gamma Produced by Activated Lymphomonocytes and Are Mediated by Cell-To-Cell Contact and Soluble Factors. *Front. Immunol.* **2020**, *11*, 54. [CrossRef]
24. Wang, Y.; Ma, J.; Du, Y.; Miao, J.; Chen, N. Human Amnion-Derived Mesenchymal Stem Cells Protect Human Bone Marrow Mesenchymal Stem Cells against Oxidative Stress-Mediated Dysfunction via ERK1/2 MAPK Signaling. *Mol. Cells* **2016**, *39*, 186–194. [CrossRef]
25. He, F.; Wang, Y.; Li, Y.; Yu, L. Human amniotic mesenchymal stem cells alleviate paraquat-induced pulmonary fibrosis in rats by inhibiting the inflammatory response. *Life Sci.* **2020**, *243*, 117290. [CrossRef]
26. Xie, C.; Jin, J.; Lv, X.; Tao, J.; Wang, R.; Miao, D. Anti-aging Effect of Transplanted Amniotic Membrane Mesenchymal Stem Cells in a Premature Aging Model of Bmi-1 Deficiency. *Sci. Rep.* **2015**, *5*, 13975. [CrossRef] [PubMed]
27. Jiao, H.; Shi, K.; Zhang, W.; Yang, L.; Yang, L.; Guan, F.; Yang, B. Therapeutic potential of human amniotic membrane-derived mesenchymal stem cells in APP transgenic mice. *Oncol. Lett.* **2016**, *12*, 1877–1883. [CrossRef] [PubMed]
28. Li, J.Y.; Ren, K.K.; Zhang, W.J.; Xiao, L.; Wu, H.Y.; Liu, Q.Y.; Ding, T.; Zhang, X.C.; Nie, W.J.; Ke, Y.; et al. Human amniotic mesenchymal stem cells and their paracrine factors promote wound healing by inhibiting heat stress-induced skin cell apoptosis and enhancing their proliferation through activating PI3K/AKT signaling pathway. *Stem Cell Res. Ther.* **2019**, *10*, 247. [CrossRef] [PubMed]
29. Kusuma, G.D.; Carthew, J.; Lim, R.; Frith, J.E. Effect of the Microenvironment on Mesenchymal Stem Cell Paracrine Signaling: Opportunities to Engineer the Therapeutic Effect. *Stem Cells Dev.* **2017**, *26*, 617–631. [CrossRef]
30. Pawitan, J.A. Prospect of stem cell conditioned medium in regenerative medicine. *Biomed. Res. Int.* **2014**, *2014*, 965849. [CrossRef]
31. Sagaradze, G.; Grigorieva, O.; Nimiritsky, P.; Basalova, N.; Kalinina, N.; Akopyan, Z.; Efimenko, A. Conditioned Medium from Human Mesenchymal Stromal Cells: Towards the Clinical Translation. *Int. J. Mol. Sci.* **2019**, *20*, 1656. [CrossRef] [PubMed]
32. Simopoulou, M.; Sfakianoudis, K.; Rapani, A.; Giannelou, P.; Anifandis, G.; Bolaris, S.; Pantou, A.; Lambropoulou, M.; Pappas, A.; Deligeoroglou, E.; et al. Considerations Regarding Embryo Culture Conditions: From Media to Epigenetics. *In Vivo* **2018**, *32*, 451–460. [CrossRef] [PubMed]
33. Leese, H.J.; Baumann, C.G.; Brison, D.R.; McEvoy, T.G.; Sturmey, R.G. Metabolism of the viable mammalian embryo: Quietness revisited. *Mol. Hum. Reprod.* **2008**, *14*, 667–672. [CrossRef] [PubMed]
34. Eisenbach, M.; Giojalas, L.C. Sperm guidance in mammals—An unpaved road to the egg. *Nat. Rev. Mol. Cell Biol.* **2006**, *7*, 276–285. [CrossRef]
35. Baak, N.A.; Cantineau, A.E.; Farquhar, C.; Brison, D.R. Temperature of embryo culture for assisted reproduction. *Cochrane Database Syst. Rev.* **2019**, *9*, CD012192. [CrossRef]
36. Higdon, H.L., 3rd; Blackhurst, D.W.; Boone, W.R. Incubator management in an assisted reproductive technology laboratory. *Fertil. Steril.* **2008**, *89*, 703–710. [CrossRef]
37. Muller, W.U. Temperature dependence of combined exposure of preimplantation mouse embryos to X-rays and mercury. *Radiat. Environ. Biophys.* **1990**, *29*, 109–114. [CrossRef]
38. Morbeck, D.E.; Paczkowski, M.; Fredrickson, J.R.; Krisher, R.L.; Hoff, H.S.; Baumann, N.A.; Moyer, T.; Matern, D. Composition of protein supplements used for human embryo culture. *J. Assist. Reprod. Genet.* **2014**, *31*, 1703–1711. [CrossRef] [PubMed]
39. Hayashi, M.; Yoshida, K.; Kitada, K.; Kizu, A.; Tachibana, D.; Fukui, M.; Morita, T.; Koyama, M. Low-dose irradiation of mouse embryos increases Smad-p21 pathway activity and preserves pluripotency. *J. Assist. Reprod. Genet.* **2018**, *35*, 1061–1069. [CrossRef]
40. Edwards, L.J.; Kind, K.L.; Armstrong, D.T.; Thompson, J.G. Effects of recombinant human follicle-stimulating hormone on embryo development in mice. *Am. J. Physiol. Endocrinol. Metab.* **2005**, *288*, E845–E851. [CrossRef]
41. Zhang, S.; Lin, H.; Kong, S.; Wang, S.; Wang, H.; Wang, H.; Armant, D.R. Physiological and molecular determinants of embryo implantation. *Mol. Aspects Med.* **2013**, *34*, 939–980. [CrossRef]
42. Hammadeh, M.E.; Fischer-Hammadeh, C.; Ali, K.R. Assisted hatching in assisted reproduction: A state of the art. *J. Assist. Reprod. Genet.* **2011**, *28*, 119–128. [CrossRef]

43. Hwang, I.S.; Kim, H.G.; Jo, D.H.; Lee, D.H.; Koo, Y.H.; Song, Y.J.; Na, Y.J.; Choi, O.H. Comparison with human amniotic membrane- and adipose tissue-derived mesenchymal stem cells. *Korean J. Obstet. Gynecol.* **2011**, *54*, 674–683. [CrossRef]
44. Kim, D.; Kyung, J.; Park, D.; Choi, E.K.; Kim, K.S.; Shin, K.; Lee, H.; Shin, I.S.; Kang, S.K.; Ra, J.C.; et al. Health Span-Extending Activity of Human Amniotic Membrane- and Adipose Tissue-Derived Stem Cells in F344 Rats. *Stem Cells Transl. Med.* **2015**, *4*, 1144–1154. [CrossRef]
45. Dizaji Asl, K.; Shafaei, H.; Soleimani Rad, J.; Nozad, H.O. Comparison of Characteristics of Human Amniotic Membrane and Human Adipose Tissue Derived Mesenchymal Stem Cells. *World J. Plast. Surg.* **2017**, *6*, 33–39.
46. Kuscu, N.; Gungor-Ordueri, N.E.; Sozen, B.; Adiguzel, D.; Celik-Ozenci, C. FoxO transcription factors 1 regulate mouse preimplantation embryo development. *J. Assist. Reprod. Genet.* **2019**, *36*, 2121–2133. [CrossRef] [PubMed]
47. Lu, J.; Wang, Z.; Cao, J.; Chen, Y.; Dong, Y. A novel and compact review on the role of oxidative stress in female reproduction. *Reprod. Biol. Endocrinol.* **2018**, *16*, 80. [CrossRef]
48. Wang, Y.; Zhou, Y.; Graves, D.T. FOXO transcription factors: Their clinical significance and regulation. *Biomed. Res. Int.* **2014**, *2014*, 925350. [CrossRef] [PubMed]
49. Greer, E.L.; Oskoui, P.R.; Banko, M.R.; Maniar, J.M.; Gygi, M.P.; Gygi, S.P.; Brunet, A. The energy sensor AMP-activated protein kinase directly regulates the mammalian FOXO3 transcription factor. *J. Biol. Chem.* **2007**, *282*, 30107–30119. [CrossRef]
50. Essers, M.A.; Weijzen, S.; de Vries-Smits, A.M.; Saarloos, I.; de Ruiter, N.D.; Bos, J.L.; Burgering, B.M. FOXO transcription factor activation by oxidative stress mediated by the small GTPase Ral and JNK. *EMBO J.* **2004**, *23*, 4802–4812. [CrossRef]
51. Brunet, A.; Bonni, A.; Zigmond, M.J.; Lin, M.Z.; Juo, P.; Hu, L.S.; Anderson, M.J.; Arden, K.C.; Blenis, J.; Greenberg, M.E. Akt promotes cell survival by phosphorylating and inhibiting a Forkhead transcription factor. *Cell* **1999**, *96*, 857–868. [CrossRef]
52. Fasano, C.; Disciglio, V.; Bertora, S.; Lepore Signorile, M.; Simone, C. FOXO3a from the Nucleus to the Mitochondria: A Round Trip in Cellular Stress Response. *Cells* **2019**, *8*, 1110. [CrossRef] [PubMed]
53. Brown, A.K.; Webb, A.E. Regulation of FOXO Factors in Mammalian Cells. *Curr. Top. Dev. Biol.* **2018**, *127*, 165–192. [CrossRef] [PubMed]
54. Tatone, C.; Di Emidio, G.; Vitti, M.; Di Carlo, M.; Santini, S., Jr.; D'Alessandro, A.M.; Falone, S.; Amicarelli, F. Sirtuin Functions in Female Fertility: Possible Role in Oxidative Stress and Aging. *Oxid. Med. Cell Longev.* **2015**, *2015*, 659687. [CrossRef]
55. Salmen, J.J.; Skufca, F.; Matt, A.; Gushansky, G.; Mason, A.; Gardiner, C.S. Role of glutathione in reproductive tract secretions on mouse preimplantation embryo development. *Biol. Reprod.* **2005**, *73*, 308–314. [CrossRef]
56. Khazaei, M.; Aghaz, F. Reactive Oxygen Species Generation and Use of Antioxidants during In Vitro Maturation of Oocytes. *Int. J. Fertil. Steril.* **2017**, *11*, 63–70. [CrossRef]
57. Zhang, T.; Andrukhov, O.; Haririan, H.; Muller-Kern, M.; Liu, S.; Liu, Z.; Rausch-Fan, X. Total Antioxidant Capacity and Total Oxidant Status in Saliva of Periodontitis Patients in Relation to Bacterial Load. *Front. Cell Infect. Microbiol.* **2015**, *5*, 97. [CrossRef]
58. Baraniak, P.R.; McDevitt, T.C. Stem cell paracrine actions and tissue regeneration. *Regen. Med.* **2010**, *5*, 121–143. [CrossRef]
59. Maguire, G. Stem cell therapy without the cells. *Commun. Integr. Biol.* **2013**, *6*, e26631. [CrossRef]
60. Gunawardena, T.N.A.; Rahman, M.T.; Abdullah, B.J.J.; Abu Kasim, N.H. Conditioned media derived from mesenchymal stem cell cultures: The next generation for regenerative medicine. *J. Tissue Eng. Regen. Med.* **2019**, *13*, 569–586. [CrossRef]
61. Grzywocz, Z.; Pius-Sadowska, E.; Klos, P.; Gryzik, M.; Wasilewska, D.; Aleksandrowicz, B.; Dworczynska, M.; Sabalinska, S.; Hoser, G.; Machalinski, B.; et al. Growth factors and their receptors derived from human amniotic cells in vitro. *Folia Histochem. Cytobiol.* **2014**, *52*, 163–170. [CrossRef] [PubMed]
62. Garcia-Fernandez, M.; Castilla-Cortazar, I.; Diaz-Sanchez, M.; Navarro, I.; Puche, J.E.; Castilla, A.; Casares, A.D.; Clavijo, E.; Gonzalez-Baron, S. Antioxidant effects of insulin-like growth factor-I (IGF-I) in rats with advanced liver cirrhosis. *BMC Gastroenterol.* **2005**, *5*, 7. [CrossRef] [PubMed]
63. Goksen, S.; Balabanli, B.; Coskun-Cevher, S. Application of platelet derived growth factor-BB and diabetic wound healing: The relationship with oxidative events. *Free Radic. Res.* **2017**, *51*, 498–505. [CrossRef] [PubMed]
64. Kalay, Z.; Cevher, S.C. Oxidant and antioxidant events during epidermal growth factor therapy to cutaneous wound healing in rats. *Int. Wound J.* **2012**, *9*, 362–371. [CrossRef]
65. Santangelo, C.; Matarrese, P.; Masella, R.; Di Carlo, M.C.; Di Lillo, A.; Scazzocchio, B.; Vecci, E.; Malorni, W.; Perfetti, R.; Anastasi, E. Hepatocyte growth factor protects rat RINm5F cell line against free fatty acid-induced apoptosis by counteracting oxidative stress. *J. Mol. Endocrinol.* **2007**, *38*, 147–158. [CrossRef] [PubMed]
66. Wei, T.; Shu, Q.; Ning, J.; Wang, S.; Li, C.; Zhao, L.; Zheng, H.; Gao, H. The Protective Effect of Basic Fibroblast Growth Factor on Diabetic Nephropathy Through Remodeling Metabolic Phenotype and Suppressing Oxidative Stress in Mice. *Front. Pharmacol.* **2020**, *11*, 66. [CrossRef]
67. McIlwain, D.R.; Berger, T.; Mak, T.W. Caspase functions in cell death and disease. *Cold Spring Harb. Perspect. Biol.* **2013**, *5*, a008656. [CrossRef]
68. Rigoulet, M.; Yoboue, E.D.; Devin, A. Mitochondrial ROS generation and its regulation: Mechanisms involved in H_2O_2 signaling. *Antioxid. Redox. Signal.* **2011**, *14*, 459–468. [CrossRef]
69. Amable, P.R.; Teixeira, M.V.; Carias, R.B.; Granjeiro, J.M.; Borojevic, R. Protein synthesis and secretion in human mesenchymal cells derived from bone marrow, adipose tissue and Wharton's jelly. *Stem Cell Res. Ther.* **2014**, *5*, 53. [CrossRef]
70. Pires, A.O.; Mendes-Pinheiro, B.; Teixeira, F.G.; Anjo, S.I.; Ribeiro-Samy, S.; Gomes, E.D.; Serra, S.C.; Silva, N.A.; Manadas, B.; Sousa, N.; et al. Unveiling the Differences of Secretome of Human Bone Marrow Mesenchymal Stem Cells, Adipose Tissue-

Derived Stem Cells, and Human Umbilical Cord Perivascular Cells: A Proteomic Analysis. *Stem Cells Dev.* **2016**, *25*, 1073–1083. [CrossRef]
71. Pervaiz, S.; Holme, A.L. Resveratrol: Its biologic targets and functional activity. *Antioxid. Redox. Signal.* **2009**, *11*, 2851–2897. [CrossRef] [PubMed]
72. Pinarli, F.A.; Turan, N.N.; Pinarli, F.G.; Okur, A.; Sonmez, D.; Ulus, T.; Oguz, A.; Karadeniz, C.; Delibasi, T. Resveratrol and adipose-derived mesenchymal stem cells are effective in the prevention and treatment of doxorubicin cardiotoxicity in rats. *Pediatr. Hematol. Oncol.* **2013**, *30*, 226–238. [CrossRef] [PubMed]
73. Okay, E.; Simsek, T.; Subasi, C.; Gunes, A.; Duruksu, G.; Gurbuz, Y.; Gacar, G.; Karaoz, E. Cross effects of resveratrol and mesenchymal stem cells on liver regeneration and homing in partially hepatectomized rats. *Stem Cell Rev. Rep.* **2015**, *11*, 322–331. [CrossRef] [PubMed]
74. Xian, Y.; Lin, Y.; Cao, C.; Li, L.; Wang, J.; Niu, J.; Guo, Y.; Sun, Y.; Wang, Y.; Wang, W. Protective effect of umbilical cord mesenchymal stem cells combined with resveratrol against renal podocyte damage in NOD mice. *Diabetes Res. Clin. Pract.* **2019**, *156*, 107755. [CrossRef]

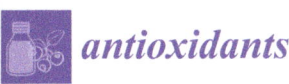

Article

Effects of *Lippia citriodora* Leaf Extract on Lipid and Oxidative Blood Profile of Volunteers with Hypercholesterolemia: A Preliminary Study

Antonella Angiolillo [1,*], Deborah Leccese [1], Marisa Palazzo [2,*], Francesco Vizzarri [3], Donato Casamassima [2], Carlo Corino [4] and Alfonso Di Costanzo [1]

1. Centre for Research and Training in Medicine of Aging, Department of Medicine and Health Sciences "V. Tiberio", University of Molise, 86100 Campobasso, Italy; d.leccese@studenti.unimol.it (D.L.); alfonso.dicostanzo@unimol.it (A.D.C.)
2. Department of Agricultural, Environmental and Food Sciences, University of Molise, 86100 Campobasso, Italy; casamassima.d@unimol.it
3. Department of Agricultural and Environmental Science, University of Bari Aldo Moro, 70126 Bari, Italy; francesco.vizzarri@uniba.it
4. Department of Veterinary Medicine, University of Milano, 26900 Lodi, Italy; carlo.corino@unimi.it
* Correspondence: angiolillo@unimol.it (A.A.); m.palazzo@unimol.it (M.P.)

Abstract: *Lippia citriodora* is a plant traditionally used for its anti-inflammatory, antioxidant and antispasmodic effects, as well as for additional biological activities proven in cell culture, animal studies and a small number of human clinical trials. The plant has also shown a marked improvement in blood lipid profile in some animal species. In the present preliminary study, we investigated the effect of a leaf extract on lipid and oxidative blood profile of hypercholesterolemic volunteers. Twelve adults received *Lippia citriodora* extract caps, containing 23% phenylpropanoids, (100 mg, once a day) for 16 weeks. Selected blood lipids and plasma oxidative markers were measured at baseline and after 4, 8 and 16 weeks of treatment. Compared with baseline, total cholesterol levels significantly decreased and high-density lipoprotein cholesterol increased, while low-density lipoprotein cholesterol and triglycerides showed only a downward trend. Oxidative status was improved due to a decrease in the concentration of total oxidant status, reactive oxygen metabolites and malondialdehyde, and a significant increase in ferric reducing ability of plasma, vitamin A and vitamin E. These preliminary results suggest that dietary supplementation with *Lippia citriodora* extract can improve the lipid profile, enhance blood antioxidant power, and could be a valuable natural compound for the management of human hypercholesterolemia.

Keywords: verbascoside; hypercholesterolemia; antioxidants

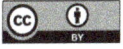

1. Introduction

Cardiovascular disease (CVD) is a pathological process that affects the arterial system as a whole and determines the progressive narrowing of the arteries, up to their complete obstruction. Therefore, it must be considered a unique disease that manifests itself clinically in different ways, depending on which arterial district is concerned. In Western countries, it still represents the main cause of death and an important contribution to disability. The prevalence of CVD cases nearly doubled from 1990 to 2019, and the number of CVD deaths in the same period has steadily increased [1].

The principal risk factors converge on an unhealthy diet, typical of industrialized countries, with consequent dyslipidemia, diabetes, obesity and hypertension. Additional factors include a sedentary lifestyle, stress and smoking, which, unfortunately, are still widespread. High levels of low-density lipoprotein cholesterol (LDL-C) are one of the main modifiable cardiovascular risk factors (CVRF) [1]. Indeed, LDL-C and other cholesterol-rich apolipoprotein-B-containing lipoproteins, including very low-density lipoproteins (VLDL) and their remnants, intermediate-density lipoproteins (IDL) and lipoprotein (a), play a pivotal role in the development of atherosclerotic plaques since, in high concentrations, they accumulate within the arterial intima [2]. At this site they are separated from plasma antioxidants and become particularly susceptible to oxidative alterations, acquiring proinflammatory and immunogenic properties. Although advanced lesions can grow enough to arrest blood flow, the main clinical complication is an acute obstruction due to a thrombus development [3,4]. LDL-C concentration is closely linked to the incidence of atherosclerotic CVD, such as myocardial infarction and ischemic stroke [2].

Evaluation of the cumulative effect of the various CVRF and estimation of atherosclerotic CVD risk is crucial to the implementation of prevention programs. Recent guidelines of the European Society of Cardiology (ESC) and the European Atherosclerosis Society (EAS) for the management of dyslipidemias provide Systematic Coronary Risk Evaluation (SCORE) charts, which indicate the risk of developing atherosclerotic CVD over the next ten years. The risk is calculated considering age, sex, smoking status, systolic blood pressure and total cholesterol (TC). They also recommend new LDL-C treatment goals based on cardiovascular risk categories (<116, 100, 70 and 55 mg/dL for low, moderate, high, and very high risk, respectively). The guidelines point out the importance of adopting and sustaining a healthy lifestyle, and preventative action for a person should be related to the total risk: the higher the risk, the more intense the action. In some cases, unfortunately, prevention is not sufficient and it is necessary to resort to the use of pharmacologic therapy [5]. The backbone drugs for hypercholesterolemia are statins. Their mechanism of action is focused on the competitive inhibition of the 3-hydroxy-3methyl-glutaryl coenzyme A (HMG-CoA) reductase, which regulates the limiting step of the synthesis of cholesterol at the level of hepatocytes; this leads to a reduction in cholesterol synthesis and an increase in LDL receptors at the level of liver cells, with a consequent further reduction in the plasma cholesterol. They produce several other effects termed as pleiotropic effects of statins [6]. If they are contraindicated, cholesterol-absorption inhibitors and bile-acid-binding resins can be used. In case of failure, an association therapy or monoclonal antibodies anti-proprotein convertase subtilisin/kexin type 9 or bempedoic acid can be assessed [5]. However, these drugs are not free of adverse effects: gastrointestinal disorders, myalgias, arthralgias, transaminases/creatine phosphokinase (CPK) elevation and rhabdomyolysis are common [7]. The guidelines also suggest a nutraceutical approach (that can or cannot include statins) which could help treat hypercholesterolemia whilst avoiding every possible side effect [8].

In the last few years attention was paid to several plants' natural molecules, some of which can improve lipid profile and oxidative status [9,10]. *Lippia citriodora* (lemon verbena) is a plant from the Verbenaceae family, which grows spontaneously in South America and is cultivated in North Africa and South Europe. It is mainly used as a spice, but also as a medicinal plant possessing digestive, antispasmodic, antipyretic, anti-inflammatory, antioxidant, anxiolytic, neuroprotective, anticancer, anesthetic, antimicrobial and sedative properties. Leaf infusions have traditionally been used to treat cold, fever, colic, diarrhea, nerve problems, acne, insomnia and rheumatism [11]. The medicinal effects are due to a large number of polar compounds present in the plant: phenylpropanoids glycosides (a large group of natural polyphenols, one of the best known is the verbascoside, also called acteoside), flavonoids, phenolic acids and iridoid glycosides. Verbascoside is structurally characterized by a caffeic acid moiety and a 3,4-hydroxyphenylethanol ethyl moiety (hydroxytyrosol), bound to β-(D)-glucopyranoside through ester and glycosidic links, respectively, with a rhamnose in sequence (1–3) to the glucose molecule [12].

The biological activities of *Lippia citriodora* were proven in cell culture, animal studies and a small number of human clinical trials [11]. The plant also showed a marked improvement in blood lipid profile in some animal species such as rabbit [13], hare [14], horse [15], sheep [16] and donkey [17]. However, the plant has not been fully assessed regarding its safety and efficacy in humans.

In the present study we investigated the effect of a *Lippia citriodora* leaf extract on lipid and oxidative blood profile of hypercholesterolemic adult volunteers, to identify its therapeutic benefits in human dyslipidemia.

2. Materials and Methods

2.1. Study Design and Participants

This was a preliminary, open-label, single-arm, phase I clinical study conducted on 12 hypercholesterolemic volunteers (average age 58 ± 9.02 years) whose characteristics are described in Table 1.

Table 1. Baseline characteristics of the analyzed subjects.

ID	SEX	AGE (Years)	SMOKE	BMI (kg/m^2)	GLU (mg/dL)	BP (mmHg)	TC (mg/dL)	LDL-C (mg/dL)	SCORE
1	M	60	No	24.8	104	135/85	212	140.00	3%
2	M	68	Yes	25.4	102	150/90	210	120.00	13%
3	M	65	Yes	23.3	124	120/80	236	131.00	7%
4	M	63	No	22.9	101	120/70	220	129.00	3%
5	F	44	No	34.2	83	120/70	261	168.00	0%
6	M	57	Yes	44.9	91	140/90	229	168.00	5%
7	F	59	Yes	26.9	106	130/80	274	180.00	3%
8	M	67	No	24.4	110	140/80	214	149.00	6%
9	M	53	Yes	23.6	93	120/80	224	134.00	2%
10	F	56	No	25.8	97	120/80	231	130.00	1%
11	F	39	No	33.3	101	125/70	332	230.00	0%
12	F	65	Yes	20.1	90	150/110	248	178.00	7%

M, male; F, female; BMI, body mass index; GLU, glucose; BP, blood pressure; TC, total cholesterol; LDL-C, low-density lipoprotein cholesterol; SCORE, Systematic Coronary Risk Evaluation.

All subjects were evaluated by an accurate anamnesis and complete physical examination. Eligibility criteria were: age from 30 to 85 years, LDL-C > 116 mg/dL, CPK and transaminases normal values, with either an intolerance or hypersensitivity to statins. The participants also had to promise not to change eating habits and not to consume products with similar activity to *Lippia citriodora* during the study period. Exclusion criteria were: triglycerides (TG) > 500 mg/dL, type 1 and type 2 diabetes, chronic kidney disease, uncontrolled hypo- or hyperthyroidism, clinical conditions affecting the absorption of the product or adherence to the study (gastrointestinal diseases, neoplastic diseases, metabolic deficits), pregnancy or breastfeeding, a history of major cardiovascular events (acute myocardial infarction or stroke), severe peripheral atherosclerotic disease and arterial revascularization, intake of immunosuppressive agents in the previous 3 months, intake of glucocorticoids or drugs for lipid profile and body weight control and intolerance or hypersensitivity, or both, to one or more of the substances in the study. For all subjects, the 10-year risk of fatal CVD based on age, gender, smoking status, systolic blood pressure and TC (SCORE chart, low-risk regions of Europe) [5] was calculated. Each subject took a capsule containing 100 mg of *Lippia citriodora* leaf extract once a day for 16 weeks. The dosage was established based on previous animal studies [15] employing up to 1.0 mg of verbascoside per kg of metabolic body weight. Considering an average weight of 70 kg for an adult (corresponding to a metabolic weight of about 24 kg) and the percentage of phenylpropanoids (23%, consisting mainly of verbascoside) contained in the leaf extract, a 100 mg/day dose was calculated.

The study was conducted in accordance with the ethical principles stated in the Declaration of Helsinki, and the approved national and international guidelines for human research. The Institutional Review Board of the University of Molise, Campobasso, Italy, reviewed and approved this study (protocol code 006-08-2018; 2 August 2018). Written informed consent was obtained from each participant. All clinical information relating to patients has been stored and processed for statistical purposes in compliance with current privacy protection legislation.

2.2. Lippia citriodora Leaf Extract

Lippia citriodora leaf extract containing 23% phenylpropanoids (PLX23) was provided by Monteloeder (Monteloeder, Ltd., Elche, Spain). The quantitative analysis of the phenolic compounds was performed by high-performance liquid chromatography (HPLC) and reported in a manufacturer's certificate of analysis. The plant is approved for use in humans by the Italian Ministry of Public Health, Rome, Italy.

2.3. Blood Collection

Blood samples were obtained from the antecubital vein, after overnight fasting, in vacutainer tubes at weeks 0, 4, 8 and 16, respectively. Timing for data collection and total treatment time were established based on previous animal studies [13,15]. The first evaluation, at 4 weeks, was carried out in order to identify any early muscular or hepatic alterations. Blood was centrifuged at $1500 \times g$ for 10 min. Serum was used to determine the following analytes: TC, high-density lipoprotein cholesterol (HDL-C), LDL-C, TG, glucose (GLU), CPK, aspartate aminotransferase (AST) and alanine aminotransferase (ALT), using a semiautomatic clinical chemistry analyzer (ARCO Biotecnica Instruments SPA, Rome, Italy). Oxidative state markers were measured in the plasma. Total oxidant status (TOS), which measures the blood antioxidant capacity, was determined using an assay based on the oxidation of ferrous ion to ferric ion in the presence of various oxidant species in acidic medium and ferric ion measurement by xylenol orange [18]. The results were expressed in μM H_2O_2 equivalent per liter. Reactive oxygen metabolites (ROM), i.e., the concentration of hydroperoxides in the plasma, were determined using a free radicals (FR) determination system (D-Roms test, Diacron International srl, Grosseto, Italy). The test is based on transition metals' ability to catalyze in the presence of peroxides with the formation of FR, which are trapped by an alchilamine. The alchilamine reacts, forming a colored radical detectable at 505 nm [19]. The results were expressed as U Carr (1 Unit Carratelli corresponds to 0.024 mmol/L of H_2O_2; the higher the value measured, the greater the oxidative stress in the blood). Ferric ion reducing antioxidant power (FRAP) test measured the ferric-reducing ability of plasma. Ferric to ferrous ion reduction at low pH led to the formation of a colored ferrous-tripyridyltriazine complex. FRAP values were obtained by comparing the absorbance change at 593 nm in test reaction mixtures with those containing ferrous ions in known concentrations [20]. One FRAP unit is expressed in mmol TEAC/L (TEAC, Trolox equivalent antioxidant capacity; the higher the value obtained, the better the blood antioxidant capacity). Malondialdehyde (MDA), the ultimate product of all oxidative processes involving polyunsaturated fatty acids, was determined spectrophotometrically, according to the thiobarbituric acid (TBA) assay [21]. Vitamin E and vitamin A were extracted from plasma samples with chloroform and analyzed on an HPLC system consisting of an autosampler (HPLC Autosampler 360, Kontron Instruments, Milan, Italy) with a 20 mL loop, a high-pressure mixing pump and a 5 µm, 250 × 4.60 mm C18 column (Phenomenex, Torrance, CA, USA). The mobile phase was 100% methanol at a flow rate of 1.0 mL/min. A fluorimeter detector (SFM) and computer with Kroma System 2000 software were used. The concentrations of vitamins A and E were determined by using an internal standard and the elution time of pure standards [22].

2.4. Statistical Analysis

Data were analyzed using SPSS (v. 17.0) statistical software package (SPSS Inc., Chicago, IL, USA). Variables were examined for outliers and extreme values using box and normal quantile-quantile plots, and Shapiro—Wilk's and Kolmogorov—Smirnov's tests. No variables needed to be transformed. Repeated measures analysis of variance (ANOVA) and post hoc pairwise comparison tests, namely least significant difference (LSD) and Bonferroni's correction (BC), were used. The assumptions of sphericity were assessed by means of Mauchly's test. The Greenhouse—Geisser or the Huynh—Feldt correction was applied if the assumption of sphericity was violated. Statistical significance was set at p value < 0.05.

3. Results

Using repeated measures ANOVA, the lipid blood profile showed a weak significant reduction in TC ($p = 0.035$) and a strong significant increase in HDL-C ($p = 0.007$) levels during treatment with *Lippia citriodora* leaf extract, as reported in Table 2.

Table 2. Blood parameters of 12 volunteers at baseline and after 4, 8 and 16 weeks of *Lippia citriodora* extract treatment.

	BASELINE	4 WEEKS	8 WEEKS	16 WEEKS	ANOVAF (df = 3, 33)	p Value
TC	240.9 ± 10.1	236.2 ± 11.4	229.2 ± 9.9 *	227.0 ± 10.2 *	3.22	0.035
HDL-C	56.6 ± 2.7	59.1 ± 2.3	62.7 ± 3.3 *	56.8 ± 3.2	4.78	0.007
LDL-C	154.7 ± 9.1	147.7 ± 9.2	143.7 ± 7.7 *	144.1 ± 7.6 *	2.56	0.072
TG	139.8 ± 11.3	121.4 ± 12.6	111.8 ± 12.3 *	119.8 ± 13.1	2.10	0.119
GLU	100.2 ± 3.1	96.3 ± 2.8 *	88.7 ± 2.3 *	89.4 ± 2.9 *	10.11	0.002
CPK	111.7 ± 12.2	107.2 ± 14.9	107.7 ± 18.9	113.7 ± 18.4	0.32	0.321
AST	25.7 ± 2.9	21.8 ± 1.6	23.2 ± 2.8	21.0 ± 1.8	0.96	0.423
ALT	30.7 ± 5.3	24.8 ± 4.2	26.9 ± 3.6	22.3 ± 1.6	1.78	0.169
TOS	13.4 ± 0.9	12.9 ± 0.7 *	12.3 ± 0.6 *	11.5 ± 0.6 *	7.42	0.012
ROM	306.5 ± 18.3	267.8 ± 7.6 *	255.3 ± 4.9 *	271.4 ± 21.3	2.99	0.069
MDA	8.1 ± 0.5	6.1 ± 0.5 *	4.4 ± 0.4 *	3.7 ± 0.2 *	35.23	<0.001
FRAP	0.8 ± 0.04	0.9 ± 0.05 *	0.9 ± 0.06 *	0.9 ± 0.06 *	8.13	0.002
Vit E	20.3 ± 1.4	23.9 ± 1.2 *	25.2 ± 1.3 *	26.2 ± 1.3 *	27.08	<0.001
Vit A	1.2 ± 0.06	1.3 ± 0.07 *	1.4 ± 0.07 *	1.8 ± 0.14 *	13.88	0.002

TC, total cholesterol (mg/dL); HDL-C, high-density lipoprotein cholesterol (mg/dL); LDL-C, low-density lipoprotein cholesterol (mg/dL); TG, triglycerides (mg/dL); GLU, glucose (mg/dL); CPK, creatine phosphokinase (U/L); AST, aspartate transaminase (U/L); ALT, alanine transaminase (U/L); TOS, total oxidant status (μmol H_2O_2 Eq/L); ROM, reactive oxygen metabolites (U Carr); MDA, malondialdehyde (nmol/mL); FRAP, ferric reducing ability of plasma (mmol TEAC/L); Vit E, vitamin E (μmol/L); Vit A, vitamin A (μmol/L). Values are mean ± standard deviation; * significantly different compared with baseline (least significant difference).

Post hoc LSD pairwise comparisons showed a weak reduction in TC at 8 weeks ($p = 0.043$), not significant after BC, and a strong reduction ($p = 0.016$, after BC) at 16 weeks of treatment (Figure 1a). HDL-C significantly increased ($p = 0.026$, after BC) only after 8 weeks of treatment (Figure 1b). LDL-C showed a reduction at the limit of significance ($p = 0.072$) during the treatment (Table 2). Post hoc LSD pairwise comparison (Figure 1c) showed a weak reduction at 8 ($p = 0.036$) and 16 weeks ($p = 0.033$), not significant after BC. TG levels showed a not significant downward trend after treatment (Table 2). However, post hoc LSD pairwise comparison (Figure 1d) showed a fairly good reduction at 8 weeks ($p = 0.016$), not significant after BC ($p = 0.098$). GLU levels showed a significant reduction ($p = 0.002$) during the treatment (Table 2), particularly at 8 and 16 weeks (Figure 1e). However, the reduction at 16 weeks was at the limit of significance ($p = 0.056$) after BC.

The results related to the oxidative state markers differences during the treatment with *Lippia citriodora* leaf extract showed a global improvement of the oxidative blood profile. In fact, TOS levels were significantly reduced ($p = 0.012$, after correction for lack of sphericity), after treatment. Post hoc LSD pairwise comparisons showed a reduction at 4, 8 and 16 weeks (Figure 2a); however, only the reduction at 16 weeks was at the limit of significance ($p = 0.068$) after BC. ROM levels were weakly reduced ($p = 0.069$, after correction for lack of sphericity), after treatment. Post hoc LSD pairwise comparisons showed a weak reduction at 4 weeks ($p = 0.021$), not significant after BC, and a stronger reduction ($p = 0.009$) at 8 weeks of treatment (Figure 2b), which was at the limit of significance ($p = 0.055$) after BC. MDA levels were significantly decreased (Table 2) at 4, 8 and 16 weeks of treatment (Figure 2c), even after BC. Conversely, FRAP, vitamin E and vitamin A levels were significantly increased (Table 2) at 4, 8 and 16 weeks of treatment (Figure 2d–f), even after BC, with the exception of FRAP and vitamin A levels at 4 weeks which were at the limit of significance ($p = 0.050$ and $p = 0.061$, respectively). LSD pairwise comparison did not show significant differences between women and men for any of the measured parameters.

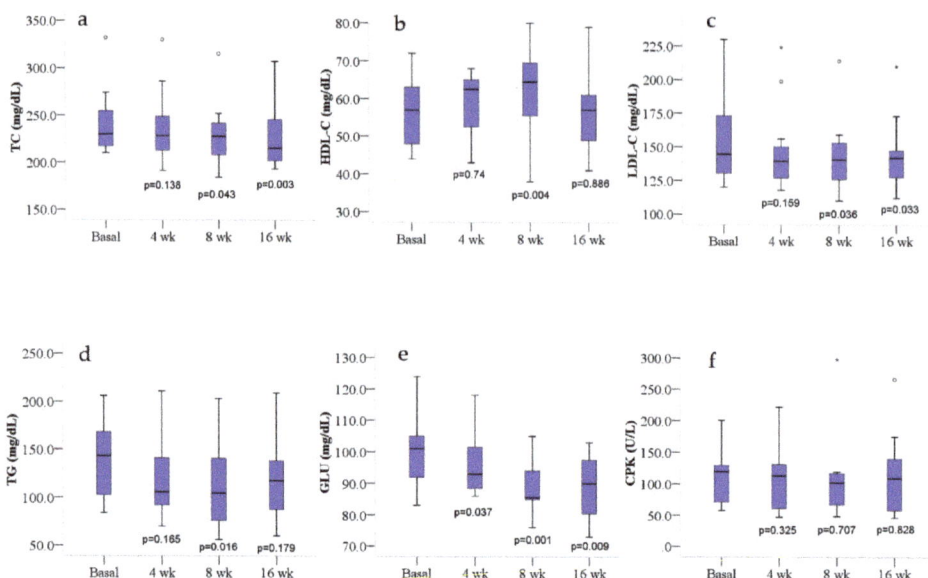

Figure 1. Lipids, glucose and CPK blood profile at basal level and after 4, 8 and 16 weeks of treatment. Box plots show median (horizontal line in the box), 25th and 75th percentiles (edges of box), maximum and minimum values (whiskers) and outliers (°, *) of: (**a**) total cholesterol (TC), (**b**) high-density lipoprotein cholesterol (HDL-C), (**c**) low-density lipoprotein cholesterol (LDL-C), (**d**) triglycerides (TG), (**e**) glucose (GLU) and (**f**) creatine phosphokinase (CPK) concentrations. *p* values measure the significance of differences compared with basal values (least significant difference); wk, weeks.

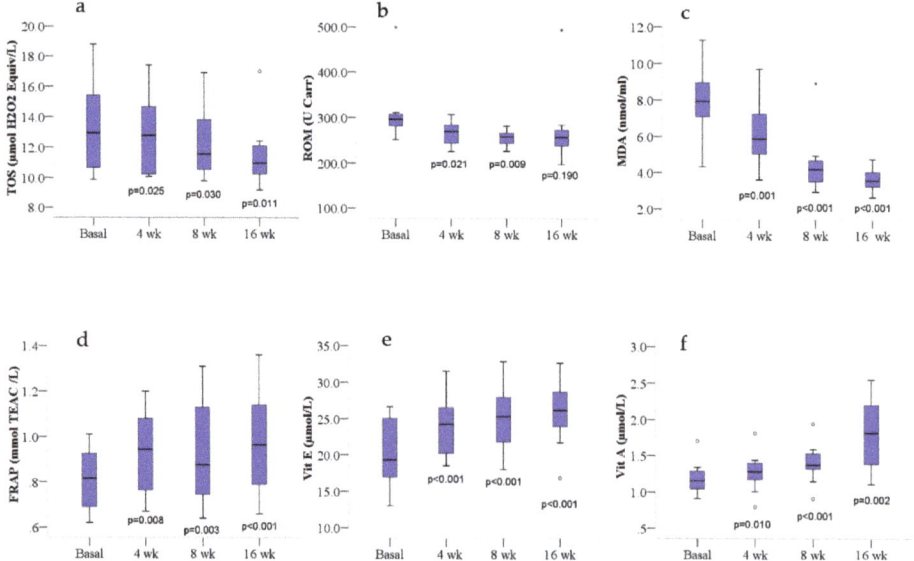

Figure 2. Blood oxidative profile at basal level and after 4, 8 and 16 weeks of treatment. Box plots show median (horizontal line in the box), 25th and 75th percentiles (edges of box), maximum and minimum values (whiskers) and outliers (°, *) of: (**a**) total oxidant status (TOS), (**b**) reactive oxygen metabolites (ROM), (**c**) malondialdehyde (MDA), (**d**) ferric reducing ability of plasma (FRAP), (**e**) vitamin E (Vit E) and (**f**) vitamin A (Vit A) concentrations. *p* values measure the significance of differences compared with basal values (least significant difference); wk, weeks.

To highlight possible adverse events concerning the intake of the extract, some analytes were also measured to check for potential organ damage (AST, ALT), as well as the serum levels of CPK (whose values increase in patients taking statins) to evaluate problems affecting skeletal muscle tissue. No significant variations were observed regarding the CPK and transaminase (AST and ALT) levels (Table 2 and Figure 1f), and no side or adverse effects were reported by participants.

4. Discussion

In the present study, we analyzed the lipid and oxidative profile changes induced by treatment with *Lippia citriodora* leaf extract (100 mg, once a day, for 16 weeks) in 12 hypercholesterolemic volunteers (7 males and 5 females). Results showed an improvement in blood lipid profile, compared with baselines, with a significant decrease in TC, particularly at 16 weeks, and a significant increase in HDL-C at 8 weeks. Additionally, TG and LDL-C showed a downward trend at 8 weeks and at both 8 and 16 weeks, respectively. These results are broadly in line with previous studies reporting significant changes on the lipid profile after dietary supplementation with a *Lippia citriodora* extract. Rabbits [13], hares [14], horses [15] and sheep [16] treated with low and high doses of verbascoside showed a decrease in TC, LDL-C, (not measured in the hare study), TG and an elevation in HDL-C compared with control groups, who received a feed without verbascoside. Higher doses of dietary supplementation with verbascoside generally produced better effects than lower doses did, but the differences were not statistically significant. Yang et al. [23] evaluated the effects of *Ligustrum robustum* Blume (LR), a plant used in Chinese folk medicine for the treatment of obesity and hyperlipidemia, in mice fed with a high-fat diet. LR leaf extracts, mainly containing phenylpropanoid glycosides with verbascoside as a major active component, produced a significant reduction in TC and a downward trend in TG levels, without a significant dose—effect relation. Kassi et al. [24] carried out a randomized placebo-controlled trial in normocholesterolemic healthy volunteers. Following the administration of an aqueous extract of *Sideritis euboea* (containing verbascoside, flavonoid diglycosides and phenolic acid), at 0.3 g/day for a month, the intervention group showed a significant reduction in TC, compared with the control group.

The hypocholesterolemic effect of the *Lippia citriodora* extract can be explained by some of the molecular mechanisms related to verbascoside, namely a downregulation of the mRNA-encoding enzymes involved in cholesterol biosynthesis, such as HMG-CoA reductase and mevalonate kinase, and an upregulation of the mRNA encoding molecules involved in lipid transport and metabolism, such as VLDL receptor, lipoprotein lipase (LPL), lipin 1, peroxisome proliferator activated receptor-alpha (PPARα), acetyl CoA acyl transferases (Acaa1a and Acaa1b) and carnitine palmitoyl transferase 1A (Cpt1a) [25]. PPARα is known to be able to modulate the production of the apoproteins ApoA-1 and ApoA-2 (the main constituents of HDL-C) and this could be directly related to HDL-C concentration [26]. Furthermore, using HepG2 cells treated with a high concentration of oleic acid as a lipid accumulation model, it has been shown that verbascoside is also able to downregulate the expression of 7-dehydrocholesterol reductase (DHCR7), lanosterol synthase (LSS) and farnesyl-diphosphate farnesyltransferase 1 (FDFT1), which are involved in cholesterol biosynthesis, and to increase the expression of HDL scavenger receptors class B member 1 and 2 (SCARB1 and SCARB2) [27]. SCARB1 is the primary receptor involved in the transfer of circulating cholesterol from HDL to the liver, termed as the reverse cholesterol transport pathway, ending with the excretion of cholesterol via bile and feces [28].

According to these findings, we can assume that the TC and LDL-C decrease seen in our study is probably due to a reduction in cholesterol biosynthesis and to an increase in lipid β-oxidation, whereas the HDL-C elevation at 8 weeks is likely related to PPARα upregulation. The return of HDL-C levels to baseline values at 16 weeks may be caused by overexpression of SCARB1, which causes an increased hepatic metabolism and clearance of HDL-C [28]. However, the reduction in circulating HDL-C seems to have a beneficial effect against atherosclerosis. Indeed, whole-body SCARB1 knockout (KO) (Sr-bl$^{-/-}$) mice showed an increase in HDL-C with a significant rise in aortic lesions, proving that SCARB1 deficiency is proatherogenic. Conversely, overexpression of SCARB1 in mouse models reduces atherosclerosis [28].

The increased PPARα and LPL expression may also explain the downward trend in TG in the present study [26].

Verbascoside also prevents the formation of oxidized LDL-C (oxLDL), lowers the expression of genes related to oxidative stress and oxLDL-mediated inflammatory response and protects endothelial cells from oxLDL-induced cytotoxicity [29]. The accumulation of oxLDL in the arterial intima contributes significantly to the recruitment of monocytes and the formation of "foam cells" (early atherosclerotic lesions composed of cholesterol-engorged macrophages) [4]. Considering the crucial role of oxLDL in the pathogenesis of atherosclerotic plaques, we can presume that circulant LDL-C in subjects treated with *Lippia citriodora* is less atherogenic as it is less oxidized.

Treatment with *Lippia citriodora* leaf extract in the present study also improved the oxidative status with a significant decrease in TOS and MDA, a downward trend in ROM and a significant increase in FRAP, vitamin E and vitamin A. Carrera-Quintanar et al. [30] underlined the benefits of *Lippia citriodora* extract on the oxidative stress induced by aerobic training in university students. Indeed, verbascoside was able to increase the activity of the main antioxidant enzymes like catalase, glutathione peroxidase and glutathione reductase [30], probably acting at the post-transcriptional level or through a Nrf2-related mechanism [29]. A marked improvement in blood oxidative status has also been detected in some animal species, such as rabbit [13], hare [14], horse [15], sheep [16] and donkey [17], resulting in a decrease in plasma ROM and thiobarbituric acid-reactive substances values, and an increase in the concentrations of plasma vitamin E and vitamin A. Generally, high doses of verbascoside produced better effects than low doses, but the differences were not statistically significant.

Similarly, a study using animal models showed a decrease in oxidative stress-correlated enzyme activity in the plasma, brain and hippocampus, as well as a decrease in cerebral MDA, after verbascoside administration [31]. The elevation of vitamin E and vitamin A, both concurring to the improvement of blood antioxidant power [32], is likely due to verbascoside influence on the stability of low molecular weight molecules such as these vitamins [15]. Vitamin A (through retinol and β-carotene) and vitamin E (through α-Tocopherol) protect cell membranes from lipid peroxidation, acting as chain-breaking antioxidants. They also act as scavengers of hydroxyl radicals, superoxide anions and peroxynitrite [32].

Flavonoids and phenolic acids present in *Lippia citriodora* may also be responsible for the antioxidant phenotype [33]. The enhanced blood antioxidant capacity is beneficial for endothelial function, since oxidant stimuli cause an imbalance in vasoconstrictor, prothrombotic, proliferative and inflammatory pathways and this phenotype is characteristic of chronic inflammatory diseases such as atherosclerosis [34]. Some studies show that verbascoside also has a vasodilator action, inhibiting the contractions induced by noradrenaline [35], and an anti-inflammatory effect since it is able to inhibit downstream proinflammatory cytokines and growth factors [29,36].

Another beneficial effect of *Lippia citriodora* treatment in the present study was the significant improvement of the glycemic profile. Indeed, verbascoside can suppress postprandial glucose peak and normalize glucose tolerance, likely due to inhibition of sodium-dependent glucose co-transporter 1 (SGLUT-1). In addition to verbascoside, iridoids present in the extract also have an antidiabetic activity [35].

Overall, the results of this study suggest that *Lippia citriodora*, through its compounds such as verbascoside, flavonoids, phenolic acids and iridoids, has pleiotropic effects similar to statins; it acts not only on lipid profile, but also on lipoprotein oxidation, endothelial function and inflammatory status. Its notable polypharmacological effects could represent a valuable nutraceutical approach for the management of hypercholesterolemia and the prevention of CVD. Unlike statins, however, the safety and tolerability profile of

Lippia citriodora treatment seems more favorable, since transaminases and CPK were not altered and no subjects reported side or adverse effects. These findings are in line with previous studies showing that supplementation with *Lippia citriodora* extract decreases the signs of muscular damage in chronic running exercise, without blocking the cellular adaptation to exercise [37].

We are aware that the present study has several limitations: the number of participants is small, the study is open-label, a control group is missing and follow-up information is lacking. This is motivated by the fact that our intention was to perform a pilot, preliminary study aimed at verifying whether the beneficial effects of *Lippia citriodora* on the lipid and oxidative blood profile demonstrated in previous animal studies were also present in humans. A randomized, placebo-controlled, multiple dose, double-blind clinical trial, eventually including sex- and age-matched participants without hypercholesterolemia, is certainly needed to evaluate the safety and efficacy of this plant extract.

5. Conclusions

In conclusion, this preliminary study demonstrated that dietary supplementation with *Lippia citriodora* extract can improve the lipid profile, particularly by reducing TC and increasing HDL-C, and enhance the blood antioxidant power, particularly by reducing TOS and MDA and increasing FRAP and vitamins A and E. These results suggest that *Lippia citriodora* could be a valuable natural compound for the management of dyslipidemia and the prevention of CVD. Clinical trials of phase II and III are necessary to confirm these findings.

Author Contributions: Conceptualization, A.D.C., D.C. and C.C.; methodology, F.V. and M.P.; formal analysis, A.D.C.; investigation, F.V. and M.P.; writing—original draft preparation, A.A. and D.L.; writing—review and editing, A.D.C., A.A. and C.C.; visualization, A.A. and D.L.; supervision, A.D.C. and D.C.; project administration, A.D.C. and D.C. All authors have read and agreed to the published version of the manuscript.

Funding: This research received no external funding.

Institutional Review Board Statement: The study was conducted according to the guidelines of the Declaration of Helsinki, and approved by the Institutional Review Board of University of Molise, Campobasso, Italy (protocol code 006-08-2018; 2 August 2018).

Informed Consent Statement: Informed consent was obtained from all subjects involved in the study.

Data Availability Statement: All data are presented in the paper.

Acknowledgments: This article is based upon work from COST Action NutRedOx-CA16112 supported by COST (European Cooperation in Science and Technology). The authors are grateful to Santina Ciccotelli for her valuable assistance.

Conflicts of Interest: The authors declare no conflict of interest.

References

1. Roth, G.A.; Mensah, G.A.; Johnson, C.O.; Addolorato, G.; Ammirati, E.; Baddour, L.M.; Barengo, N.C.; Beaton, A.Z.; Benjamin, E.J.; Benziger, C.P.; et al. Global Burden of Cardiovascular Diseases and Risk Factors, 1990–2019: Update From the GBD 2019 Study. *J. Am. Coll. Cardiol.* **2020**, *76*, 2982–3021. [CrossRef] [PubMed]
2. Ference, B.A.; Ginsberg, H.N.; Graham, I.; Ray, K.K.; Packard, C.J.; Bruckert, E.; Hegele, R.A.; Krauss, R.M.; Raal, F.J.; Schunkert, H.; et al. Low-density lipoproteins cause atherosclerotic cardiovascular disease. 1. Evidence from genetic, epidemiologic, and clinical studies. A consensus statement fromthe European Atherosclerosis Society Consensus Panel. *Eur. Heart J.* **2017**, *38*, 2459–2472. [CrossRef] [PubMed]
3. Lusis, A.J. Atherosclerosis. *Nature* **2000**, *407*, 233–241. [CrossRef] [PubMed]
4. Libby, P.; Buring, J.E.; Badimon, L.; Hansson, G.K.; Deanfield, J.; Bittencourt, M.S.; Tokgözoğlu, L.; Lewis, E.F. Atherosclerosis. *Nat. Rev. Dis. Prim.* **2019**, *5*, 1–18. [CrossRef] [PubMed]
5. Mach, F.; Baigent, C.; Catapano, A.L.; Koskinas, K.C.; Casula, M.; Badimon, L.; Chapman, M.J.; De Backer, G.G.; Delgado, V.; Ference, B.A.; et al. 2019 ESC/EAS Guidelines for the management of dyslipidaemias: Lipid modification to reduce cardiovascular risk. *Eur. Heart J.* **2020**, *41*, 111–188. [CrossRef] [PubMed]

6. Oesterle, A.; Laufs, U.; Liao, J.K. Pleiotropic Effects of Statins on the Cardiovascular System. *Circ. Res.* **2017**, *120*, 229–243. [CrossRef] [PubMed]
7. Golomb, B.A.; Evans, M.A. Statin adverse effects: A review of the literature and evidence for a mitochondrial mechanism. *Am. J. Cardiovasc. Drugs* **2008**, *8*, 373–418. [CrossRef] [PubMed]
8. Santini, A.; Novellino, E. Nutraceuticals in hypercholesterolaemia: An overview. *Br. J. Pharmacol.* **2017**, *174*, 1450–1463. [CrossRef] [PubMed]
9. Pronin, A.V.; Danilov, L.L.; Narovlyansky, A.N.; Sanin, A.V. Plant polyisoprenoids and control of cholesterol level. *Arch. Immunol. Ther. Exp.* **2014**, *62*, 31–39. [CrossRef] [PubMed]
10. Cabral, C.E.; Klein, M.R.S.T. Phytosterols in the treatment of hypercholesterolemia and prevention of cardiovascular diseases. *Arq. Bras. Cardiol.* **2017**, *109*, 475–482. [CrossRef] [PubMed]
11. Bahramsoltani, R.; Rostamiasrabadi, P.; Shahpiri, Z.; Marques, A.M.; Rahimi, R.; Farzaei, M.H. Aloysia citrodora Paláu (Lemon verbena): A review of phytochemistry and pharmacology. *J. Ethnopharmacol.* **2018**, *222*, 34–51. [CrossRef]
12. D'Imperio, M.; Cardinali, A.; D'Antuono, I.; Linsalata, V.; Minervini, F.; Redan, B.W.; Ferruzzi, M.G. Stability-activity of verbascoside, a known antioxidant compound, at different pH conditions. *Food Res. Int.* **2014**, *66*, 373–378. [CrossRef]
13. Casamassima, D.; Palazzo, M.; Vizzarri, F.; Ondruska, L.; Massanyi, P.; Corino, C. Effect of dietary Lippia citriodora extract on reproductive and productive performance and plasma biochemical parameters in rabbit does. *Anim. Prod. Sci.* **2017**, *57*, 65–73. [CrossRef]
14. Palazzo, M.; Vizzarri, F.; Cinone, M.; Corino, C.; Casamassima, D. Assessment of a natural dietary extract, titrated in phenylpropanoid glycosides, on blood parameters and plasma oxidative status in intensively reared Italian hares (Lepus corsicanus). *Animal* **2011**, *5*, 844–850. [CrossRef]
15. Palazzo, M.; Vizzarri, F.; Cinone, M.; D'Alessandro, A.G.; Martemucci, G.; Casamassima, D. Dietary effect of lemon verbena extract on selected blood parameters and on plasma oxidative profile in Avelignese horses. *Anim. Sci. J.* **2019**, *90*, 222–228. [CrossRef] [PubMed]
16. Casamassima, D.; Palazzo, M.; Martemucci, G.; Vizzarri, F.; Corino, C. Effects of verbascoside on plasma oxidative status and blood and milk production parameters during the peripartum period in Lacaune ewes. *Small Rumin. Res.* **2012**, *105*, 1–8. [CrossRef]
17. D'Alessandro, A.G.; Vizzarri, F.; Palazzo, M.; Martemucci, G. Dietary verbascoside supplementation in donkeys: Effects on milk fatty acid profile during lactation, and serum biochemical parameters and oxidative markers. *Animal* **2017**, *11*, 1505–1512. [CrossRef]
18. Erel, O. A new automated colorimetric method for measuring total oxidant status. *Clin. Biochem.* **2005**, *38*, 1103–1111. [CrossRef] [PubMed]
19. Cesarone, M.R.; Belcaro, G.; Carratelli, M.; Cornelli, U.; De Sanctis, M.T.; Incandela, L.; Barsotti, A.; Terranova, R.; Nicolaides, A. A simple test to monitor oxidative stress. *Int. Angiol.* **1999**, *18*, 127–130.
20. Benzie, I.F.F.; Strain, J.J. The ferric reducing ability of plasma (FRAP) as a measure of "antioxidant power": The FRAP assay. *Anal. Biochem.* **1996**, *239*, 70–76. [CrossRef] [PubMed]
21. Esterbauer, H.; Zollern, H. Methods for determination of aldehydic lipid peroxidation products. *Free Radic. Biol. Med.* **1989**, *7*, 197–203. [CrossRef]
22. Zhao, B.; Tham, S.Y.; Lu, J.; Lai, M.H.; Lee, L.K.H.; Moochhala, S.M. Simultaneous determination of vitamins C, E and β-carotene in human plasma by high-performance liquid chromatography with photodiode-array detection. *J. Pharm. Pharm. Sci.* **2004**, *7*, 200–204.
23. Yang, R.M.; Liu, F.; He, Z.D.; Ji, M.; Chu, X.X.; Kang, Z.Y.; Cai, D.Y.; Gao, N.N. Anti-obesity effect of total phenylpropanoid glycosides from Ligustrum robustum Blume in fatty diet-fed mice via up-regulating leptin. *J. Ethnopharmacol.* **2015**, *169*, 459–465. [CrossRef] [PubMed]
24. Kassi, E.; Dimas, C.; Dalamaga, M.; Panagiotou, A.; Papoutsi, Z.; Spilioti, E.; Moutsatsou, P. Sideritis euboea extract lowers total cholesterol but not LDL cholesterol in humans: A randomized controlled trial. *Clin. Lipidol.* **2013**, *8*, 627–634. [CrossRef]
25. Shimoda, H.; Tanaka, J.; Takahara, Y.; Takemoto, K.; Shan, S.J.; Su, M.H. The hypocholesterolemic effects of Cistanche tubulosa extract, a chinese traditional crude medicine, in mice. *Am. J. Chin. Med.* **2009**, *37*, 1125–1138. [CrossRef] [PubMed]
26. Duval, C.; Müller, M.; Kersten, S. PPARα and dyslipidemia. *Biochim. Biophys. Acta Mol. Cell Biol. Lipids* **2007**, *1771*, 961–971. [CrossRef]
27. Sun, L.; Yu, F.; Yi, F.; Xu, L.; Jiang, B.; Le, L.; Xiao, P. Acteoside From Ligustrum robustum (Roxb.) Blume Ameliorates Lipid Metabolism and Synthesis in a HepG2 Cell Model of Lipid Accumulation. *Front. Pharmacol.* **2019**, *10*, 1–9. [CrossRef] [PubMed]
28. Kent, A.P.; Stylianou, I.M. Scavenger receptor class B member 1 protein: Hepatic regulation and its effects on lipids, reverse cholesterol transport, and atherosclerosis. *Hepatic Med. Evid. Res.* **2011**, 29–44. [CrossRef]
29. Alipieva, K.; Korkina, L.; Orhan, I.E.; Georgiev, M.I. Verbascoside—A review of its occurrence, (bio)synthesis and pharmacological significance. *Biotechnol. Adv.* **2014**, *32*, 1065–1076. [CrossRef] [PubMed]
30. Carrera-Quintanar, L.; Funes, L.; Viudes, E.; Tur, J.; Micol, V.; Roche, E.; Pons, A. Antioxidant effect of lemon verbena extracts in lymphocytes of university students performing aerobic training program. *Scand. J. Med. Sci. Sport.* **2012**, *22*, 454–461. [CrossRef]
31. Li, M.; Zhu, Y.; Li, J.; Chen, L.; Tao, W.; Li, X.; Qiu, Y. Effect and mechanism of verbascoside on hypoxic memory injury in plateau. *Phyther. Res.* **2019**, *33*, 2692–2701. [CrossRef]

32. Koekkoek, W.A.C.; Van Zanten, A.R.H. Antioxidant Vitamins and Trace Elements in Critical Illness. *Nutr. Clin. Pract.* **2016**, *31*, 457–474. [CrossRef] [PubMed]
33. de Camargo, A.C.; Regitano-d'Arce, M.A.B.; Rasera, G.B.; Canniatti-Brazaca, S.G.; do Prado-Silva, L.; Alvarenga, V.O.; Sant'Ana, A.S.; Shahidi, F. Phenolic acids and flavonoids of peanut by-products: Antioxidant capacity and antimicrobial effects. *Food Chem.* **2017**, *237*, 538–544. [CrossRef] [PubMed]
34. Daiber, A.; Chlopicki, S. Revisiting pharmacology of oxidative stress and endothelial dysfunction in cardiovascular disease: Evidence for redox-based therapies. *Free Radic. Biol. Med.* **2020**, *157*, 15–37. [CrossRef] [PubMed]
35. Morikawa, T.; Xie, H.; Pan, Y.; Ninomiya, K.; Yuan, D.; Jia, X.; Yoshikawa, M.; Nakamura, S.; Matsuda, H.; Muraoka, O. A review of biologically active natural products from a desert plant cistanche tubulosa. *Chem. Pharm. Bull.* **2019**, *67*, 675–689. [CrossRef] [PubMed]
36. Nigro, O.; Tuzi, A.; Tartaro, T.; Giaquinto, A.; Vallini, I.; Pinotti, G. Biological effects of verbascoside and its anti-inflammatory activity on oral mucositis: A review of the literature. *Anticancer Drugs* **2020**, *31*, 1–5. [CrossRef]
37. Funes, L.; Carrera-Quintanar, L.; Cerdán-Calero, M.; Ferrer, M.D.; Drobnic, F.; Pons, A.; Roche, E.; Micol, V. Effect of lemon verbena supplementation on muscular damage markers, proinflammatory cytokines release and neutrophils' oxidative stress in chronic exercise. *Eur. J. Appl. Physiol.* **2011**, *111*, 695–705. [CrossRef]

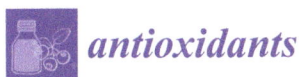

Article

Bioprospection of Natural Sources of Polyphenols with Therapeutic Potential for Redox-Related Diseases

Regina Menezes [1,2,3,†], Alexandre Foito [4,†], Carolina Jardim [2,3], Inês Costa [2,3], Gonçalo Garcia [2,3], Rita Rosado-Ramos [1,2,3], Sabine Freitag [4], Colin James Alexander [5], Tiago Fleming Outeiro [6,7,8], Derek Stewart [4,9] and Cláudia N. Santos [1,2,3,*]

1. CEDOC, Chronic Diseases Research Centre, NOVA Medical School/Faculdade de Ciências Médicas, Universidade NOVA de Lisboa, Campo dos Mártires da Pátria, 130, 1169-056 Lisboa, Portugal; regina.menezes@nms.unl.pt (R.M.); rita.ramos@nms.unl.pt (R.R.-R.)
2. iBET, Instituto de Biologia Experimental e Tecnológica, Apartado 12, 2781-901 Oeiras, Portugal; cjardim@medicina.ulisboa.pt (C.J.); inescosta.bms@gmail.com (I.C.); ggarcia@campus.ul.pt (G.G.)
3. Instituto de Tecnologia Química e Biológica, Universidade Nova de Lisboa, Av. da República, 2780-157 Oeiras, Portugal
4. Environmental and Biochemical Science Group, The James Hutton Institute, Dundee DD2 5DA, UK; alex.foito@hutton.ac.uk (A.F.); Sabine.Freitag@hutton.ac.uk (S.F.); Derek.Stewart@hutton.ac.uk (D.S.)
5. Biomathematics and Statistics Scotland, Invergowrie, Dundee DD2 5DA, UK; Colin.Alexander@hutton.ac.uk
6. Department of Experimental Neurodegeneration, Center for Biostructural Imaging of Neurodegeneration, University Medical Center Goettinge, 37073 Göttingen, Germany; touteir@gwdg.de
7. Max Planck Institute for Experimental Medicine, 37075 Göttingen, Germany
8. Translational and Clinical Research Institute, Faculty of Medical Sciences, Newcastle University, Framlington Place, Newcastle Upon Tyne NE2 4HH, UK
9. School of Engineering and Physical Sciences, Institute of Mechanical, Process and Energy Engineering, Heriot-Watt University, Edinburgh EH14 4AS, UK
* Correspondence: claudia.nunes.santos@nms.unl.pt
† These authors contributed equally to this work.

Received: 22 July 2020; Accepted: 18 August 2020; Published: 26 August 2020

Abstract: Plants are a reservoir of high-value molecules with underexplored biomedical applications. With the aim of identifying novel health-promoting attributes in underexplored natural sources, we scrutinized the diversity of (poly)phenols present within the berries of selected germplasm from cultivated, wild, and underutilized *Rubus* species. Our strategy combined the application of metabolomics, statistical analysis, and evaluation of (poly)phenols' bioactivity using a yeast-based discovery platform. We identified species as sources of (poly)phenols interfering with pathological processes associated with redox-related diseases, particularly, amyotrophic lateral sclerosis, cancer, and inflammation. In silico prediction of putative bioactives suggested cyanidin–hexoside as an anti-inflammatory molecule which was validated in yeast and mammalian cells. Moreover, cellular assays revealed that the cyanidin moiety was responsible for the anti-inflammatory properties of cyanidin–hexoside. Our findings unveiled novel (poly)phenolic bioactivities and illustrated the power of our integrative approach for the identification of dietary (poly)phenols with potential biomedical applications.

Keywords: bioactivity-based assays; cyanidin; metabolomics; *Rubus* genus; (poly)phenols; yeast-based discovery platform

1. Introduction

Plants synthesize a staggering variety of secondary metabolites that provide a chemically diverse pool of high-value small molecules with potential application for human health that cannot be matched by any synthetic libraries [1]. The use of plants in traditional medicine dates back to antiquity and is still, despite huge investments into combinatorial chemistry and high-throughput screens, an important source of novel drugs and metabolites with a myriad of underexplored pharmacological and biotechnological applications [2]. From conventional folk medicine to the scientific validation of protective properties, (poly)phenolic compounds have been implicated and/or identified as underpinning the beneficial health properties of several plants.

Rubus is a large and diverse genus of the Rosaceae family comprising more than 250 species with the most commonly known being red and black raspberries and blackberries. These fruits are characterized by their high polyphenolic content and diversity, which make them a major source of (poly)phenols with potential importance for human health. This includes redox-related diseases, such as neurodegeneration and cancer, which is consistent with the well-described role of (poly)phenols in targeting signaling pathways regulating redox homeostasis. Besides sharing oxidative stress and chronic inflammation as common pathological processes, neurodegenerative diseases (NDs) are also known as conformational disorders, as they are associated with protein misfolding and aggregation [3,4] in a process thought to lead to neuronal death. Alzheimer's disease (AD) pathology is associated to the accumulation of Aβ42 amyloid plaques [5] and hyperphosphorylated tau neurofibrillary tangles [6]. The accumulation of concentric hyaline cytoplasmic inclusions of α-synuclein (αSyn), known as Lewy bodies (LBs), is the major pathological hallmark of Parkinson's disease (PD) and other LB diseases [7,8]. Proteotoxic aggregates in neuronal cells of Huntington's disease (HD) patients are formed by N-terminal polyglutamine (polyQ)-expanded huntingtin (HTT) [9]. In amyotrophic lateral sclerosis (ALS), fused in sarcoma or translocated in liposarcoma (FUS/TLS) protein has been implicated in the formation of toxic aggregates and neuronal demise [10,11].

With the goal of harnessing the diversity of *Rubus* (poly)phenols for the discovery of new phenolic compounds of value, we developed an integrative approach that combined the power of metabolomics, for polyphenolic content characterization, and a Simple Molecular Architecture Research Tool (SMART) discovery platform for filtering potential bioactivities to be further explored in advanced pre-clinical models [12–14]. The platform is composed of yeast strains expressing human disease genes associated with the most-studied NDs as cited before (*Aβ42* [15], *SNCA* [16], *HTTpQ103* [17], *FUS/TLS* [18]), cancer (*RAS* and *RAF* [19]), and inflammation (*CRZ1* [20], the yeast orthologue of human Nuclear Factor of Activated T-cell—NFAT). This is possible due to the high degree of evolutionary conservation of fundamental biological processes among eukaryotes, which has established the budding yeast as a powerful model for the identification of molecular targets amenable for therapeutic intervention and lead molecules with health-promoting potential [21,22]. Benefiting from the easy and low-cost handling, facile genetic manipulation and the possibility to search against specific molecular targets, yeast-based screening technologies have proved to be very useful for the identification of promising drug candidates [12,13,23–25] including the flavonoids quercetin and epigallocatechin gallate [26].

2. Materials and Methods

2.1. Plant Material and Extraction Procedure

A range of different cultivars and species from the *Rubus* genus cultivated in Portugal (Odemira) and UK (Dundee) (Table S1) were manually harvested in the field at full ripeness as assessed by picker. Samples were kept in a cool box until they were transferred to −20 °C storage. Samples were extracted as described by Dudnik et al. [12]. In summary, approximately 50 g of frozen fruit from each species/cultivar was weighted and transferred into a solvent-proof blender containing 150 mL of pre-cooled 50 ng/mL Morin (Sigma–Aldrich, Gillingham, UK) solution prepared with 0.2% formic acid methanolic solution. Samples were then blended with three pulses of 10 s duration and subsequently filtered using Whatman filter paper grade 1. The filtrate was aliquoted and solvent-dried using a speed-vac (VWR, Lutterworth, UK) and subsequently lyophilized. Dried extracts were flushed with N_2 and stored at −20 °C until analysis by Liquid Chromatography coupled to a Time-of-Flight Mass Spectrometer (LC-ToF-MS). The filtrates to be used in the cell assays were solvent-dried using speed-vac, resuspended in CH_3COOH/H_2O (50/50), and subjected to solid-phase extraction [27].

2.2. Total Phenolic Quantification

Total phenolic content of the eluates were determined using the Folin–Ciocalteu method adapted to a microplate reader [27]. The eluates were aliquoted, freeze-dried, and frozen at −20 °C.

2.3. Phenolic Profile Determination by LC-ToF-MS

Analysis of sample extracts was performed as described by Dudnik et al. [12]. Briefly, dried extracts from each species/cultivar were resolubilized in triplicate using 2 mL of a 75% methanol solution with 0.1% formic acid. Five hundred microliters of the extract were decanted into filter vials, sealed with 0.45 mm Polytetrafluoroethylene-lined screwcap (Thomson Instrument Company, London, UK) and transferred into the autosampler. The analysis was achieved using an Agilent LC-ToF-MS system consisting of a quaternary pump (Agilent 1260, Cheadle, UK), a diode-array-detector (DAD) (Agilent 1260), a temperature control device (Agilent 1260), and a thermostat (Agilent 1290) coupled to an Agilent 6224 time-of-flight (ToF) instrument. Five microliters of the sample were injected onto a 2 × 150 mm (4 µm) C18 column (Phenomenex, Torrance, CA, USA) fitted with a C18 4 × 2 mm Security Guard™ cartridge (Phenomenex, Torrance, CA, USA). Sample and column temperature were maintained at 4 °C and 30 °C, respectively. The samples were eluted at a flow rate of 0.3 mL/min using two mobile phases (A: 0.1% formic acid in ultrapure water; B: 0.1% formic acid in 50:50 ultrapure water:acetonitrile) with the following gradient: 0 min 5% B; 4 min 5% B; 32.00 min 100% B; 34.00 min 100% B; 36.00 min 5% B; 40.00 min 5% B.

For optimal electrospray ionization conditions, the nebulizer pressure, drying gas temperature, and drying gas were set to 45 psi, 350 °C, and 3 L/min, respectively. In addition, the DAD was performed at 254, 280, and 520 nm. Morin levels (internal standard) were integrated in Agilent Mass Hunter Quan software (v. B.06.00, Cheadle, UK), and all samples with deviations larger than 10% relative to the dataset mean were reinjected. For all samples, three aliquots were analyzed across three different analytical batches.

2.4. Component Detection, Peak Alignment, and Integration

All chromatograms were evaluated in the same manner using the Agilent Software Profinder v. B.06.00, as previously described by Dudnik et al. [12], which integrates peak findings in an automated and unbiased way with a peak integration user interface that allows user-driven curation of individual peaks. For positive mode data, the batch recursive molecular feature was used with peak extraction restricted to 2.1–38.00 min of the chromatography and peaks with levels higher than 15,000 counts with potential adducts of +H, +Na^+, +K^+, and +NH_4^+ (−H and +Cl^- in negative mode) and a maximum of one charge state. The compound ion count threshold was set at two or more ions, and for alignment purposes the RT window was set at 0.70% + 0.60 min and the mass window was set at 25 ppm + 2 mDa. A post-processing filter to restrict analysis to compounds with more than 15,000 counts and present in at least 3 of the files in at least one sample group (species/line). The find-by-ion options were set to limit the extracted ion chromatogram (EIC) to the expected retention time +/− 0.40 min. The "Agile" algorithm was used for the integration of EIC, with a Gaussian smoothing of 9 points applied before the integration and a Gaussian width of 3 points. Additionally, peak filters were set at over 15,000 counts and the chromatogram formats were set to centroid when available and otherwise profile. The spectrum was extracted at 10% of peak height and excluded if the spectra within the m/z range used was above 20% of the saturation. Finally, a post-processing filter was applied and compounds with less than 15,000 counts or present in less than 3 files in at least one sample group (species/line) were excluded.

The output of automated peak finding and integration resulted in 542 and 210 molecular features found in the positive and negative modes, respectively. Manual curation resulted in the narrowing down of the molecular features found to 366 and 169 in the positive and negative modes, respectively. These were subsequently used in the statistical analysis.

2.5. Multivariate Analysis

GenStat for Windows, 16th Edition (VSN international Ltd., Hemel Hempstead, UK) was used for all the multivariate analysis performed. A principal component analysis (PCA), based on the correlation matrix, was applied to all the QC samples to ensure that the blank, reference samples, and berry samples were well separated (data not shown). The positive and negative metabolite datasets were analyzed separately and PCA plots were generated for the first 4 principal components. These were subsequently used for selecting the species with the greatest phytochemical differences.

2.6. Yeast Strains, Plasmids, and Transformation

Strains and plasmids used in this study are listed in Tables S3 and S4, respectively. The W303-1A_FUS and W303-1A_T strains were obtained by transformation of the W303-1A strain with plasmids pAG303_GAL1pr-FUS and pAG303_ GAL1pr-ccdB previously linearized with *BstZ17*I. Yeast transformation procedures were carried out as indicated using the lithium acetate standard method [28].

2.7. Yeast Growth Conditions

Synthetic complete (SC) medium (0.67% yeast nitrogen base without amino acids (YNB) (Difco™ Thermo Scientific Inc., Waltham, MA, USA) and 0.79 g/L complete supplement mixture (CSM) (MP Biomedicals, Inc.—Fisher Scientific, Irvine, CA, USA)), containing 1% raffinose was used for growth of PD and ALS integrative yeast models. Synthetic dropout CSM_{URA} medium (0.67% YNB and 0.77 g/L single amino acid dropout CSM_{-URA} (MP Biomedicals, Inc.—Fisher Scientific, Irvine, CA, USA)) containing 1% raffinose was used for growth of AD and ALS episomal yeast models. For growth of the HD model, a synthetic dropout SC-LEU medium was used (0.67 % YNB and 0.54 g/L 6-amino acid dropout $CSM_{-ADE-HIS-LEU-LYS-TRP-URA}$ (MP Biomedicals, Inc.—Fisher Scientific, Irvine, CA, USA), supplemented with standard concentrations of the required amino acids and containing 1% (w/v) raffinose. For growth of the RAS–RAF interaction yeast model, $CSM_{-HIS-URA-TRP}$ media was used (0.67% YNB and 0.54 g/L 6-amino acid dropout $CSM_{-ADE-HIS-LEU-LYS-TRP-URA}$ (MP Biomedicals, Inc.—Fisher Scientific, Irvine, CA, USA), supplemented with standard concentrations of the required amino acids and containing 1% raffinose. In all conditions, medium containing glucose (control, disease-protein OFF) and galactose (disease-protein ON), at a final concentration of 2%, were used for the repression or induction of disease protein expression, respectively. Growth of Crz1 activation yeast model was performed in SC medium containing 2% (w/v) glucose, and Crz1 activation was induced with 1.8 mM $MnCl_2$ [29]. Radicicol (Sigma, Gillingham, UK) and FK506 (Cayman Chemicals, Ann Arbor, MI, USA) were used as positive controls for the yeast models of RAS–RAF interaction and Crz1 activation, respectively.

A pre-inoculum was prepared in raffinose or glucose (for Crz1 activation model) medium. Cultures were incubated overnight at 30 °C under orbital shaking, diluted in fresh medium, and incubated under the same conditions until the optical density at 600 nm (OD_{600}) reached 0.5 ± 0.05 (log growth phase). Cultures were then diluted according to the equation: $ODi \times Vi = (ODf/(2^{(t/gt)})) \times Vf$, where ODi = initial optical density of the culture, Vi = initial volume of culture, ODf = final optical density of the culture, t = time (usually 16 h), gt = generation time of the strain, and Vf = final volume of culture. Readings were performed in a 96 well microtiter plate using a Biotek Power Wave XS plate spectrophotometer (Biotek® Instruments, Winooski, VT, USA). Dried extracts of *Rubus* species/cultivar obtained after total phenolic compounds determination were re-solubilized in adequate growth medium for the cellular assays.

2.8. Growth Assays

For the phenotypic growth assays, the strains were grown as described to OD_{600} 0.1 ± 0.01 and were inoculated (OD_{600} 0.2 ± 0.02) in medium supplemented or not with the indicated concentrations of *Rubus* extracts. After 6 h, $OD_{600\,nm}$ was adjusted to 0.05 ± 0.005, serial dilutions were performed with a ratio of 1:3, and 5 µL of each dilution was spotted onto solid medium containing glucose or galactose as the sole carbon sources. Growth was recorded after 48 h incubation at 30 °C. Images were acquired using Chemidoc$_{TM}$ XRS and Image-Lab® 6.0.1 software (Biorad, Hercules, CA, USA). For the growth curves, yeast cultures were diluted to OD_{600} 0.12 ± 0.012 in fresh medium supplemented or not with the indicated concentrations of the extracts in a 96 well microtiter plate. After 2 h incubation at 30 °C, cultures were further diluted to OD_{600} 0.03 ± 0.003 in repressing (glucose) or inducing (galactose) media supplemented or not with the extracts. The cultures were incubated at 30 °C with shaking for 24 h or 48 h (for the AD model) and cellular growth was monitored hourly by measuring OD_{600} using a Biotek Power Wave XS Microplate Spectrophotometer (Biotek® Instruments, Winooski, VT, USA). The areas under the curve (AUC) were integrated using the Origin 6 software (OriginLab, Northampton, MA, USA). For the RAS/RAF interaction model, final biomass was calculated by normalizing OD_{600} of cultures after 48 h incubation at 30 °C to the initial OD_{600}.

2.9. Flow Cytometry

Cell cultures at OD_{600} 0.2 ± 0.02 were exposed or not to the indicated concentrations of *Rubus* extracts for 6 h. Cultures were further diluted to OD_{600} 0.2 ± 0.02 in glucose and galactose supplemented or not with the indicated concentrations of *Rubus* extracts for 12 h. Flow cytometry was performed in a FACS BD Calibur equipped with a blue solid-state laser (488 nm) and green fluorescence channel 530/30 nm. Data analysis was performed using FlowJo software (BD, San Jose, CA, USA), and the cell doublets exclusion was performed based on Forward-A and -W scatter parameters. A minimum of 30,000 events were analyzed for each experiment. Results are expressed as the percentage of GFP positive cells as compared to the control.

2.10. Fluorescence Microscopy

Yeast cells subjected to the same treatment as above were monitored for the formation of disease-protein intracellular inclusions or nuclear translocation of Crz1 by fluorescence microscopy using a Leica DMRA2 fluorescence microscope (Leica, Wetzlar, Germany) equipped with a CoolSNAP HQ CCD camera (1.3MPx monochrome). Images were analyzed using ImageJ 1.8.0 software (NIH, Bethesda, MD, USA).

2.11. Protein Extraction

Tris-based buffer (TBS) [30] or trichloroacetic acid (TCA)/MURB (50 mM sodium phosphate, 25 mM MES pH 7.0, 1% SDS, 3 M urea, 0.5% 2-mercaptoethanol, 1 mM sodium azide) [31] were used for total protein extraction. Aliquots corresponding to OD_{600} 1–2 of cultured cells were harvested by centrifugation at 5000× *g* for 3 min. For TBS extraction, cells were resuspended in TBS supplemented with protease and phosphatase inhibitors, disrupted with glass beads (3 cycles of 30 s in the vortex and 5 min on ice), and cell debris were removed by centrifugation at 700× *g* for 3 min. Total protein was quantified using the MicroBCA kit (Thermo Fisher Scientific, Waltham, MA, USA) according the manufacturer's instructions. Samples were incubated at 95 °C for 10 min before SDS-PAGE.

For the TCA/MURB protocol, cells were first resuspended in TCA to a 10% final concentration, and the samples were incubated for 20 min at −20 °C. The cells were harvested by centrifugation at 15,000× *g* for 3 min, washed twice with acetone, and the air-dried cell pellet was resuspended in MURB supplemented with protease and phosphatase inhibitor cocktails. Cells suspensions were disrupted with glass beads (3 cycles of 30 s in the vortex and 5 min on ice), the samples were incubated at 70 °C for 10 min, and unlysed cells were removed by centrifugation at 10,000× *g* for 1 min.

2.12. Immunoblotting

Equal volumes of protein extract, normalized to the OD_{600} of cell cultures (for TCA/MURB protocol), or equal concentrations of total proteins (for TBS protocol) were loaded in a 15% SDS-PAGE. The Trans-Blot Turbo transfer system (BioRad, Hercules, CA, USA) was used to transfer proteins to a 0.22 µm nitrocellulose membrane according to the manufacturer's specifications. Membranes were washed with TBS, blocked with 5% skim milk in TBS-Tween for 1 h at room temperature, and incubated overnight at 4 °C with antibodies against GFP (1:5000, Neuromab, Davis, CA, USA), FUS/TLS (1:1000, Millipore, Burlington, MA, USA), and PgK1 (1:5000, Life Technologies Corporation, Carlsbad, CA, USA). Membranes were washed three times with TBS-Tween and incubated with horseradish peroxidase-conjugated secondary antibodies (1:10,000, Pierce, Waltham, MA, USA) for 2 h at room temperature. Protein signals were detected using Amersham ECL Prime Detection Reagent (GE Healthcare, Chicago, IL, USA) and signal intensity was estimated using the ImageJ 1.8.0 software (NIH, Bethesda, MD, USA).

2.13. β–Galactosidase Assays

For monitoring of RAS/RAF interaction, cell cultures at OD_{600} 1 ± 0.1 were exposed or not to the indicated concentrations of *Rubus* extracts for 90 min. The extracts were removed, cells were patched at a density of 4.5×10^7 onto solid medium containing glucose or galactose, and incubated 3 h at 30 °C. The assay was revealed by overlaying the cells with 5-Bromo-4-Chloro-3-Indolyl β-D-Galactopyranoside (X-Gal) solution (0.5% agarose, 50% LacZ buffer, 0.2% SDS, 2 mg X-Gal/mL and at 70 °C). Plates were maintained at 30 °C and monitored until the development of the blue color [32].

For quantitative measurements of β–galactosidase activity, cell cultures at OD_{600} 0.5 ± 0.05 were diluted to OD_{600} 0.1 ± 0.01 and challenged or not with extracts and the pure compounds for 90 min. Just before cell lysis, OD_{600} of cultures were recorded. Cells were incubated with Y-PER Yeast Protein Extraction Reagent (ThermoFisher Scientific) in 96 well microtiter plates for 20 min at 37 °C, LacZ buffer containing 4 mg/L 2-Nitrophenyl β-D-galactopyranoside (ONPG) was added, and plates were incubated at 30 °C [32]. The OD_{420} and OD_{550} were monitored using a Biotek Power Wave XS Microplate Spectrophotometer (Biotek® Instruments, Winooski, VT, USA). Miller units were calculated as described previously [33].

2.14. Quantitative Real-Time PCR

The qRT-PCR analyses were performed according to the MIQE guidelines (Minimum Information for Publication of Quantitative Real-Time PCR Experiments) [34]. Total RNA was extracted using the ENZA yeast RNA extraction kit (OMEGA, Norcross, GA, USA). After cleaning, 200–300 ng of total RNA was used for reverse-transcription with qScript™ cDNA superMix kit (Quanta Biosciences Inc., Gaithersburg, MD, USA). The qRT-PCR was performed in a LightCycler 480 Instrument (Roche, Basel, Switzerland), using LightCycler 480 SYBR Green I Master (Roche, Basel, Switzerland) to evaluate expression of the *FUS–GFP* (5′-ACGGACACTTCAGGCTATGG-3′; 5′-CCCGTAAGACGATTGGGAGC-3′) (GeneID: 2521), *PMR1* (5′-CACCTTGGTTCCTGGTGATT-3′; 5′-CCGGTTCATTTTCACCAGTT-3′) (GeneID: 852709), *PMC1* (5′-GTGGCGCACCATTTTCTATT-3′; 5′-TACTTCATCGGGGCAGATTC-3′) (GeneID: 852878), and *GSC2* (5′-CCCGTACTTTGGCACAGATT-3′; 5′-GACCCTTTTGTGCTTTGGAA-3′) (GeneID: 852920) genes. Standard curves were constructed for each gene and expression was calculated by the relative quantification method with efficiency correction using LightCycler 480 Software version 1.5.0.39 (Roche, Basel, Switzerland). Both *ACT1* (5′-GATCATTGCTCCTCCAGAA-3′; 5′-ACTTGTGGTGAACGATAGAT-3′) and *PDA1* (5′-TGACGAACAAGTTGAATTAGC-3′; 5′-TCTT AGGGTTGGAGTTTCTG-3′) were used as reference genes. The results were expressed as fold-change mRNA levels relative to the control (mRNA fold change) of at least three independent biological replicates.

2.15. Microglia-Induced Inflammation Model

Microglial N9 cells were cultured in EMEM (Eagle Minimum Essential Media, Sigma–Aldrich, Gillingham, UK) media, supplemented with 1% (v/v) L-glutamine (Biochrom AG, Berlin, Germany), 1% (v/v) penicillin/streptomycin, and 10% FBS (Fetal Bovine Serum, Gibco, Waltham, MA, USA). Cell cultures were maintained at 37 °C in 5% (v/v) CO_2, and split at sub-confluent cultures (about 60–80%). Cells were then detached by agitation before suspension of the culture media with a pipette (no cellular detaching agent was used). For immunostaining, cells were grown at 5×10^4 cell/well in 24 well plates containing coated coverslips and cultured overnight. Cells were pre-incubated or not with 5 mM of the indicated compounds for 6 h in culture media with reduced FBS to 0.5% (v/v). The medium was discarded, and cells were washed with PBS. Fresh culture media containing 300 ng/mL of LPS (Lipopolysaccharide) or 3 mM ATP (Sigma-Aldrich–Poole, Gillingham, UK) was added and cell cultures were incubated for 1 h to induce transcription factor nuclear localization. For nitric oxide (NO) and tumor necrosis factor alpha (TNF-α) quantifications, cells were seeded at 5×10^5 cells/well in 6 well plates, cultured overnight, and pre-incubated or not with 5 mM of the indicated compounds for 6 h in culture media with reduced FBS to 0.5% (v/v). The medium was discarded, cells were washed with PBS, and incubated in fresh culture media containing 300 ng/mL of LPS for 24 h.

2.16. Immunofluorescence

Immunostaining was performed as described by Figueira et al. [35], using rabbit polyclonal anti-NF-κB p65 (C-20) (1:200, Santa Cruz Biotechnology, Santa Cruz, CA, USA) or rabbit polyclonal anti-NFAT1c (1:200, Cell Signalling, Danvers, MA, USA) as primary antibodies and Alexa 594 anti-rabbit IgG (1:500) (Invitrogen, Carlsbad, CA, USA) as the secondary antibody. Nuclei were counterstained with DAPI. Cells were washed three times with PBS between each incubation. Widefield images were acquired on a Leica DMRA2 upright microscope, equipped with a CoolSNAP HQ CCD camera, using a 63× 1.4NA oil immersion objective, DAPI + TRITC fluorescence filter sets. Post-acquiring treatment was performed using ImageJ 1.8.0 software (NIH, Bethesda, MD, USA).

2.17. Nitric Oxide (NO) Quantification

The NO release to media was quantified as described by Ii et al. [36] using the Griess Reagent (Sigma–Aldrich, Gillingham, UK), according to manufacturer's instructions. After incubation with LPS, cell media were removed and immediately analyzed for nitrite quantification. Standard curves of sodium nitrite (0–25 µmol/L) were prepared and absorbance was acquired in a Synergy HT microplate reader (Biotek® Instruments, Winooski, VT, USA).

2.18. TNF-α Quantification

The TNF-α release was assayed by ELISA according to the manufacturer's instructions (PeproTech®; Princeton Business Park, Rocky Hill, NJ, USA). All reagents and plates used were provided in the kit. For the standard curve, recombinant murine TNF-α (PeproTech®) was diluted from 0–2 µg/L. The plate was incubated at room temperature in a Synergy HT microplate reader (Biotek® Instruments, Winooski, VT, USA) for 35 min, with 5 min intervals Abs_{405} readings.

2.19. Statistical Analysis

The results reported in this study are the average of at least independent biological triplicates and are represented as the mean ± SEM. Analysis of variance with Tukey's HSD (Honest Significant Difference) multiple comparison test ($\alpha = 0.05$) using SigmaStat 3.10 (Systat, Chicago, IL, US) was used to assess the differences among treatments.

3. Results

3.1. Selection of Most Chemically Diverse Species

(Poly)phenol-enriched extracts were prepared from a *Rubus* germplasm collection composed of 36 species/cultivars (Table S1). These were analyzed by LC-ToF-MS with the goal of selecting the most phytochemically diverse species. This was achieved using an untargeted analysis of extracts in both positive and negative modes which produced a total of 535 distinct molecular features for the entire dataset and subsequently combined with multivariate statistical analysis. There was no significant effect caused by instrument variability (see Figures S1 and S2), and principal component analysis (PCA) on the correlation matrix of the *Rubus* molecular features showed groupings of samples, with the majority of samples clustered according to their species/cultivar, reflecting their phytochemical similarity (Figure 1).

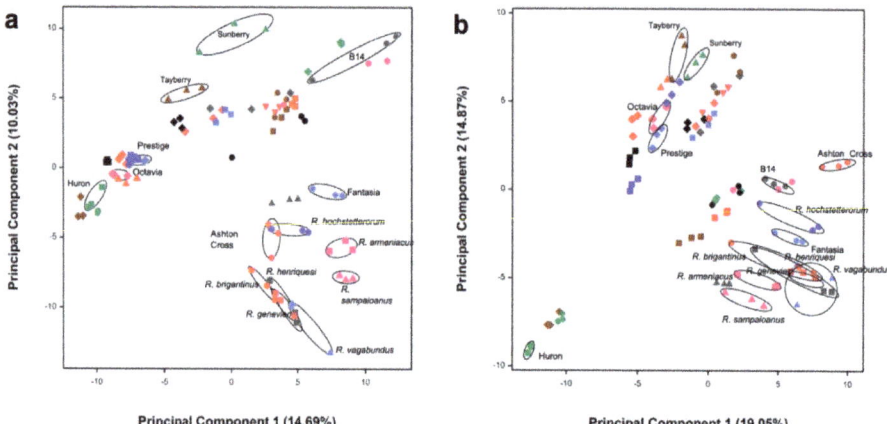

Figure 1. Principal component analysis (PCA) plots of the first two principal components (PCs) for the untargeted analysis acquired in positive (**a**) and negative (**b**) modes. These plots illustrate the phytochemical diversity present within the *Rubus* germplasm collection analyzed which included 36 species/cultivars. In positive mode, it was possible to identify three major groups comprising black and red raspberries (negative values for principal component 1, PC1), hybrid berries (high positive values for principal component 2, PC2), and wild and some domesticated blackberries (positive for PC1 and negative for PC2). In negative mode, three main groups were also observed, although they comprised black raspberries (negative for PC1 and PC2), red raspberries and hybrid species (high positive values for PC2), and wild and domesticated blackberries clustering with some hybrid species (positive values for PC1). The species selected for evaluation of bioactivity are circled in both plots.

We selected for further bioactivity assessment the species/samples showing the largest separation on the PCA plots (the first four principal components) generated from the positive and negative modes, as they were likely to represent the highest variability in phytochemical composition. Therefore, a total of 15 cultivars/species extracts were selected for screening in the SMART discovery platform: *Rubus vagabundus* Samp. *Rubus brigantinus* Samp., *Rubus sampaioanus* Sudre ex Samp., *Rubus genevieri* Boreau., *Rubus hochstetterorum* Seub, *Rubus henriquesii* Samp., *Rubus loganobaccus* L.H. Bailey (var. Tayberry and var. Sunberry), *Rubus fruticosus* L. *agg* (var. Fantasia, var. Ashton cross), *Rubus idaeus* L. (var. Prestige, var. Octavia), *Rubus occidentalis* L. (var. Huron), *Rubus armeniacus* Focke (var. Himalayan giant), and *Rubus* spp. (James Hutton Institute accession number B14).

3.2. Identification of Bioactivities Using a SMART Discovery Platform

Our approach involved the exploitation of a yeast-based screening platform, which was used to assess the potential of bioactives to modulate specific pathological pathways associated with redox-related diseases, particularly, neurodegenerative diseases, cancer, and inflammation (Figures S3–S8).

The most chemically diverse samples were screened in this discovery platform, and the protection factor for each pathological process was determined (Table 1). Protection factors above 10% were considered positive. The protection assays were preceded by cytotoxicity assays using control strains to determine the maximum useable extract concentration that caused less than 20% toxicity. Only the R. idaeus (var. Octavia) extract slightly improved the growth of αSyn-expressing cells (Parkinson's disease-PD-model), whereas R. loganocaccus (var. Sunberry) efficiently rescued the growth of yeast cells expressing Aβ (Alzheimer's disease-AD-model).

Table 1. Bioactivity of *Rubus* polyphenol-enriched extracts towards pathological processes of redox-related diseases as determined by the estimation of the protection factor.

Rubus Samples	Protective Factor in Each Disease Model					
	αSyn Toxicity [a]	Aβ42 Toxicity [a]	HTT Toxicity [a]	FUS Toxicity [a]	KRAS/RAF Interaction [b,c]	Crz1 Activation [b,d]
R. vagabundus	0	0	0	0	0	0
R. brigantinus	0	0	10.5 ± 10.1	0	0	35.2 ± 13.1
R. sampaioanus	0	0	0	0	0	15.7 ± 9.2
R. genevieri	0	0	0	39.0 ± 13.9	0	0
R. hochstetterorum	0	0	17.0 ± 10.7	0	0	12.2 ± 8.3
R. henriquesii	0	0	16.0 ± 10.1	0	0	10.3 ± 2.9
R. loganobaccus var. Tayberry	0	0	0	0	52.5 ± 1.2	0
R. loganobaccus var. Sunberry	0	90.3 ± 6.2	87.6 ± 30.7	0	0	6.4 ± 2.6
R. fruticosus var. Fantasia	0	0	0	0	0	0
R. fruticosus var. Ashton cross	0	0	0	0	0	41.2 ± 5.3
R. idaeus var. Prestige	0	0	98.7 ± 28.8	49.4 ± 24.0	15.4 ± 2.0	19.5 ± 0.9
R. idaeus var. Octavia	12.3 ± 6.6	0	0	22.4 ± 30.0	0	60.8 ± 8.5
R. occidentalis var. Huron	0	0	0	0	57.7 ± 1.2	57 ± 4.9
R. armeniacus var. Himalayan giant	0	0	0	0	27.1 ± 6.2	46.4 ± 3.4
Rubus sp. B14	0	0	0	0	35.9 ± 6.0	0

a—Protection factor (P%) = 100 × ((AUC$_{sample}$ − AUC$_{disease}$)/(AUC$_{control}$ − AUC$_{disease}$)); b—protection factor (P%) = 100 × (100 − (MU$_{disease}$ − MU$_{sample}$)/(MU$_{disease}$ − MU$_{control}$)); c—KRAS/BRAF interaction; d—Crz1 activation; AUC—area under the curve; MU—Miller units. The darker the green, the greater the bioactivity.

Several bioactivities for cellular pathologies associated with Huntington's disease (HD) and amyotrophic lateral sclerosis (ALS) were identified. *R. idaeus* (var. Prestige), and *R. loganobaccus* (var. Sunberry) extracts almost restored the growth of cells expressing mutant HTT (HD model) to values comparable to those of control cells. In cells expressing FUS (ALS model), the Portuguese endemic species *R. genevieri* and *R. idaeus* (var. Prestige) yielded the most potent extracts. *R. occidentalis* (var. Huron) conferred similar levels of protection (~57%) in KRAS/BRAF and Crz1–lacZ models. Remarkably, inflammation was the pathological process with a higher number of positive hits, as 10 out of 15 extracts tested conferred protection in the Crz1–lacZ model.

As the most potent extract among the Portuguese endemic species against FUS-mediated toxicity and conferring the highest level of protection in the KRAS/BRAF model, R. genevieri and R. occidentalis (var. Huron) extracts were chosen to obtain further insight into their mode of action towards ALS and cancer, respectively. Because inflammation is a central pathological process of neurodegenerative diseases, such as HD, and R. idaeus (var. Prestige) was previously shown by us to confer protective activities against this disease [13], we also included the characterization of the anti-inflammatory potential of this extract in the present study.

3.3. Bioactivity Towards the Mitigation of FUS Proteotoxicity

Rubus genevieri extracts conferred significant protection for the FUS-expressing model at the final concentration of 250 µg GAE/mL (Table 1), the higher non-toxic concentration tolerated by cells as defined in the cytotoxicity assays (data not shown). We then performed phenotypic growth assays to evaluate extract bioactivity as a pre-treatment. This condition contrasts with those used in the discovery platform, where cells were exposed to the extracts simultaneously with the induction of FUS expression. Cells expressing FUS displayed reduced growth in comparison with the control strain (Figure 2a and Figure S4b,c). Pre-treatment with R. genevieri (poly)phenol-enriched extracts partially rescued cellular growth, consistent with the screening assays, even when half the concentration (125 µg GAE/mL) was used (Figure 2a). Extracts from R. henriquesii slightly protected cells from FUS toxicity when applied as a pre-treatment (Figure 2a) in contrast to the screening assays where no protection was detected. Growth improvement mediated by R. genevieri phenolics was neither associated with alterations in the percentage of GFP positive cells (Figure 2b) nor FUS–GFP mRNA levels (Figure 2c). Analysis of protein levels by immunoblotting indicated that treatment with R. genevieri phenolics decreased FUS–GFP levels as compared to the control condition (Figure 2d, upper panels). As flow cytometry showed no variation of GFP signals among conditions, we assessed whether treatment with R. genevieri phenolics affected FUS biochemical status using a detergent solubility assay. In agreement with the flow cytometry results, no differences in FUS–GFP levels were observed under these conditions (Figure 2d, lower panels). These data suggest that R. genevieri phenolics may induce the formation of insoluble intracellular FUS structures.

3.4. Bioactives Modulating RAS/RAF Pathological Interactions

Rubus occidentalis (var. Huron) was the most potent in reducing the KRAS/BRAF interaction (Table 1). We performed a dose–response analysis to determine the concentration range of R. occidentalis (var. Huron) phenolics that conferred protective activity. Radicicol and R. sampaioanus extract (Table 1) were used as positive [37,38] and negative controls, respectively. Radicicol inhibited KRAS/BRAF interaction to levels comparable to the control strain bearing the empty plasmids (Figure 3a, left panel). Extracts from R. occidentalis (var. Huron) prevented KRAS/BRAF interaction at a concentration range of 125–250 µg GAE/mL, whereas R. sampaioanus had no significant effect on the interactions among these proteins. Similar results were obtained when β-galactosidade activity was measured in liquid medium (Figure 3a, right panel), except that only the lower concentration of R. occidentalis exhibited inhibitory activity on KRAS/BRAF interactions. Evaluation of BRAF interaction with the HRAS isoform revealed that R. occidentalis (var. Huron) bioactivity was maintained (Figure 3b), further supporting the protective role of (poly)phenolics present in this extract towards pathological RAS/RAF interactions. Notably, R. occidentalis (var. Huron) blocked RAS/RAF to a similar level to that of radicicol. No effects were observed in cells where the expression of BRAF-B42 fusion was turned off (Figure S9a,b).

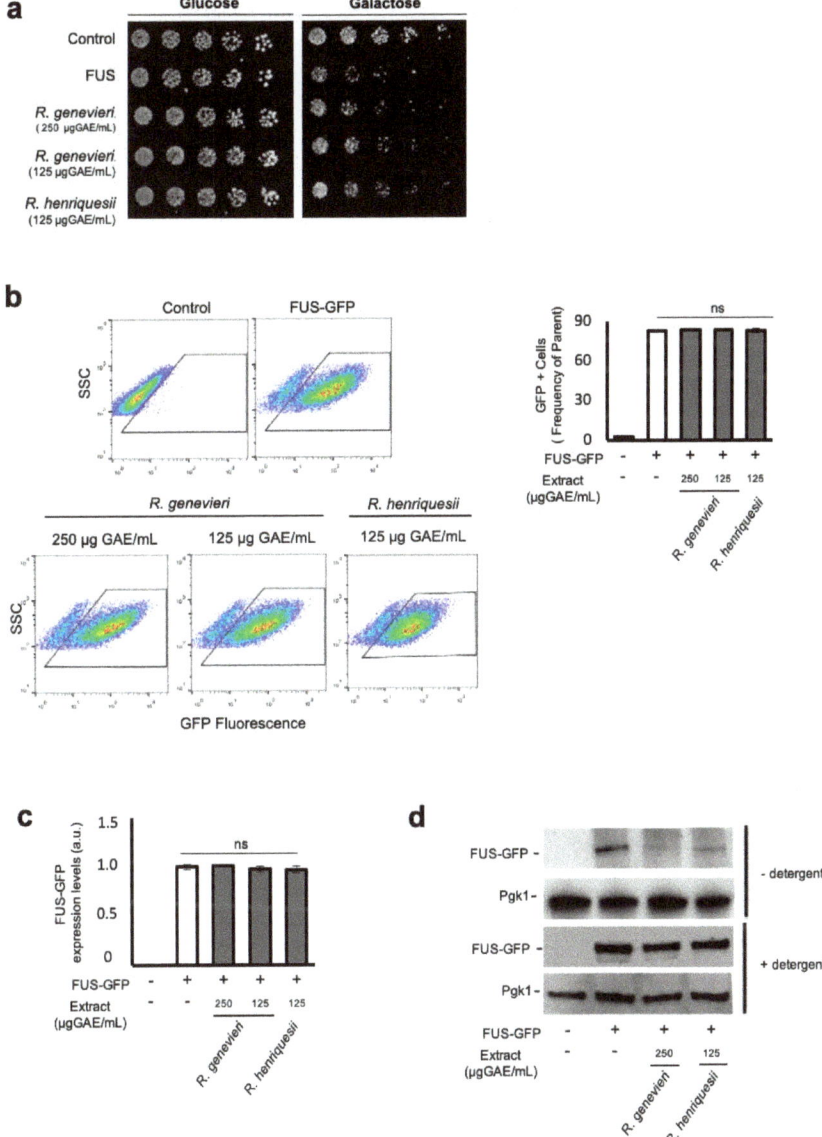

Figure 2. Bioactivity towards Amyotrophic lateral sclerosis is associated with the reduction of soluble FUS levels by *R. genevieri*. W303-1A recombinant cells expressing FUS were pre-grown in synthetic complete raffinose medium, and cells encoding the empty vector were used as the control. (**a**) The viability of cells exposed or not to the indicated concentrations of phenolic compound-enriched extracts was assessed by phenotypic growth assays on synthetic complete glucose and synthetic complete galactose media. (**b**) FUS expression evaluated by side scatter (SSC) versus FUS–GFP fluorescence, assessed by flow cytometry (left panel). The percentage of FUS–GFP-positive cells is shown (right panel). (**c**) FUS–GFP expression levels as evaluated by qRT-PCR. (**d**) FUS–GFP protein levels upon extraction in the presence or absence of detergent as evaluated by immunoblotting. Representative images are shown, and the values represent the mean ± SEM of at least three biological replicates.

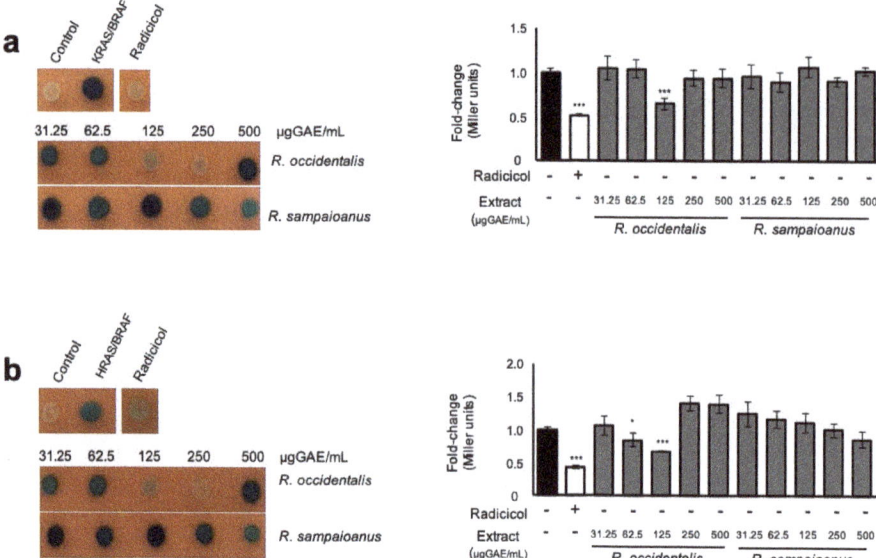
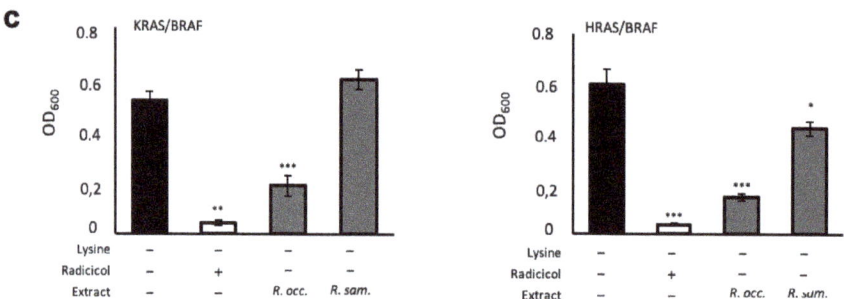

Figure 3. Mitigation of the pathological interaction between RAS and RAF by *R. occidentalis* (var. Huron). SKY197 recombinant cells expressing *ADH1pr-λCI-RAS GAL1pr-B42-BRAF* from 2μ vectors were pre-grown in synthetic dropout raffinose medium and exposed or not to the indicated concentrations of phenolic compounds-enriched extracts. Radicicol was used as a positive control. Cells containing the empty vectors were used as control. KRAS/BRAF (**a**) and HRAS/BRAF (**b**) interaction was assessed by monitoring β-galactosidase activity in SD galactose medium using 5-Bromo-4-Chloro-3-Indolyl β-D-Galactopyranoside (X-Gal) (left panels) and 2-Nitrophenyl β-D-galactopyranoside (ONPG) (right panels). (**c**) RAS/RAF interaction assessed by monitoring the final biomass of cell cultures grown in SD galactose medium without lysine and supplemented with 125 μg GAE/mL of the indicated phenolic compounds-enriched extracts. Representative images are shown, and the values represent the mean ± SEM of at least three biological replicates, * $p < 0.05$, ** $p < 0.01$, *** $p < 0.001$. *R. occ.*—*R. occidentalis*; *R. sam.*—*R. sampaioanus*.

The RAS/BRAF interaction was also assessed using *LYS2* as a reporter (Figure S7e). For that, cells co-expressing the control constructs, KRAS/BRAF and HRAS/BRAF were treated with the indicated extracts and the final biomass of cultures were monitored after 48 h incubation at 30 °C. As depicted in Figure 3c, the *R. occidentalis* (var. Huron) extracts mediated a strong protection towards BRAF interaction with both RAS isoforms, whereas *R. sampaioanus* had only a marginal effect on HRAS/BRAF interaction. Modulation of RAS/RAF interaction by *R. occidentalis* (var. Huron) (poly)phenolics occurred under subtoxic concentrations when the final biomass of cultures grown in galactose or glucose medium supplemented with lysine was measured (Figure S9c). Similar results were observed for the control cells expressing the empty plasmids (Figure S9d).

3.5. Attenuation of Crz1 Activation

(Poly)phenolic-enriched extracts were also tested for their potential to reduce Crz1 activation (Figure S8). *Rubus occidentalis* (var. Huron) extract was one of the most potent at inhibiting Crz1 activation (Table 1). The dose–response analysis indicated that this protection was restricted to the concentration range of 62.5–125 µg GAE/mL. Lower (31.25 µg GAE/mL) and higher (250 µg GAE/mL) concentrations had no effect on Crz1 activation and neither did the extract from *R. genevieri* at all concentrations tested (31.25–500 µg GAE/mL) (Figure 4a). These results emphasize the specificity of *R. occidentalis* (var. Huron) (poly)phenolics. The immunosuppressant FK506, which inhibits calcineurin activation thereby preventing Crz1 activation, was used as a positive control. In contrast to FK506, which was shown to reduce Crz1 basal activity, *R. occidentalis* (var. Huron) protection is specific for conditions in which cells were exposed to $MnCl_2$, a well-known inducer of Ca^{2+}-signaling pathway and Crz1 activity (Figure S10).

In a conserved mechanism to NFAT, Crz1 is dispersed throughout the cell under non-inducing conditions. Upon external stimuli leading to the increase of Ca^{2+} cytosolic levels, dephosphorylated Crz1 (and NFAT) accumulates in the nucleus where it binds to calcineurin-dependent response element (CDRE) and activates transcription of the target genes. The Crz1–GFP construct was used to further evaluate the potential of *R. occidentalis* (var. Huron) (poly)phenolics to modulate Crz1 activation by controlling its subcellular localization. As expected, GFP fluorescence signals were observed throughout the cell under physiological conditions. Exposure to $MnCl_2$, a well-known inducer of Ca^{2+}-signaling pathway and Crz1 activity, led to the rapid translocation of Crz1 into the nucleus (Figure 4b and Figure S8d), which was partially abolished by treatment with FK506 as indicated by the reduced number of cells displaying nuclear GFP signals (Figure 4b). *Rubus occidentalis* (var. Huron), but not *R. genevieri* extracts, reduced the percentage of cells with nuclear GFP indicating that this extract controls Crz1 activity by preventing its accumulation in the nucleus. If (poly)phenolics from *R. occidentalis* (var. Huron) prevent Crz1 nuclear translocation, it can be hypothesized that activation of Crz1 regulon should also be affected. Thus, we monitored by qPCR the mRNA levels of *PMR1*, *PMC1*, and *GSC2* Crz1-regulated genes. Fully supporting our hypothesis, the treatment of cells with *R. occidentalis* (var. Huron) extract downregulated expression of the three genes to a similar extent of that of FK506, whereas *R. genevieri* extracts had only a minor effect on the expression of *GSC2* (Figure 4c).

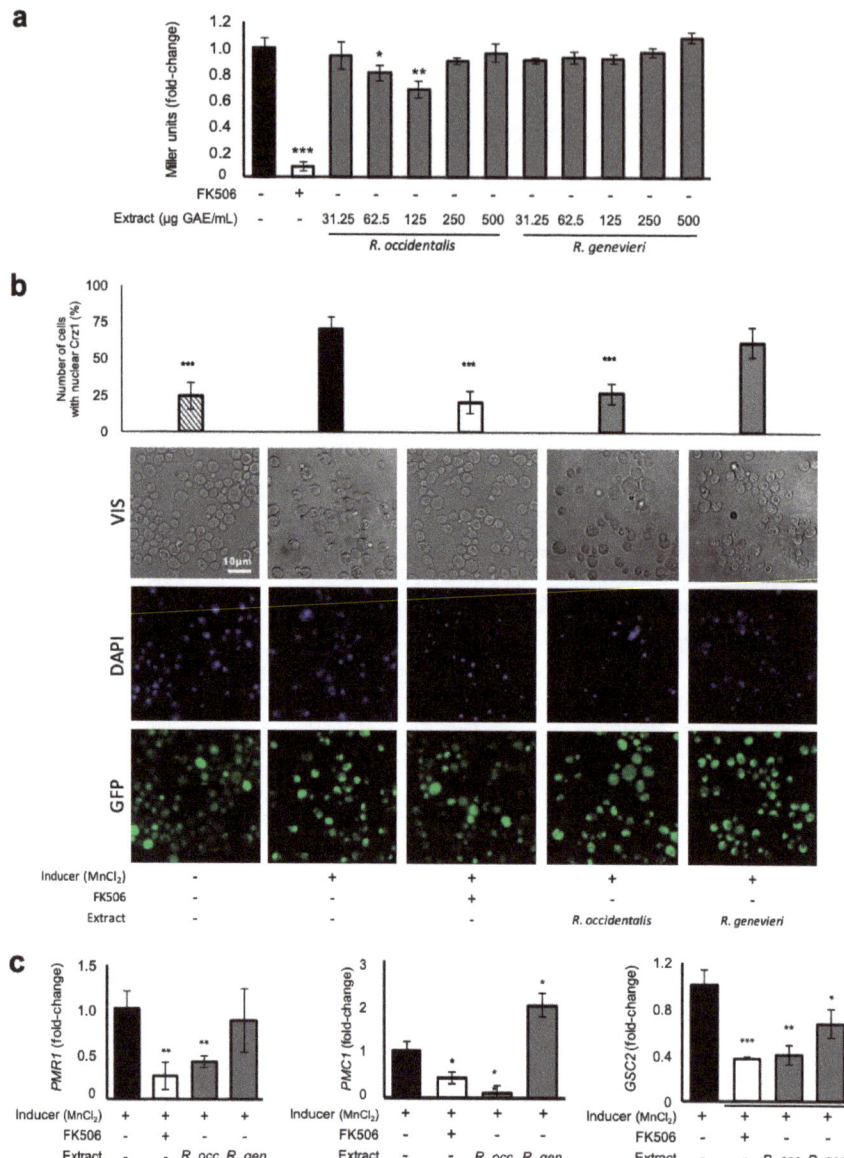

Figure 4. Attenuation Crz1 activation by *Rubus occidentalis* (var. Huron). BY4741 yeast strains encoding $CRZ1^{promoter}$–*lacZ* or *CRZ1*–*GFP* were subjected or not to the indicated concentrations of phenolic compounds-enriched extracts and induced with 1.8 mM $MnCl_2$. (**a**) Crz1 activation was assessed by monitoring β-galactosidase activity using 2-Nitrophenyl β-D-galactopyranoside (ONPG). (**b**) Crz1 subcellular dynamics evaluated by fluorescence microscopy in cells treated with 125 µg GAE/mL of the indicated phenolic compounds-enriched extracts. (**c**) Activation of Crz1 target genes *PMR1*, *PMC1*, and *GSC2* in cells treated as above by means of qRT-PCR. The immunosuppressant FK506, which inhibits calcineurin and prevents Crz1 activation, was used as a positive control. Representative images are shown, and the values represent the mean ± SEM of at least three biological replicates, * $p < 0.05$, ** $p < 0.01$, *** $p < 0.001$.

3.6. Runs Test for the Selection of Potential Components with Bioactivities

The qualitative and quantitative diversity present in the extracts ultimately translated into differences in the specificity and efficacy of the extracts in modulating bioactivity in the described disease models. Although an association between phytochemical composition and bioactivity is apparent, few studies have studied the association between bioactivities and the phytochemical composition of phylogenetically related species [39]. While correlation analysis approaches using metabolite and activity levels have been previously used in models of cytotoxicity or enzymatic activity where a dose-response is often observed between metabolite and bioactivity, it may result in false negative errors in the analysis of cell-based bioactivity models, which may experience additional cytotoxic effects at high metabolite concentrations. Similarly, a test of means of metabolite concentrations in bioactive extracts versus non-bioactive extracts may result in false negative results when there is a toxicity response at higher metabolite concentrations. To mitigate this, for each molecular feature the species were ordered according to their levels and a runs test was used on the bioactivity levels (+/−) of this order to test the randomness of the conditional distribution (molecular feature levels) given the observations of bioactivity (+) or lack of bioactivity (−) (Figure S11). This detects any significantly larger than expected number of runs of the same level of bioactivity as molecular feature levels increase. Out of the 535 molecular features in the metabolite dataset, the runs test yielded 48 molecular features with potential effects on whether a berry extract is active or inactive ($p < 0.05$). These results were further filtered in order to match two expected models of response for bioactivity: (a) higher molecular feature levels associated with bioactive extracts or (b) higher levels of molecular features associated to bioactivity and a lack of bioactivity observed at the highest levels due to the cytotoxic effects (Figure S11). This allowed the reduction of 48 potential molecular features to 15 tentatively annotated metabolites with potential bioactivities for four disease models (Table S2). This analysis provided three potential bioactives for HTT toxicity, nine hits for KRAS/RAF interaction, one hit for FUS toxicity, and two hits for Crz1 activation (Table S2). As there is only one extract each with reported bioactivity for Aβ42 and αSyn toxicity (Table 1), the statistical analysis returned no significant compounds ($p < 0.05$).

3.7. Unveiling Cyanidin as the Anti-Inflammatory Molecule

Cyanidin-hexoside was one of the potential hits selected for anti-inflammatory properties. As a proof of concept, we first evaluated the protective activity of cyanidin-3-O-glucoside, the most common cyaniding-hexoside in the *Rubus* species, in the Crz1 activation model. Pelargonidin-3-O-glucoside, another common anthocyanin hexoside present in the studied species, was used for comparative purposes. Only cyanidin-3-O-glucoside, but not pelargonidin-3-O-glucoside, decreased Crz1 activation, validating the prediction from the runs test (Figure 5a). Remarkably, cyanidin aglycone caused similar protection levels to cyanidin-3-O-glucoside, whereas pelargonidin aglycone did not, suggesting that the cyanidin moiety is the protective structure.

In a conserved mechanism to Crz1, activated NFAT translocates into the nucleus of immune cells. Therefore, we tested cyanidin and cyanidin-3-O-glucoside bioactivity in microglia cells (the immune cells resident in the brain) after stimulation with ATP as a pro-inflammatory insult. The anti-inflammatory activity of both compounds was evaluated in the N9 microglia cell line by following NFATc1 subcellular localization in cells exposed to cyanidin and cyanidin-3-O-glucoside before ATP insult. As shown in Figure 5b, NFATc1 was dispersed throughout the cells in control cells, and treatment with ATP led to its nuclear accumulation which is accompanied by cell morphological changes associated with microglia activation. Pre-treatment with both cyanidin-3-O-glucoside and cyanidin aglycone prevented NFATc1 accumulation in the nucleus, validating the results obtained using the yeast model of Crz1 activation.

The NF-kB pathway represents a central pathway in inflammatory responses, and the NF-kB regulatory activity is also controlled at the level of subcellular localization. Thus, the anti-inflammatory potential of cyanidin and cyanidin-3-O-glucoside towards p65, a subunit of the NF-kB complex, was further investigated in cells pre-treated with both compounds before stimulation with LPS. Similar to NFATc1, both compounds prevented p65 nuclear accumulation (Figure 5c). Notably, only cyanidin aglycone mediated a significant decrease of nitric oxide levels and TNF-α release (Figure 5d,e).

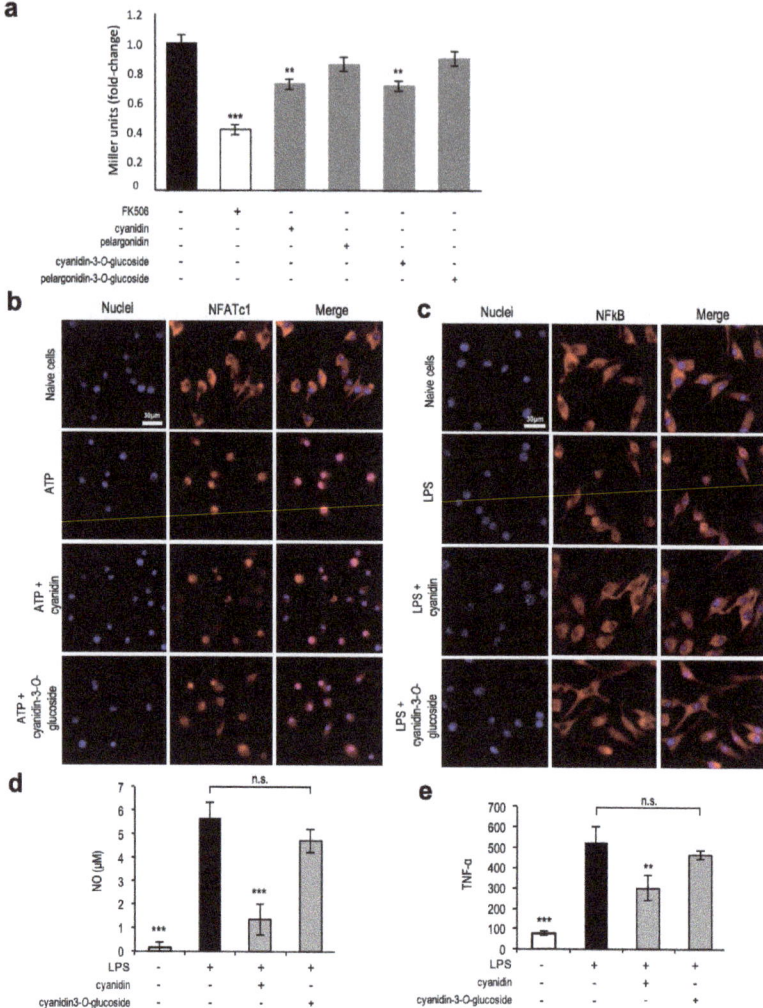

Figure 5. Cyanidin modulates Crz1 activation in yeast and NFAT and NF-kB in microglia. (**a**) BY4741 yeast strain encoding $CRZ1^{promoter}$-$lacZ$ was subjected or not to 50 µM of the indicated compounds, induced with 1.8 mM $MnCl_2$, and Crz1 activation was assessed by monitoring β-galactosidase activity using 2-Nitrophenyl β-D-galactopyranoside (ONPG). The immunosuppressant FK506 was used as a positive control. (**b**) NFATc1 and (**c**) NF-kB translocation to the nucleus in N9 cells pre-treated with 5 µM cyanidin or cyanidin-3-O-glucoside for 6 h before 1 h ATP stimulation (NFATc1) or LPS stimulation (NF-kB). NFATc1 and NF-kB were immunostained with Alexa Fluor 594 (red) and nuclei were stained with DAPI (blue). (**d**) NO and TNF-α release in N9 cells pre-treated with 5 µM cyanidin or cyanidin-3-O-glucoside for 6 h before LPS stimulation (NF-kB). Representative images are shown, and the values represent the mean ± SEM of at least three biological replicates, ** $p < 0.01$, *** $p < 0.001$.

4. Discussion

4.1. Cell-Based Assays for Discovery of Health-Promoting Attributes in the Rubus Germplasm

Soft fruit from the *Rubus* genus have been described as important sources of phenolic compounds with health-promoting activities. This study describes an integrated approach combining the power of metabolomics with the exploitation of a facile, reliable and cost-effective yeast-based discovery platform. The aim was to mine the diversity of (poly)phenolic compounds in selected berry germplasm of cultivated, wild, and underutilized *Rubus* species for bioactives able to modulate pathological processes associated with major chronic diseases. We have previously used a similar approach to systematically analyze *Rubus idaeus* (var. Prestige) extracts for the identification of bioactive compounds conferring protection against HD. The extract was fractionated, re-tested in the yeast platform; salidroside—a glycosylated phenol—was identified as the bioactive compound [13].

In this study, the untargeted metabolomics analysis identified the 15 most chemically diverse polyphenol-enriched extracts from a *Rubus* germplasm collection composed of 35 species/cultivars. With a minimum number of bioactivity screening efforts in the yeast-based discovery platform, this approach fast-tracked the identification of *R. genevieri* as novel source of potential bioactive compounds for ALS and *R. occidentalis* (var. Huron) conferring potential anti-cancer and anti-inflammatory properties, among other bioactivities indicated in Table 1.

Mechanistic studies were performed and suggest that *R. genevieri* (poly)phenolics led FUS to be trapped into insoluble intracellular structures thereby reducing its pathological activity. This is a well-known route of cellular protection against the toxic effect of several oligomerization-prone proteins described for several diseases [40]. It remains to identify the major molecular players in this process and to evaluate whether this mechanism is conserved in higher eukaryotes.

One-third of human tumors are driven by RAS mutations, especially the KRAS isoform [41], whereas approximately 8% of tumors express an activated form of BRAF [42], accounting together for almost 40% of cancers. Given the impact of deregulated RAS–RAF–MEK–ERK signaling cascade in cancer, the identification of compounds targeting its components has improved clinical outcomes [43]. The model used in the present study relies on the expression of mutant versions of *RAS* and *RAF* genes, encoding hyperactivated proteins of the RAS–RAF–MEK–ERK cell proliferation signaling pathway, in human cells. *Rubus occidentalis* (var. Huron) extracts were identified as a potent inhibitor of RAS/RAF interaction, thus potentially modulating cell proliferation in contexts of dysregulated signaling in cancer. Curiously, protection against pathological cancer processes was concentration dependent and exhibited a hormetic pattern with concentrations higher than 250 µg GAE/mL exerting the opposite effect, i.e., inducing the interaction between HRAS/BRAF above the levels observed for the untreated condition via a mechanism that still remains to be elucidated.

Chronic activation of immune responses is a common link between neurodegeneration and cancer [44]. Therefore, the identification of molecules targeting inflammatory process may impact both pathologies. Modulation of inflammatory processes is driven by persistent activation of key transcription factors, such as NFAT and NF-κB, which in turn upregulate transcription of pro-inflammatory genes creating a positive feedback loop further amplifying initial stimuli. CRZ1 is the yeast homologue of NFAT, a transcription factor controlling inflammatory responses in humans. Similarly to NFAT, Crz1 regulation is modulated by the calcium (Ca^{2+})-signaling pathway, which culminates in calcineurin (CaN) activation by calmodulin, Crz1 dephosphorylation, and nuclear translocation [29,32]. The same concentration range of *R. occidentalis* (var. Huron) polyphenol-enriched extracts driving potential anti-cancer effects also mediated the anti-inflammatory properties of this extract. A mechanistic insight into the molecular targets of *R. occidentalis* (var. Huron) (poly)phenols was obtained by showing that it inhibits Crz1 nuclear accumulation thereby preventing the expression of the reporter gene *lacZ* as well as its endogenous targets genes.

4.2. Exploring Statistical Tools to Expedite Compounds Bioactivity Identification

Discrete differences observed among the metabolite profiles of the extracts analyzed may be responsible for the bioactivity against a range of different disease processes. The literature presented in the last decade clearly indicates that the potential therapeutic effect of some phytochemical components of fruit is determined by qualitative compositional differences and gross measurements, such as total phenol content and total antioxidant potential, do not fully explain the bioactivity of some extracts [45]. While the major phytochemical components present in the extracts are usually well characterized, there is a limited amount of research on the bioactivity associated with the minor phytocomponents. To ensure the optimization of the discovery of novel bioactives, it is of paramount importance that the metabolomics approach used should be untargeted thereby avoiding introducing bias into the analysis.

A traditional approach for the discovery of novel components from bioactive extracts is an iterative process which includes the fractionation of bioactive extracts, re-testing the bioactivity of the various fractions, and subsequent fractionation and testing until a single component is isolated. This is an extremely labor- and time-intensive process with a number of pitfalls often including the lack of available material for performing an extensive number of iterations and the loss of potential synergistic effects. The statistical approach (i.e., the runs test) used in this resulted in the identification of 15 compounds with potential bioactivities for 4 disease models.

A total of three compounds had significance for Huntington's disease (HD) model including quercetin 3-O-glucuronide and a triterpenoid isomer. The supplementation of rodent models with quercetin derivatives attenuated symptoms of HD [46], while recent in vitro and in vivo evidence indicated that quercetin-3-O-glucuronide modulated neurogenesis [47]. Additionally, triterpenoids such as celastrol, onjisaponin B, and ginsenosides from various plant sources have provided encouraging evidence of their preclinical efficacy in modulating HD [48].

The runs test for the ALS model resulted in the identification of a unique significant molecular feature tentatively identified as a leucine isomer. Interestingly, ALS has been associated with abnormal glutamate metabolism, and since branched-chain amino acids (BCAAs; e.g., L-leucine, L-isoleucine, and L-valine) can modify glutamate metabolism, these have been evaluated with respect to their therapeutic potential [49]. However, clinical studies have provided conflicting evidence with some studies reporting negative effects or a lack of efficacy [49–51], whereas others reported amelioration of ALS symptoms [52,53]. More recently, in vivo preclinical evidence suggests that BCAA, tryptophan, and particularly arginine and proline metabolic pathways are associated with disease progression [54].

The runs test for the RAS/RAF interaction model (cancer model) indicated a total of nine compounds with potential bioactivities that included (−)-epicatechin, various anthocyanins, an unidentified triterpenoid, a hydroxysphingosine isomer, and a benzoic acid di-hexoside. The potential of berry extracts to modulate cancer disease progression have been shown both via in vitro and in vitro models and anthocyanins have been found to be major contributors towards inhibiting cell proliferation and inducing apoptosis [55]. Dietary triterpenoids, which are often found in *Rubus* species, are able to survive in vivo digestion [56] and have shown promising results in pre-clinical trials in colorectal cancer models [57]. Interestingly, (−)-epicatechin has been found to provide synergistic effects in modulating growth and apoptosis in human cancerous cell cultures when combined with other phytochemicals such as curcumin [58] and EGCG [59], whereas epidemiological evidence found association between dietary intake of catechin-derived compounds and reduced colorectal cancer incidence [60,61]. Finally, MS-based fingerprint analyses of biofluids have reported significant lower levels of hydroxysphingosine in the plasma of patients with multiple myeloma, chronic lymphocytic leukemia [62], and urine of patients with prostate cancer [63] in comparison with control healthy individuals.

4.3. Identification of a Single Compound—Cyanidin—with Anti-Inflammatory Properties towards NFAT and NF-kB Transcription Factors

The runs test of the Crz1 activation model (inflammation model) indicated two potential bioactive compounds including an anthocyanin hexoside. Anthocyanins have been associated with anti-inflammatory properties in various in vitro and in vivo studies [64], whereas epidemiological evidence has suggested that higher anthocyanin intakes were also associated with increased anti-inflammatory effects [65]. Interestingly, anthocyanin-rich fractions of *Rubus* fruits have also shown anti-inflammatory properties in vitro [66]. In our study, we validated the bioactivity of cyanidin-3-O-glucoside for inflammation in yeast and mammalian cells models whereas no activity was found for pelargonidin-3-O-glucoside. In addition, our findings unveil the health-promoting attributes of cyanidin-3-O-glucoside not only for the target identified in the yeast discovery platform (NFAT), but also for the canonical inflammatory NF-kB pathway as revealed in mammalian in vitro model. This is in agreement with previous studies showing that cyanidin 3-O-glucoside exerts inhibitory roles towards the NF-kB proinflammatory pathway in several cell models [67–71]. As for NFAT, little is known, with little evidence indicating that cyanidin 3-O-glucoside downregulates NFATc1 thereby inhibiting RANKL-mediated osteoclastogenesis [72]. In contrast, we did not report a significant effect of pelargonidin and pelargonidin 3-O-glucoside despite evidence of its role in the inhibition of the NF-kB pathway [73]. The cellular assays extended the predictions made by the runs test and proved that the cyanidin moiety, rather than cyanindin-3-O-glucoside, was responsible for the detected bioactivity. This finding illustrates the power of combining metabolomics, in silico analysis, and cellular assays for the identification of single bioactive compounds.

As mentioned before, this study was designed to fast-track potential bioactives to be further explored in more robust pre-clinical models. As such, and also taking into account the limited uptake of certain compounds due to the yeast cell wall, the criteria was using non-toxic concentrations of (poly)phenol-enriched extracts for bioactivity determination. Once a single compound was identified —the cyanidin— and the bioactivity confirmed in yeast, physiologically relevant concentrations (5 µM) [74] were tested in mammalian cell models for study validation in a nutritional point of view.

In brief, our approach revealed potential bioactive compounds for pathological processes associated with redox-related diseases. With regard to cyanidin, the protective effect was validated at levels in the range of described bioavailable concentrations. However, even in the scenario of a compound fails to be active under concentrations in the physiological range, nutraceutical/therapeutical applications could be ensured by the development of formulations for controlled delivery to target tissues

5. Conclusions

This study described the use of an integrative approach, combining the power of metabolomics, cellular assays and potent statistical analysis, to identify novel health-promoting attributes in underexplored (poly)phenol sources. The rationale involved the selection of the most chemically diverse samples of an extensive *Rubus* collection followed by the determination of health-promoting activities using a SMART discovery platform.

Overall, the study allowed the identification of (poly)phenol-enriched extracts and single compounds from *Rubus* modulating pathological processes of redox-related diseases responsible for major societal and economic impacts as well as provided some clues regarding the possible molecular mechanisms underlying their protective activity. Our objective was to deliver novel plant (poly)phenolic bioactives with the potential to be exploited either in food engineering and in the pharmaceutical and biotechnological sector as nutraceutical/therapeutic alternatives for redox-related chronic diseases. Of course, in therapeutic applications, development of formulations for controlled delivery to target tissues should further be developed to ensure that physiologically relevant concentrations of bioactive compounds reach their target sites.

Although the number of novel plant (poly)phenolics with potential bioactivity is limited, we tentatively identified several phytochemicals in *Rubus*, such as triterpenoids, benzoyl di-hexoside, hydroxysphingosine, and a leucine isomer, which have not been extensively studied such as *Rubus*-derived bioactive compounds. Interestingly, (−)-epicatechin has previously been described as possessing synergistic effects [58,59], and while our model does not tackle synergistic and antagonistic effects, it is possible that significant results from the runs test could be associated with synergistic effects rather than intrinsically high bioactivity.

While more work is necessary in compound annotation, development of the statistical model in order to cope with synergistic and antagonistic effects and validation of bioactivities in advanced models, this report highlights the feasibility of this strategy for the replication and identification of novel bioactive lead molecules from crude extracts from berry fruits.

Supplementary Materials: The following are available online at http://www.mdpi.com/2076-3921/9/9/789/s1. Table S1: *Rubus* species/varieties used in this study, Table S2: Significant compounds from runs test for all disease models tested, Table S3: Yeast strains used in this study, Table S4: Plasmids used in this study, Figure S1: PCA analysis of the entire positive mode dataset, Figure S2: PCA analysis of the entire negative mode dataset, Figure S3: Yeast model of Parkinson's disease, Figure S4: Yeast model of amyotrophic lateral sclerosis, Figure S5: Yeast model of Huntington's disease, Figure S6: Yeast model of Alzheimer's disease, Figure S7: Yeast model of RAS/RAF interaction, Figure S8: Yeast model of Crz1 activation, Figure S9: Supplementary data for the cancer (HRAS/KRAS) model, Figure S10: Supplementary data for the Crz1 activation model, Figure S11: Visual representation of the runs test.

Author Contributions: R.M. and A.F. contributed equally to this study. Conceptualization, C.N.S.; methodology, R.M., A.F., D.S., C.N.S.; validation, R.M., A.F., C.N.S.; formal analysis, S.F., C.J.A.; investigation, R.M., A.F., C.J., I.C., G.G., R.R.-R.; resources, R.M., T.F.O., D.S., C.N.S.; data curation, R.M., A.F., D.S., C.N.S.; writing—original draft preparation, R.M., A.F.; writing—review and editing, R.M., A.F., T.F.O., D.S., C.N.S.; visualization, R.M., A.F.; supervision, R.M., D.S., C.N.S.; project administration, C.N.S., D.S.; funding acquisition, C.N.S., D.S. All authors have read and agreed to the published version of the manuscript.

Funding: iNOVA4Health-UID/Multi/04462/2013, a program financially supported by Fundação para a Ciência e Tecnologia/Ministério da Educação e Ciência, through national funds and co-funded by FEDER under the PT2020 Partnership Agreement is acknowledged. This work was supported by Fundação para a Ciência e Tecnologia (IF/01097/2013 to C.N.S.), by The Scottish Government Rural and Environment Science and Analytical Services Division (A.F. and D.S.), and BacHBerry FP7-KBBE-2013-613793 (R.M., A.F., C.J., I.C., G.G., R.R.-R., J.P., A.M., C.D., D.S. and C.N.S.). T.F.O. was supported by the Deutsche Forschungsgemeinschaft (DFG, German Research Foundation) Center for Nanoscale Microscopy and Molecular Physiology of the Brain (CNMPB), and is currently supported by the DFG under Germany's Excellence Strategy—EXC 2067/1-390729940.

Acknowledgments: Both pAG303_GAL1pr-FUS and pAG303_ GAL1pr-ccdB were kindly provided by Gregory Petsko (Weill Cornell Medical College, US), while p425GAL1_HTT103Q was kindly provided by Flavino Giorgini (University of Leicester, UK), and p416_GPDpr-GFP-Aβ42 was kindly provided by Ian Macraedie (RMIT University, AU). Strain SKY197 and plasmids pGKS5_ADH1pr-acKRAS V12, pGKS5_ADH1pr-HRAS V12, pGKS5, pJG4-5_ GAL1pr-BRAF, and pJG4-5 were kindly provided by Vladimir Khazak (NEXUSPHARMA INC.). The Microglia N9 cell line was kindly provided by Teresa Pais (Institute Calouste Gulbenkian, Portugal).

Conflicts of Interest: The authors declare no conflict of interest.

References

1. Shen, B. A New Golden Age of Natural Products Drug Discovery. *Cell* **2015**, *163*, 1297–1300. [CrossRef]
2. Newman, D.J.; Cragg, G.M. Natural Products as Sources of New Drugs from 1981 to 2014. *J. Nat. Prod.* **2016**, *79*, 629–661. [CrossRef] [PubMed]
3. Soto, C. Unfolding the role of protein misfolding in neurodegenerative diseases. *Nat. Rev. Neurosci.* **2003**, *4*, 49–60. [CrossRef] [PubMed]
4. Quist, A.; Doudevski, I.; Lin, H.; Azimova, R.; Ng, D.; Frangione, B.; Kagan, B.; Ghiso, J.; Lal, R. Amyloid ion channels: A common structural link for protein-misfolding disease. *Proc. Natl. Acad. Sci. USA* **2005**, *102*, 10427–10432. [CrossRef] [PubMed]
5. O'Brien, R.J.; Wong, P.C. Amyloid precursor protein processing and Alzheimer's disease. *Annu. Rev. Neurosci.* **2011**, *34*, 185–204. [CrossRef]
6. Lee, V.M.; Goedert, M.; Trojanowski, J.Q. Neurodegenerative tauopathies. *Annu. Rev. Neurosci.* **2001**, *24*, 1121–1159. [CrossRef]
7. Nalls, M.A.; Pankratz, N.; Lill, C.M.; Do, C.B.; Hernandez, D.G.; Saad, M.; DeStefano, A.L.; Kara, E.; Bras, J.; Sharma, M.; et al. Large-scale meta-analysis of genome-wide association data identifies six new risk loci for Parkinson's disease. *Nat. Genet.* **2014**, *46*, 989–993. [CrossRef]
8. Shults, C.W. Lewy bodies. *Proc. Natl. Acad. Sci. USA* **2006**, *103*, 1661–1668. [CrossRef]

9. DiFiglia, M.; Sapp, E.; Chase, K.O.; Davies, S.W.; Bates, G.P.; Vonsattel, J.P.; Aronin, N. Aggregation of huntingtin in neuronal intranuclear inclusions and dystrophic neurites in brain. *Science* **1997**, *277*, 1990–1993. [CrossRef]
10. Kwiatkowski, T.J., Jr.; Bosco, D.A.; Leclerc, A.L.; Tamrazian, E.; Vanderburg, C.R.; Russ, C.; Davis, A.; Gilchrist, J.; Kasarskis, E.J.; Munsat, T.; et al. Mutations in the FUS/TLS gene on chromosome 16 cause familial amyotrophic lateral sclerosis. *Science* **2009**, *323*, 1205–1208. [CrossRef]
11. Vance, C.; Rogelj, B.; Hortobagyi, T.; De Vos, K.J.; Nishimura, A.L.; Sreedharan, J.; Hu, X.; Smith, B.; Ruddy, D.; Wright, P.; et al. Mutations in FUS, an RNA processing protein, cause familial amyotrophic lateral sclerosis type 6. *Science* **2009**, *323*, 1208–1211. [CrossRef] [PubMed]
12. Dudnik, A.; Almeida, A.F.; Andrade, R.; Avila, B.; Banados, P.; Barbay, D.; Bassard, J.E.; Benkoulouche, M.; Bott, M.; Braga, A.; et al. BacHBerry: BACterial Hosts for production of Bioactive phenolics from bERRY fruits. *Phytochem. Rev.* **2018**, *17*, 291–326. [CrossRef]
13. Kallscheuer, N.; Menezes, R.; Foito, A.; Henriques da Silva, M.D.; Braga, A.; Dekker, W.; Mendez Sevillano, D.; Rosado-Ramos, R.; Jardim, C.; Oliveira, J.; et al. Identification and microbial production of the raspberry phenol salidroside that is active against Huntington's disease. *Plant Physiol.* **2018**, *179*, 969–985. [CrossRef] [PubMed]
14. Rencus-Lazar, S.; DeRowe, Y.; Adsi, H.; Gazit, E.; Laor, D. Yeast Models for the Study of Amyloid-Associated Disorders and Development of Future Therapy. *Front. Mol. Biosci.* **2019**, *6*, 15. [CrossRef]
15. Bharadwaj, P.; Martins, R.; Macreadie, I. Yeast as a model for studying Alzheimer's disease. *FEMS Yeast Res.* **2010**, *10*, 961–969. [CrossRef]
16. Outeiro, T.F.; Lindquist, S. Yeast cells provide insight into alpha-synuclein biology and pathobiology. *Science* **2003**, *302*, 1772–1775. [CrossRef]
17. Willingham, S.; Outeiro, T.F.; DeVit, M.J.; Lindquist, S.L.; Muchowski, P.J. Yeast genes that enhance the toxicity of a mutant huntingtin fragment or alpha-synuclein. *Science* **2003**, *302*, 1769–1772. [CrossRef]
18. Ju, S.; Tardiff, D.F.; Han, H.; Divya, K.; Zhong, Q.; Maquat, L.E.; Bosco, D.A.; Hayward, L.J.; Brown, R.H., Jr.; Lindquist, S.; et al. A yeast model of FUS/TLS-dependent cytotoxicity. *PLoS Biol.* **2011**, *9*, e1001052. [CrossRef]
19. Khazak, V.; Kato-Stankiewicz, J.; Tamanoi, F.; Golemis, E.A. Yeast screens for inhibitors of Ras-Raf interaction and characterization of MCP inhibitors of Ras-Raf interaction. *Methods Enzym.* **2006**, *407*, 612–629. [CrossRef]
20. Araki, Y.; Wu, H.; Kitagaki, H.; Akao, T.; Takagi, H.; Shimoi, H. Ethanol stress stimulates the Ca^{2+}-mediated calcineurin/Crz1 pathway in Saccharomyces cerevisiae. *J. Biosci. Bioeng.* **2009**, *107*, 1–6. [CrossRef]
21. Menezes, R.; Tenreiro, S.; Macedo, D.; Santos, C.N.; Outeiro, T.F. From the baker to the bedside: Yeast models of Parkinson's disease. *Microb. Cell* **2015**, *2*, 18. [CrossRef] [PubMed]
22. Tenreiro, S.; Munder, M.C.; Alberti, S.; Outeiro, T.F. Harnessing the power of yeast to unravel the molecular basis of neurodegeneration. *J. Neurochem.* **2013**, *127*, 438–452. [CrossRef] [PubMed]
23. Tardiff, D.F.; Jui, N.T.; Khurana, V.; Tambe, M.A.; Thompson, M.L.; Chung, C.Y.; Kamadurai, H.B.; Kim, H.T.; Lancaster, A.K.; Caldwell, K.A.; et al. Yeast reveal a "druggable" Rsp5/Nedd4 network that ameliorates alpha-synuclein toxicity in neurons. *Science* **2013**, *342*, 979–983. [CrossRef] [PubMed]
24. Tardiff, D.F.; Lindquist, S. Phenotypic screens for compounds that target the cellular pathologies underlying Parkinson's disease. *Drug Discov. Today Technol.* **2013**, *10*, e121–e128. [CrossRef] [PubMed]
25. Vincent, B.M.; Tardiff, D.F.; Piotrowski, J.S.; Aron, R.; Lucas, M.C.; Chung, C.Y.; Bacherman, H.; Chen, Y.; Pires, M.; Subramaniam, R.; et al. Inhibiting Stearoyl-CoA Desaturase Ameliorates alpha-Synuclein Cytotoxicity. *Cell Rep.* **2018**, *25*, 2742–2754. [CrossRef] [PubMed]
26. Griffioen, G.; Duhamel, H.; Van Damme, N.; Pellens, K.; Zabrocki, P.; Pannecouque, C.; van Leuven, F.; Winderickx, J.; Wera, S. A yeast-based model of alpha-synucleinopathy identifies compounds with therapeutic potential. *Biochim. Biophys. Acta* **2006**, *1762*, 312–318. [CrossRef]
27. Tavares, L.F.S.; Carrilho, C.; McDougall, G.J.; Stewart, D.; Ferreira, R.B.; Santos, C.N. Antioxidant and antiproliferative properties of strawberry tree tissues. *J. Berry Res.* **2010**, *1*, 3–12. [CrossRef]
28. Gietz, R.D.; Schiestl, R.H. Applications of high efficiency lithium acetate transformation of intact yeast cells using single-stranded nucleic acids as carrier. *Yeast* **1991**, *7*, 253–263. [CrossRef]
29. Stathopoulos, A.M.; Cyert, M.S. Calcineurin acts through the CRZ1/TCN1-encoded transcription factor to regulate gene expression in yeast. *Genes Dev.* **1997**, *11*, 3432–3444. [CrossRef]

30. Tenreiro, S.; Rosado-Ramos, R.; Gerhardt, E.; Favretto, F.; Magalhaes, F.; Popova, B.; Becker, S.; Zweckstetter, M.; Braus, G.H.; Outeiro, T.F. Yeast reveals similar molecular mechanisms underlying alpha- and beta-synuclein toxicity. *Hum. Mol. Genet.* **2016**, *25*, 275–290. [CrossRef]
31. Miller-Fleming, L.; Cheong, H.; Antas, P.; Klionsky, D.J. Detection of Saccharomyces cerevisiae Atg13 by western blot. *Autophagy* **2014**, *10*, 514–517. [CrossRef] [PubMed]
32. Garcia, G.; Santos, C.N.; Menezes, R. High-Throughput Yeast-Based Reporter Assay to Identify Compounds with Anti-inflammatory Potential. *Methods Mol. Biol.* **2016**, *1449*, 441–452. [CrossRef] [PubMed]
33. Miller, J. *Experiments in Molecular Genetics*; Cold Spring Harbor Laboratory: Cold Spring Harbor, NY, USA, 1972; pp. 352–355.
34. Bustin, S.A.; Benes, V.; Garson, J.A.; Hellemans, J.; Huggett, J.; Kubista, M.; Mueller, R.; Nolan, T.; Pfaffl, M.W.; Shipley, G.L.; et al. The MIQE guidelines: Minimum information for publication of quantitative real-time PCR experiments. *Clin. Chem.* **2009**, *55*, 611–622. [CrossRef] [PubMed]
35. Figueira, I.; Garcia, G.; Pimpao, R.C.; Terrasso, A.P.; Costa, I.; Almeida, A.F.; Tavares, L.; Pais, T.F.; Pinto, P.; Ventura, M.R.; et al. Polyphenols journey through blood-brain barrier towards neuronal protection. *Sci. Rep.* **2017**, *7*, 11456. [CrossRef] [PubMed]
36. Ii, M.; Sunamoto, M.; Ohnishi, K.; Ichimori, Y. beta-Amyloid protein-dependent nitric oxide production from microglial cells and neurotoxicity. *Brain Res.* **1996**, *720*, 93–100. [CrossRef]
37. Ki, S.W.; Kasahara, K.; Kwon, H.J.; Eishima, J.; Takesako, K.; Cooper, J.A.; Yoshida, M.; Horinouchi, S. Identification of radicicol as an inhibitor of in vivo Ras/Raf interaction with the yeast two-hybrid screening system. *J. Antibiot. (Tokyo)* **1998**, *51*, 936–944. [CrossRef]
38. Soga, S.; Kozawa, T.; Narumi, H.; Akinaga, S.; Irie, K.; Matsumoto, K.; Sharma, S.V.; Nakano, H.; Mizukami, T.; Hara, M. Radicicol leads to selective depletion of Raf kinase and disrupts K-Ras-activated aberrant signaling pathway. *J. Biol. Chem.* **1998**, *273*, 822–828. [CrossRef]
39. Lee, S.; Oh, D.G.; Lee, S.; Kim, G.R.; Lee, J.S.; Son, Y.K.; Bae, C.H.; Yeo, J.; Lee, C.H. Chemotaxonomic Metabolite Profiling of 62 Indigenous Plant Species and Its Correlation with Bioactivities. *Molecules* **2015**, *20*, 19719–19734. [CrossRef]
40. Carija, A.; Navarro, S.; de Groot, N.S.; Ventura, S. Protein aggregation into insoluble deposits protects from oxidative stress. *Redox Biol.* **2017**, *12*, 699–711. [CrossRef]
41. Pang, X.; Liu, M. A combination therapy for KRAS-mutant lung cancer by targeting synthetic lethal partners of mutant KRAS. *Chin. J. Cancer* **2016**, *35*, 92. [CrossRef]
42. Pratilas, C.A.; Xing, F.; Solit, D.B. Targeting oncogenic BRAF in human cancer. *Curr. Top. Microbiol. Immunol.* **2012**, *355*, 83–98. [CrossRef] [PubMed]
43. Santarpia, L.; Lippman, S.M.; El-Naggar, A.K. Targeting the MAPK-RAS-RAF signaling pathway in cancer therapy. *Expert Opin. Targets* **2012**, *16*, 103–119. [CrossRef] [PubMed]
44. Heneka, M.T.; Kummer, M.P.; Latz, E. Innate immune activation in neurodegenerative disease. *Nat. Rev. Immunol.* **2014**, *14*, 463–477. [CrossRef] [PubMed]
45. Foito, A.; Stewart, D. Metabolomics: A high-throughput screen for biochemical and bioactivity diversity in plants and crops. *Curr. Pharm. Des.* **2018**, *24*, 2043–2054. [CrossRef]
46. Suganthy, N.; Devi, K.P.; Nabavi, S.F.; Braidy, N.; Nabavi, S.M. Bioactive effects of quercetin in the central nervous system: Focusing on the mechanisms of actions. *Biomed. Pharm.* **2016**, *84*, 892–908. [CrossRef]
47. Baral, S.; Pariyar, R.; Kim, J.; Lee, H.S.; Seo, J. Quercetin-3-O-glucuronide promotes the proliferation and migration of neural stem cells. *Neurobiol. Aging* **2017**, *52*, 39–52. [CrossRef]
48. Dey, A.; De, J.N. Neuroprotective therapeutics from botanicals and phytochemicals against Huntington's disease and related neurodegenerative disorders. *J. Herb. Med.* **2015**, *5*, 19. [CrossRef]
49. Testa, D.; Caraceni, T.; Fetoni, V. Branched-chain amino acids in the treatment of amyotrophic lateral sclerosis. *J. Neurol.* **1989**, *236*, 445–447. [CrossRef]
50. Tandan, R.; Bromberg, M.B.; Forshew, D.; Fries, T.J.; Badger, G.J.; Carpenter, J.; Krusinski, P.B.; Betts, E.F.; Arciero, K.; Nau, K. A controlled trial of amino acid therapy in amyotrophic lateral sclerosis: I. Clinical, functional, and maximum isometric torque data. *Neurology* **1996**, *47*, 1220–1226. [CrossRef]
51. The Italian ALS Study Group. Branched-chain amino acids and amyotrophic lateral sclerosis: A treatment failure. *Neurology* **1993**, *43*, 2466–2470. [CrossRef]
52. Plaitakis, A.; Smith, J.; Mandeli, J.; Yahr, M.D. Pilot trial of branched-chain aminoacids in amyotrophic lateral sclerosis. *Lancet* **1988**, *1*, 1015–1018. [CrossRef]

53. Mori, N.; Adachi, Y.; Takeshima, T.; Kashiwaya, Y.; Okada, A.; Nakashima, K. Branched-chain amino acid therapy for spinocerebellar degeneration: A pilot clinical crossover trial. *Intern. Med.* **1999**, *38*, 401–406. [CrossRef] [PubMed]
54. Patin, F.; Corcia, P.; Vourc'h, P.; Nadal-Desbarats, L.; Baranek, T.; Goossens, J.F.; Marouillat, S.; Dessein, A.F.; Descat, A.; Madji Hounoum, B.; et al. Omics to Explore Amyotrophic Lateral Sclerosis Evolution: The Central Role of Arginine and Proline Metabolism. *Mol. Neurobiol.* **2017**, *54*, 5361–5374. [CrossRef] [PubMed]
55. Nunez-Sanchez, M.A.; Gonzalez-Sarrias, A.; Romo-Vaquero, M.; Garcia-Villalba, R.; Selma, M.V.; Tomas-Barberan, F.A.; Garcia-Conesa, M.T.; Espin, J.C. Dietary phenolics against colorectal cancer—From promising preclinical results to poor translation into clinical trials: Pitfalls and future needs. *Mol. Nutr. Food Res.* **2015**, *59*, 1274–1291. [CrossRef] [PubMed]
56. McDougall, G.J.; Allwood, J.W.; Pereira-Caro, G.; Brown, E.M.; Verrall, S.; Stewart, D.; Latimer, C.; McMullan, G.; Lawther, R.; O'Connor, G.; et al. Novel colon-available triterpenoids identified in raspberry fruits exhibit antigenotoxic activities in vitro. *Mol. Nutr. Food Res.* **2017**, *61*, 1600327. [CrossRef] [PubMed]
57. Sharma, S.H.; Thulasingam, S.; Nagarajan, S. Terpenoids as anti-colon cancer agents—A comprehensive review on its mechanistic perspectives. *Eur. J. Pharm.* **2017**, *795*, 169–178. [CrossRef]
58. Saha, A.; Kuzuhara, T.; Echigo, N.; Suganuma, M.; Fujiki, H. New role of (-)-epicatechin in enhancing the induction of growth inhibition and apoptosis in human lung cancer cells by curcumin. *Cancer Prev. Res. (Phila)* **2010**, *3*, 953–962. [CrossRef]
59. Suganuma, M.; Okabe, S.; Kai, Y.; Sueoka, N.; Sueoka, E.; Fujiki, H. Synergistic effects of (−)-epigallocatechin gallate with (−)-epicatechin, sulindac, or tamoxifen on cancer-preventive activity in the human lung cancer cell line PC-9. *Cancer Res.* **1999**, *59*, 44–47.
60. Arts, I.C.; Jacobs, D.R., Jr.; Gross, M.; Harnack, L.J.; Folsom, A.R. Dietary catechins and cancer incidence among postmenopausal women: The Iowa Women's Health Study (United States). *Cancer Causes Control* **2002**, *13*, 373–382. [CrossRef]
61. Theodoratou, E.; Kyle, J.; Cetnarskyj, R.; Farrington, S.M.; Tenesa, A.; Barnetson, R.; Porteous, M.; Dunlop, M.; Campbell, H. Dietary flavonoids and the risk of colorectal cancer. *Cancer Epidemiol. Biomark. Prev.* **2007**, *16*, 684–693. [CrossRef]
62. Piszcz, J.; Lemancewicz, D.; Dudzik, D.; Ciborowski, M. Differences and similarities between LC-MS derived serum fingerprints of patients with B-cell malignancies. *Electrophoresis* **2013**, *34*, 2857–2864. [CrossRef] [PubMed]
63. Struck-Lewicka, W.; Kordalewska, M.; Bujak, R.; Yumba Mpanga, A.; Markuszewski, M.; Jacyna, J.; Matuszewski, M.; Kaliszan, R.; Markuszewski, M.J. Urine metabolic fingerprinting using LC-MS and GC-MS reveals metabolite changes in prostate cancer: A pilot study. *J. Pharm. Biomed. Anal.* **2015**, *111*, 351–361. [CrossRef] [PubMed]
64. Morais, C.A.; De Rosso, V.V.; Estadella, D.; Pisani, L.P. Anthocyanins as inflammatory modulators and the role of the gut microbiota. *J. Nutr. Biochem.* **2016**, *33*, 1–7. [CrossRef] [PubMed]
65. Cassidy, A.; Rogers, G.; Peterson, J.J.; Dwyer, J.T.; Lin, H.; Jacques, P.F. Higher dietary anthocyanin and flavonol intakes are associated with anti-inflammatory effects in a population of US adults. *Am. J. Clin. Nutr.* **2015**, *102*, 172–181. [CrossRef]
66. Jung, H.; Lee, H.J.; Cho, H.; Lee, K.; Kwak, H.K.; Hwang, K.T. Anthocyanins in Rubus fruits and antioxidant and anti-inflammatory activities in RAW 264.7 cells. *Food Sci. Biotechnol.* **2015**, *24*, 1879–1886. [CrossRef]
67. Fratantonio, D.; Speciale, A.; Ferrari, D.; Cristani, M.; Saija, A.; Cimino, F. Palmitate-induced endothelial dysfunction is attenuated by cyanidin-3-O-glucoside through modulation of Nrf2/Bach1 and NF-kappaB pathways. *Toxicol. Lett.* **2015**, *239*, 152–160. [CrossRef]
68. Ferrari, D.; Speciale, A.; Cristani, M.; Fratantonio, D.; Molonia, M.S.; Ranaldi, G.; Saija, A.; Cimino, F. Cyanidin-3-O-glucoside inhibits NF-kB signalling in intestinal epithelial cells exposed to TNF-alpha and exerts protective effects via Nrf2 pathway activation. *Toxicol. Lett.* **2016**, *264*, 51–58. [CrossRef]
69. Ajit, D.; Simonyi, A.; Li, R.; Chen, Z.; Hannink, M.; Fritsche, K.L.; Mossine, V.V.; Smith, R.E.; Dobbs, T.K.; Luo, R.; et al. Phytochemicals and botanical extracts regulate NF-kappaB and Nrf2/ARE reporter activities in DI TNC1 astrocytes. *Neurochem. Int.* **2016**, *97*, 49–56. [CrossRef]
70. Serra, D.; Paixao, J.; Nunes, C.; Dinis, T.C.; Almeida, L.M. Cyanidin-3-glucoside suppresses cytokine-induced inflammatory response in human intestinal cells: Comparison with 5-aminosalicylic acid. *PLoS ONE* **2013**, *8*, e73001. [CrossRef]

71. Cimino, F.; Ambra, R.; Canali, R.; Saija, A.; Virgili, F. Effect of cyanidin-3-O-glucoside on UVB-induced response in human keratinocytes. *J. Agric. Food Chem.* **2006**, *54*, 4041–4047. [CrossRef]
72. Park, K.H.; Gu, D.R.; So, H.S.; Kim, K.J.; Lee, S.H. Dual Role of Cyanidin-3-glucoside on the Differentiation of Bone Cells. *J. Dent. Res.* **2015**, *94*, 1676–1683. [CrossRef] [PubMed]
73. Duarte, L.J.; Chaves, V.C.; Nascimento, M.; Calvete, E.; Li, M.; Ciraolo, E.; Ghigo, A.; Hirsch, E.; Simoes, C.M.O.; Reginatto, F.H.; et al. Molecular mechanism of action of Pelargonidin-3-O-glucoside, the main anthocyanin responsible for the anti-inflammatory effect of strawberry fruits. *Food Chem.* **2018**, *247*, 56–65. [CrossRef] [PubMed]
74. Manach, C.; Williamson, G.; Morand, C.; Scalbert, A.; Remesy, C. Bioavailability and bioefficacy of polyphenols in humans. I. Review of 97 bioavailability studies. *Am. J. Clin. Nutr.* **2005**, *81*, 230S–242S. [CrossRef] [PubMed]

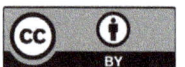

© 2020 by the authors. Licensee MDPI, Basel, Switzerland. This article is an open access article distributed under the terms and conditions of the Creative Commons Attribution (CC BY) license (http://creativecommons.org/licenses/by/4.0/).

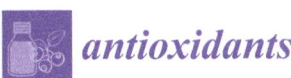

Article

Activation of NRF2 and ATF4 Signaling by the Pro-Glutathione Molecule I-152, a Co-Drug of *N*-Acetyl-Cysteine and Cysteamine

Rita Crinelli [1,*], Carolina Zara [1], Luca Galluzzi [1], Gloria Buffi [1], Chiara Ceccarini [1], Michael Smietana [2], Michele Mari [1], Mauro Magnani [1] and Alessandra Fraternale [1]

[1] Department of Biomolecular Sciences, University of Urbino Carlo Bo, 61029 Urbino, Italy; c.zara@campus.uniurb.it (C.Z.); luca.galluzzi@uniurb.it (L.G.); g.buffi@campus.uniurb.it (G.B.); c.ceccarini2@campus.uniurb.it (C.C.); michele.mari@uniurb.it (M.M.); mauro.magnani@uniurb.it (M.M.); alessandra.fraternale@uniurb.it (A.F.)
[2] Institut des Biomolécules Max Mousseron, Université de Montpellier UMR 5247 CNRS, ENSCM, 34095 Montpellier, France; michael.smietana@umontpellier.fr
* Correspondence: rita.crinelli@uniurb.it; Tel./Fax:+39-0722-305288; Fax: +39-0722-304578

Abstract: I-152 combines two pro-glutathione (GSH) molecules, namely N-acetyl-cysteine (NAC) and cysteamine (MEA), to improve their potency. The co-drug efficiently increases/replenishes GSH levels in vitro and in vivo; little is known about its mechanism of action. Here we demonstrate that I-152 not only supplies GSH precursors, but also activates the antioxidant kelch-like ECH-associated protein 1/nuclear factor E2-related factor 2 (KEAP1/NRF2) pathway. The mechanism involves disulfide bond formation between KEAP1 cysteine residues, NRF2 stabilization and enhanced expression of the γ-glutamil cysteine ligase regulatory subunit. Accordingly, a significant increase in GSH levels, not reproduced by treatment with NAC or MEA alone, was found. Compared to its parent compounds, I-152 delivered NAC more efficiently within cells and displayed increased reactivity to KEAP1 compared to MEA. While at all the concentrations tested, I-152 activated the NRF2 pathway; high doses caused co-activation of activating transcription factor 4 (ATF4) and ATF4-dependent gene expression through a mechanism involving Atf4 transcriptional activation rather than preferential mRNA translation. In this case, GSH levels tended to decrease over time, and a reduction in cell proliferation/survival was observed, highlighting that there is a concentration threshold which determines the transition from advantageous to adverse effects. This body of evidence provides a molecular framework for the pro-GSH activity and dose-dependent effects of I-152 and shows how synergism and cross reactivity between different thiol species could be exploited to develop more potent drugs.

Keywords: GSH; Cysteamine; N-acetyl cysteine; KEAP1; NRF2; ATF4

Citation: Crinelli, R.; Zara, C.; Galluzzi, L.; Buffi, G.; Ceccarini, C.; Smietana, M.; Mari, M.; Magnani, M.; Fraternale, A. Activation of NRF2 and ATF4 Signaling by the Pro-Glutathione Molecule I-152, A Co-Drug of *N*-Acetyl-Cysteine and Cysteamine. *Antioxidants* **2021**, *10*, 175. https://doi.org/10.3390/antiox10020175

Academic Editor: Ana Sofia Fernandes

Received: 7 January 2021
Accepted: 22 January 2021
Published: 26 January 2021

Publisher's Note: MDPI stays neutral with regard to jurisdictional claims in published maps and institutional affiliations.

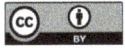

Copyright: © 2021 by the authors. Licensee MDPI, Basel, Switzerland. This article is an open access article distributed under the terms and conditions of the Creative Commons Attribution (CC BY) license (https://creativecommons.org/licenses/by/4.0/).

1. Introduction

Reduced glutathione is the most abundant non-protein thiol specie within the cell, where it plays a crucial role in controlling redox homeostasis, metabolism, detoxification, and signal transduction [1]. Maintenance of adequate GSH levels is fundamental to proper cell functioning, proliferation and survival under physiological and stress conditions.

Glutathione is synthesized in a two-step process consisting of enzymatic reactions catalysed by γ-glutamyl-cysteine ligase (GCL, EC 6.3.2.2) and glutathione synthase (GS, EC 6.3.2.3). The rate of glutathione synthesis is essentially dependent on cysteine levels and GCL activity. GCL is composed of a catalytic (GCLC) and modifier (GCLM) subunit; the catalytic monomer functions autonomously, but its association with the regulatory subunit greatly increases the Km for glutamate and ATP and the Ki for GSH [2].

Notably, GCL activity is mainly regulated at the level of transcription, although other levels of regulation may occur post-translationally [3]. Both GCL subunits are under the transcriptional control of NRF2, which is activated by many oxidants and electrophilic compounds [4,5]. The classical mechanism of activation involves alkylation and/or oxidation of redox-sensitive cysteine residues on KEAP1, an E3 ligase adaptor protein, which, under basal conditions, targets NRF2 to proteasome-mediated degradation, keeping NRF2 levels low [6]. Upon oxidation/alkylation, KEAP1 becomes non-functional with the consequent stabilization and translocation of NRF2 to the nucleus, where the factor drives the transcription of a set of genes involved in glutathione synthesis and recycling, xenobiotic metabolism and transport, and antioxidant genes [7].

ATF4 is a cAMP-response element binding protein that belongs to the activating transcription factor/cAMP response element-binding protein family (ATF/CREB) [8]. ATF4 is known as the main effector of the integrated stress response (IRS), an adaptive pathway where different stress stimuli signal disturbance in cell homeostasis, converging on a common transducer, namely the eukaryotic translation initiation factor 2α (eIF2α). In this pathway, phosphorylation of eIF2α leads to global attenuation of Cap-dependent translation, while concomitantly initiating the preferential translation of specific mRNAs such as the ATF4 mRNA [9]. Under stressful conditions, elevated translation of ATF4 facilitates transcriptional upregulation of protective or pro-apoptotic stress-responsive genes, depending on the nature, intensity, and duration of the stress stimuli.

A growing body of evidence suggests that simultaneous activation of NRF2 and ATF4 potentiates the expression of cytoprotective genes and increases GSH levels under both basal and oxidative stress conditions [10,11]. Although the NRF2 and ATF4 signaling pathways have independent mechanisms of activation, they do indeed share some downstream target genes [12,13]. Moreover, NRF2 and ATF4 cooperate on the level of glutathione, where ATF4 promotes the uptake of glutathione amino acid building blocks, including glutamine and cysteine, and promotes glutamate production via induction of asparagine synthetase [14,15]. On the other hand, ATF4 is also involved in the degradation of GSH under stress conditions by inducing the expression of the cation transport regulator-like protein 1 (CHAC1; EC 4.3.2.7) [16]. CHAC1 belongs to a family of enzymes responsible for the degradation of intracellular glutathione in response to different types of stresses to provide three vital amino acids and help cells to cope with stress [17].

Disturbances in glutathione homeostasis have been implicated in the etiology and/or progression of several human diseases, including cancer, cardiovascular, and neurodegenerative disorders [18]. Attempts to replenish GSH levels in chronic and transient depletion states have focused on the use of GSH or GSH analogues and biosynthetic precursors such as L-cysteine. More recently, approaches related to the possibility of manipulating the activity of the enzymes involved in GSH homeostasis have also been taken into consideration [19,20]. These approaches involve the use of natural or chemically synthesized compounds able to activate antioxidant signalling pathways, although for most of these substances a clear mechanism of action has not been provided.

I-152 is a conjugate of NAC and S-acetyl-MEA (SMEA) linked together by an amide bond [21]. The molecule is deacetylated on the MEA moiety and hydrolyzed within the cells to release NAC and MEA, two well-known pro-glutathione compounds. I-152 has been shown to efficiently boost GSH both in vivo and in vitro, under physiological and pathological conditions characterized by GSH depletion (i.e., viral infection) (reviewed in [22]). Little is known about the mechanism of action of I-152. To date, its beneficial effects on GSH metabolism have been attributed to its ability to provide cysteine precursors.

In this investigation, we show that I-152 activates the NRF2 signaling pathway in RAW 264.7 cells by inducing KEAP-1 oxidation and NRF2 stabilization, leading to GCLM expression and increased intracellular GSH levels. The same effects could not be reproduced using equimolar concentrations of NAC or MEA. Notably, while I-152 dose-dependently activated NRF2 at all the doses tested, only high doses induced transcriptional activation of ATF4 and ATF4-dependent gene expression. Under this condition, GSH levels did not change, but rather tended to decrease over time. This paradoxical effect and the possible consequences of the concomitant activation of NRF2 and ATF4 are discussed.

2. Materials and Methods

2.1. Cell Culture and Treatment

The murine macrophage cell line RAW 264.7 was cultured in Dulbecco's Modified Eagle's Medium (DMEM) high glucose supplemented with 10% heat-inactivated fetal bovine serum, 2 mM L-glutamine, 100 µg/mL streptomycin and 100 U/mL penicillin. Cells were plated in 35 mm dishes at a density of 0.1×10^6 cells/well two days before the treatment. I-152 was synthesized as previously described [21], while cysteamine and N-acetyl cysteine were purchased from Sigma-Aldrich. The chemicals were directly dissolved into the cell culture medium, which was then filtered through a sterile 0.22 µm pore size membrane. On the day of the treatment, the culture medium was removed and replaced with a fresh one containing or not containing the indicated molecules.

2.2. Cell Lysates

Cells were washed on ice with cold Phosphate-Buffered Saline (PBS) and directly lysed in Sodium Dodecyl Sulfate (SDS) buffer (50 mM Tris-HCl, pH 7.8, 0.25 M sucrose, 2% (w/v) SDS, 10 mM N-ethylmaleimide-NEM) supplemented with a cocktail of protease (Complete, Roche) and phosphatase inhibitors (1 mM Na_3VO_4, 1 mM NaF). Whole cell lysates were boiled for 5 min, sonicated at 70 Watts for 40 s to shear nucleic acids and centrifuged at $14,000 \times g$ at room temperature (RT) to remove debris. Protein content was determined in the supernatant by the Lowry Assay using bovine serum albumin (BSA) as a reference standard.

2.3. SDS-PAGE and Western Immunoblotting

Proteins were resolved by SDS polyacrylamide gel electrophoresis (SDS-PAGE) and electroblotted onto polyvinylidene difluoride (PVDF) membranes (0.2 µm pore size). After blocking in 5% (w/v) nonfat dry milk (Cell Signaling Technologies, #9999), membranes were incubated with the following primary antibodies: anti NRF2 (D1Z9C, XP #12721), anti KEAP1 (D1G10, #7705), anti p53 (1C12, #2524), anti ATF4 (D4B8, #11815), anti [P]eIF2α (Ser51) (D9G8, XP #3398) and anti β-ACTIN (#4967) from Cell Signaling Technologies; anti HMOX1 (F-4, sc-390991) and anti GADD153 (CHOP) (B-3, sc-7351) (from Santa Cruz Biotechnology; anti GCLC (VPA00695) from BioRad; anti GCLM (A5314) from ABclonal; anti CHAC1 (N1C3, GTX120775) from GeneTex. After overnight incubation at +4 °C, a horseradish peroxidase (HRP)-conjugated secondary antibody (Bio-Rad, Hercules, CA, USA) was used to detect immunoreactive bands. Bands were visualized with the enhanced chemiluminescence detection kit WesternBright ECL (Advansta, San Jose, CA, USA) in a ChemiDoc MP Imaging System and quantified by using the Image Lab software (Bio-Rad, Hercules, CA, USA).

2.4. Cycloheximide (CHX) Chase Assay and Relative Half-Life Determination

Cells were left untreated or treated with 1 mM I-152. CHX (50 µg/mL) was added to the culture medium of both untreated and I-152-treated cells at the beginning of the incubation (co-treatment) or after 30 min of pre-incubation with medium containing or not containing the I-152 molecule. Cells were collected immediately (time 0) and at specific time points (10, 20, 30, and 60 min) following CHX administration. Whole cell lysates were obtained as described above and separated by SDS-PAGE for Western blotting analysis. To determine the relative half-life, the intensity of the immunoreactive bands was measured and expressed as the percent of the time 0 sample value (initial value). The Log_{10} of the percentage values was plotted versus time (min). After linear regression analysis, the time required for degradation of 50% of the protein from its initial value (half-life) was calculated from the equation by replacing y with Log_{10} of 50 and solving for x.

2.5. NEM-Alkylated Redox Western Blotting

Cells were washed with cold PBS and scraped in 10% (w/v) trichloroacetic acid (TCA). After 30 min on ice, samples were centrifuged at $14,000 \times g$ + 4 °C, and the pellets were washed twice in ice-cold acetone. Protein pellets were dissolved by vortexing in 100 mM Tris-HCl, pH 6.8, 2% (w/v) SDS, 40 mM NEM. NEM was used to block free sulfhydryl groups and avoid Cys oxidation during extraction. Protein extracts were centrifuged again to remove insoluble debris, and protein concentration was determined by the Lowry Method. Protein samples were separated by non-reducing SDS-PAGE. Parallel runs were performed under reducing conditions to demonstrate the specificity of the signal.

2.6. RNA Isolation and cDNA Synthesis

RAW 264.7 cells were directly lysed with 700 µL of QIAzol® Lysis Reagent (Qiagen, Hilden, Germany). Total RNA was isolated using the miRNeasy Mini Kit (Qiagen, Hilden, Germany) and eluted in 40 µL of RNase-free water. The extracted RNA was quantified using a NanoVue PlusTM spectrophotometer (GE Healthcare Life Sciences, Piscataway, NJ, USA). Total RNA (500 ng) was reverse transcribed using PrimeScriptTM RT Master Mix (Perfect Real Time) (Takara Bio Europe, Saint-Germain-en-Laye, France) according to the manufacturer's instructions.

2.7. Quantitative Real-Time PCR

The expression of *Atf4*, *Chac1*, *Chop*, *Gclc*, *Gclm*, *Hmox1* and *Nrf2* (*Nfe2l2*) genes was monitored by qPCR as previously described [23] with slight modifications. Briefly, the qPCR reactions were performed in duplicate in a final volume of 20 µL using TB Green PreMix ex Taq II Master Mix (Takara Bio Europe, France) and 200 nM primers (Table 1), in a RotorGene 6000 instrument (Corbett life science, Sydney, Australia). The amplification conditions were 95 °C for 10 min, 40 cycles at 95 °C for 10 s and 60 °C for 50 s. To confirm the absence of non-specific products or primer dimers, a melting curve analysis was performed from 65 to 95 °C at the end of each run, with a slope of 1 °C/s, and 5 s at each temperature. A duplicate non-template control was included for each target as a negative control. *Gapdh* (glyceraldchydes-3-phosphate dehydrogenase) and *Gusb* (β-D-glucuronidase) were used as reference genes. The relative expression levels were calculated using the $2^{-\Delta\Delta Ct}$ method [24].

Table 1. Primers used for gene expression analysis in RAW 264.7 cells.

Target mRNA	Accession Number	Forward Primer (5′–3′)	Reverse Primer (5′–3′)
Atf4	NM_001287180	GCAGTGTTGCTGTAACGGAC	ATCTCGGTCATGTTGTGGGG
Chac1	NM_026929	TATAGTGACAGCCGTGTGGG	GCTCCCCTCGAACTTGGTAT
Chop	NM_007837	GAGTCCCTGCCTTTCACCTT	TTCCTCTTCGTTTCCTGGGG
Gclc	NM_010295	GGAGAGGACAAACCCCAACC	CTCAGACATCGTTCCTCCGT
Gclm	NM_008129	GGAACCTGCTCAACTGGGG	GGTCTTTTGGATACAGTCCCGA
Hmox1	NM_010442	TTAAGCTGGTGATGGCTTCCT	AGTGGGGCATAGACTGGGTT
Nrf2	NM_010902	CACATTCCCAAACAAGATGCCT	TATCCAGGGCAAGCGACTCA
Gusb	NM_010368	GGGTGTGGTATGAACGGGAA	CCATTCACCCACACAACTGC
Gapdh	NM_001289726	TGCCCCCATGTTTGTGATG	TGTGGTCATGAGCCCTTCC

Atf4, Mus musculus activating transcription factor 4; *Chac1*, Mus musculus ChaC, cation transport regulator 1; *Chop*, Mus musculus DNA-damage inducible transcript 3; *Gclc*, Mus musculus glutamate-cysteine ligase, catalytic subunit; *Gclm*, Mus musculus glutamate-cysteine ligase, modifier subunit; *Hmox1*, Mus musculus heme oxygenase 1; *Nrf2*, Mus musculus nuclear factor, erythroid derived 2, like 2; *Gapdh*, Mus musculus glyceraldehyde-3-phosphate dehydrogenase; *Gusb*, Mus musculus β-D-glucuronidase. *Atf4*, *Chac1* and *Chop* primers were described in [23]; *Nrf2* primers were taken from [25] and *Gapdh* primers from [26].

2.8. Thiol Content Determination by High Performance Liquid Chromatography (HPLC)

Thiol content was assayed as previously described [27]. Briefly, after treatment, cells were lysed with 100 µL of a buffer consisting of 0.1% (v/v) Triton X-100, 0.1 M Na_2HPO_4, 5 mM EDTA, pH 7.5. Fifteen µL of 0.1 N HCl and 140 µL of precipitating solution (100 mL containing 1.67 g of glacial metaphosphoric acid, 0.2 g of disodium EDTA, 30 g of NaCl) were then added. After centrifugation, the pellet was dissolved in 0.1 M NaOH and protein concentration was determined by the Bradford assay; the supernatant was mixed with 25% (v/v) 0.3 M Na_2HPO_4, and 10% (v/v) 5,5'-dithio-bis-(2-nitrobenzoic acid) (DTNB) was then immediately added. The mixture was stirred for 1 min at RT, then left at RT for another 5 min, and finally used for determination of GSH and other thiols by a high-performance liquid chromatography (HPLC) method. Quantitative measurements were obtained by injection of standards of known concentrations and values were normalized on protein concentration.

2.9. Lactate Dehydrogenase (LDH)-Based Cytotoxicity Assay

Cell growth inhibition and cell death were assessed by using a modified version of the assay described by Smith et al. [28]. Briefly, 10,000 cells/well were seeded in 96 well tissue culture plates for two days and then treated with different concentrations of I-152. Untreated cells were used as controls (CTR). Each condition was assayed in octuplicate. After 24 h and 48 h of treatment, the medium deriving from four wells for each condition was recovered and pooled in a tube; care was taken not to disturb the underlying cell layer. Two % (v/v) Triton X-100 was added to the remaining four wells and mixed thoroughly using a pipette to ensure complete cell lysis. The pooled media (S) and the pooled extracts (cell lysate + medium, TOT) were then centrifuged at 1000× g for 10 min at 4 °C and the supernatants transferred in fresh tubes. Lactate dehydrogenase (EC 1.1.1.27) activity (LDH_{act}) was assayed spectrophotometrically following the protocol described in Beutler et al. [29]. Since the culture medium contained low levels of LDH, this basal activity was subtracted from the LDH_{act} determined in the samples before calculation.

$$\text{Percent killing: } (LDH_{act}\ S/LDH_{act}\ TOT) \times 100 \quad (1)$$

$$\text{Percent total effect: } [1-(LDH_{act}\ I\text{-}152\ TOT/LDH_{act}\ CTR\ TOT)] \times 100 \quad (2)$$

Percent growth inhibition: Percent total effect (Equation (2))—percent killing (Equation (1)).

2.10. Statistical Analysis

Data were analyzed using Prism software version 5.0 (GraphPad, San Diego, CA, USA). The *t*-test was performed to compare two groups of data, whereas one-way ANOVA was used to compare more than two groups. The Tukey posttest was used when every mean was compared to every other mean, whereas the Dunnet posttest was used to compare every mean to the control mean. Asterisks indicate significance versus control (denoted by 0 or CTR) unless otherwise specified, and $p \leq 0.05$ were considered significant.

3. Results

3.1. I-152 Increases the Levels of NRF2

The ability of I-152 to increase intracellular GSH levels has been previously demonstrated in vivo, in a murine model of retroviral infection [30] and in vitro, in human monocyte-derived macrophages, peritoneal murine macrophages and RAW 264.7 cells [21,27]. Since overlapping results have been obtained in primary and immortalized cells, the latter were selected as an experimental model to study how I-152 influences GSH homeostasis at the molecular level.

Previous evidence indicates that 10 mM I-152 causes GSH depletion in RAW 264.7 cells but yields a high content of thiol species in the form of NAC, MEA and I-152. By contrast, 1 mM I-152 increases cellular GSH content [27]. Thus, this range of concentrations was initially used to test whether the molecule is able to activate the NRF2 signaling pathway, considering that both MEA and NAC have been reported as potential NRF2 activators [31,32].

As shown in Figure 1A, 10 mM I-152 did not affect NRF2 levels, while 5 and 1 mM significantly increased NRF2 expression.

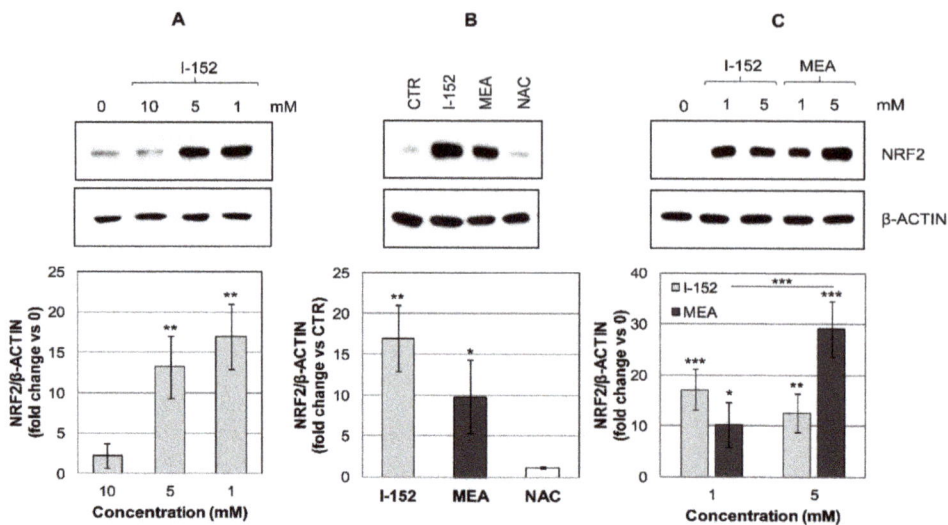

Figure 1. NRF2 levels in cells treated with I-152 and its metabolites NAC and MEA. RAW 264.7 cells were treated with: (**A**) different concentrations of I-152; (**B**) 1 mM I-152 compared to equimolar concentrations of NAC or MEA; (**C**) I-152 or MEA at two different concentrations. Cells were incubated with the molecules for 2 h while control cells (denoted by 0 or controls (CTR)) were incubated with fresh medium. Whole cell lysates (10 μg) were separated on 8% (w/v) SDS-polyacrylamide gels, blotted onto PVDF membranes and probed with an antibody against NRF2. β-ACTIN was stained as a control. Immunoreactive bands were quantified with the Image Lab software and NRF2 levels, normalized on β-ACTIN, expressed as fold-change relative to CTR (0). Values are the mean ± S.D. of at least three independent experiments. * $p < 0.05$; ** $p < 0.01$, *** $p < 0.001$.

When NAC and MEA were tested singularly, only MEA activated NRF2; by contrast, NAC had no effect (Figure 1B). Notably, MEA increased NRF2 levels dose-dependently; by contrast, the efficacy of I-152 was inversely correlated with its concentration (Figure 1C). Overall, these results suggest that I-152 may activate the NRF2 pathway, probably by delivering MEA.

To compare the potency of I-152 and MEA we subsequently performed dose-dependent experiments at concentrations equal to and below 1 mM. MEA is typically used in vitro at concentrations ranging from 1 mM to 0.05 mM [33,34], while doses up to 10 mM of NAC can be found in literature [35]. A stronger activation of NRF2 was observed in I-152-treated cells than in those incubated with MEA (Figure 2). Indeed, after 2 h, only 1 mM MEA significantly increased NRF2 levels over the basal level, while I-152 was effective at concentrations as low as 0.125 mM. Moreover, the effects of I-152 were still evident after 24 h incubation, while MEA was no longer effective.

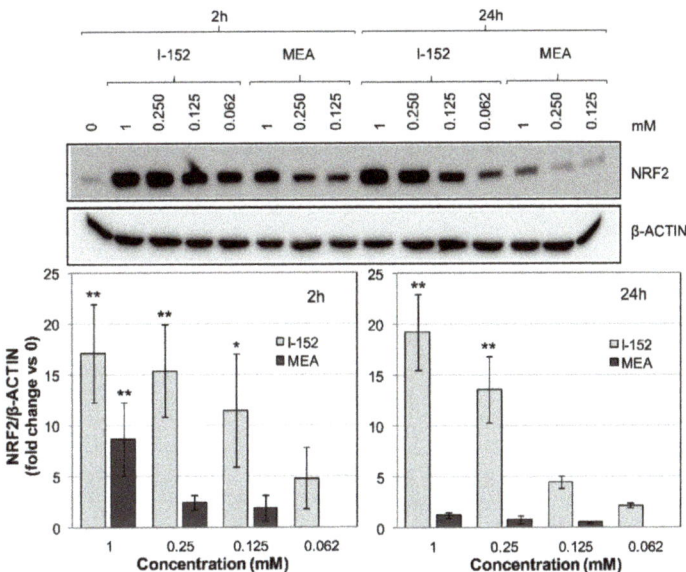

Figure 2. NRF2 levels in I-152- versus MEA-treated RAW 264.7 cells. Cells were treated with different concentrations of I-152 and MEA for 2 h and 24 h; control cells received only fresh medium (0). Whole cell lysates (10 µg) were separated on 8% (w/v) SDS-polyacrylamide gels and analyzed by immunoblotting using an antibody against NRF2. β-ACTIN was stained as a control. Immunoreactive bands were detected in a Molecular Imager and quantified with the Image Lab software. NRF2 levels, normalized to β-ACTIN content, are reported in the graph as fold change relative to control (0). Values are the mean ± SD of at least three independent experiments. * $p < 0.05$, ** $p < 0.01$.

3.2. I-152 Induces KEAP1 Oxidation and NRF2 Stabilization

To shed light on the mechanism(s) of I-152-mediated NRF2 intracellular accumulation, *Nrf2* gene expression and the rate of protein degradation were determined. After incubation with I-152, *Nrf2* mRNA levels were substantially unchanged compared to the control (Figure 3A), allowing us to exclude transcriptional induction. By contrast, co-treatment with cycloheximide, a well-known translational inhibitor, followed by Western blotting analysis revealed that NRF2 protein degradation was significantly reduced in I-152-treated cells compared to untreated cells receiving only CHX (0) (Figure 3B). More marked differences were obtained when CHX was added to the culture medium after 30 min pre-incubation with I-152 (Figure 3C).

The relative NRF2 half-life was 16.7 min and 28.4 min in I-152-treated cells depending on whether CHX was added together with I-152 or after pre-incubation with I-152, respectively versus 8.2 ± 0.47 min in untreated cells (Figure S1A,B). By contrast, degradation of p53, another short half-life protein, was unaffected, suggesting that the effect of I-152 is specific for NRF2 (Figure 3D).

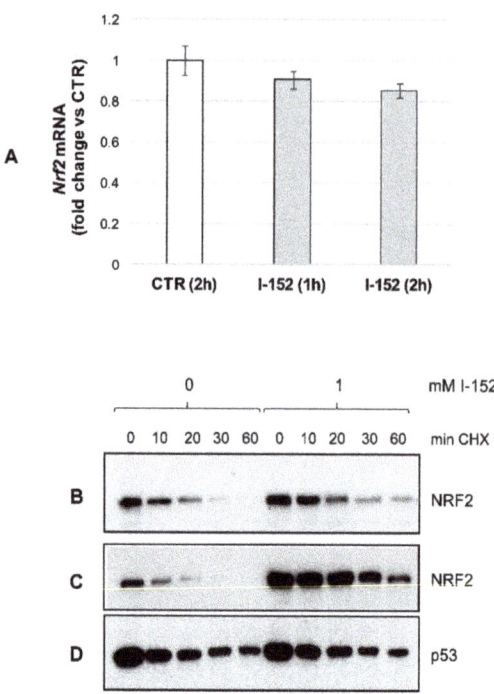

Figure 3. Nrf2 mRNA levels and NRF2 protein degradation after I-152 treatment. (**A**) RTqPCR analysis of *Nrf2* mRNA levels in cells treated with 1 mM I-152 for 1 h and 2 h. Expression levels were normalized to the housekeeping genes *Gapdh* and *Gusb* and expressed as fold-change versus untreated cells (CTR). The values are the mean ± SD of two independent experiments with two technical replicates (**B**) Western immunoblotting analysis of NRF2 levels in extracts obtained from cells treated with 1 mM I-152 together with cycloheximide (CHX) for different times. Control cells were left untreated and incubated only with CHX (0). In some experiments, CHX was added after 30 min pre-incubation with I-152 and NRF2 (**C**) and p53 (**D**) protein levels were determined by western blotting. Ten µg of total proteins were loaded on 8% (*w/v*) SDS polyacrylamide gels.

In light of this evidence, we then investigated the redox state of endogenous KEAP1 by NEM-alkylated redox western, which makes it possible to detect protein oxidation by monitoring changes in electrophoretic mobility under non-reducing conditions. After treatment, cell extracts were resolved by SDS-PAGE under non-reducing and reducing conditions and stained with an antibody against KEAP1. In all the reduced samples, KEAP1 migrated as a single band of the expected molecular weight (about 70 kDa) (Figure 4A), although a faint band of lower molecular weight could be detected in all the samples.

When reduction was omitted, KEAP1 still migrated as a major band of the same molecular mass (denoted by Red for reduced), but a second less intense band with faster mobility (denoted by Ox1 for oxidized form 1) appeared in I-152- and MEA-treated samples, but not in lysates from untreated cells (0) (Figure 4B). Moreover, a 75 kDa immunoreactive species was present in all the samples, independently of the treatment. Finally, two bands (denoted by Ox2 and Ox3) with a much slower mobility than red KEAP1 were evident in the upper part of the non-reducing gel, while they were absent in reduced samples. The intensity of the Ox1, Ox2, and Ox3 bands increased with the I-152 dose and was more pronounced in cells treated with 1 mM I-152 than in those treated with an equimolar concentration of MEA, suggesting that I-152 is a more potent KEAP1 oxidant than MEA (Figure 4B). Notably, NRF2 staining indicated that there was a good correlation between KEAP1 oxidation and NRF2 stabilization, pointing to a cause and effect relationship. The link between KEAP1 oxidation and NRF2 stabilization was further demonstrated by a time course analysis. As shown in Figure 4C, KEAP1 was already strongly oxidized after 15 min incubation with 1 mM I-152, while NRF2 levels were significantly increased over the control levels at 30 min, a time lag which is consistent with the estimated NRF2 half-life between 15 and 30 min [36,37].

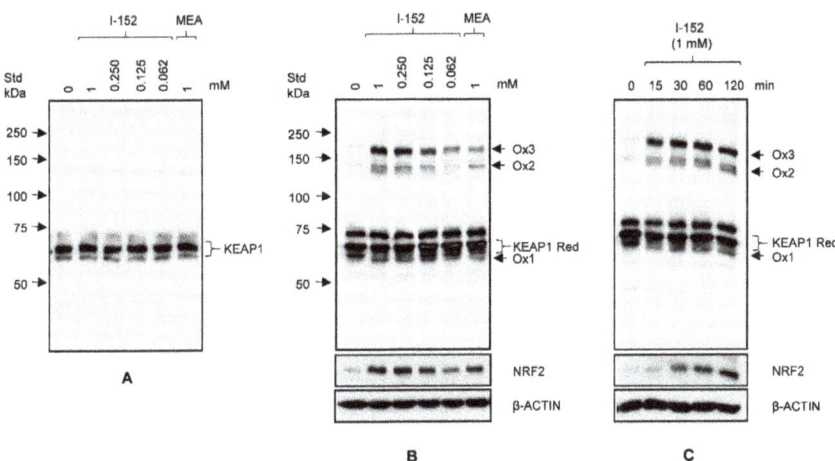

Figure 4. KEAP1 oxidation in cells treated with I-152 and MEA. RAW 264.7 cells were exposed to different concentrations of I-152 and to 1 mM MEA for 2 h. The cells were then lysed in the presence of NEM to block free sulfhydryl groups. The lysates were separated by reducing (**A**) and non-reducing (**B**) SDS-PAGE, and KEAP1 was revealed by western immunoblotting analysis using an anti-KEAP1 antibody. Ten μg of total proteins were loaded on 8% (*w/v*) polyacrylamide gel. (**C**) Raw 264.7 cells were treated with 1 mM I-152 for different times and lysates, obtained as in A, were separated under non-reducing conditions. In panels B and C, the blots were re-probed with anti NRF2 antibody and β-ACTIN was stained as a control. Arrows on the right side indicate the oxidized faster migrating (Ox1) and the oxidized slower migrating (Ox2 and Ox3) KEAP1 species, while brackets show the position of reduced (Red) KEAP1.

3.3. I-152 Activates NRF2-Dependent Gene Transcription and Increases GCLM Protein Levels

To assess whether accumulation of NFR2 resulted in increased transcriptional activity, the mRNA levels of heme oxygenase-1 (*Hmox1*), a prototypical NRF2 target gene, *Gclc* and *Gclm* were determined by RTqPCR. At 6 h of treatment, all the genes were activated by all the I-152 doses tested and by 1 mM MEA (Figure S2A, Figure 5A,B). The most relevant induction was observed in the case of the *Gclm* gene (Figure 5B).

Analysis of the protein levels reveals that no changes occurred in GCLC intracellular concentrations (Figure 5C and Figure S2C), while both HMOX1 (Figure S2B) and GCLM (Figure 5C,D) protein levels were increased at 6 h incubation and rose further at 24 h in the case of GCLM. In agreement with mRNA induction, GCLM protein accumulated only in cells treated with 1 mM MEA (Figure 5C,D).

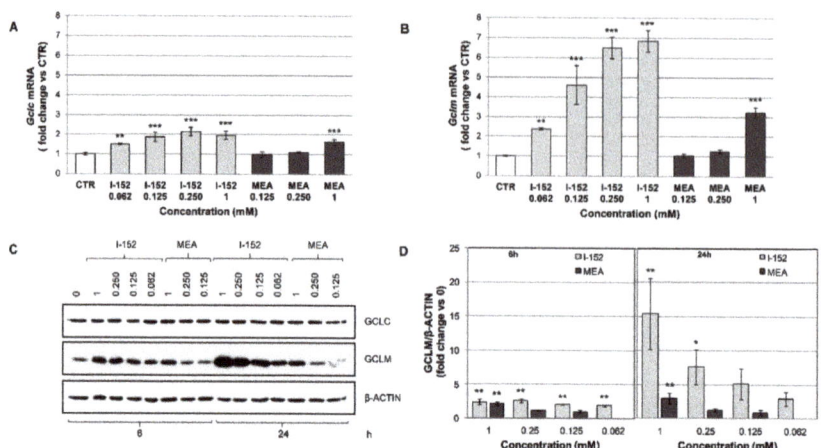

Figure 5. NRF2-dependent gene transcription and protein expression. RAW 264.7 cells were exposed to different concentrations of I-152 and MEA for 6 h and 24 h. (**A,B**) RTqPCR analysis of *Gclc* and *Gclm* mRNA levels after 6 h of treatment. mRNA levels were normalized to the housekeeping genes *Gapdh* and *Gusb* and expressed as fold-change versus untreated cells (CTR). The values are the mean ± SD of at least two independent experiments with two technical replicates. (**C**) Western immunoblotting analysis of GCLC and GCLM protein expression. Cell lysates (5 μg) were separated on 10% (*w/v*) gels and immunoblotted with specific antibodies against the target proteins. β-ACTIN was stained as a loading control. (**D**) Immunoreactive bands were quantified with the Image Lab software. GCLM levels, normalized to β-ACTIN content, are reported in the graphs as fold change relative to control (0). Values are the mean ± SD of at least three independent experiments. * $p < 0.05$; ** $p < 0.01$, *** $p < 0.001$.

3.4. I-152 Increases Intracellular Thiol Content and Dose-Dependently Modulates GSH Levels

At 2 h incubation, analysis of the free thiol pools showed that cysteine represented the most abundant thiol species, GSH excluded, except in cells treated with 1 mM I-152, where NAC was predominant (Figure 6A). Notably, at 24 h incubation, a predominance of NAC was observed at all the I-152 doses tested. Although I-152 is expected to liberate equimolar concentrations of its metabolites, intracellular MEA levels were markedly lower than those of NAC, suggesting that MEA could be partially converted into cystamine upon oxidation of its sulfhydryl group and/or form mixed disulfides. Such disulfides could not be revealed by the chromatographic analysis used here since it was specific for the identification of –SH carrying molecules. Within the time frame 2–24 h, GSH content dose-dependently increased over the physiological level in cells treated with I-152 (Figure 6B). However, significant depletion of intracellular GSH was observed at 24 h, but only at the highest doses tested (i.e., 0.25 and 1 mM). Thus, I-152 dose-dependently increased intracellular thiol levels: (i) By delivering I-152, NAC and MEA; (ii) by providing high levels of cysteine and (iii) by elevating GSH content.

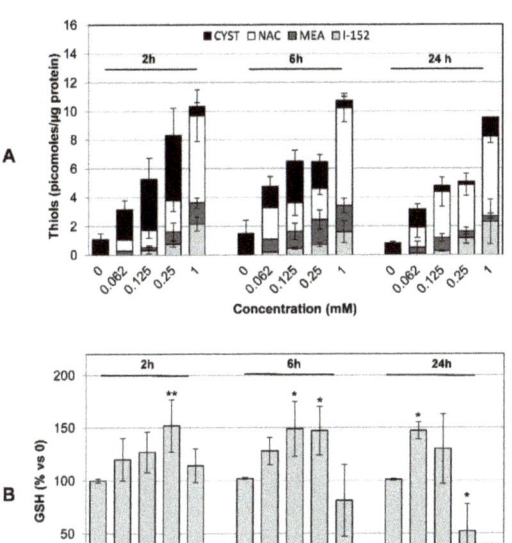

Figure 6. Thiol species in I-152 treated cells. MEA, NAC, I-152, cysteine (**A**) and GSH (**B**) content in RAW 264.7 cells treated with different concentrations of I-152 for 2, 6, and 24 h. After incubation, cells were washed and lysed; the lysate was then treated with precipitating solution and centrifuged. Thiol species and GSH levels were determined in the lysate supernatant by HPLC, while protein content was quantified spectrophotometrically in the lysate pellet. Quantification of thiol species was obtained by injection of standards of known concentrations and values were normalized on protein concentration. GSH content is expressed as the percent of the value obtained in untreated cells (0). Values are the mean ± SD of five independent experiments. * $p < 0.05$; ** $p < 0.01$, *** $p < 0.001$.

Increased cysteine levels together with MEA were found within the cells upon MEA administration (Figure S3A). Cysteine content was also elevated in NAC-treated cells, but NAC was detectable only when delivered at the highest dose and/or for longer times (Figure S4A). Despite higher cysteine availability, both MEA and NAC only modestly affected GSH cellular content (Figures S3B and S4B).

3.5. I-152 Activates the ATF4 Signaling Pathway

Like any other biological molecule, GSH levels largely depend on its rate of synthesis and degradation. Thus, we reasoned that at the highest I-152 concentrations tested, GSH overproduction might lead to reductive stress and result in the activation of degradative pathways to rebalance redox homeostasis [38]. GSH depletion has often been associated with ATF4 activation and CHAC1 expression, the latter of which controls intracellular GSH degradation under stressful conditions. ATF4 was indeed strongly activated by 1 mM I-152 and modestly activated by 0.25 mM via a signaling pathway not dependent on eIF2α phosphorylation, which was unaffected by the treatment (Figure 7A), but dependent on *Atf4* transcriptional induction (Figure 7B).

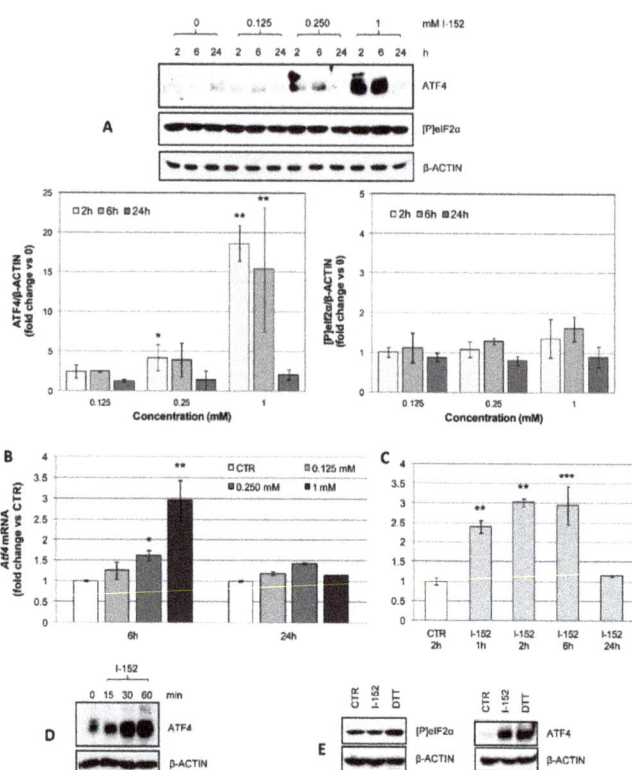

Figure 7. Activating transcription factor 4 (ATF4) transcriptional activation and protein accumulation in I-152-treated cells. (**A**) Cells were incubated with different concentrations of I-152 for 2 h, 6 h, and 24 h and whole lysates corresponding to 10 µg of proteins were separated on 10% (*w/v*) polyacrylamide gels. The blots were probed with anti ATF4 and anti [P]eIF2α antibodies. β-ACTIN was stained as a control. Untreated cells receiving only fresh medium served as a control (denoted by 0). Immunoreactive bands were quantified with the Image Lab software. ATF4 and [P]eIF2α levels, normalized to β-ACTIN content, are reported in the graphs as fold change relative to control (0). Values are the mean ± SD of at least three independent experiments. * $p < 0.05$, ** $p < 0.01$. (**B**) RTqPCR analysis of *Atf4* mRNA levels in cells treated with different concentrations of I-152 for 6 h and 24 h. (**C**) RTqPCR analysis of *Atf4* mRNA levels in cells treated with 1 mM I-152 for different times. mRNA levels were normalized to the housekeeping genes *Gapdh* and *Gusb* and expressed as fold-change versus untreated cells (CTR). The values are the mean ± SD of at least two independent experiments with two technical replicates. * $p < 0.05$, ** $p < 0.01$, *** $p < 0.001$. (**D**) Cells were incubated with 1 mM I-152 for different times and lysates were resolved by SDS-PAGE, immunoblotted and stained with anti ATF4. (**E**) Western immunoblotting analysis of cell extracts obtained from CTR cells and cells treated with 1 mM I-152 and 1 mM DTT for 30 min (left panel) and 1 h (right panel). ATF4 and [P]eIF2α were detected using specific antibodies, while β-ACTIN was stained as a loading control.

At 6 h, both the mRNA and protein levels were still high to return to basal levels at 24 h (Figure 7A,B). Time course analysis of *Atf4* mRNA expression revealed that at 1 h, the transcription was fully activated (Figure 7C). Subsequent analysis of the kinetics of protein accumulation demonstrated that ATF4 protein levels started to increase as soon as 15 min after I-152 treatment (Figure 7D), highlighting an unexpectedly fast activation of the ATF4 signaling. To further exclude the involvement of the ISR pathway, cells were treated in parallel with I-152 and dithiotreitol (DTT), which is known to induce ER stress, leading to eIF2α phosphorylation and sustained ATF4 translation [39]. As expected, levels of [P]eIF2α were increased after exposure to DTT, but not to I-152, although ATF4 accumulation was observed in both cases (Figure 7E). This clearly demonstrates that the two thiol species induce distinct signaling cascades to activate ATF4.

Chac1 mRNA induction followed the same trend reported for *Atf4* (Figure 8A), but no changes in protein expression could be observed using two different antibodies (one from GeneTex, as reported in Material and Methods, and one from Biorbyt orb100972) specifically recognizing a band of the expected molecular weight (Figure 8B and data not shown).

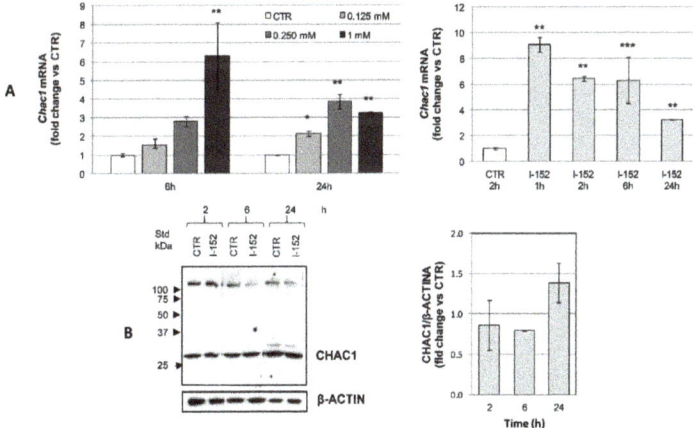

Figure 8. CHAC1 transcriptional activation and protein levels in I-152-treated cells. (**A**) RTqPCR analysis of *Chac1* mRNA levels in cells treated with different concentrations of I-152 for 6 h and 24 h and in cells treated with 1 mM I-152 for different times. mRNA levels were normalized to the housekeeping genes *Gapdh* and *Gusb* and expressed as fold-change versus untreated cells (CTR). The values are the mean ± SD of two independent experiments with two technical replicates (**B**) Cells were incubated with different concentrations of I-152 for 2 h, 6 h and 24 h, and whole lysates corresponding to 10 µg of proteins were separated on 12% (w/v) polyacrylamide gels. The blots were probed with anti CHAC1 antibody. β-ACTIN was stained as a control. Untreated cells receiving only fresh medium served as a control (CTR). Immunoreactive bands were quantified with the Image Lab software. CHAC1 levels, normalized to β-ACTIN content, are reported in the graph as fold change relative to CTR. Values are the mean ± SD of at least three independent experiments. * $p < 0.05$, ** $p < 0.01$, *** $p < 0.001$.

By contrast, the ATF4 gene target *GADD153* (*Chop*) was induced both at the transcriptional and protein level consistently with ATF4 activation, indicating that ATF4 was transcriptionally competent (Figure 9A,B).

Since CHOP is a well-known mediator of apoptosis, LDH-based cytotoxicity assays were performed at 24 h and 48 h of incubation with the molecule. The use of the classical MTS assay was avoided because I-152 per se induced a strong reduction of the MTS tetrazolium compound. As shown in Figure 10, only 1 mM I-152 promoted a block in cell proliferation and caused cell death. The effects were very mild at 24 h, with only 10% of the cells being affected. By contrast, these effects became more evident at 48 h, although more cells appeared to be inhibited in their growth rather than killed by the molecule.

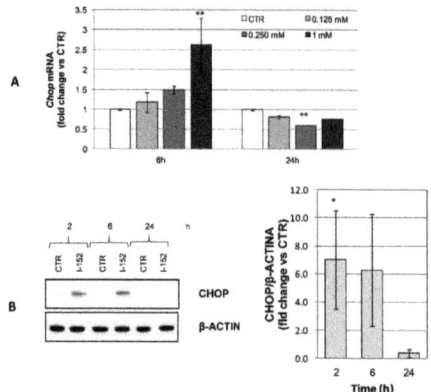

Figure 9. CHOP transcriptional activation and protein expression in I-152-treated cells. (**A**) RTqPCR analysis of *Chop* mRNA levels in cells treated with different concentrations of I-152 for 6 h and 24 h. mRNA levels were normalized to the housekeeping genes *Gapdh* and *Gusb* and expressed as fold-change versus untreated cells (CTR). The values are the mean ± SD of two independent experiments with two technical replicates (**B**) Cells were incubated with 1 mM I-152 for 2 h, 6 h, and 24 h and whole lysates corresponding to 20 µg of proteins were separated on 12% (w/v) polyacrylamide gels. The blots were probed with anti CHOP antibody. β-ACTIN was stained as a control. Untreated cells receiving only fresh medium served as a control (CTR). Immunoreactive bands were quantified with the Image Lab software. GHOP levels, normalized to β-ACTIN content, are reported in the graphs as fold change relative to CTR. Values are the mean ± SD of at least three independent experiments. * $p < 0.05$; ** $p < 0.01$.

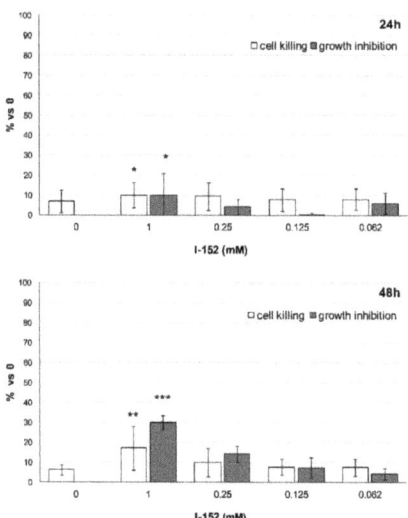

Figure 10. Cell killing and growth inhibition after I-152 treatment. Cells were incubated with different doses of I-152 for 24 h and 48 h. Untreated cells receiving only fresh medium served as a control (denoted by 0). LDH activity was measured for each condition in the cell culture medium and, in parallel, in the medium after complete cell lysis with Triton-X100. This method makes it possible to distinguish cell death versus growth inhibition as described in materials and methods. Data are reported in the graph as fold change relative to control (0). The values are the mean ± SD of two independent experiments with four technical replicates. * $p < 0.05$, ** $p < 0.01$, *** $p < 0.001$.

4. Discussion

I-152 increases physiological GSH levels and replenishes intracellular GSH content under conditions of depletion; however, the molecular mechanisms underlying its pro-GSH activity have only been partially elucidated.

Data reported in this paper demonstrate that I-152 is a potent pro-GSH molecule since it can stimulate GSH biosynthesis by forcing GSH production through the combined delivery of NAC, which provides the rate limiting building block cysteine, and MEA, which induces NRF2 activation and GCLM protein expression. It has been shown that GCLM levels are limiting within cells, thus upregulation of GCLM alone is sufficient to increase GCL catalytic activity by increasing holoenzyme formation. The heterodimeric enzyme is more efficient in catalysing the reaction and less sensitive to feedback inhibition by GSH [2,40].

The potency of I-152 in terms of its ability to increase GSH content was far superior than that of NAC or MEA administered alone. This difference in potency can be accounted for by the different uptake mechanisms of the molecules together with the inability or low capacity of NAC and MEA, respectively, to activate the NRF2 pathway. When used alone, NAC was available early intracellularly only when used at the highest concentration tested and for long periods of incubation. This is because NAC enters by passive diffusion, but its permeability is low since it is mostly negatively charged at physiological pH. Thus, high doses and longer treatments are required to favor its cell penetration [41]. Conversely, high cysteine levels were detected in NAC-treated cells, supporting the notion that NAC may also reduce extracellular cystine to cysteine, which then enters the cells [42]. Compared to the administration of NAC alone, I-152-treated cells contained a significantly higher amount of NAC, which was also detectable at the lower doses, suggesting that I-152 enters as such and it is mostly metabolized intracellularly. Unlike NAC, MEA was readily detectable at all the doses and times tested, together with high cysteine levels. MEA uptake is thought to occur very quickly through a mechanism involving thiol-disulphide interchange with extracellular cystine to form cysteamine–cysteine mixed disulphides that enter cells through amino acid transporters and are then reduced back to cysteamine and cysteine [43]. The ability of MEA to increase GSH levels has been attributed to its capacity to release cysteine from cystine pools, but other molecular mechanisms might be involved [34]. Calkins et al. [31] provided evidence that MEA is a weak activator of the NRF2 pathway in neuronal cells. In this system, however, the oxidized form of MEA, cystamine (here named MEA_{S-S} for simplicity), displayed a much higher potency, suggesting that MEA_{S-S} rather than MEA activates NRF2. In circulation and within cells, MEA is partially converted into MEA_{S-S} after the oxidation of its sulfhydryl group. It has been widely documented that both MEA and MEA_{S-S} can affect the activity of different proteins, including transglutaminase, whose mechanism(s) of inactivation has been thoroughly studied. In particular, MEA_{S-S} but not MEA, has been shown to inhibit transglutaminase activity by an oxidative mechanism where MEA_{S-S} promotes the formation of a physiologically relevant disulfide bond between Cys370 and Cys371 [44]. A similar mechanism of disulfide interchange may be responsible for the formation of the three oxidized KEAP1 species (Ox1, 2 and 3) in cells treated with I-152. Using KEAP1 mutants, Fourquet et al. [45] demonstrated that in cells exposed to oxidants, KEAP1 is oxidized generating three byproducts: One oxidized species, corresponding to Ox1, which carries an intramolecular Cys226–Cys613 disulfide, and two high molecular weight oxidized species, corresponding to Ox2 and Ox3, involving Cys151-Cys151 mixed disulfide between two KEAP1 molecules, and KEAP1 and another polypeptide. While intramolecular disulfide formation was not essential to NRF2 activation, Cys151-Cys151 intermolecular disulfide was critical to relieving KEAP1-mediated NRF2 degradation [45]. Different conclusions were drawn when two NRF2 inducers, namely sulphoraphane and trinitrobenzene sulphonate, were tested and found to promote intra- and intermolecular disulphides, respectively [46], suggesting that KEAP-1 function might be affected by both types of modifications. It is worth noting that the above-mentioned studies were performed in cells ectopically expressing KEAP1; by contrast, our observations concern the endogenously expressed protein, highlighting the biological relevance of these oxidizing mechanisms.

I-152 is expected to release equimolar amounts of NAC and MEA; however, analysis of the thiol species revealed that MEA levels were markedly lower than those of NAC. Based on this observation, it could be speculated that the MEA moiety, released after I-152 metabolization, may be partly oxidized into MEA$_{S-S}$, although we cannot exclude conjugation to other thiol species. Moreover, since cells also contain a certain amount of non-hydrolyzed I-152, a direct/indirect role for the I-152 molecule in NRF2 activation cannot be excluded.

The intracellular delivery of high amounts of thiol species as well as the overproduction of GSH may induce reductive stress, which, in turn, may enhance mitochondrial oxidation with the production of ROS [47]. Thus, I-152 and/or its metabolites could act as antioxidants or pro-oxidants depending on the dose used: At low doses, I-152 stimulates the expression of antioxidant enzymes, while at high doses it leads to GSH depletion and reduced cell proliferation and death. It is worth noting that NAC is also known to behave differently according to its concentration and the redox status of the cells in which it is used [48,49].

Interestingly, it has recently been shown that NAC displays powerful mitochondrial and antioxidant effects, not only as a glutathione precursor, but also by triggering mitohormesis [50]. Mitohormesis assumes that a moderate increase in ROS production during mitochondrial activity leads to the activation of cellular defense systems, leading to a long-term increase in the levels of mitochondria and antioxidant enzymes. Thus, future studies might investigate these mechanisms in cells treated with I-152. On the other hand, an excessive production of ROS could deplete GSH levels, thus damaging cells. Interestingly, at I-152 concentrations promoting GSH depletion, NRF2 activation was paralleled or even preceded by transcriptional induction of the bZIP factor ATF4. Similar results were obtained by Mimura et al. [11], who demonstrated that low-dose carnosinic acid (CA) activates the NRF2 pathway only, exhibiting moderate anti-oxidative effects; by contrast, high-dose CA activates both NRF2 and ATF4 to potentiate the NRF2 antioxidative pathway. Cooperation between NRF2 and ATF4 in modulating antioxidant gene expression has also been shown to occur in response to treatment with fisetin, a flavonoid able to stimulate GSH production [10]. In the case of fisetin, no mechanistic explanation for ATF4 induction was provided, whereas for CA, activation of the ISR pathway was shown. Moreover, GSH levels were increased by low doses of CA, whereas they were unchanged by high dose administration, despite induction of GCLM and GCLC mRNA levels. Since the authors found induction of CHAC1 mRNA expression, they speculated that higher concentrations of CA could deplete GSH by ATF4-mediated induction of CHAC1 to reestablish homeostasis.

In our experimental system, I-152 did not induce ISR activation, as demonstrated by the fact that eIF2α phosphorylation was unaffected by the treatment. Moreover, despite strong induction of CHAC1 mRNA levels, protein levels were unchanged, allowing us to exclude the activation of compensatory degradative GSH pathways. At present, the reason why CHAC1 mRNA induction does not result in higher protein expression is unknown. Difficulty in detecting the CHAC1 protein despite high mRNA expression has been reported [51]. On the contrary, ATF activation was accompanied by the expression of its target gene CHOP, as well as by the inhibition of cell proliferation together with a small percentage of dead cells observed at 24 h and 48 h treatment with 1 mM I-152. ATF4 controls life-death decisions after stress, switching from adaptive to pro-apoptotic gene expression [52]. This switch has been attributed in part to the formation of different ATF4 heterodimers that control the expression of specific sets of gene targets. It has been proposed that dimerization with its target gene CHOP signals apoptosis [53,54], although ATF4 and CHOP may cooperate to induce genes mediating stress relief and cell survival such as genes encoding for proteins involved in autophagy [55]. Thus, further experiments will aim to assess the consequence of ATF4/CHOP co-activation in terms of pro-survival/pro-apoptotic gene expression. Another aspect that warrants investigation is the mechanism underlying transcriptional induction of ATF4. ATF4 gene transcription is induced in response to different stresses and is mediated by different transcription factors, including NRF2 and ATF4 itself [56,57]. Since NRF2 was activated by all the I-152 doses tested, while ATF4 was induced only at the highest concentrations, its involvement appears unlikely. Moreover, the increase in ATF4 protein levels preceded NRF2 protein accumulation in time course experiments again allowing us to exclude a cause and effect relationship between NRF2 activation and ATF4 transcriptional induction. Finally, the half-life of ATF4 was unchanged in the presence of I-152 (unpublished data), thus excluding the possibility that the factor, which is intrinsically unstable, could become stabilized by I-152 treatment, activating its own expression.

5. Conclusions

In conclusion, the data presented herein provide evidence that I-152 efficiently delivers NAC and MEA within the cells, exerting unique effects which are also dependent on the dose applied. At high and low doses (0.062-1 mM), KEAP1 is oxidized and NRF2 is stabilized, leading to transcriptional induction of its target genes, including GCLM. GCLM overexpression together with co-delivery of cysteine precursors boosts GSH production. At high I-152 doses (0.25–1 mM), however, GSH levels tend to decrease over time, leading to reduced proliferation and ultimately resulting in cell death (1 mM I-152). Interestingly, this effect was accompanied by an early activation of ATF4 and ATF4-dependent gene transcription (i.e., CHOP and CHAC1), as part of a stress response which is not mediated by the classical ISR pathway. Although NRF2 and ATF4 have been reported to concur in enhancing GSH levels and mounting the antioxidant response, in this context, the co-activation of ATF4 is probably necessary to switch from the adaptive response to pro-apoptotic signaling. ATF4 has been described as a redox-regulated pro-death transcription factor in neuronal cells where it seems to positively influence ROS levels and increase glutathione consumption [58].

I-152 represents the very first attempt to combine two pro-GSH molecules to improve their potency. The co-drug approach, which involves linking two drugs via a cleavable covalent bond, represents a novel strategy for enhancing GSH levels [59]. The approach makes it possible to improve membrane permeability and antioxidant activity compared to parent compounds [60]. Moreover, because of the potential synergism and cross-reactivity between the released compounds, the co-delivery of different thiol species may lead to unpredictable outcomes warranting further investigation.

Supplementary Materials: The following are available online at https://www.mdpi.com/2076-3921/10/2/175/s1, Figure S1: NRF2 relative half-life, Figure S2: HMOX1 and GCLC expression, Figure S3: NAC, cysteine and GSH content in NAC-treated cells, Figure S4: MEA, cysteine and GSH content in MEA-treated cells.

Author Contributions: Conceptualization, R.C. and A.F.; Data curation, C.Z., G.B., and C.C.; Formal analysis, R.C., L.G., and A.F.; Funding acquisition, R.C. and A.F.; Investigation, R.C., C.Z., G.B., C.C., and A.F.; Resources, M.S., M.M. (Michele Mari) and M.M. (Mauro Magnani); Visualization, R.C., L.G., and A.F.; Writing—original draft, R.C.; Writing—review and editing, L.G., M.S., M.M. (Michele Mari), M.M. (Mauro Magnani), and A.F. All authors have read and agreed to the published version of the manuscript.

Funding: This research was funded by the Ministero dell'Università e della Ricerca (MIUR) Fondo per il finanziamento delle attività base di ricerca [grant DISB_CRINELLI_FFABR_CTC]; the Università degli Studi di Urbino Carlo Bo (UNIURB) [grant DISB_CRINELLI_PROGETTI_VALORIZZAZIONE_2017/2018; grant DISB_FRATERNALE_ATENEO_PRIN 2015].

Institutional Review Board Statement: Not applicable.

Informed Consent Statement: Not applicable.

Data Availability Statement: The data presented in this study are available within the article and in supplementary material.

Conflicts of Interest: The authors declare no conflict of interest.

Abbreviations

ATF4	activating transcription factor 4
CA	carnosinic acid
CHAC1	cation transport regulator-like protein 1
CHOP	C/EBP-homologous protein (CHOP10/GADD153)
CHX	cycloheximide
DTT	dithiothreitol
eIF2α	eukaryotic translation initiation factor 2α
GAPDH	glyceraldehyde-3-phosphate dehydrogenase
GCLC	γ-glutamyl-cysteine ligase catalytic subunit
GCLM	γ-glutamyl-cysteine ligase modifier subunit
GSH	glutathione
GUSB	β-D-glucuronidase
HMOX1	heme oxygenase 1
HPLC	high performance liquid chromatography
IRS	integrated stress response
KEAP1	kelch-like ECH-associated protein 1
LDH	lactate dehydrogenase
MEA	cysteamine/β-mercaptoethylamine
MEAs-s	cystamine
NAC	N-acetyl-cysteine
NEM	N-ethylmaleimide
NRF2	nuclear factor E2-related factor 2
SMEA	S-acetyl-cysteamine

References

1. Forman, H.J.; Zhang, H.; Rinna, A. Glutathione: Overview of its protective roles, measurement, and biosynthesis. *Mol. Asp. Med.* **2009**, *30*, 1–12. [CrossRef] [PubMed]
2. Chen, Y.; Shertzer, H.G.; Schneider, S.N.; Nebert, D.W.; Dalton, T.P. Glutamate cysteine ligase catalysis: Dependence on ATP and modifier subunit for regulation of tissue glutathione levels. *J. Biol. Chem.* **2005**, *280*, 33766–33774. [CrossRef] [PubMed]
3. Franklin, C.C.; Backos, D.S.; Mohar, I.; White, C.C.; Forman, H.J.; Kavanagh, T.J. Structure, function, and post-translational regulation of the catalytic and modifier subunits of glutamate cysteine ligase. *Mol. Asp. Med.* **2009**, *30*, 86–98. [CrossRef]
4. Wild, A.C.; Moinova, H.R.; Mulcahy, R.T. Regulation of gamma-glutamylcysteine synthetase subunit gene expression by the transcription factor Nrf2. *J. Biol. Chem.* **1999**, *274*, 33627–33636. [CrossRef] [PubMed]
5. Moinova, H.R.; Mulcahy, R.T. Up-regulation of the human gamma-glutamylcysteine synthetase regulatory subunit gene involves binding of Nrf-2 to an electrophile responsive element. *Biochem. Biophys. Res. Commun.* **1999**, *261*, 661–668. [CrossRef]
6. He, X.; Ma, Q. NRF2 cysteine residues are critical for oxidant/electrophile-sensing, Kelch-like ECH-associated protein-1-dependent ubiquitination-proteasomal degradation, and transcription activation. *Mol. Pharmacol.* **2009**, *76*, 1265–1278. [CrossRef]
7. Tonelli, C.; Chio, I.; Tuveson, D.A. Transcriptional Regulation by Nrf2. *Antioxid. Redox Signal.* **2018**, *29*, 1727–1745. [CrossRef] [PubMed]
8. Karpinski, B.A.; Morle, G.D.; Huggenvik, J.; Uhler, M.D.; Leiden, J.M. Molecular cloning of human CREB-2: An ATF/CREB transcription factor that can negatively regulate transcription from the cAMP response element. *Proc. Natl. Acad. Sci. USA* **1992**, *89*, 4820–4824. [CrossRef] [PubMed]
9. Pakos-Zebrucka, K.; Koryga, I.; Mnich, K.; Ljujic, M.; Samali, A.; Gorman, A.M. The integrated stress response. *EMBO Rep.* **2016**, *17*, 1374–1395. [CrossRef] [PubMed]
10. Ehren, J.L.; Maher, P. Concurrent regulation of the transcription factors Nrf2 and ATF4 mediates the enhancement of glutathione levels by the flavonoid fisetin. *Biochem. Pharmacol.* **2013**, *85*, 1816–1826. [CrossRef]
11. Mimura, J.; Inose-Maruyama, A.; Taniuchi, S.; Kosaka, K.; Yoshida, H.; Yamazaki, H.; Kasai, S.; Harada, N.; Kaufman, R.J.; Oyadomari, S.; et al. Concomitant Nrf2- and ATF4-activation by Carnosic Acid Cooperatively Induces Expression of Cytoprotective Genes. *Int. J. Mol. Sci.* **2019**, *20*, 1706. [CrossRef] [PubMed]
12. Ye, P.; Mimura, J.; Okada, T.; Sato, H.; Liu, T.; Maruyama, A.; Ohyama, C.; Itoh, K. Nrf2- and ATF4-dependent upregulation of xCT modulates the sensitivity of T24 bladder carcinoma cells to proteasome inhibition. *Mol. Cell. Biol.* **2014**, *34*, 3421–3434. [CrossRef] [PubMed]

13. He, C.H.; Gong, P.; Hu, B.; Stewart, D.; Choi, M.E.; Choi, A.M.; Alam, J. Identification of activating transcription factor 4 (ATF4) as an Nrf2-interacting protein. Implication for heme oxygenase-1 gene regulation. *J. Biol. Chem.* **2001**, *276*, 20858–20865. [CrossRef] [PubMed]
14. Sato, H.; Nomura, S.; Maebara, K.; Sato, K.; Tamba, M.; Bannai, S. Transcriptional control of cystine/glutamate transporter gene by amino acid deprivation. *Biochem. Biophys. Res. Commun.* **2004**, *325*, 109–116. [CrossRef]
15. Siu, F.; Bain, P.J.; LeBlanc-Chaffin, R.; Chen, H.; Kilberg, M.S. ATF4 is a mediator of the nutrient-sensing response pathway that activates the human asparagine synthetase gene. *J. Biol. Chem.* **2002**, *277*, 24120–24127. [CrossRef]
16. Crawford, R.R.; Prescott, E.T.; Sylvester, C.F.; Higdon, A.N.; Shan, J.; Kilberg, M.S.; Mungrue, I.N. Human CHAC1 Protein Degrades Glutathione, and mRNA Induction Is Regulated by the Transcription Factors ATF4 and ATF3 and a Bipartite ATF/CRE Regulatory Element. *J. Biol. Chem.* **2015**, *290*, 15878–15891. [CrossRef]
17. Bachhawat, A.K.; Kaur, A. Glutathione Degradation. *Antioxid. Redox Signal.* **2017**, *27*, 1200–1216. [CrossRef]
18. Ballatori, N.; Krance, S.M.; Notenboom, S.; Shi, S.; Tieu, K.; Hammond, C.L. Glutathione dysregulation and the etiology and progression of human diseases. *Biol. Chem.* **2009**, *390*, 191–214. [CrossRef]
19. Kode, A.; Rajendrasozhan, S.; Caito, S.; Yang, S.R.; Megson, I.L.; Rahman, I. Resveratrol induces glutathione synthesis by activation of Nrf2 and protects against cigarette smoke-mediated oxidative stress in human lung epithelial cells. *Am. J. Physiol. Lung Cell. Mol. Physiol.* **2008**, *294*, L478–L488. [CrossRef]
20. Wei, Y.; Lu, M.; Mei, M.; Wang, H.; Han, Z.; Chen, M.; Yao, H.; Song, N.; Ding, X.; Ding, J.; et al. Pyridoxine induces glutathione synthesis via PKM2-mediated Nrf2 transactivation and confers neuroprotection. *Nat. Commun.* **2020**, *11*, 941. [CrossRef]
21. Oiry, J.; Mialocq, P.; Puy, J.Y.; Fretier, P.; Clayette, P.; Dormont, D.; Imbach, J.L. NAC/MEA conjugate: A new potent antioxidant which increases the GSH level in various cell lines. *Bioorg. Med. Chem. Lett.* **2001**, *11*, 1189–1191. [CrossRef]
22. Crinelli, R.; Zara, C.; Smietana, M.; Retini, M.; Magnani, M.; Fraternale, A. Boosting GSH Using the Co-Drug Approach: I-152, a Conjugate of N-acetyl-cysteine and β-mercaptoethylamine. *Nutrients* **2019**, *11*, 1291. [CrossRef] [PubMed]
23. Galluzzi, L.; Diotallevi, A.; De Santi, M.; Ceccarelli, M.; Vitale, F.; Brandi, G.; Magnani, M. Leishmania infantum Induces Mild Unfolded Protein Response in Infected Macrophages. *PLoS ONE* **2016**, *11*, e0168339. [CrossRef] [PubMed]
24. Pfaffl, M.W. A new mathematical model for relative quantification in real-time RT-PCR. *Nucleic Acids Res.* **2001**, *29*, e45. [CrossRef] [PubMed]
25. Amatore, D.; Celestino, I.; Brundu, S.; Galluzzi, L.; Coluccio, P.; Checconi, P.; Magnani, M.; Palamara, A.T.; Fraternale, A.; Nencioni, L. Glutathione increase by the n-butanoyl glutathione derivative (GSH-C4) inhibits viral replication and induces a predominant Th1 immune profile in old mice infected with influenza virus. *FASEB Bioadv.* **2019**, *1*, 296–305. [CrossRef] [PubMed]
26. Pal, S.; Wu, J.; Murray, J.K.; Gellman, S.H.; Wozniak, M.A.; Keely, P.J.; Boyer, M.E.; Gomez, T.M.; Hasso, S.M.; Fallon, J.F.; et al. An antiangiogenic neurokinin-B/thromboxane A2 regulatory axis. *J. Cell Biol.* **2006**, *174*, 1047–1058. [CrossRef]
27. Fraternale, A.; Crinelli, R.; Casabianca, A.; Paoletti, M.F.; Orlandi, C.; Carloni, E.; Smietana, M.; Palamara, A.T.; Magnani, M. Molecules altering the intracellular thiol content modulate NF-kB and STAT-1/IRF-1 signalling pathways and IL-12 p40 and IL-27 p28 production in murine macrophages. *PLoS ONE* **2013**, *8*, e57866. [CrossRef]
28. Smith, S.M.; Wunder, M.B.; Norris, D.A.; Shellman, Y.G. A simple protocol for using a LDH-based cytotoxicity assay to assess the effects of death and growth inhibition at the same time. *PLoS ONE* **2011**, *6*, e26908. [CrossRef]
29. Beutler, E. Lactate Deydrogenase (LDH). In *Red Cell Metabolism. A Manual of Biochemical Method*, 3th ed.; Beutler, E., Ed.; Grune and Stratton, Inc.: New York, NY, USA, 1984; pp. 65–66.
30. Brundu, S.; Palma, L.; Picceri, G.G.; Ligi, D.; Orlandi, C.; Galluzzi, L.; Chiarantini, L.; Casabianca, A.; Schiavano, G.F.; Santi, M.; et al. Glutathione Depletion Is Linked with Th2 Polarization in Mice with a Retrovirus-Induced Immunodeficiency Syndrome, Murine AIDS: Role of Proglutathione Molecules as Immunotherapeutics. *J. Virol.* **2016**, *90*, 7118–7130. [CrossRef]
31. Calkins, M.J.; Townsend, J.A.; Johnson, D.A.; Johnson, J.A. Cystamine protects from 3-nitropropionic acid lesioning via induction of nf-e2 related factor 2 mediated transcription. *Exp. Neurol.* **2010**, *224*, 307–317. [CrossRef]
32. Wang, L.L.; Huang, Y.H.; Yan, C.Y.; Wei, X.D.; Hou, J.Q.; Pu, J.X.; Lv, J.X. N-acetylcysteine Ameliorates Prostatitis via miR-141 Regulating Keap1/Nrf2 Signaling. *Inflammation* **2016**, *39*, 938–947. [CrossRef] [PubMed]
33. Mao, Z.; Choo, Y.S.; Lesort, M. Cystamine and cysteamine prevent 3-NP-induced mitochondrial depolarization of Huntington's disease knock-in striatal cells. *Eur. J. Neurosci.* **2006**, *23*, 1701–1710. [CrossRef]
34. Wilmer, M.J.; Kluijtmans, L.A.; van der Velden, T.J.; Willems, P.H.; Scheffer, P.G.; Masereeuw, R.; Monnens, L.A.; van den Heuvel, L.P.; Levtchenko, E.N. Cysteamine restores glutathione redox status in cultured cystinotic proximal tubular epithelial cells. *Biochim. Biophys. Acta* **2011**, *1812*, 643–651. [CrossRef] [PubMed]
35. Ezeriņa, D.; Takano, Y.; Hanaoka, K.; Urano, Y.; Dick, T.P. N-Acetyl Cysteine Functions as a Fast-Acting Antioxidant by Triggering Intracellular H_2S and Sulfane Sulfur Production. *Cell Chem. Biol.* **2018**, *25*, 447–459. [CrossRef]
36. Stewart, D.; Killeen, E.; Naquin, R.; Alam, S.; Alam, J. Degradation of transcription factor Nrf2 via the ubiquitin-proteasome pathway and stabilization by cadmium. *J. Biol. Chem.* **2003**, *278*, 2396–2402. [CrossRef] [PubMed]
37. Itoh, K.; Wakabayashi, N.; Katoh, Y.; Ishii, T.; O'Connor, T.; Yamamoto, M. Keap1 regulates both cytoplasmic-nuclear shuttling and degradation of Nrf2 in response to electrophiles. *Genes Cells* **2003**, *8*, 379–391. [CrossRef]
38. Xiao, W.; Loscalzo, J. Metabolic Responses to Reductive Stress. *Antioxid. Redox Signal.* **2020**, *32*, 1330–1347. [CrossRef]
39. Oslowski, C.M.; Urano, F. Measuring ER stress and the unfolded protein response using mammalian tissue culture system. *Methods Enzymol.* **2011**, *490*, 71–92. [CrossRef]

40. Lee, J.I.; Kang, J.; Stipanuk, M.H. Differential regulation of glutamate-cysteine ligase subunit expression and increased holoenzyme formation in response to cysteine deprivation. *Biochem. J.* **2006**, *393*, 181–190. [CrossRef]
41. Samuni, Y.; Goldstein, S.; Dean, O.M.; Berk, M. The chemistry and biological activities of N-acetylcysteine. *Biochim. Biophys. Acta* **2013**, *1830*, 4117–4129. [CrossRef]
42. Whillier, S.; Raftos, J.E.; Chapman, B.; Kuchel, P.W. Role of N-acetylcysteine and cystine in glutathione synthesis in human erythrocytes. *Redox Rep.* **2009**, *14*, 115–124. [CrossRef] [PubMed]
43. Khomenko, T.; Kolodney, J.; Pinto, J.T.; McLaren, G.D.; Deng, X.; Chen, L.; Tolstanova, G.; Paunovic, B.; Krasnikov, B.F.; Hoa, N.; et al. New mechanistic explanation for the localization of ulcers in the rat duodenum: Role of iron and selective uptake of cysteamine. *Arch. Biochem. Biophys.* **2012**, *525*, 60–70. [CrossRef] [PubMed]
44. Palanski, B.A.; Khosla, C. Cystamine and Disulfiram Inhibit Human Transglutaminase 2 via an Oxidative Mechanism. *Biochemistry* **2018**, *57*, 3359–3363. [CrossRef] [PubMed]
45. Fourquet, S.; Guerois, R.; Biard, D.; Toledano, M.B. Activation of NRF2 by nitrosative agents and H_2O_2 involves KEAP1 disulfide formation. *J. Biol. Chem.* **2010**, *285*, 8463–8471. [CrossRef]
46. Chen, Y.T.; Shi, D.; Yang, D.; Yan, B. Antioxidant sulforaphane and sensitizer trinitrobenzene sulfonate induce carboxylesterase-1 through a novel element transactivated by nuclear factor-E2 related factor-2. *Biochem. Pharmacol.* **2012**, *84*, 864–871. [CrossRef] [PubMed]
47. Liu, Y.; Liu, K.; Wang, N.; Zhang, H. N-acetylcysteine induces apoptosis via the mitochondria-dependent pathway but not via endoplasmic reticulum stress in H9c2 cells. *Mol. Med. Rep.* **2017**, *16*, 6626–6633. [CrossRef] [PubMed]
48. Alam, K.; Ghousunnissa, S.; Nair, S.; Valluri, V.L.; Mukhopadhyay, S. Glutathione-redox balance regulates c-rel-driven IL-12 production in macrophages: Possible implications in antituberculosis immunotherapy. *J. Immunol.* **2010**, *184*, 2918–2929. [CrossRef]
49. Finn, N.A.; Kemp, M.L. Pro-oxidant and antioxidant effects of N-acetylcysteine regulate doxorubicin-induced NF-kappa B activity in leukemic cells. *Mol. Biosyst.* **2012**, *8*, 650–662. [CrossRef]
50. Singh, F.; Charles, A.L.; Schlagowski, A.I.; Bouitbir, J.; Bonifacio, A.; Piquard, F.; Krähenbühl, S.; Geny, B.; Zoll, J. Reductive stress impairs myoblasts mitochondrial function and triggers mitochondrial hormesis. *Biochim. Biophys. Acta* **2015**, *1853*, 1574–1585. [CrossRef]
51. Perra, L.; Balloy, V.; Foussignière, T.; Moissenet, D.; Petat, H.; Mungrue, I.N.; Touqui, L.; Corvol, H.; Chignard, M.; Guillot, L. CHAC1 Is Differentially Expressed in Normal and Cystic Fibrosis Bronchial Epithelial Cells and Regulates the Inflammatory Response Induced by Pseudomonas aeruginosa. *Front. Immunol.* **2018**, *9*, 2823. [CrossRef]
52. Wortel, I.; van der Meer, L.T.; Kilberg, M.S.; van Leeuwen, F.N. Surviving Stress: Modulation of ATF4-Mediated Stress Responses in Normal and Malignant Cells. *Trends Endocrinol. Metab.* **2017**, *28*, 794–806. [CrossRef] [PubMed]
53. Matsumoto, H.; Miyazaki, S.; Matsuyama, S.; Takeda, M.; Kawano, M.; Nakagawa, H.; Nishimura, K.; Matsuo, S. Selection of autophagy or apoptosis in cells exposed to ER-stress depends on ATF4 expression pattern with or without CHOP expression. *Biol. Open* **2013**, *2*, 1084–1090. [CrossRef] [PubMed]
54. Teske, B.F.; Fusakio, M.E.; Zhou, D.; Shan, J.; McClintick, J.N.; Kilberg, M.S.; Wek, R.C. CHOP induces activating transcription factor 5 (ATF5) to trigger apoptosis in response to perturbations in protein homeostasis. *Mol. Biol. Cell* **2013**, *24*, 2477–2490. [CrossRef] [PubMed]
55. B'chir, W.; Maurin, A.C.; Carraro, V.; Averous, J.; Jousse, C.; Muranishi, Y.; Parry, L.; Stepien, G.; Fafournoux, P.; Bruhat, A. The eIF2α/ATF4 pathway is essential for stress-induced autophagy gene expression. *Nucleic Acids Res.* **2013**, *41*, 7683–7699. [CrossRef]
56. Afonyushkin, T.; Oskolkova, O.V.; Philippova, M.; Resink, T.J.; Erne, P.; Binder, B.R.; Bochkov, V.N. Oxidized phospholipids regulate expression of ATF4 and VEGF in endothelial cells via NRF2-dependent mechanism: Novel point of convergence between electrophilic and unfolded protein stress pathways. *Arterioscler. Thromb. Vasc. Biol.* **2010**, *30*, 1007–1013. [CrossRef]
57. Cho, H.; Wu, M.; Zhang, L.; Thompson, R.; Nath, A.; Chan, C. Signaling dynamics of palmitate-induced ER stress responses mediated by ATF4 in HepG2 cells. *BMC Syst. Biol.* **2013**, *7*, 9. [CrossRef]
58. Lange, P.S.; Chavez, J.C.; Pinto, J.T.; Coppola, G.; Sun, C.W.; Townes, T.M.; Geschwind, D.H.; Ratan, R.R. ATF4 is an oxidative stress-inducible, prodeath transcription factor in neurons in vitro and in vivo. *J. Exp. Med.* **2008**, *205*, 1227–1242. [CrossRef]
59. Cacciatore, I.; Cornacchia, C.; Pinnen, F.; Mollica, A.; Di Stefano, A. Prodrug approach for increasing cellular glutathione levels. *Molecules* **2010**, *15*, 1242–1264. [CrossRef]
60. Kals, J.; Starkopf, J.; Zilmer, M.; Pruler, T.; Pulges, K.; Hallaste, M.; Kals, M.; Pulges, A.; Soomets, U. Antioxidant UPF1 attenuates myocardial stunning in isolated rat hearts. *Int. J. Cardiol.* **2008**, *125*, 133–135. [CrossRef]

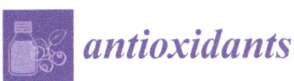

Article

In Vivo Bioavailability of Selenium in Selenium-Enriched *Streptococcus thermophilus* and *Enterococcus faecium* in CD IGS Rats

Gabriela Krausova [1,*], Antonin Kana [2], Marek Vecka [3], Ivana Hyrslova [1], Barbora Stankova [3], Vera Kantorova [2], Iva Mrvikova [1], Martina Huttl [4] and Hana Malinska [4]

1. Department of Microbiology and Technology, Dairy Research Institute, Ltd., Ke Dvoru 12a, 160 00 Prague, Czech Republic; hyrslova@milcom-as.cz (I.H.); mrvikova@milcom-as.cz (I.M.)
2. Department of Analytical Chemistry, Faculty of Chemical Engineering, University of Chemistry and Technology Prague, Technicka 5, 166 28 Prague, Czech Republic; Antonin.Kana@vscht.cz (A.K.); Vera.Kantorova@vscht.cz (V.K.)
3. 4th Department of Medicine Department of Gastroenterology and Hepatology, First Faculty of Medicine, Charles University in Prague, U Nemocnice 2, 128 00 Prague, Czech Republic; marek.vecka@lf1.cuni.cz (M.V.); barbora.stankova@lf1.cuni.cz (B.S.)
4. Centre for Experimental Medicine, Institute for Clinical and Experimental Medicine (IKEM), Videnska 1958/9, 140 21 Prague, Czech Republic; martina.huttl@ikem.cz (M.H.); hana.malinska@ikem.cz (H.M.)
* Correspondence: krausova@milcom-as.cz; Tel.: +420-773-088-810

Abstract: The selenium (Se) enrichment of yeasts and lactic acid bacteria (LAB) has recently emerged as a novel concept; the individual health effects of these beneficial microorganisms are combined by supplying the essential micronutrient Se in a more bioavailable and less toxic form. This study investigated the bioavailability of Se in the strains *Enterococcus faecium* CCDM 922A (EF) and *Streptococcus thermophilus* CCDM 144 (ST) and their respective Se-enriched forms, SeEF and SeST, in a CD (SD-Sprague Dawley) IGS rat model. Se-enriched LAB administration resulted in higher Se concentrations in the liver and kidneys of rats, where selenocystine was the prevalent Se species. The administration of both Se-enriched strains improved the antioxidant status of the animals. The effect of the diet was more pronounced in the heart tissue, where a lower glutathione reductase content was observed, irrespective of the Se fortification in LAB. Interestingly, rats fed diets with EF and SeEF had higher glutathione reductase activity. Reduced concentrations of serum malondialdehyde were noted following Se supplementation. Diets containing Se-enriched strains showed no macroscopic effects on the liver, kidneys, heart, and brain and had no apparent influence on the basic parameters of the lipid metabolism. Both the strains tested herein showed potential for further applications as promising sources of organically bound Se and Se nanoparticles.

Keywords: selenium-enriched *Enterococcus faecium*; selenium-enriched *Streptococcus thermophilus*; antioxidant capacity; glutathione reductase; glutathione peroxidase; CD IGS rats; oxidative stress; lactic acid bacteria

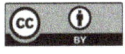

1. Introduction

In recent years, natural antioxidants have attracted interest from researchers because of the diseases caused by free radicals and reactive oxygen species (ROS), including heart disease, atherosclerosis, neurological disorders, and type II diabetes. The World Health Organization (WHO) expects cardiovascular disease to be the leading cause of mortalities by 2030, affecting approximately 23.3 million people [1]. Enrichment of the diet with antioxidants is a basic prerequisite for maintaining good health. In addition to synthetic antioxidants, natural antioxidants, including probiotic microorganisms and their metabolic products, are also available. Probiotic bacteria are defined as living microorganisms that, when consumed in sufficient quantities, confer health benefits to the host, such as the modulation of the immune system, maintenance of healthy intestinal microbiota, and lowering of cholesterol or prevention of diarrhea [2]. Probiotic microorganisms can act as antioxidants in several ways, such as by trapping ROS, chelating metal ions, inhibiting enzymes, and reducing or inhibiting ascorbate autooxidation. Furthermore, the metabolic activities of probiotics can have antioxidant effects, such as the capturing of oxidative compounds or prevention of their formation in the intestine [3]. One of the ways to increase the antioxidant activities of probiotic strains is their enrichment with selenium (Se), an essential microelement for humans found in a number of protein-based enzymes, including glutathione peroxidases, thioredoxin reductases, and iodothyronine deiodinases; in humans, these enzymes are associated with the responses to oxidative stress resulting from various biological activities [4]. The antioxidant enzymes glutathione peroxidase (GPx), glutathione (GSH), and superoxide dismutase (SOD) protect cells from oxidative damage by eliminating superoxide-free radicals [5]. Malondialdehyde (MDA), formed during lipoxidation, indicates cell or tissue injury and is an indicator of lipid peroxidation [6]. Furthermore, Se supplementation has beneficial effects in cancer, inflammation, immune responses, cardiovascular disease, thyroiditis, and male fertility [7]. On the contrary, low Se levels have been associated with an increased risk of mortality, poor immune function, and cognitive decline [8]. Se is involved in the immune responses of the body [9,10], similar to other natural substances such as probiotics. The positive effects of probiotics and Se co-supplementation on human mental health, hormonal profiles, and biomarkers of inflammation and oxidative stress have been documented [5,11,12]. For example, Se-enriched *Bifidobacterium longum* has a hepatoprotective effect in mice fed a high-fat diet [9]. Furthermore, Se-enriched probiotics exhibit antibacterial activity against pathogenic *Escherichia coli* [13]. The selenization of probiotics and lactic acid bacteria (LAB), a recently suggested concept, may provide multiple health benefits to the host. The selenization of yeasts and LAB confers benefits such as the following: (i) the delivery of Se for biological processes; (ii) increased bioavailability of Se in its less toxic organic form; (iii) individual health benefits of LAB and yeasts in live or inactivated forms (e.g., organic acid production, probiotic function, production of antimicrobial compounds, bacteriocins, etc.); and (iv) less burden on the environment due to the organic form of Se.

Selenized strains of yeasts and LAB represent sources of the more bioavailable organic forms of Se, making them more suitable application forms compared to food supplements containing Se in its inorganic form, such as sodium selenite [14]. Additionally, there is evidence suggesting that selenized cells of some LABs show a higher resistance to various stress conditions compared to the parental cells [15–17].

Se deficiency is as dangerous as its overdose. Despite the recognition of Se as an important microelement, discussion on the mode of its supplementation remains controversial. The main concern of Se supplementation is selenium nephrotoxicity, because this element accumulates in the kidneys, liver, and respiratory organs [18]. The most toxic forms of Se are the inorganic species SeIV and SeVI, which are permitted as food supplements in the form of sodium selenite, sodium hydrogen sulfite, and sodium selenate by Commission Regulation No. 1170/2009. However, selenium-enriched yeast containing this element in the organic form is also permitted for use in foodstuffs and food supplements under this regulation in the European Union. Some strains of LAB, bifidobacteria, and yeast can biotransform inorganic selenium present in the growth medium [19] into organic forms such as selenocysteine, selenomethionine, or methylselenocysteine [20,21]. Additionally, probiotics containing organic selenium species have shown negligible liver and kidney toxicity [18]. To obtain products that are well-defined in terms of health benefits and, more importantly, the safety of consumers, it is necessary to map selenium metabolism, its accumulation, and biotransformation in each Se-enriched strain individually.

In our previous study [22], an in vitro assessment of the properties of the selenized LAB strains *Streptococcus thermophilus* CCDM 144 and *Enterococcus faecium* CCDM 922A revealed that both strains could tolerate sodium selenite and accumulate, as well as biotransform Se into its organic form. These strains were further studied for their beneficial properties and potential to improve the host health. As previously reported [23], the strain CCDM 922A exhibits immunomodulatory abilities and the capacity to reduce low-density lipoprotein and very low-density lipoprotein cholesterol in rats. Good adhesion properties and the presence of the gene encoding the bacteriocin enterocin A were also observed in the strain CCDM 922A. *Streptococcus thermophilus* CCDM 144 is an exopolysaccharide (EPS)-producing strain used in the production of fermented dairy products, as part of the yogurt culture, to improve their texture. Both strains are commercially used in dairy processing plants, and the CCDM 922A strain is also used in animal nutrition. However, additional information is needed to evaluate the safety, functionality, and properties of their selenized forms. Overall, further studies are required to obtain legislative approval for the use of selenized LAB in food and food supplements. Hence, with the intention to jumpstart this process, this study aimed to evaluate the effects of the two promising Se-enriched candidates of LAB, the strains *S. thermophilus* CCDM 144 and *E. faecium* CCDM 922A, on the biological functions of rats in vivo.

2. Materials and Methods

2.1. Bacterial Strains and Their Selenium Enrichment

The two LAB strains, *S. thermophilus* CCDM 144 (ST) and *E. faecium* CCDM 922A (EF), used for selenization in this study were provided by the Culture Collection of Dairy Microorganisms Laktoflora® (Tábor, Czech Republic). M17 broth and M17 agar, according to Terzaghi (Merck, Darmstadt, Germany), were used for precultivation and storage. Both strains were cultured under aerobic conditions at 37 °C for 48 h. For enumeration of the bacterial cells, 10-fold dilutions of the cultures were plated, and the resultant colony-forming units were counted. For selenization, 50-mg/L sodium selenite (Sigma-Aldrich, Steinheim, Germany) was added to the M17 broth, and fresh overnight grown cultures of each strain were inoculated into the M17 medium at a final concentration of 10^5 colony-forming units (CFU)/mL and cultivated for 24 h at 37 °C under aerobic conditions. As controls, the strains CCDM 144 and CCDM 922A were grown in selenite-free M17 cultivation medium. After cultivation, the cells were centrifuged repeatedly at $4100\times g$ for 10 min (Spectrafuge 6C, Labnet International Inc., Edison, NJ, USA) and washed twice with sterile saline to remove unbound selenium. Subsequently, 1% inoculum of each bacterial suspension was added to skimmed (1.5% fat) and Ultra-heat treatment (UHT)-treated milk and incubated aerobically at 37 °C for 16–18 h. The pH was adjusted to 5.5–6.0 using 15% NaOH. Following this, the obtained samples were lyophilized (Lyobeta 35; Telstar, Barcelona, Spain) with the addition of 20% lactose as the cryoprotective medium, and the total amount of Se bound to the bacterial cells and Se species were determined in the samples. In this manner, the Se-enriched biomass of both strains, SeST and SeEF, were used for further application as foodstuffs. The final counts (colony-forming units (CFU)) of the strains EF, ST, SeEF, and SeST after lyophilization were also determined.

2.2. Animal Model and Study Design

All experiments with laboratory animals were conducted in compliance with the laws of the Czech Republic (311/1997 column.) and the European Community Council recommendations (86/609/EEC) regarding the protection of animals used for experimental and other scientific purposes. This experimental study was approved by the committee of the Ministry of Education, Youth, and Sports of the Czech Republic, approval No. MSMT-11197/2020-2. A total of 48 adult cesarian derived (CD) (SD-Sprague Dawley) International Genetic Standardization (IGS) male rats (Velaz, Prague, Czech Republic)—outbred multipurpose breed of albino rat—were used in this study. Six-week-old rats were randomly divided into six groups (A–F) ($n = 8$) and fed a standard maintenance diet and tap water for two weeks to acclimatize. Rats were housed in cages in a room with controlled temperature (22–24 °C), humidity (55–60%), and natural light conditions (12-h light/dark cycle). Following acclimatization, the experimental diets were administered to the animals for 58 days. Group A was fed a standard maintenance diet of Altromin 1324, control group B was fed a Se-deficient diet of Altromin C 1045, group C was fed Altromin C 1045 with added *S. thermophilus* (ST), group D was fed Altromin C 1045 with added selenized *S. thermophilus* (SeST), group E was fed Altromin C 1045 with added *E. faecium* (EF), and group F was fed Altromin C 1045 with added selenized *E. faecium* (SeEF).

Twenty-two grams of the appropriate diet was administered daily to the animals. Tap water was supplied ad libitum. After 58 days, rats were euthanized by decapitation following anesthetization (zoletil 5 mg/kg body weight) in the postprandial state. Aliquots of the serum and tissue samples were collected and stored at −80 °C for further analyses.

2.3. Experimental Diets

The following six types of diets were administered to the rats: (a) standard maintenance diet of Altromin 1324 (Altromin Spezialfutter GmbH & Co, Lage, Germany), (b) Altromin C 1045 as the Se-deficient diet (control group), (c) Altromin C 1045 with added *S. thermophilus* CCDM 144 (ST), (d) Altromin C 1045 with added selenized *S. thermophilus* CCDM 144 (SeST), (e) Altromin C 1045 with added *E. faecium* CCDM 922A (EF), and (f) Altromin C 1045 with added selenized *E. faecium* CCDM 922A (SeEF). All diets were processed into 10-mm pellets. The special diets were manufactured by Altromin Spezialfutter GmbH & Co, and the lyophilized strains ST, EF, SeST, and SeEF in the milk matrix were processed into the feedstuff by the manufacturer. Based on the measurements of the total Se concentrations in the lyophilized matrices, the dosage in the feed mixture was determined. Detailed information about the Se content and its chemical form in the individual diets is presented in Table 1. The Se concentrations used in this study were safe in terms of toxicity, as the diets of groups D and F, which were supplemented with selenized strains, had only slightly higher Se concentrations than that in the standard maintenance diet.

Table 1. Selenium concentrations and its forms in the experimental groups; data are presented as the mean ± expanded uncertainty with coverage factor $k = 2$.

	Se Concentration (mg/kg)	Added Se Form
A—Altromin 1324	0.408 ± 0.086	inorganic
B—Altromin C 1045	0.183 ± 0.039	-
C—Altromin C 1045 + ST	0.233 ± 0.076	-
D—Altromin C 1045 + SeST	0.439 ± 0.016	Organically bound
E—Altromin C 1045 + EF	0.185 ± 0.032	-
F—Altromin C 1045 + SeEF	0.445 ± 0.078	Organically bound

ST, *Streptococcus thermophilus*, SeST, selenium-enriched *Streptococcus thermophilus*, EF, *Enterococcus faecium*, and SeEF, selenium-enriched *Enterococcus faecium*.

2.4. Antioxidant and Oxidative Stress Parameters

Blood samples were collected gravitationally following the decapitation of the rats, and the serum was isolated from the blood by centrifugation at 1500× g at 4 °C for 10 min. Tissues were removed and immediately weighed, washed with cold phosphate-buffered saline (PBS) (0.02 mol/L, pH 7.1), and aliquoted in PBS (300–500-mg tissue in 0.5-mL PBS; 0.6–1.0 g in 1-mL PBS). The resulting suspension was subjected to two freeze/thaw cycles. The homogenate was centrifuged (1500× g for 15 min), and the supernatant was divided into three minimal aliquots, which were stored at −80 °C. Concentrations of total cholesterol, high-density lipoprotein (HDL) cholesterol, and triacylglycerols were assessed by enzymatic-colorimetric methods (CHOD/PAP, direct homogeneous enzymatic-colorimetric reaction without precipitation, GPO/PAP; Lab Mark a.s., Prague, Czech Republic) using an automatic biochemical analyzer modular (Roche, Prague, Czech Republic). The concentrations and activities of the antioxidants glutathione peroxidase (GPx), glutathione reductase (GR), and malondialdehyde (MDA) in the serum, brain, and heart tissue were evaluated by the sandwich heterogenous enzymatic immunoassay using commercial Enzyme-Linked ImmunoSorbent Assay (ELISA) kits for rat GPx, GR, and MDA (MyBioSource Inc., San Diego,

CA, USA). Lipoperoxidation products were assessed based on the levels of thiobarbituric acid-reactive substances (TBARS) by assaying the reaction with thiobarbituric acid.

2.5. Determining Total Selenium and Se Species Contents

The total contents of Se, Cu, Zn, Cr, and Fe in the liver and kidneys, as well as in the feedstuff, were determined using inductively coupled plasma mass spectrometry (ICP-MS) after microwave-assisted acid digestion. Three microliters of concentrated nitric acid (67% Analpure®, Analytika spol. s r.o., Prague, Czech Republic) was added to the homogenized feedstuff and tissue samples that were placed in a Teflon® digestion vessel (Berghof, Germany). The mixture was then mineralized in a closed vessel in a microwave digestion system (Speedwave 4; Berghof, Germany) for 15 min at 200 °C. After cooling, the decomposed samples were transferred to 50-mL volumetric flasks, spiked with rhodium solution (Astasol®, Analytika spol. s r.o., Czech Republic) as an internal standard to obtain a final concentration of 20-µg/L Rh after adjusting the volume with demineralized water (Milli-Q, Millipore, Billerica, MA, USA). The ICP-MS (DRC-e; Perkin-Elmer, Concord, ON, Canada) measurement conditions were as follows: RF (radio-frequency) power, 1.4 kW; nebulizer gas flow rate, 0.76 L/min; auxiliary gas flow rate, 1 L/min; plasma gas flow rate, 11 L/min; and measured isotopes ^{80}Se, ^{63}Cu, ^{66}Zn, ^{53}Cr, ^{57}Fe (analytes), and ^{103}Rh (internal standard). The spectral interference of ^{40}Ar$_2{}^+$ was eliminated using a dynamic reaction cell with methane as the reaction gas (methane flow rate 0.3 mL/min, rejection parameter q 0.3).

The selenium species were identified using ion-pair liquid chromatography (HPLC) coupled with ICP-MS, as described previously [22]. Briefly, reversed-phase column (Purospher® STAR RP-8 endcapped, 250 × 4.6 mm, 5 µm, Merck, Germany) and the mobile phase consisting of 1.0-g/L sodium butane-1-sulfonate, 0.22-g/L tetramethylammonium hydroxide pentahydrate, 0.42-g/L malonic acid, and 0.05% (v/v) methanol (Sigma Aldrich, Steinheim, Germany) were used for Se species separation. To extract the samples by enzymatic hydrolysis, 0.25 g of the tissue sample or 0.1 g of the feedstuff sample was weighed in 15-mL polypropylene tubes and homogenized for 1 min at 20,500 rpm using a disperser Ultra-Turrax® with 2 mL of 20-mmol/L tris-(hydroxymethyl)-aminomethane (Fluka, Buchs, Switzerland) solution buffered (pH = 7.0) using HCl (Suprapur®, Merck, Germany). Thereafter, 25 mg of protease XIV (Sigma-Aldrich, Tokyo, Japan) was added, and the sample was extracted for 18 h at 37 °C. The reaction mixture was then filtered through a 0.45-µm syringe nylon filter (Whatman, Maidstone, UK) and analyzed. The standards of the selenium species, selenate (SeVI), selenite (SeIV), selenomethionine (SeMet), selenocystine (SeCys2), and Se-methylselenocysteine (MeSeCys) were obtained from Sigma Aldrich (Germany). Calibration solutions of the selenium species containing 1-, 5-, 10-, 50-, and 100-µg/L Se were prepared by diluting the stock solutions of the selenium species with water.

2.6. Detection of Se Nanoparticles Using Transmission Electron Microscope (TEM)

Images of nanoparticles (NPs) were acquired using a TEM Jeol 2200 FS (Jeol, Tokyo, Japan). Elemental mapping of the selected region was conducted using an energy-dispersive X-ray spectrometer (EDX) attached to the TEM. The TEM images were evaluated using ImageJ 1.50i software (Wayne Rasband, National Institutes of Health, College Park, MD, USA). Fresh bacterial suspensions of the strains CCDM 144 and CCDM 922A grown overnight in M17 broth supplemented with 10 mg/L of sodium selenite were centrifuged (6000× g, 5 min) and resuspended in water. Samples for TEM imaging were prepared by evaporating (3 h at 24 ± 1 °C) a drop of culture placed onto a 300-mesh lacey carbon copper grid.

2.7. Microbiota Composition

Samples of the distal part of the colon with feces were taken into sterile samplers containing Wilkins-Chalgren Anaerobe broth (Oxoid Limited, Basingstoke, Hampshire, UK) and frozen at −20 °C immediately after collection until further analyses. Differences in the composition of the gut microbiota among the experimental groups were observed by the detection of selected bacterial genera and species. Viable counts were determined by the plate count enumeration method with 10-fold dilutions. Fecal samples were stored in Wilkins-Chalgren anaerobic broth at $-20\,°C$. Prior to analyses, 1 g of the feces was weighed and properly homogenized (vortex VELP Scientifica; Usmate, Italy) in 9 mL of physiological saline, serially diluted, and plated on Petri dishes. Each concentration gradient was measured in triplicate. The family *Enterobacteriaceae* and the genera *Clostridium and Lactobacillus*, as well as *E. coli* in fecal matter, were enumerated using the following selective cultivation media and conditions: for *Enterobacteriaceae*, VRBG agar (crystal-violet, neutral-red, bile, glucose agar; MILCOM, Tábor, Czech Republic) was used at 37 °C for 72 h; for *Clostridium*, RCM (Reinforced Clostridial Medium; MILCOM, Tábor, Czech Republic) was used at 37 °C for 72 h under anaerobic conditions after the previous inactivation of samples at 85 °C for 10 min; *E. coli* chromogenic TBX agar (tryptone, bile, X-glucuronide; MILCOM, Tábor, Czech Republic) was used at 37 °C for 72 h; and *Lactobacillus*, MRS 5.7 agar (de Man, Rogosa, and Sharpe; MILCOM, Tábor, Czech Republic) was used at 37 °C for 72 h under anaerobic conditions.

2.8. Statistical Analyses

For the data evaluation, Statgraphics® Centurion XV (StatPoint, Inc., Warrenton, VA, USA) was used with two-way ANOVA for multiple comparisons, and the post hoc least significance difference test (LSD) was performed, considering the statistical significance at $p < 0.05$ (evaluation of the microbial counts).

Homoscedasticity and normality of data distribution were tested by the Levene and Shapiro-Wilk tests, respectively, as assumptions for the use of an analysis of variance (ANOVA). ANOVA followed by Tukey's honestly significant difference (HSD) test was used for comparison of the data groups, and Dunnett's test was used for comparison of the experimental groups with the control group. Statistica 13.1 software (StatSoft, Inc., Tulsa, OK, USA) and Real Statistics Resource Pack software (Release 7.2, Charles Zaiontz) were used for testing.

3. Results

3.1. Selenium Enrichment and Diets

Following lyophilization, viable counts (CFU) of the strains EF, ST, SeEF, and SeST were 10^9 CFU/g. Both strains remained sufficiently viable, even after being processed into feed, and their counts reached approximately 10^4 CFU/g in the final diet. Their presence in the live form confirms their desirable technological properties and ability to survive the heat treatment process.

Based on the contents of the selected biogenic elements, Table 2 shows the differences in the nutritional compositions of the experimental diets based on Altromin 1324 and Altromin C 1045. The selenium content in group A was determined by the addition of sodium selenite during the production of Altromin 1324 (producer information). Moreover, the addition of selenized LAB resulted in increased total Se contents (as expected) in groups D and F. The contents of the other elements remained unchanged in groups B–F after the addition of non-selenized/selenized LAB. The differences in contents of the elements between group A and groups B–F are shown in the diet matrix; maintenance diet Altromin 1324 is based on raw materials from cereal, while Se-deficient diet Altromin C 1045 is based on purified raw materials such as casein, starch, and sugars.

In addition to the total selenium content, Se speciation was analyzed in the feedstuff pellets (Figure 1). The efficiency of the enzymatic extraction was 40–85%. The speciation analyses revealed no significant differences in Se species abundances among groups B–F. The most abundant species was SeCys2, which accounted for 30–40% of total Se species. A smaller proportion was found for SeMet (8–16%), and minor species were represented by the inorganic Se forms, SeVI, and SeIV, with an average proportion of 2%. The rest of the selenium contents in the extract consisted of unidentified species. The chromatographic patterns obtained for the extract of diet A differed from each other. Although sodium selenite was added to this diet by the manufacturer, a higher proportion of inorganic selenium compounds was not found. It can thus be assumed that SeCys2 is a major selenium species in this diet; however, owing to the insufficient separation of the peaks in the chromatogram range of 3–5 min, this cannot be proven and evaluated.

Table 2. Total contents of the elements in the feedstuff (mg/kg wet weight, $n = 3$). The averages marked by the same letter do not significantly differ at $p < 0.05$ within the individual columns; data are presented as the mean ± expanded uncertainty with a coverage factor $k = 2$.

Sample	Cu (mg/kg)	Zn (mg/kg)	Cr (mg/kg)	Fe (mg/kg)
A—Altromin 1324	26.0 ± 9.0 [a]	63.7 ± 9.9 [a]	51.4 ± 8.4 [a]	418 ± 43 [a]
B—Altromin C 1045	14.4 ± 5.4 [b]	48.7 ± 2.3 [b]	37.8 ± 2.9 [b]	125 ± 11 [b]
C—Altromin C 1045 + ST	13.8 ± 4.8 [b]	47.7 ± 1.2 [b]	37.3 ± 6.4 [b]	123 ± 28 [b]
D—Altromin C 1045 + SeST	13.2 ± 2.3 [b]	47.8 ± 6.8 [b]	37.4 ± 5.6 [b]	117 ± 16 [b]
E—Altromin C 1045 + EF	13.3 ± 3.3 [b]	46.8 ± 3.9 [b]	38.2 ± 7.4 [b]	119 ± 13 [b]
F—Altromin C 1045 + SeEF	15.8 ± 5.5 [b]	47.1 ± 2.0 [b]	36.4 ± 6.8 [b]	122 ± 11 [b]

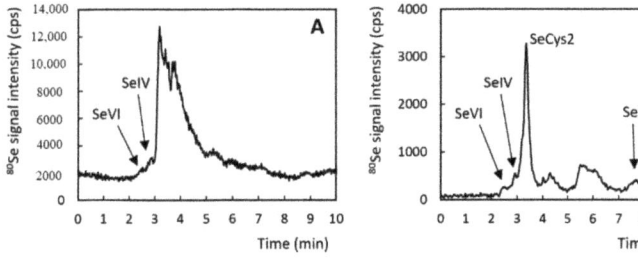

Figure 1. Chromatogram of the extracts of diet A (**A**) and diet B (**B**).

Besides the selenium species mentioned above, selenium NPs were found in both selenized strains and characterized by TEM (Figure 2). TEM demonstrated the localization of the NPs outside of the cells. Se NPs inside the cells or cell membrane-bound NPs were not observed. The images showed that individual selenium NPs had approximately spherical shapes. The CCDM 144 strain produced NPs with a broad size distribution of 98–236 nm (average value of 171 nm), while the CCDM 922A strain produced NPs with sizes in the range of 42–185 nm (average value of 122 nm).

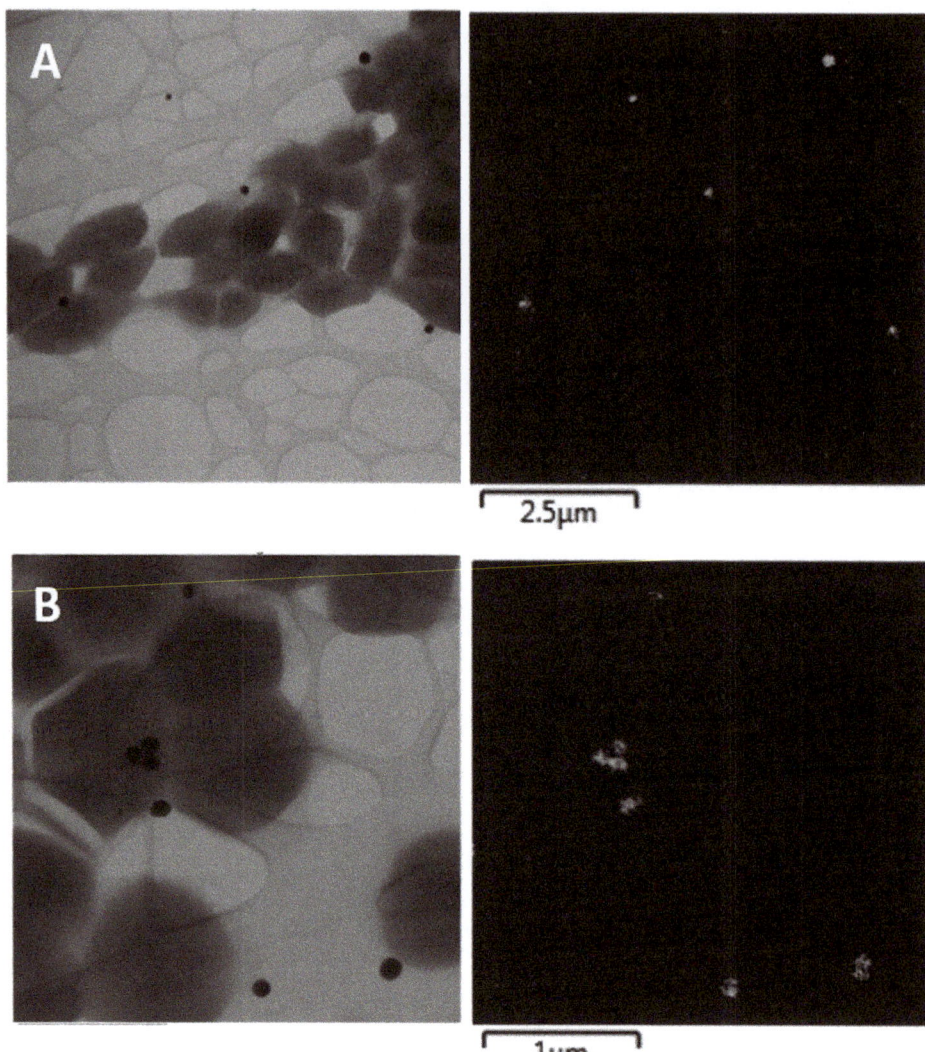

Figure 2. Bright field TEM images (**left**) of the CCDM 144 (**A**) and CCDM 922A (**B**) selenized strains with the corresponding energy-dispersive X-ray (EDX) maps of the signal intensity of selenium Se $K\alpha_1$ spectral line (**right**).

3.2. Effects of Selenium-Enriched Strains on Biochemical Parameters and Enzyme Activities in Tissue Homogenates and Blood

The diets had negligible effects on the body weight gains and weights of selected organs, except for lower brain weights in the Altromin 1324 group. In this group, the weights of the other organs also tended to be lower (Table 3).

Similarly, the serum concentrations of the total cholesterol, HDL cholesterol, and triacylglycerols (TAG) did not differ between the control and other groups (Table 4). The Altromin 1324 group tended to have higher lipid concentrations, which was consistent with the higher weight gain in this group.

Table 3. The body weights and weights of organs in grams ($n = 8$). Data are presented as the mean (standard deviation). [a,b]–values in columns with different supercase letters significantly differ ($p < 0.05$).

Group	Body Weight Gain (g)	Heart (g)	Brain (g)	Liver (g)	Kidneys (g)
A—Altromin 1324	102 (60) [a]	1.04 (0.13) [a]	1.58 (0.20) [b]	13.7 (4.8) [a]	2.86 (0.46) [a]
B—Altromin C 1045	85 (41) [a]	1.25 (0.11) [a]	2.12 (0.08) [a]	14.3 (2.7) [a]	3.27 (0.34) [a]
C—Altromin C 1045 + ST	89 (67) [a]	1.34 (0.25) [a]	2.15 (0.10) [a]	14.8 (2.7) [a]	3.38 (0.29) [a]
D—Altromin C 1045 + SeST	68 (35) [a]	1.27 (0.15) [a]	2.14 (0.06) [a]	14.3 (1.4) [a]	3.32 (0.24) [a]
E—Altromin C 1045 + EF	75 (42) [a]	1.25 (0.14) [a]	2.13 (0.06) [a]	15.1 (1.8) [a]	3.40 (0.46) [a]
F—Altromin C 1045 + SeEF	65 (50) [a]	1.21 (0.11) [a]	2.09 (0.13) [a]	14.6 (2.0) [a]	3.30 (0.32) [a]

Table 4. Serum concentrations of the basic lipid parameters (mmol/L, $n = 8$). Data are presented as the mean (standard deviation). [a]–values in columns with the same superscript letter do not significantly differ ($p < 0.05$).

Group	Cholesterol mmol/L	TAG (mmol/L)	HDL Cholesterol (mmol/L)
A—Altromin 1324	1.69 (0.23) [a]	1.01 (0.44) [a]	1.25 (0.26) [a]
B—Altromin C 1045	1.55 (0.25) [a]	0.79 (0.45) [a]	1.16 (0.22) [a]
C—Altromin C 1045 + ST	1.46 (0.22) [a]	0.49 (0.38) [a]	1.04 (0.12) [a]
D—Altromin C 1045 + SeST	1.44 (0.18) [a]	0.59 (0.49) [a]	1.03 (0.14) [a]
E—Altromin C 1045 + EF	1.49 (0.27) [a]	0.87 (0.43) [a]	1.09 (0.23) [a]
F—Altromin C 1045 + SeEF	1.53 (0.24) [a]	0.66 (0.38) [a]	1.10 (0.19) [a]

TAG–triacylglycerols; HDL–high-density lipoprotein cholesterol.

Next, the activities (U/mL of the homogenate or serum) and concentrations (in ng/mL of the homogenate or serum) of the two antioxidant enzymes were measured. To gain more information on the oxidative stress status, the concentrations of MDA in the serum and heart were analyzed (Table 5). The effects of the diets were more pronounced in the heart, where a lower GR content was observed in all groups with added strains irrespective of Se fortification, with the activity of GR being higher in both diets with EF and SeEF (groups E and F). Notably, GPx was significantly less influenced by the diets. The MDA concentrations were also changed by both diets with EF/SeEF, especially in the heart, where the MDA concentrations were higher in the respective groups (E and F), unlike the changes in the serum (serum MDA was significantly lower only in group F, with SeEF).

Table 5. The levels of the selected parameters of oxidative stress in the serum and tissues ($n = 8$). Data are presented as the mean (standard deviation). [a,b]–values in columns with different superscript letters significantly differ ($p < 0.05$).

(A)

Group	Heart GPx (ng/mL)	Heart GPx (U/mL)	Brain GPx (ng/mL)	Brain GPx (U/mL)	Serum GPx (ng/mL)	Serum GPx (U/mL)
A—Altromin 1324	45.7 (8.7) [a]	13.3 (3.7) [a]	51.8 (7.0) [a]	15.3 (2.3) [a]	27.9 (2.09) [b]	0.34 (0.39) [a]
B—Altromin C 1045	41.9 (4.1) [a]	14.6 (1.3) [a]	49.8 (5.3) [a]	14.5 (3.3) [a]	25.1 (2.58) [a]	1.49 (2.27) [a]
C—Altromin C 1045 + ST	28.6 (12.0) [b]	14.8 (2.3) [a]	49.8 (4.6) [a]	14.7 (4.2) [a]	24.6 (1.84) [a]	0.15 (0.09) [a]
D—Altromin C 1045 + SeST	34.7 (8.3) [a]	12.1 (6.1) [a]	50.9 (3.3) [a]	12.0 (2.7) [a]	25.0 (1.90) [a]	0.12 (0.07) [a]
E—Altromin C 1045 + EF	39.3 (5.7) [a]	15.7 (2.2) [a]	50.1 (4.5) [a]	11.3 (1.4) [a]	25.5 (1.16) [a]	0.90 (1.63) [a]
F—Altromin C 1045 + SeEF	40.4 (6.1) [a]	14.5 (2.7) [a]	51.8 (1.8) [a]	9.4 (1.3) [b]	24.2 (1.69) [a]	0.16 (0.29) [a]

(B)

Group	Heart GR (ng/mL)	Heart GR (U/mL)	Brain GR (ng/mL)	Brain GR (U/mL)	Serum MDA (ng/mL)	Brain MDA (ng/mL)	Heart MDA (ng/mL)
A—Altromin 1324	88.8 (11.9) [a]	138.8 (5.0) [a]	0.67 (0.46) [a]	158.9 (23.5) [a]	280 (97) [a]	469 (86) [a]	348 (89) [a]
B—Altromin C 1045	75.5 (10.9) [a]	135.7 (6.5) [a]	0.35 (0.23) [a]	178.1 (67.1) [a]	305 (182) [a]	454 (49) [a]	288 (144) [a]
C—Altromin C 1045 + ST	43.9 (15.2) [b]	138.6 (12.2) [a]	0.48 (0.23) [a]	156.8 (8.3) [a]	296 (35) [a]	414 (63) [a]	348 (61) [a]
D—Altromin C 1045 + SeST	43.2 (7.9) [b]	136.0 (13.7) [a]	0.60 (0.13) [a]	150.0 (10.1) [a]	260 (81) [a]	432 (48) [a]	358 (92) [a]
E—Altromin C 1045 + EF	49.2 (14.8) [b]	149.4 (7.6) [b]	0.31 (0.13) [a]	144.4 (18.8) [a]	201 (59) [a]	445 (39) [a]	570 (100) [b]
F—Altromin C 1045 + SeEF	38.3 (10.1) [b]	155.3 (3.9) [b]	0.38 (0.28) [a]	139.0 (8.0) [a]	164 (51) [b]	485 (79) [a]	460 (65) [b]

GPx–glutathione peroxidase; GR–glutathione reductase; MDA–malondialdehyde.

3.3. Effects of Selenium-Enriched Strains on Total Selenium and Selenium-Species Contents in Tissue Homogenates

The concentrations of Se in the kidneys and liver of rats are higher than that in other organs [24]. Therefore, the total selenium content and selenium species in these tissues were analyzed. A higher selenium content (Table 6) was found in the kidneys of rats in groups A, D, and F, which were fed a Se-fortified diet. The contents of the other monitored elements were not affected by the diet, with the exception of the copper content, which was higher in group A. In the case of the liver samples (Table 7), the differences in the total Se contents between the groups with Se-fortified diets and non-selenized groups were significantly greater than those in the kidney samples. Moreover, the total Se content in group A was higher than those in groups D and F, where selenium was added in the form of selenized LAB. The contents of the other monitored elements were also not affected by the diet.

Table 6. Total contents of the elements in rat kidneys (mg/kg wet weight, $n = 8$). The averages marked by the same letter do not significantly differ at $p < 0.05$ within the individual columns; data are presented as the mean (standard deviation).

Sample	Se (mg/kg)	Cu (mg/kg)	Zn (mg/kg)	Cr (mg/kg)	Fe (mg/kg)
A—Altromin 1324	1.22 (0.17) [a]	12.0 (3.4) [a]	16.6 (2.9) [a]	0.233 (0.039) [a]	88 (27) [a]
B—Altromin C 1045	0.79 (0.15) [b]	6.2 (1.5) [b]	17.3 (2.7) [a]	0.254 (0.045) [a]	131 (69) [a]
C—Altromin C 1045 + ST	0.79 (0.07) [b]	6.4 (1.4) [b]	17.4 (1.8) [a]	0.205 (0.046) [a]	132 (84) [a]
D—Altromin C 1045 + SeST	1.08 (0.18) [ac]	7.4 (2.9) [b]	17.5 (1.4) [a]	0.221 (0.026) [a]	94 (47) [a]
E—Altromin C 1045 + EF	0.81 (0.16) [b]	6.7 (2.2) [b]	17.2 (2.1) [a]	0.243 (0.076) [a]	90 (54) [a]
F—Altromin C 1045 + SeEF	0.89 (0.12) [bc]	5.0 (0.7) [b]	16.1 (2.4) [a]	0.200 (0.027) [a]	77 (38) [a]

Table 7. Total contents of the elements in rat livers (mg/kg wet weight, $n = 8$). The averages marked by the same letter do not significantly differ at $p < 0.05$ within the individual columns; data are presented as the mean (standard deviation).

Sample	Se (mg/kg)	Cu (mg/kg)	Zn (mg/kg)	Cr (mg/kg)	Fe (mg/kg)
A—Altromin 1324	0.383 (0.058) [a]	2.25 (0.26) [a]	11.9 (1.7) [a]	0.070 (0.017) [a]	131 (37) [a]
B—Altromin C 1045	0.137 (0.018) [b]	2.43 (0.25) [a]	11.9 (1.5) [a]	0.067 (0.011) [a]	113 (17) [ab]
C—Altromin C 1045 + ST	0.152 (0.023) [b]	2.42 (0.27) [a]	11.5 (1.1) [a]	0.074 (0.015) [a]	119 (13) [ab]
D—Altromin C 1045 + SeST	0.252 (0.055) [c]	2.37 (0.31) [a]	11.2 (2.1) [a]	0.072 (0.015) [a]	110 (14) [ab]
E—Altromin C 1045 + EF	0.142 (0.029) [b]	2.44 (0.21) [a]	10.5 (1.1) [a]	0.066 (0.016) [a]	104 (28) [ab]
F—Altromin C 1045 + SeEF	0.213 (0.039) [c]	2.31 (0.12) [a]	11.1 (1.3) [a]	0.072 (0.013) [a]	105 (23) [b]

The aim of the speciation analysis was to determine whether the Se speciation varied with the Se and LAB contents in the diet. The efficiency of the enzymatic extraction of the selenium species from the kidney samples was $80 \pm 6\%$. The HPLC column recovery for the kidney samples was $98\% \pm 8\%$, indicating that all selenium species in the extract were eluted from the column. The extraction efficiency of the selenium species from the liver samples was $74 \pm 16\%$, and the column recovery was $103 \pm 7\%$. These data indicate that a major part of the total Se was extracted, and no selenium species were captured on the HPLC column. The performed analysis thus provided a reliable overview of the distribution of selenium between the individual species.

The speciation analysis revealed differences between the liver and kidney samples. SeCys2 was the major species and SeMet the minor species in both samples (Figure 3). The kidney samples also contained MeSeCys. The other minor Se species were unidentified. The species with retention times of 4.1, 4.3, and 5.0 min seemed to be specific for the liver, and the species with a retention time of 5.4 min were specific for the kidney samples. Unidentified species with a retention time of 6.6 min were observed in both sample types. No inorganic forms (SeVI or SeIV) were observed in the tissue samples.

The average content of SeCys2 in the kidney samples (Figure 4) was the lowest in group A (51%) and the highest in control group B (80%). The SeCys2 percentages in the groups with added LAB in the diet (groups C–F) were similar (63–69%), regardless of their Se fortification. In the liver, as well as in the kidneys, SeCys2 was the most abundant species; however, the abundance in the liver (42–58%) was slightly lower than that in the kidneys. The SeCys2 percentages did not differ significantly for the individual groups, although higher average values were observed for groups D and F (57% and 58%, respectively), and the lowest average value was observed for control group B (42%). Besides SeCys2, SeMet was also found in the extracts. The proportions of SeMet were similar in all groups and reached values of 1–7% in the kidney samples and 6–16% in the liver samples. The last identified species, MeSeCys, was only found in the kidney extracts. The lowest content of MeSeCys (8%) was observed in control group B, while the other groups contained higher amounts (13–19%) of MeSeCys. Although the unidentified species constituted a minor portion (8–24%) of the total selenium content in the kidneys, a significant proportion (34–49%) was detected in the liver. All percentage values were based on an analysis of only two samples for each group. Due to the low number of analyzed samples, the actual variability or mean values may vary slightly.

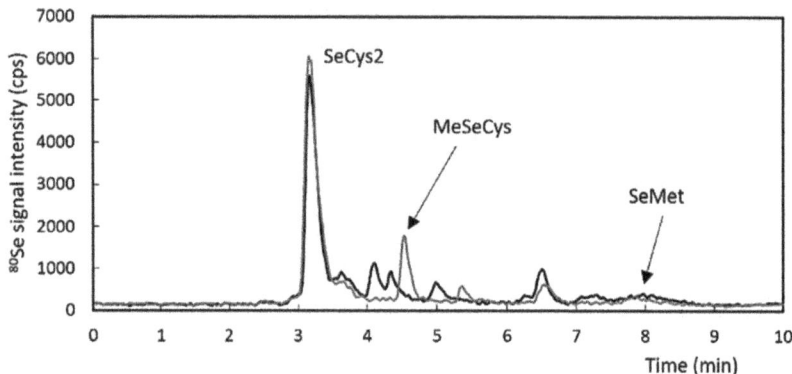

Figure 3. Chromatogram of the liver extract (black) and kidney extract (grey); both organ types were collected from group D rats (Altromin C 1045 + Se-enriched *Streptococcus thermophilus* (SeST)).

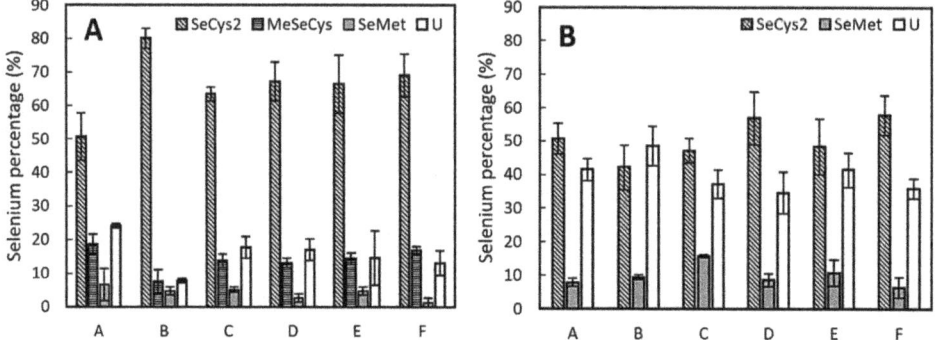

Figure 4. Selenium species representation expressed as a percentage of the total selenium content: (**A**) kidneys and (**B**) liver. The error bars indicate the standard deviation (n = 2). SeCys2 (selenocysteine), MeSeCys (Se-methylselenocysteine), SeMet (selenomethionine), and U (sum of unidentified species).

3.4. Effect of Selenium-Enriched Strains on Bacterial Populations in Fecal Matter

Four different bacterial groups were subjected to analyses and were enumerated in the fecal matter collected from rat colons. The results are presented in Table 8. Compared with the group fed a standard maintenance diet (group A), the total counts (CFU/g) of *Clostridium* sp. decreased significantly ($p < 0.05$) in all other experimental groups, whereas their reduction was even more apparent in the groups supplemented with the strain *Enterococcus faecium* (groups E and F). In group E, the counts of *Clostridium* sp. were reduced by more than two logarithmic orders. The *Enterobacteriaceae* and *E. coli* groups were slightly reduced in the supplemented groups (C, D, E, and F) and, also, in the Se-deficient group (B); however, this decrease was significant only in the group administered Se-enriched *Enterococcus faecium* ($p < 0.05$), both in terms of *Enterobacteriaceae* and *E. coli*. In contrast, high viable counts of *Lactobacillus* sp. as a beneficial bacterial group were observed (ranging from 7.64 to 8.34 log CFU/g), which was a desirable count. The total counts of the *Lactobacillus* sp. were minimally affected among the experimental groups compared to the rats fed the standard maintenance diet (group A), although, in groups D and E, the viable counts were found to be slightly higher.

Table 8. Effects of the experimental diets on the intestinal bacterial groups.

Groups	Total Counts (log CFU/g)			
	Clostridium	*Enterobacteriaceae*	*Escherichia coli*	*Lactobacillus*
A—Altromin 1324	3.04 (0.46) [d]	5.01 (0.67) [b]	4.98 (0.72) [b]	7.78 (0.64) [ab]
B—Altromin C 1045	1.99 (0.43) [c]	4.42 (0.57) [b]	4.37 (0.62) [b]	7.87 (0.62) [ab]
C—Altromin C 1045 + ST	1.85 (0.60) [bc]	4.74 (0.51) [b]	4.58 (0.42) [b]	7.98 (0.48) [ab]
D—Altromin C 1045 + SeST	1.51 (0.80) [bc]	4.79 (0.77) [b]	4.73 (0.64) [b]	8.29 (0.61) [b]
E—Altromin C 1045 + EF	0.96 (0.32) [a]	4.68 (0.92) [b]	4.40 (0.53) [b]	8.34 (0.55) [b]
F—Altromin C 1045 + SeEF	1.39 (0.38) [ab]	3.39 (0.77) [a]	3.25 (1.04) [a]	7.64 (0.61) [a]

ST, *Streptococcus thermophilus*, SeST, selenium-enriched *Streptococcus thermophilus*, EF, *Enterococcus faecium*, and SeEF, selenium-enriched *Enterococcus faecium*. Data are presented as the mean (standard deviation) from triplicate determination. Values within columns with different superscripts indicate a significant difference at $p < 0.05$. CFU: colony-forming units.

4. Discussion

In our previous study [22], we highlighted the abilities of S. *thermophilus* CCDM 144 and E. *faecium* CCDM 922A to accumulate up to 7.3 mg/g Se and 6.5 mg/g Se, respectively. Therefore, these strains were used for selenium enrichment of the SeST (group D) and SeEF (group F) diets in this study. The Se content in the diet of group A was derived from the natural Se contents in the ingredients of the diet and the added sodium selenite (according to the information provided by the producer). The diets were designed to obtain a difference of approximately 0.25-mg/kg Se between the Se-deficient diets (groups B, C, and E) and Se-enriched diets (groups A, D, and F). The speciation analysis revealed a different Se speciation in the diet of group A compared to the diets of the other groups. However, the differences in speciation may not represent the efficacies of the Se supplementation. Takahashi et al. [25] demonstrated an increased rapid absorption of SeMet and MeSeCys compared to the other Se species; however, at the same time, they also reported a lower efficiency of assimilation into selenoproteins. Moreover, although dietary Se amino acids are not directly incorporated into selenoproteins, all dietary forms of Se must be metabolized and enzymatically converted into selenide, which serves as a Se source for Se amino acids and for the subsequent protein synthesis [26]. The Se bioavailability in terms of selenoprotein production is thus similar for all Se species, with the main advantage of using organically bound Se to lower the toxicity. Se supplementation via LAB (groups D and F) is also supported by the fact that, in addition to organic Se species, LABs also contain nanoparticles that are considered to have a low toxicity [18].

In the presence of selenite, the bacterial cultivation medium was found to be red in color, which indicates the reduction of added selenite to elemental Se; this has been documented in previous studies as well [16,27]. Both strains used in this study produced spherical-shaped Se nanoparticles, as confirmed by the TEM results. *Streptococcus thermophilus* produced nanoparticles of sizes ranging from 98 to 236 nm, whereas *Enterococcus faecium* produced smaller nanoparticles with sizes ranging from 42 to 185 nm. In lactobacilli, a wider range of particle sizes, from 25 to 370 nm, was documented by Pescuma et al. [16]. Differences in particle sizes were also observed among the particles produced by different species of the same genus [28]. Moreover, differences were observed in terms of the location at which the NPs were produced. Although, in our case, Se NPs were located outside the cells, references to extracellular Se NPs are less common in the literature [29], and intracellular production is mostly described for LAB [27,30]. However, the presence of extracellular Se NPs could be advantageous over intracellular production because of their ease of accessibility and bioavailability. Moreover, Se NP formation is not a common feature of all LAB strains. Martínez et al. [31] demonstrated that Se NPs were produced in only eight (*Lactococcus lactis*, *Lactobacillus brevis* and *Lactobacillus plantarum*, *Fructobacillus tropaeola*, *Enterococcus casseliflavus*, and *Weissella cibaria*) out of 96 tested LAB strains. The binding of Se to the cell wall of LAB and their storage in the cell are mediated by complex processes that depend on factors such as the characteristics of the element (Se) and the specific physiological properties of individual LAB strains, as well as the cultivation media in which the bacteria are grown [19].

The LAB production of Se nanoparticles has been previously studied [16,28,32,33], and the NPs produced were found to be less toxic than other inorganic Se forms. The particle size depends on the strain used. In LABs, the sizes of the NPs produced ranged between 40 and 500 nm. According to Nagy et al. [28], smaller Se nanoparticles could be more toxic to the producing bacteria themselves. *Streptococcus thermophilus* tested in the aforementioned study produced Se nanoparticles of sizes ranging from 60 to 280 nm, which was followed by necrotic cell disruption. It has been reported that NPs are toxic to the cell, because they disrupt cell membranes. Therefore, the extracellular NPs produced by the two strains tested in this study could be advantageous, because they were not toxic to the cells themselves, in addition to their high bioavailability. Nevertheless, elemental Se is referred to as one of the least toxic Se forms with high bioavailability [18]. The absorption of Se NPs smaller than 100 nm in the gastrointestinal tract was proved to be 15–250 times higher than that of large-sized NPs [34]. Xu et al. [27] showed that *L. casei* with intracellularly accumulated Se NPs maintains an intestinal microbiota balance in response to oxidative stress and infection and exhibits an improved integrity of the intestinal epithelial barrier.

The antioxidant parameters were evaluated in the serum by measuring the GPx, GR enzyme activity, and MDA, a parameter of lipoperoxidation. In a recent study [5], a significant increase in GPx and SOD activities, along with reduced MDA concentrations and GSH activities, was observed in the serum of rats fed with Se- and Zn-enriched probiotics. Accordingly, the beneficial effects of Se-enriched strains improving the antioxidant status in comparison with the control group were observed in this study as well. The MDA values provide a rough estimate of the oxidative stress in the tissue. We observed lower concentrations of serum MDA following Se supplementation, as in the study of Malyar et al. [5], which was accompanied by higher serum activities of antioxidative enzymes. This association, however, is not supported by the results of our study, as the serum and heart GPx activities did not change between the observed groups. The activity of GPx was lower in the rat heart and brain tissues than that in the other tissues. These tissues differed by both concentrations of Se (app. three-fold higher in the heart) and the relative amount of Se bound to GPx (20% in the heart vs. 3% in the brain) [35]. In another study, the supplementation with SeMet revealed no effect on the GPX heart activity in rodents [36]. Following Se supplementation, we observed the changes in the heart GR activity. This enzyme is not Se-dependent but reduces glutathione to maintain a reduced glutathione pool [37].

In the rat hearts of all the groups in which LAB strains were administered, changes in the oxidative stress parameters were observed. In heart tissues of the groups with added ST and SeST strains (groups C and D), the concentration of MDA only tended to increase; therefore, lower amounts of GR (reduced glutathione-forming enzyme), together with its sustained activity, were most likely sufficient to maintain an acceptable level of oxidative stress. In contrast, the higher indices of oxidative stress in the heart following the diets with EF and SeEF (groups E and F)—observed as high heart MDA concentrations—were associated with the increased activity of GR despite its lower amounts. We can speculate that it may be a result of the efforts to maintain a reduced pool of GSH capable of inactivating elevated lipoperoxide levels, which is reflected in the increased MDA concentrations in the heart tissue of these rats. At the moment, we can only hypothesize why this happened in just the EF and SeEF groups. The effect of the strain *Enterococcus faecium* CCDM 922A remains speculative itself, since it has been reported to interfere with the lipid metabolism and exhibits the capacity to reduce low-density lipoprotein and very low-density lipoprotein cholesterol in rats [23]. The two diets, standard Altromin 1234 and

Se-deficient Altromin C 1045, differed both in vitamin E content (75 mg/kg vs. 150 mg/kg) and Se concentration (408 µg/kg vs. 108 µg/kg). The parameters of the antioxidative system did not differ between these two groups; thus, no effect or sum of opposite effects can be expected. In rats, Se and vitamin E exhibited dietary compensatory relationships and were found to act synergistically [38,39]. Moreover, various additional interactions between Se and other trace elements or nutrients have been described [40]. The content of Cu, Fe, Cr, and Zn in the liver and kidneys did not differ in the EF/SeEF groups compared to the B–D groups, and for this reason, the influence of other elements may be ruled out. To consider all the possible parameters, we also can speculate the stress response to hunger/conditions before decapitation, given that groups E and F were euthanized last. It is known that different selenoproteins are involved in the cardiovascular stress response; among them, the GPx family is one of the best characterized. Nevertheless, the exact role of the other selenoproteins involved (e.g., thioredoxin reductase, thyroid hormone deiodinases, selenoprotein R, and selenoprotein K) remains only partly understood, and further investigation of the Se-dependent effects at the molecular level is needed [41].

The Se levels were monitored in the liver and kidney samples, as these organs are involved in Se regulation, the production of excretory selenium forms, and generally accumulate a higher amount of selenium in comparison to other organs [42]. The total observed selenium levels in the liver (0.14–0.38 mg/kg) and kidneys (0.8–1.2 mg/kg) agreed with those observed in other studies focusing on animals fed with Se-enriched foodstuffs [38,43–45]. In these studies, the Se contents in the liver samples were found to be in the range of 0.25–5.0 mg/kg, while those in the kidney samples were in the range of 1.0–6.7 mg/kg.

Higher Se levels in Se-enriched diets resulted in increased Se contents in the kidneys and liver. Although the Se contents in the kidney samples of the groups fed with Se-enriched diets were similar, and the differences were not significant ($p < 0.05$) in all cases, the highest average Se content was observed in the kidney samples from group A, the diets of which contained both inorganic and organic Se. The highest Se content in group A was also observed in the liver samples; this value was significantly higher than the Se content in groups D and F with diets containing organically bound Se only. However, the knowledge on whether the addition of inorganic Se into diet leads to higher Se contents in rat liver and kidneys compared to the addition of organic forms is sporadic in the literature. Rýdlová et al. [38] confirmed that the intake of Se-enriched defatted rapeseed (0.2 mg/kg Se) added had no effect on the Se content in the liver and kidneys of Wistar and spontaneously hypertensive rats in comparison to the control group. The opposite trend has been described more often; Zhou et al. [46] highlighted that Se accumulation from organic Se supplements was higher than that from inorganic supplements in most biological tissues of Sprague–Dawley rats. The Se content in the liver of rats fed a diet fortified with Se-enriched *Bifidobacterium longum* or selenized yeast was much higher than that of rats fed a selenite-enriched diet. The Se content in the kidneys showed the same trend, but the differences were smaller for all three groups. Similarly, Zhang et al. [47] found higher Se levels in the kidneys and liver of rats administered a diet fortified with Se-enriched garlic and a mixture of non-selenized garlic and selenite than in the kidneys and liver of rats administered a selenite-enriched diet only. Qin et al. [43] observed a higher Se content in the kidneys and liver of lambs fed Se-enriched yeast and Se-enriched probiotics (a mixture of *Lactobacillus* and *Saccharomyces cerevisiae*) than in the kidneys and liver of lambs fed a selenite-fortified diet. Marounek et al. [48] observed the same effect in rabbits fed Se-enriched yeast, Se-enriched algae, and selenite-fortified diets. Some studies also showed no difference between the organic and inorganic Se sources in terms of their accumulation in organs. Sobeková et al. [45] confirmed in the case of lambs that an increased dietary Se intake in the form of selenite and Se-enriched yeast led to significantly higher Se contents in the liver and kidneys in comparison to the control; however, no significant difference between diets enriched with selenite and Se-enriched yeast was observed. These findings were supported by Han et al. [44], who fed hens a Se-fortified diet (selenite and Se-enriched yeasts).

Due to the importance of the liver and kidneys in the metabolism of Se, many studies also focused on Se speciation in these organs. SeCys2 or SeCys are described as the major Se species in the kidneys and liver, followed by SeMet as the second-most abundant species for various animal species, e.g., broiler chicks [49], rain trout [50], rats [51], or lambs [52]. However, in some animals—for example, sheep [42] and lambs [53]—similar percentages of SeMet, SeCys2, and MeSeCys were observed. SeCys2 thus appears to be the dominant species in the liver and kidneys of most animals, although, in some cases, SeMet and MeSeCys may be on par with SeCys2. Our results were consistent with the published data. SeCys2 was found to be the major Se species in the liver samples (42–58%) and kidney samples (51–80%). Instead of SeCys2, only SeMet was identified in the liver, and its percentage ranged from 6% to 16%. In the kidneys, although SeMet was only found in trace amounts (1–7%), MeSeCys was present in larger amounts (8–19%). Other species in the liver and kidneys were unidentified. A statistically significant difference ($p < 0.05$) was observed only in the proportion of SeCys2 and MeSeCys in the kidneys between groups A and B, but the differences were not significant. Thus, the addition of Se to the diet, whether in its organic or inorganic form, did not alter the Se speciation. Similar results were obtained by Juniper et al. [52] in the case of lambs fed a Se-enriched yeast diet. The kidney and liver samples were comprised of a large proportion of the total Se as SeCys, and no change in speciation was observed in comparison to the control group. Small changes in Se speciation were observed in the study of Zhao et al. [49], who fed broiler chicks with the inorganic and organic forms of Se. SeCys2 and SeMet were found to be the major and minor species in the livers of chicks, respectively. In the case of Se-enriched yeast diets, a larger proportion of SeMet (3.5–7.3-fold) was observed in comparison to the diets containing selenite.

The composition of the intestinal microbiota can be affected by numerous factors that alter the microbial homeostasis. These factors include stress, dietary changes, the overuse of antibiotics, and gastrointestinal or other infections. The intestinal redox status and inflammatory levels are also strongly associated with alterations in the gut microbiota [54]. The Se status has been reported as a regulator of intestinal microbiota, especially when the Se availability is limited [55]. Individual bacterial species and strains are differently sensitive to Se concentrations; a concentration of Se that is tolerable by one strain may be toxic to another. The tolerance of strains to Se can be attributed to the differences in their individual capabilities to uptake, store, use, and remove Se from cells [56]. Recent studies have supported the theory that the gut microbiota also plays a role in Se metabolism in the host by metabolizing bioselenocompounds [57], whereas both organic and inorganic Se have been proven to have an effect on the community structure of the gut microbiota [54]. Additionally, a Se-deficient diet has been associated with damaged intestinal barrier function and imbalanced gut microbiota [54].

Following feedstuff processing, sufficient counts of viable cells (approximately 10^4 CFU/g) of LAB were observed in the pellets of the experimental diet. Due to the technological properties of the strains CCDM 144 and CCDM 922A and their survival during processing, they are widely employed in industrial applications. The presence of live bacteria by itself provides benefits—for example, in the production of acids, bacteriocins, and other antimicrobial compounds and the competitive exclusion of pathogens that are well-known in LAB strains [12]. Provided that the LABs are additionally enriched with Se, Zn, or other essential minerals, the delivery of these nutrients can also positively affect the gut microbiota and, hence, multiply the overall beneficial effect of the LAB or probiotic LAB administration. Dietary Se supplementation, whether in organic or inorganic forms via Se-enriched LAB or yeasts, was associated with modulation of the gut microbiota, as demonstrated in several previous studies [56,58–60]. For example, Se nanoparticles have been documented to increase the abundance of *Lactobacillus* sp. or *Faecalibacterium prausnitzii* and reduce the abundances of harmful strains—for example *Enterococcus cecorum* in poultry [61,62]. *Lactobacillus* sp. is an important LAB species, which includes many important strains with probiotic functions contributing to the maintenance of healthy and balanced gut ecosystems. In this study, we observed desirable high levels of *Lactobacillus* sp. (10^7–10^8 CFU/g) in the fecal matter of rats in all experimental groups, regardless of the final Se concentration in the diet and regardless of supplementation with LAB or Se-enriched LAB. In contrast, the highest influence of the supplementation was observed in the *Clostridium* sp. The highest counts of *Clostridium* sp. were detected in group A, which was administered a standard maintenance diet, whereas lower counts were observed in the remaining groups—that is, groups administered both Se-enriched LAB and LAB without Se-enrichment, as well as in groups administered the Se-deficient diet (groups B–F). Consistent with our results, *Clostridiaceae* were also more enhanced in the group of normal diet-fed rats compared to the low-Se diet-fed group in the study by Cheng et al. [54]. Notably, with the exception of the group fed a standard diet (group A), in all other groups, the levels of *Clostridium* sp. diminished, even in the groups (D and F) in which Se-enriched LAB were supplemented; thus, the final Se contents in the groups fed these two diets were comparable with those in the groups fed a standard diet (group A). We can therefore assume that the growth decrease is most probably not caused by Se itself. Among the other elements, the Fe content was more than three-fold higher in the group administered the standard Altromin 1324-based diet (group A) in comparison with that in the group administered the Altromin C1045-based diet (groups B–F). This is an important fact, because iron is known to play an important role in bacteria, especially in clostridial metabolism. Iron is involved in the active metal sites of enzymes or proteins such as ferredoxin, hydrogenase, and cytochrome, as well as participates in microbial energy conversion [63]. The *Clostridium* sp. belongs to fermentative-type iron reducers with a robust dissimilatory iron reduction capacity, efficiently stimulating cell growth and enhancing nutrient uptake [63,64]. This could explain the enhanced *Clostridium* counts in the group administered with the standard diet (group A), where the clostridia had higher amounts of available iron. The genus *Clostridium* includes species such as *C. butyricum* and *C. perfringens*, which are often associated with the development of necrotizing enterocolitis [65]. In contrast, nonpathogenic butyrate-producing strains belong to this group of bacteria [66]. Other bacterial groups analyzed in the fecal matter were the family *Enterobacteriaceae* and, within it, the *E. coli* group as a representative fecal coliform bacterium present in the colon of humans and warm-blooded animals. Only in group F, where the Se-enriched *Enterococcus faecium* strain was supplemented, the total counts of both *Enterobacteriaceae* and *E. coli* decreased significantly. In a canine model [12], following the oral administration of selenium/zinc-enriched probiotics, similar to our results, a decrease of *E. coli* in the feces was reported, along with an increase in *Lactobacillus* sp. and *Bifidobacterium* sp.

The gut microbiota may also utilize Se for the expression of its own selenoproteins. In the well-described yeast *Saccharomyces cerevisiae* model, the addition of inorganic Se into the cultivation media led to the production of SeMet [67]. SeMet and MeSeCys, two of the most common organic Se forms, were shown to be absorbed more efficiently than other selenocompounds [25]. Thus, the gut microbiota plays a role in Se metabolism. The gut microbiota form a complex ecosystem and multispecies environment where many different relationships, including commensalism, mutualism, or cross-feeding, exist between the resident gut microbiotas. Microbiota self-metabolizes Se and, thus, by Se supplementation, improves its own state; concomitantly, it helps to make dietary Se more available to the host organism.

This is the first report on the supplementation of selenized forms of the commercially used strains *Enterococcus faecium* CCDM 922A and *Streptococcus thermophilus* CCDM 144 in an in vivo model and the effect of their supplementation on the biological functions of rats. The limitations of the study included missing more extensive speciation patterns and mineral contents in other tissues, such as brain/heart tissues, which may shed more light into the findings in heart tissues. As Se is known to accumulate primarily in the liver and kidney tissues, other organs were not subjected to the Se content analysis, nor to the determination of the Se species in these tissues. Additionally, due to numerous parameters having an affinity towards oxidative stress, such as superoxide dismutase, catalase, oxidized/reduced glutathione ratio, isoprostanes, and others, we were not able to thoroughly analyze all of them and, thus, give a more definitive picture of the influence of all the possible biomarkers involved. Overall, the existing in vivo studies supplementing Se in the form of Se-enriched LAB are hardly comparable due to variables such as the different supplementation strategies, possible effects of other nutrients, vitamins and antioxidants, differences in the administered Se forms, etc.

5. Conclusions

Selenized forms of the strains *Streptococcus thermophilus* CCDM 144 and *Enterococcus faecium* CCDM 922A were proven to represent a source of organically bound Se, SeCys2 being the most abundant Se species, followed by SeMet. These species were also found in the liver and kidney tissues of rats. In addition, MeSeCys was also detected but only in the kidneys. Moreover, the production of extracellular Se NPs of different sizes was confirmed by TEM EDX in both the strains. We showed that the administration of Se-enriched LAB caused no significant changes in the basic metabolic characteristics of the experimental animals. Rats fed a standard maintenance diet and those fed the experimental diet fortified with the Se-enriched LAB diet showed similar total Se concentrations and Se speciation patterns in both the kidneys and livers. Furthermore, in the Se-enriched LAB tested in this study, no macroscopic effects on the liver, kidneys, heart, and brain were observed, with no apparent influence on the basic parameters of the lipid metabolism. The antioxidative system capacity was altered only in the heart tissue of rats fed the experimental diet. Together, both the strains—*Streptococcus thermophilus* CCDM 144 and *Enterococcus faecium* CCDM 922A—may have the potential for the production of Se-enriched LAB, representing a source of organic forms of Se and Se NPs. No adverse effects on the biological functions of the rats were observed. Our findings provide a foundation to further develop and establish their safety for industrial application in foods and food supplements.

Author Contributions: Conceptualization, G.K., A.K., and M.V.; methodology, B.S., A.K., and I.H.; formal analysis, M.H., H.M., and A.K.; investigation, A.K., G.K., and M.V.; resources, G.K.; data curation, B.S., I.M., and V.K.; writing—original draft preparation, G.K., A.K., and M.V.; writing—review and editing, M.H. and H.M.; supervision, G.K., A.K., and B.S.; project administration, I.H., I.M., and V.K.; and funding acquisition, G.K. All authors have read and agreed to the published version of the manuscript.

Funding: This research was funded by the Ministry of Agriculture of the Czech Republic, Institutional support, No. MZE-RO1421 and by the Ministry of Education, Youth and Sports of the Czech Republic, COST LTC20014 (COST Action No. CA18113).

Institutional Review Board Statement: This study was conducted in compliance with the laws of the Czech Republic (311/1997 column.) and the European Community Council recommendations (86/609/EEC) regarding the protection of animals used for experimental and other scientific purposes. This experimental study was approved by the committee of the Ministry of Education, Youth, and Sports of the Czech Republic, approval No. MSMT-11197/2020-2.

Informed Consent Statement: Not applicable.

Data Availability Statement: All data are presented in the paper.

Conflicts of Interest: The authors declare no conflict of interest.

References

1. WHO. *Cardiovascular Diseases (CVDs): Fact. Sheet N 317*; WHO: Geneva, Switzerland, 2015.
2. Chua, K.J.; Kwok, W.C.; Aggarwal, N.; Sun, T.; Chang, M.W. Designer Probiotics for the Prevention and Treatment of Human diseases. *Curr. Opin. Chem. Biol.* **2017**, *40*, 8–16. [CrossRef]
3. Amaretti, A.; Di Nunzio, M.; Pompei, A.; Raimondi, S.; Rossi, M.; Bordoni, A. Antioxidant Properties of Potentially Probiotic Bacteria: In Vitro and in Vivo Activities. *Appl. Microbiol. Biotechnol.* **2013**, *97*, 809–817. [CrossRef] [PubMed]

4. Steinbrenner, H.; Speckmann, B.; Klotz, L.O. Selenoproteins: Antioxidant Selenoenzymes and Beyond. *Arch. Biochem. Biophys.* **2016**, *595*, 113–119. [CrossRef]
5. Malyar, R.M.; Li, H.; Liu, D.; Abdulrahim, Y.; Farid, R.A.; Gan, F.; Ali, W.; Enayatullah, H.; Banuree, S.A.H.; Huang, K.; et al. Selenium/Zinc-Enriched Probiotics Improve Serum Enzyme Activity, Antioxidant Ability, Inflammatory Factors and Related Gene Expression of Wistar Rats Inflated Under Heat Stress. *Life Sci.* **2020**, *248*, 117464. [CrossRef] [PubMed]
6. Samarghandian, S.; Farkhondeh, T.; Samini, F.; Borji, A. Protective Effects of Carvacrol Against Oxidative Stress Induced by Chronic Stress in Rat'S Brain, Liver and Kidney. *Biochem. Res. Int.* **2016**, *2016*, 2645237. [CrossRef]
7. Brigelius-Flohé, R. Selenium in Human Health and Disease: An Overview. *Mol. Integr. Toxicol.* **2018**, 3–26.
8. Rayman, M.P. Selenium and Human Health. *Lancet* **2012**, *379*, 1256–1268. [CrossRef]
9. Yi, H.W.; Zhu, X.X.; Huang, X.L.; Lai, Y.Z.; Tang, Y. Selenium-Enriched Bifidobacterium Longum Protected Alcohol and High Fat Diet Induced Hepatic Injury in Mice. *Chin. J. Nat. Med.* **2020**, *18*, 169–177. [CrossRef]
10. Sun, Z.; Xu, Z.; Wang, D.; Yao, H.; Li, S. Selenium Deficiency Inhibits Differentiation and Immune Function and Imbalances the Th_1/Th_2 of Dendritic Cells. *Metallomics* **2018**, *10*, 759–767. [CrossRef] [PubMed]
11. Jamilian, M.; Mansury, S.; Bahmani, F.; Heidar, Z.; Amirani, E.; Asemi, Z. The Effects of Probiotic and Selenium Co-Supplementation on Parameters of Mental Health, Hormonal Profiles, and Biomarkers of Inflammation and Oxidative Stress in Women with Polycystic Ovary Syndrome. *J. Ovarian Res.* **2018**, *11*, 80. [CrossRef] [PubMed]
12. Ren, Z.; Zhao, Z.; Wang, Y.; Huang, K. Preparation of Selenium/Zinc-Enriched Probiotics and Their Effect on Blood Selenium and Zinc Concentrations, Antioxidant Capacities, and Intestinal Microflora in Canine. *Biol. Trace Elem. Res.* **2011**, *141*, 170–183. [CrossRef]
13. Yang, J.; Huang, K.; Qin, S.; Wu, X.; Zhao, Z.; Chen, F. Antibacterial Action of Selenium-Enriched Probiotics against Pathogenic *Escherichia coli*. *Dig. Dis. Sci.* **2009**, *54*, 246–254. [CrossRef] [PubMed]
14. Oraby, M.M.; Allababidy, T.; Ramadan, E.M. The Bioavailability of Selenium in *Saccharomyces cerevisiae*. *Ann. Agric. Sci.* **2015**, *60*, 307–315. [CrossRef]
15. Lamberti, C.; Mangiapane, E.; Pessione, A.; Mazzoli, R.; Giunta, C.; Pessione, E. Proteomic Characterization of a Selenium-Metabolizing Probiotic *Lact. Reuteri* Lb2 BM for Nutraceutical Applications. *Proteomics* **2011**, *11*, 2212–2221. [CrossRef] [PubMed]
16. Pescuma, M.; Gomez-Gomez, B.; Perez-Corona, T.; Font, G.; Madrid, Y.; Mozzi, F. Food Prospects of Selenium Enriched-*Lactobacillus acidophilus* CRL 636 and *Lactobacillus reuteri* CRL 1101. *J. Funct. Foods* **2017**, *35*, 466–473. [CrossRef]
17. Pusztahelyi, T.; Kovács, S.; Pócsi, I.; Prokisch, J. Selenite-Stress Selected Mutant Strains of Probiotic Bacteria for Se Source Production. *J. Trace Elem. Med. Biol.* **2015**, *30*, 96–101. [CrossRef]
18. Nagy, G.; Benko, I.; Kiraly, G.; Voros, O.; Tanczos, B.; Sztrik, A.; Takács, T.; Pocsi, I.; Prokisch, J.; Banfalvi, G. Cellular and Nephrotoxicity of Selenium Species. *J. Trace Elem. Med. Biol.* **2015**, *30*, 160–170. [CrossRef]
19. Mrvčić, J.; Stanzer, D.; Solić, E.; Stehlik-Tomas, V. Interaction of Lactic Acid Bacteria with Metal Ions: Opportunities for Improving Food Safety and Quality. *World J. Microbiol. Biotechnol.* **2012**, *28*, 2771–2782. [CrossRef] [PubMed]
20. Rother, M.; Hatfield, D.; Berry, M.; Gladyshev, V. Selenium Metabolism in Prokaryotes. In *Selenium*; Springer: New York, NY, USA, 2011. [CrossRef]
21. Zhang, B.; Zhou, K.; Zhang, J.; Chen, Q.; Liu, G.; Shang, N.; Qin, W.; Li, P.; Lin, F. Accumulation and Species Distribution of Selenium in Se-Enriched Bacterial Cells of the *Bifidobacterium animalis* 01. *Food Chem.* **2009**, *115*, 727–734. [CrossRef]
22. Krausova, G.; Kana, A.; Hyrslova, I.; Mrvikova, I.; Kavkova, M. Development of Selenized Lactic Acid Bacteria and Their Selenium Bioaccummulation Capacity. *Fermentation* **2020**, *6*, 91. [CrossRef]
23. Hyrslova, I.; Krausova, G.; Bartova, J.; Kolesar, L.; Jaglic, Z.; Stankova, B.; Curda, L. Characterization of *Enterococcus Faecium* CCDM 922 in Respect of its Technological and Probiotic Properties. *Int. J. Curr. Microbiol. Appl. Sci.* **2016**, *5*, 474–482. [CrossRef]
24. Shiobara, Y.; Ogra, Y.; Suzuki, K.T. Exchange of Endogenous Selenium for Dietary Selenium as 82 Se-Enriched Selenite in Brain, Liver, Kidneys and Testes. *Life Sci.* **2000**, *67*, 3041–3049. [CrossRef]
25. Takahashi, K.; Suzuki, N.; Ogra, Y. Bioavailability Comparison of Nine Bioselenocompounds In Vitro and In Vivo. *Int. J. Mol. Sci.* **2017**, *18*, 506. [CrossRef]
26. Shini, S.; Sultan, A.; Bryden, W.L. Selenium Biochemistry and Bioavailability: Implications for Animal Agriculture. *Agriculture* **2015**, *5*, 1277–1288. [CrossRef]
27. Xu, C.; Guo, Y.; Qiao, L.; Ma, L.; Cheng, Y.; Roman, A. Biogenic Synthesis of Novel Functionalized Selenium Nanoparticles by *Lactobacillus casei* ATCC 393 and its Protective Effects on Intestinal Barrier Dysfunction Caused by Enterotoxigenic *Escherichia coli* K88. *Front. Microbiol.* **2018**, *9*, 1129. [CrossRef]
28. Nagy, G.; Pinczes, G.; Pinter, G.; Pocsi, I.; Prokisch, J.; Banfalvi, G. In Situ Electron Microscopy of Lactomicroselenium Particles in Probiotic Bacteria. *Int. J. Mol. Sci.* **2016**, *17*, 1047. [CrossRef] [PubMed]
29. Alam, H.; Khatoon, N.; Khan, M.A.; Husain, S.A.; Saravanan, M.; Sardar, M. Synthesis of Selenium Nanoparticles Using Probiotic Bacteria *Lactobacillus acidophilus* and their Enhanced Antimicrobial Activity Against Resistant Bacteria. *J. Clust. Sci.* **2020**, *31*, 1003–1011. [CrossRef]
30. Pieniz, S.; Andreazza, R.; Mann, M.B.; Camargo, F.; Brandelli, A. Bioaccumulation and Distribution of Selenium in Enterococcus durans. *J. Trace Elem. Med. Biol.* **2017**, *40*, 37–45. [CrossRef] [PubMed]
31. Martínez, F.G.; Moreno-Martin, G.; Pescuma, M.; Madrid-Albarrán, Y.; Mozzi, F. Biotransformation of Selenium by Lactic Acid Bacteria: Formation of Seleno-Nanoparticles and Seleno-Amino Acids. *Front. Bioeng. Biotechnol.* **2020**, *8*, 506. [CrossRef] [PubMed]

32. Yang, J.; Li, Y.; Zhang, L.; Fan, M.; Wei, X. Response Surface Design for Accumulation of Selenium by Different Lactic Acid Bacteria. *3 Biotech* **2017**, *7*, 52. [CrossRef] [PubMed]
33. Eszenyi, P.; Sztrik, A.; Babka, B.; Prokisch, J. Elemental, Nano-Sized (100–500 nm) Selenium Production by Probiotic Lactic Acid Bacteria. *Int. J. Biosci. Biochem. Bioinformatics* **2011**, *1*, 148–152. [CrossRef]
34. Hosnedlova, B.; Kepinska, M.; Skalickova, S.; Fernandez, C.; Ruttkay-Nedecky, B.; Peng, Q.; Baron, M.; Melcova, M.; Opatrilova, R.; Zidkova, J.; et al. Nano-Selenium and its Nanomedicine Applications: A Critical Review. *Int. J. Nanomed.* **2018**, *13*, 2107–2128. [CrossRef]
35. Behne, D.; Wolters, W. Distribution of Selenium and Glutathione Peroxidase in the Rat. *J. Nutr.* **1983**, *113*, 456–461. [CrossRef] [PubMed]
36. Gu, Q.P.; Xia, Y.M.; Ha, P.C.; Butler, J.A.; Whanger, P.D. Distribution of Selenium Between Plasma Fractions in Guinea Pigs and Humans with Various Intakes of Dietary Selenium. *J. Trace Elem. Med. Biol.* **1998**, *12*, 8–15. [CrossRef]
37. Arteel, G.E.; Sies, H. The Biochemistry of Selenium and the Glutathione System. *Environ. Toxicol. Pharmacol.* **2001**, *10*, 153–158. [CrossRef]
38. Rýdlová, M.; Růnová, K.; Száková, J.; Fučíková, A.; Hakenová, A.; Mlejnek, P.; Zídek, V.; Tremlová, J.; Mestek, O.; Kaňa, A.; et al. The Response of Macro- and Micronutrient Nutrient Status and Biochemical Processes in Rats Fed on a Diet with Selenium-Enriched Defatted Rapeseed and/or Vitamin E Supplementation. *BioMed Res. Int.* **2017**, *2017*, 1–13. [CrossRef]
39. Fujihara, T.; Orden, E.A. The Effect of Dietary Vitamin E Level on Selenium Status in Rats. *J. Anim. Physiol. Anim. Nutr.* **2014**, *98*, 921–927. [CrossRef]
40. Arnaud, J.; van Dael, P.; Michalke, B. Selenium Interactions with Other Trace Elements, with Nutrients (And Drugs) in Humans. In *Selenium. Molecular and Integrative Toxicology*; Springer: Cham, Switzerland, 2018.
41. Benstoem, C.; Goetzenich, A.; Kraemer, S.; Borosch, S.; Manzanares, W.; Hardy, G.; Stoppe, C. Selenium and its Supplementation in Cardiovascular Disease—What do We Know? *Nutrients* **2015**, *7*, 3094–3118. [CrossRef]
42. Kurek, E.; Ruszczynska, A.; Wojciechowski, M.; Czauderna, M.; Bulska, E. Study on Speciation of Selenium in Animal Tissues Using High Performance Liquid Chromatography with on-line Detection by Liquid Coupled Plasma Mass Spectrometry. *Chem. Anal.* **2009**, *54*, 43–57.
43. Qin, S.; Gao, J.; Huang, K. Effects of Different Selenium Sources on Tissue Selenium Concentrations, Blood gsh-px Activities and Plasma Interleukin Levels in Finishing Lambs. *Biol. Trace Elem. Res.* **2007**, *116*, 91–102. [CrossRef]
44. Han, X.J.; Qin, P.; Li, W.X.; Ma, Q.G.; Ji, C.; Zhang, J.Y.; Zhao, L.H. Effect of Sodium Selenite and Selenium Yeast on Performance, Egg Quality, Antioxidant Capacity, and Selenium Deposition of Laying Hens. *Poult. Sci.* **2017**, *96*, 3973–3980. [CrossRef] [PubMed]
45. Sobeková, A.; Holovská, K.; Lenártová, V.; Holovská, K., Jr.; Javorský, P.; Boldižárová, K.; Grešáková, L.; Leng, L. Effects of Feed Supplemented with Selenite or Se-Yeast on Antioxidant Enzyme Activities in Lamb Tissues. *J. Anim. Feed Sci.* **2006**, *15*, 569–577. [CrossRef]
46. Zhou, Y.; Zhu, H.; Qi, Y.; Wu, C.; Zhang, J.; Shao, L.; Tan, J.; Chen, D. Absorption and Distribution of Selenium Following Oral Administration of Selenium-Enriched Bifidobacterium Longum DD98, Selenized Yeast, or Sodium Selenite in Rats. *Biol. Trace Elem. Res.* **2020**, *197*, 599–605. [CrossRef] [PubMed]
47. Zhang, B.; Piao, J.; Gu, L. Effects of selenium-enriched garlic on blood lipids and lipid peroxidation in Experimental Hyperlipidemic Rats. *Wei Sheng Yan Jiu* **2002**, *31*, 93–96.
48. Marounek, M.; Dokoupilová, A.; Volek, Z.; Hoza, I. Quality of Meat and Selenium Content in Tissues of Rabbits Fed Diets Supplemented with Sodium Selenite, Selenized Yeast and Selenized Algae. *World Rabbit Sci.* **2009**, *17*, 207–212. [CrossRef]
49. Zhao, L.; Sun, L.H.; Huang, J.Q.; Briens, M.; Qi, D.S.; Xu, S.W.; Lei, X.G. A Novel Organic Selenium Compound Exerts Unique Regulation of Selenium Speciation, Selenogenome, and Selenoproteins in Broiler Chicks. *J. Nutr.* **2017**, *147*, 789–797. [CrossRef] [PubMed]
50. Misra, S.; Peak, D.; Chen, N.; Hamilton, C.; Niyogi, S. Tissue-Specific Accumulation and Speciation of Selenium in Rainbow Trout (*Oncorhynchus mykiss*) Exposed to Elevated Dietary Selenomethionine. *Comp. Biochem. Physiol. C Toxicol. Pharmacol.* **2012**, *155*, 560–565. [CrossRef]
51. Sánchez-Martínez, M.; Pérez-Corona, T.; Martínez-Villaluenga, C.; Frías, J.; Peñas, E.; Porres, J.M.; Urbano, G.; Cámara, C.; Madrid, Y. Synthesis of 77Se-Methylselenocysteine when Preparing Sauerkraut in the Presence of 77Se-Selenite. Metabolic Transformation of 77Se-Methylselenocysteine in Wistar Rats Determined by LC–IDA–ICP–MS. *Anal. Bioanal. Chem.* **2014**, *406*, 7949–7958. [CrossRef]
52. Juniper, D.T.; Phipps, R.H.; Ramos-Morales, E.; Bertin, G. Selenium Persistency and Speciation in the Tissues of Lambs Following the Withdrawal of Dietary High-Dose Selenium-Enriched Yeast. *Animal* **2008**, *2*, 375–380. [CrossRef]
53. Gawor, A.; Ruszczynska, A.; Czauderna, M.; Bulska, E. Determination of Selenium Species in Muscle, Heart, and Liver Tissues of Lambs Using Mass Spectrometry Methods. *Animals* **2020**, *10*, 808. [CrossRef] [PubMed]
54. Cheng, Y.; Huang, Y.; Liu, K.; Pan, S.; Qin, Z.; Wu, T.; Xu, X. Cardamine Hupingshanensis Aqueous Extract Improves Intestinal Redox Status and Gut Microbiota in Se-deficient Rats. *J. Sci. Food Agric.* **2021**, *101*, 989–996. [CrossRef]
55. Hrdina, J.; Banning, A.; Kipp, A.; Loh, G.; Blaut, M.; Brigelius-Flohé, R. The Gastrointestinal Microbiota Affects the Selenium Status and Selenoprotein Expression in Mice. *J. Nutr. Biochem.* **2009**, *20*, 638–648. [CrossRef]

56. Kasaikina, M.V.; Kravtsova, M.A.; Lee, B.C.; Seravalli, J.; Peterson, D.A.; Walter, J.; Legge, R.; Benson, A.K.; Hatfield, D.L.; Gladyshev, V.N. Dietary Selenium Affects Host Selenoproteome Expression by Influencing the Gut Microbiota. *FASEB J.* **2011**, *25*, 2492–2499. [CrossRef] [PubMed]
57. Takahashi, K.; Suzuki, N.; Ogra, Y. Effect of Gut Microflora on Nutritional Availability of Selenium. *Food Chem.* **2020**, *319*, 126537. [CrossRef]
58. Zhai, Q.; Cen, S.; Li, P.; Tian, F.; Zhao, J.; Zhang, H.; Chen, W. Effects of Dietary Selenium Supplementation on Intestinal Barrier and Immune Responses Associated with its Modulation of Gut Microbiota. *Environ. Sci. Technol. Lett.* **2018**, *5*, 724–730. [CrossRef]
59. Zhu, H.; Zhou, Y.; Qi, Y.; Ji, R.; Zhang, J.; Qian, Z.; Wu, C.; Tan, J.; Shao, L.; Chen, D. Preparation and Characterization of Selenium Enriched-*Bifidobacterium Longum* DD98 and its Repairing Effects on Antibiotic-Induced Intestinal Dysbacteriosis in Mice. *Food Funct.* **2019**, *10*, 4975–4984. [CrossRef] [PubMed]
60. Yang, S.; Li, L.; Yu, L.; Sun, L.; Li, K.; Tong, C.; Xu, W.; Cui, G.; Long, M.; Li, P. Selenium-Enriched Yeast Reduces Caecal Pathological Injuries and Intervenes Changes of the Diversity of Caecal Microbiota Caused by Ochratoxin-A in broilers. *Food Chem. Toxicol.* **2020**, *137*, 111139. [CrossRef]
61. Gangadoo, S.; Dinev, I.; Chapman, J.; Hughes, R.J.; Van, T.T.H.; Moore, R.J.; Stanley, D. Selenium Nanoparticles in Poultry Feed Modify Gut Microbiota and Increase Abundance *Faecalibacterium Prausnitzii*. *Appl. Microbiol. Biotechnol.* **2018**, *102*, 1455–1466. [CrossRef] [PubMed]
62. Gangadoo, S.; Bauer, B.W.; Bajagai, Y.S.; Van, T.T.H.; Moore, R.J.; Stanley, D. In Vitro Growth of Gut Microbiota with Selenium Nanoparticles. *Anim. Nutr.* **2019**, *5*, 424–431. [CrossRef] [PubMed]
63. Zhang, Y.; Xiao, L.; Hao, Q.; Li, X.; Liu, F. Ferrihydrite Reduction Exclusively Stimulated Hydrogen Production by *Clostridium* with Community Metabolic Pathway Bifurcation. *ACS Sustain. Chem. Eng.* **2020**, *8*, 7574–7580. [CrossRef]
64. List, C.; Hosseini, Z.; Lederballe Meibom, K.; Hatzimanikatis, V.; Bernier-Latmani, R. Impact of Iron Reduction on the Metabolism of *Clostridium Acetobutylicum*. *Environ. Microbiol.* **2019**, *21*, 3548–3563. [CrossRef] [PubMed]
65. Butel, M.J.; Roland, N.; Hibert, A.; Popot, F.; Favre, A.; Tessedre, A.C.; Bensaada, M.; Rimbault, A.; Szylit, O. Clostridial Pathogenicity in Experimental Necrotising Enterocolitis in Gnotobiotic Quails and Protective Role of Bifidobacteria. *J. Med. Microbiol.* **1998**, *47*, 391–399. [CrossRef] [PubMed]
66. Rada, V.; Nevoral, J.; Trojanová, I.; Tománková, E.; Smehilová, M.; Killer, J. Growth of Infant Faecal Bifidobacteria and Clostridia on Prebiotic Oligosaccharides in in vitro Conditions. *Anaerobe* **2008**, *14*, 205–208. [CrossRef] [PubMed]
67. Zare, H.; Vahidi, H.; Owlia, P.; Khujin, M.H.; Khamisabadi, A. Yeast Enriched with Selenium: A Promising Source of Selenomethionine and Seleno-Proteins. *Trends Pept. Protein Sci.* **2017**, *1*, 130–134.

MDPI
St. Alban-Anlage 66
4052 Basel
Switzerland
Tel. +41 61 683 77 34
Fax +41 61 302 89 18
www.mdpi.com

Antioxidants Editorial Office
E-mail: antioxidants@mdpi.com
www.mdpi.com/journal/antioxidants

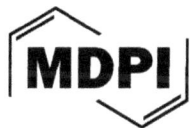